Uniquest Series
ANATOMY

Uniquest Series
ANATOMY

A Compilation of All India University Questions 2003–2021

Second Edition

Editors

Sheela Grace Jeevamani MBBS MS (Anatomy)
Formerly, Professor and Head
Department of Anatomy
Karpagam Faculty of Medical Sciences and Research
Coimbatore, Tamil Nadu, India
and
Formerly, Professor and Head
Government Mohan Kumaramangalam Medical College
Salem, Tamil Nadu, India

T Preethi Ramya MBBS MD (Anatomy)
Senior Lecturer
Clinical Anatomy Coordinator
School of Medicine
University of Notre Dame, Australia

Casual Academic Tutor
Discipline of Anatomy and Histology
University of Sydney and University of Technology Sydney, Australia

Formerly, Associate Professor
Government Kilpauk Medical College
Chennai, Tamil Nadu, India

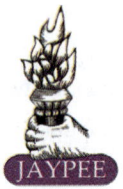

JAYPEE BROTHERS MEDICAL PUBLISHERS
The Health Sciences Publisher
New Delhi | London

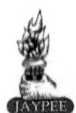 **Jaypee Brothers Medical Publishers (P) Ltd**

Headquarter

Jaypee Brothers Medical Publishers (P) Ltd
EMCA House, 23/23-B
Ansari Road, Daryaganj
New Delhi - 110 002, India
Landline: +91-11-23272143,+91-11-23272703,
+91-11-23282021,+91-11-23245672
Email: jaypee@jaypeebrothers.com

Corporate Office

Jaypee Brothers Medical Publishers (P) Ltd
4838/24, Ansari Road, Daryaganj
New Delhi 110 002, India
Phone: +91-11-43574357
Fax: +91-11-43574314
Email: jaypee@jaypeebrothers.com

Website: www.jaypeebrothers.com
Website: www.jaypeedigital.com

Overseas Office

J.P. Medical Ltd
83 Victoria Street, London
SW1H 0HW (UK)
Phone: +44 20 3170 8910
Fax: +44 (0)20 3008 6180
Email: info@jpmedpub.com

© 2023, Jaypee Brothers Medical Publishers

The views and opinions expressed in this book are solely those of the original contributor(s)/author(s) and do not necessarily represent those of editor(s) and publishers of the book.

All rights reserved. No part of this publication may be reproduced, stored or transmitted in any form or by any means, electronic, mechanical, photocopying, recording or otherwise, without the prior permission in writing of the publishers/editors.

All brand names and product names used in this book are trade names, service marks, trademarks or registered trademarks of their respective owners. The publisher is not associated with any product or vendor mentioned in this book.

Medical knowledge and practice change constantly. This book is designed to provide accurate, authoritative information about the subject matter in question. However, readers are advised to check the most current information available on procedures included and check information from the manufacturer of each product to be administered, to verify the recommended dose, formula, method and duration of administration, adverse effects and contraindications. It is the responsibility of the practitioner to take all appropriate safety precautions. Neither the publisher nor the author(s)/editor(s) assume any liability for any injury and/or damage to persons or property arising from or related to use of material in this book.

This book is sold on the understanding that the publisher is not engaged in providing professional medical services. If such advice or services are required, the services of a competent medical professional should be sought.

Every effort has been made where necessary to contact holders of copyright to obtain permission to reproduce copyright material. If any have been inadvertently overlooked, the publisher will be pleased to make the necessary arrangements at the first opportunity.

Inquiries for bulk sales may be solicited at: jaypee@jaypeebrothers.com

Uniquest Series: Anatomy

First Edition: 2019

Second Edition: **2023**

ISBN: 978-93-5465-618-7

Printed at: Sterling Graphics Pvt. Ltd.

PREFACE TO THE SECOND EDITION

The success of first edition encouraged us to bring the next edition. The new edition comprises of present curriculum as per NMC—syllabus and questions, along with previous years question papers. Answers for 19 years question papers are present, which will cover more than 80% of the portions of Anatomy. Multiple choice questions are included, decoded and explained with references. This will be useful for the first MBBS students and the students preparing for postgraduate entrance—NEET examination.

The answers are simple with bullet points, simple illustrations, and student friendly. The errors of previous edition are corrected. Anatomy is common for all medical students, so it will be of use throughout India.

Sheela Grace Jeevamani
T Preethi Ramya

PREFACE TO THE FIRST EDITION

We feel a sense of enthusiasm in presenting the first edition of the book *Uniquest Series: Anatomy*. We feel grateful to our students, who had been the sole source of motivation to start writing this book. They always had come with problem saying, they had understood and studied the subject well but found it always a challenge to score marks in the examination because they could not reproduce the exact content for the questions. This made us solve few question papers and the students found it more fruitful.

Fifteen years of question papers are decoded in this book, which took nearly 2 years to get completed. The book covers most of the portions of anatomy, and the answers are written effectively with bullet points along with corresponding simple illustrations. The answers for all the questions are precise and comprehensive. It is student-friendly for a quick reading and write the examinations. We concentrated on labeling the illustrations clearly and made it easy for the students to correlate with the theory.

We also express our gratitude for the eminent authors of the books in anatomy, which served as an excellent resource in preparing this book. We are sure that this cannot replace the textbooks, but still we hope and wish, this book will serve as a handy tool for the medico students in the years to come.

Sheela Grace Jeevamani
T Preethi Ramya

ACKNOWLEDGMENTS

With God all things are possible. Our talent is God's gift. Our gratitude to our Almighty God, who always guided our way in our project, without Him, we would not have completed.

It is our pleasure to sincerely thank Dr TP Kalaniti, Dean, Karpagam Faculty of Medical Sciences and Research, Coimbatore, Tamil Nadu, India, who gave the idea and inspired us to write the answers for the questions of university examination.

We also thank our staff Mr Anil Kumar and Dr Vidya, who helped in the initial stage in preparing the manuscript.

We are very grateful to the whole team of M/s Jaypee Brothers Medical Publishers (P) Ltd, New Delhi, India, who helped and guided us, especially Shri Jitendar P Vij (Group Chairman), Mr Ankit Vij (Managing Director), Mr MS Mani (Group President), Dr Madhu Choudhary (Director-Educational Publishing), Ms Pooja Bhandari (Production Head), Ms Sunita Katla (Executive Assistant to Group Chairman and Publishing Manager), Ms Samina Khan (Executive Assistant to Director-Content Strategy), Ms Seema Dogra (Cover Visualizer), Mr Rajesh Sharma (Production Coodinator), Mr Ankush Sharma (Graphic Designer), Mr Dinesh Bhardwaj (Typesetter) and Mr Rahul Jadli (Proofreader), for all their support to work in this project and make it a success. Without their cooperation, we could not have completed this project.

Finally, we would like to acknowledge with gratitude the support of our family members. They all kept us going.

CONTENTS

1. MBBS Examination 2003 — 1
2. MBBS Examination 2004 — 43
3. MBBS Examination 2005 — 88
4. MBBS Examination 2006 — 143
5. MBBS Examination 2007 — 186
6. MBBS Examination 2008 — 227
7. MBBS Examination 2009 — 271
8. MBBS Examination 2010 — 306
9. MBBS Examination 2011 — 339
10. MBBS Examination 2012 — 381
11. MBBS Examination 2013 — 409
12. MBBS Examination 2014 — 443
13. MBBS Examination 2015 — 476
14. MBBS Examination 2016 — 503
15. MBBS Examination 2017 — 522
16. MBBS Examination 2018 — 533
17. MBBS Examination 2019 — 545
18. MBBS Examination 2020 — 554
19. MBBS Examination 2021 — 562
    Topic-wise University Questions — 593

MBBS Examination 2003

ANSWER ALL QUESTIONS

I. Essay questions (15/10 Marks)

1. Describe the arches of foot under the following headings: Types, factors responsible for their maintenance, functions and applied anatomy.
2. Describe the urinary bladder under the following headings: External and internal features, relations, nerve supply, and applied anatomy.
3. Describe the pleura under the following headings.
   Parts and recesses, nerve supply, blood supply, and lymphatic drainage, surface marking and applied anatomy.
4. Describe the temporomandibular joint under the following headings. Articular surfaces, ligaments, relations, movements and muscles producing the movements and applied anatomy.

II. Short notes (2 Marks each)

1. Microscopic structure of bone in transverse section.
2. Intraembryonic mesoderm.
3. Brachial artery.
4. Muscles of rotator cuff shoulder.
5. Tibial collateral ligament.
6. Rectus sheath.
7. Spleen.
8. Ischiorectal fossa.
9. Development of testis.
10. Microscopic structure of pancreas.
11. Superior vena cava.
12. Third ventricle of the brain.
13. Metathalamus.
    MGB for Music – hearing (auditory pathway). LGB for Light – vision (visual pathway).
14. Submandibular salivary gland.
15. Facial nerve.
16. Esophagus.
17. Nasal septum.
18. Microscopic structure of cerebral cortex.
19. Development of palate.
20. Development of tongue.

I. ESSAY QUESTIONS

1. Describe the arches of foot under the following headings: Types, factors responsible for their maintenance, functions and applied anatomy.

Types

- Longitudinal arches—medial and lateral
- Transverse arches—anterior and posterior.

Constituents and Supports of Arches

Longitudinal Arch

Medial longitudinal arch (Fig. 1)

- Higher, more mobile and resilient
- It is made of calcaneus, head of talus, navicular, three cuneiforms, first three metatarsal bones
- Anterior end—by heads of 1st, 2nd and 3rd metatarsals
- Posterior end—by medial tubercle of the calcaneum

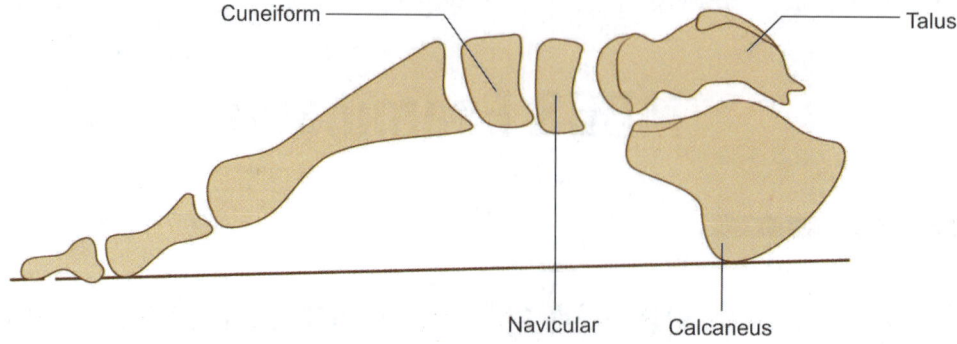

Fig. 1: Medial longitudinal arch.

- Summit—by superior articular surface of body of talus
- Pillars
  - Anterior pillar is long and weak, formed by talus, navicular, the three cuneiform bones and the first 3 metatarsals
  - Posterior pillar is short and strong, formed by medial part of calcaneum.
- Main joint of the arch is the talo-calcaneonavicular joint.

Maintenance (supports) of medial longitudinal arch (Fig. 2):

- **Shape of bones:** Bones are wedge shaped, contribute for stability
- **Intersegmental ties:** Plantar calcaneo navicular ligament (spring ligament), to support the head of talus. Talocalcaneal ligament helps for stability
- **Tie beams:** Plantar aponeurosis, medial part of flexor digitorum brevis, abductor hallucis, tendons of flexor hallucis longus and medial part of the tendon of flexor digitorum longus and flexor hallucis brevis. The plantar aponeurosis is the main tie beam
- **Suspending from above (as sling):** Tendons of tibialis anterior and deltoid ligament. Tibialis posterior helps to raise the medial border.

Lateral longitudinal arch (Fig. 3)

- Low, with limited mobility. It transmits the weight to the ground
- Bones forming are calcaneus, the cuboid and the fourth and fifth metatarsal bones
- Anterior end—by the heads of 4th and 5th metatarsals
- Posterior end—by lateral tubercle of the calcaneum
- Summit—by superior surface of calcaneum at the subtalar joint.

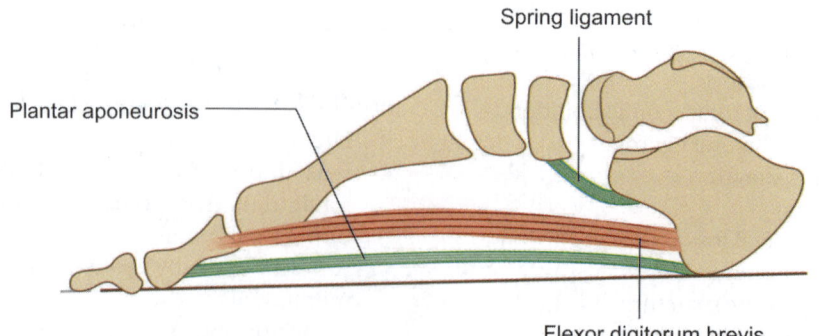

Fig. 2: Supports of medial arch.

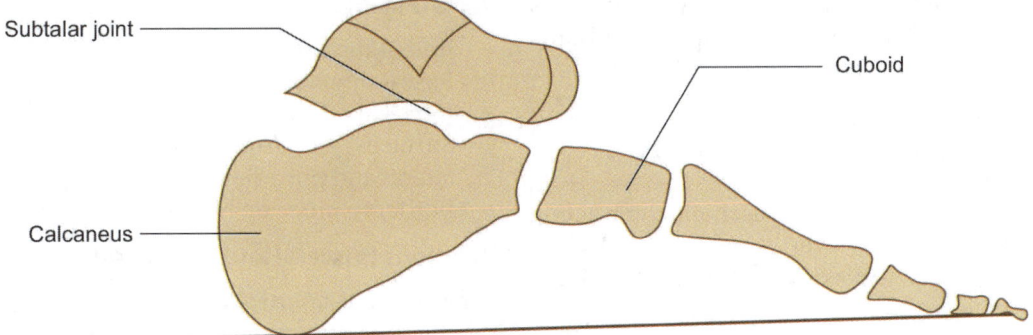

Fig. 3: Lateral longitudinal arch.

- Pillars
  - Anterior pillar is long and weak, formed by the cuboid bone and 4th and 5th metatarsals
  - Posterior pillar is short and strong formed by the lateral half of the calcaneum
- Main joint—calcaneocuboid joint.

Maintenance of lateral longitudinal arch (Fig. 4):

- **Shape of bones:** Bones are wedge shaped
- **Intersegmental ties:** The long and short plantar ligaments bind the arch
- **Tie beams:** Lateral part of plantar aponeurosis, lateral part of flexor digitorum brevis and longus tendons, abductor digiti minimi, flexor digiti minimi brevis
- **Suspending from above (as sling):** Tendons of peroneus longus, brevis and tertius.

Transverse Arches

- **Anterior transverse arch:** By heads of the 5 metatarsals. It is complete, the heads of the 1st and 5th metatarsals touch the ground
- **Posterior transverse arch:** By the cuneiform and cuboid and bases of metatarsal bones. It is incomplete as lateral end alone touches the ground (Half dome completed by the similar half dome of the opposite side).

Factors supporting the transverse arch

- **Shape:** Bones are wedge shaped, especially the intermediate and lateral cuneiform bones
- **Intersegmental ties:** Deep transverse ligaments, dorsal interossei, oblique and transverse heads of adductor hallucis
- **Tie beams:** Tendons of peroneus longus and tibialis posterior

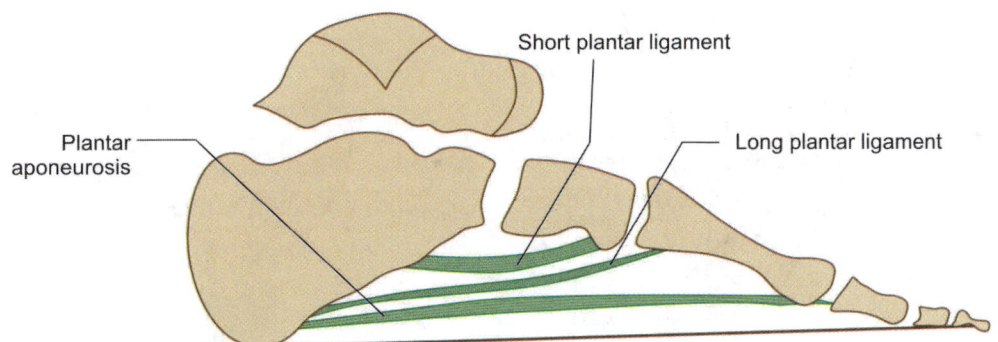

Fig. 4: Supports of lateral arch.

- **Slings:** The tendons of the peroneus brevis and tertius on lateral side and tibialis anterior on medial side.

Functions of arches of foot
- Helps in proportional distribution of body weight
- Helps in propulsive mechanism by acting as segmented lever
- Protects the vessels and nerves from compression
- Acts as spring board and helps in jumping and jolting
- Helps to adopt the foot on uneven surface.

Applied Anatomy
- **Pes planus:** Flat foot—absence or collapse of the arches. It is due to tarsal arthritis, rupture of spring ligament
- **Pes cavus:** High arched foot—due to exaggeration of the longitudinal arches, it will produce claw foot. It may be fore foot, mid foot, or hind foot cavus
- **Talipes varus:** Patient walks on the outer border of the foot
- **Talipes valgus:** Patient walks on the inner border of the foot.

---

2. Describe the urinary bladder under the following headings: External and internal features, relations, nerve supply and applied anatomy.

External Features
- An empty bladder is tetrahedral in shape; when filled up it becomes ovoid in shape

Parts (Fig. 5)
- Apex—directed forwards
- Base—directed backwards
- Neck—the lowest and most fixed part
- Surfaces—superior, right and left inferolateral and posterior (base)
- Borders—anterior, two lateral, posterior.

Relations (Visceral and Peritoneal)
- **Apex:** It is connected to the umbilicus by the median umbilical ligament (urachus) which is the remnant of the allantoic diverticulum
- **Base**
  - In female—is related to the supra vaginal part of cervix and the anterior wall of vagina **(Fig. 7A)**
  - In male—ampulla of rectum separated by rectovesical pouch, seminal vesicles and vas deferens, separated by rectovesical fascia (Denonvillier's fascia). The upper part of this surface is covered with peritoneum **(Figs. 6 and 7B)**.
- **Neck**
  - Lowest and the most fixed part—situated 3 to 4 cm posterior to the lower part of pubic symphysis
  - In male it rests and is continuous with base of prostate
  - In female is related to pelvic fascia
  - It is pierced by internal urethral orifice.
- **Superior surface**
  - Covered by peritoneum
  - Related to sigmoid colon and coils of ileum

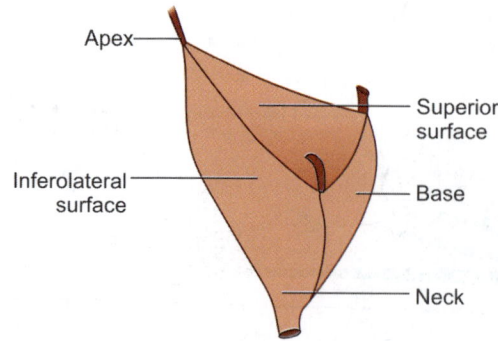

Fig. 5: Parts of bladder.

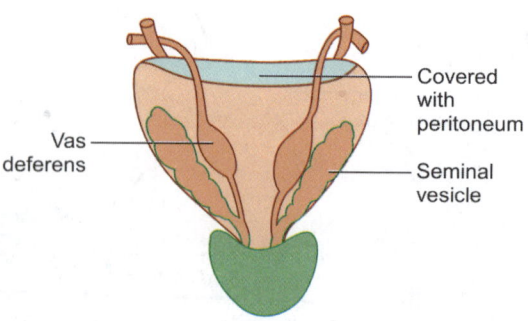

Fig. 6: Relations of base of bladder in male.

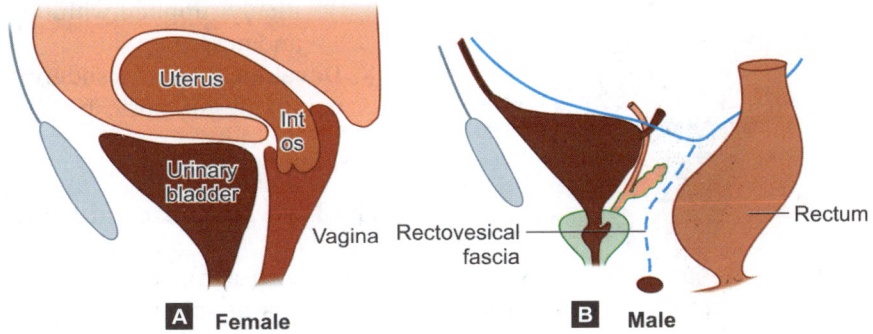

Figs. 7A and B: Peritoneal relation.

- In female, anterior surface of anteverted uterus. The posterior part of this surface is not covered with peritoneum. The peritoneum is reflected to uterus at the level of internal os.
- **Inferolateral surface (Fig. 8)**
  - Devoid of peritoneum
  - Related to body of pubis, fascia covering levator ani and obturator internus, retropubic space of Retzius with retropubic pad of fat and venous plexus
  - In male related to puboprostatic ligament and in female pubovesical ligament
  - When the bladder is full, this surface is related to the anterior abdominal muscles.
- **Anterior border:** Extends from apex to neck of bladder
- **Lateral borders:** From apex to entry of ureters.

- **Interior (internal) of bladder**
  - Many temporary mucous folds are present in the entire bladder except trigonum vesicae
  - **Trigonum vesicae (internal trigone)**
    - Triangular area on the inner side of base of the bladder
    - Mucous membrane is tense and glistening
    - Richly supplied with blood vessels and nerves.
  - **Boundaries (Fig. 9):**
    - **Apex:** Directed downwards and forwards. Formed by internal urethral orifice. In male, an elevation is formed by median lobe of prostate called **uvula vesicae**
    - **Base:** Interureteric ridge (**Mercier's bar**) extending between the orifices of the ureters. Interureteric ridge acts

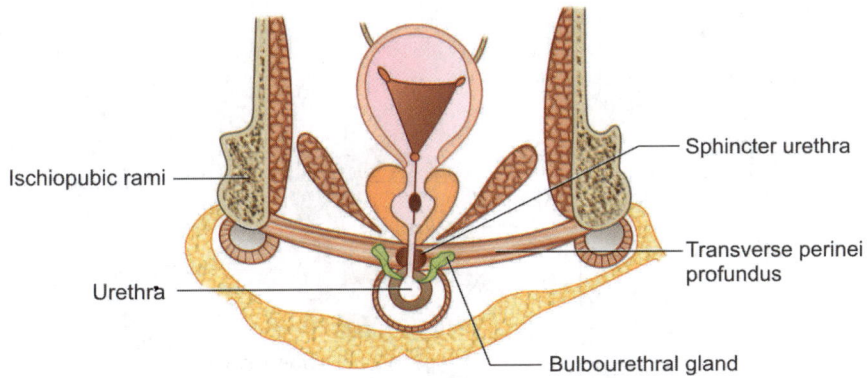

Fig. 8: Inferolateral surface.

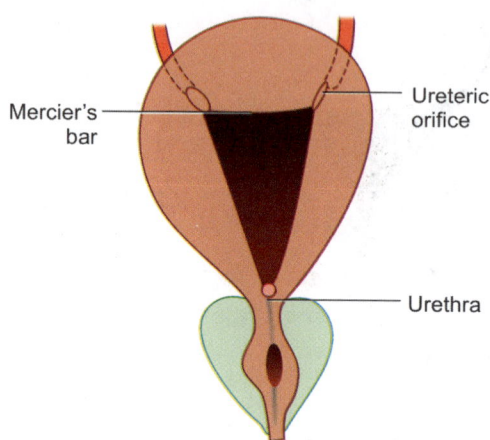

Fig. 9: Trigone of bladder.

as a **guide for the surgeons** to identify the ureteric orifices in cystoscopy
- **Posterolateral angle:** Ureteric orifices are 2.5 cm from each other when bladder is empty and 5 cm when distended
- **Laterally:** Uretero - urethral folds.
- **Importance of trigone**
  - Most fixed and dependent part
  - Trigonal muscle of Bell replaces the submucous coat and is adherent to mucous membrane
- Richly supplied with blood vessels and nerves.
- **Developed** from mesoderm (absorbed part of mesonephric duct).

Nerve Supply (Fig. 10)

Supplied by sympathetic and parasympathetic nerves.
- **Parasympathetic:** From S_2, S_3, S_4, segments of spinal cord stimulates the detrusor, called **nerve of emptying**
- **Sympathetic fibers:** From T_{11} to L_2 segments of spinal cord inhibits detrusor and stimulates the sphincter vesicae called **nerve of filling**
- **Sensory fibers:** Pain fibers are carried mainly by parasympathetic and partly by sympathetic fibers.

Applied Anatomy

- **Cystoscopy:** Instrument passed through the urethra to visualize the interior of the bladder
- **Exstrophy of bladder:** Failure of development of the entire anterior wall of bladder and anterior abdominal wall in the lower part and the trigone of bladder is exposed.

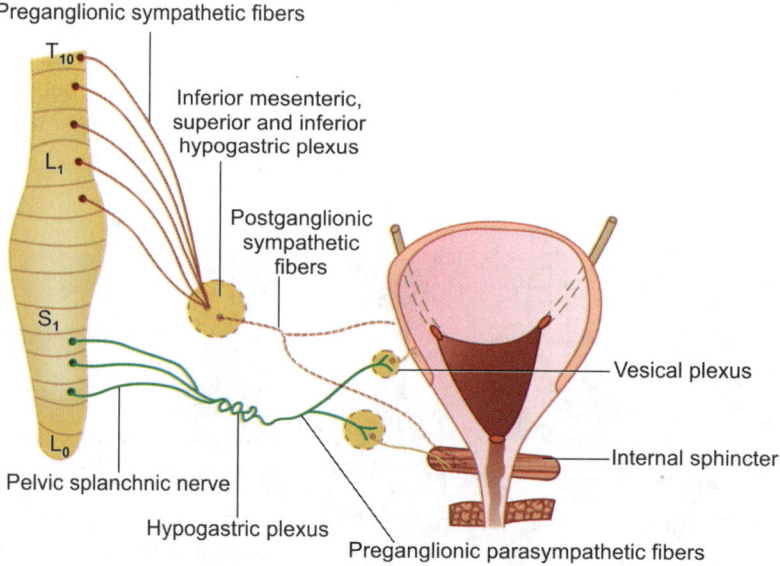

Fig. 10: Nerve supply of bladder.

- **Diverticulae:** May be seen at the margins of the trigone of bladder. May lead to infection
- Median lobe of prostate grows into the bladder.

---

3. **Describe the pleura under the following headings. Parts and recesses, nerve supply, blood supply, and lymphatic drainage, surface marking and applied anatomy.**

- The right and the left pleurae are thin serous membranes
- They line the corresponding lungs and the thoracic wall.

Parts

- An inner or visceral layer—it is adherent to the surface of the lung
- An outer or parietal layer—it covers the wall of the thoracic cavity
- The parietal and visceral layers of pleura are in contact with each other. They are separated by a potential space called the pleural cavity.

The parietal pleura is subdivided into the following parts:
- **Cervical pleura:** The apex of lung is covered by it
- **Costal pleura:** Covers the inner aspect of the thoracic cavity
- The **diaphragmatic pleura** lines the superior surface of the diaphragm
- The **mediastinal pleura** lines the structures on the corresponding side of the mediastinum.

Cervical Pleura (Fig. 11A)

- Covers the apex of lung and extends from inner border of 1st rib
- The summit of the pleura is 3 to 4 cm above the 1st costal cartilage
- It is covered by suprapleural membrane called **Sibson's fascia (Fig. 11B)**
- Fascia is attached, above to the tip of 7th cervical vertebra and below to the inner border of 1st rib.

Mediastinal Pleura

- It covers the lung root and below the root a tubular sheath of pleura extends to form a fold called **pulmonary ligament**
- Pulmonary ligament is a dead space containing loose areolar tissue and few lymphatics
- The space helps for the expansion of the inferior pulmonary veins during increased venous return.

Costal Pleura

- It covers the inner surface of the sternum, ribs and their costal cartilages, intercostal spaces and the sides of the vertebral bodies
- The endothoracic fascia seperates the costal layer from the above structures.

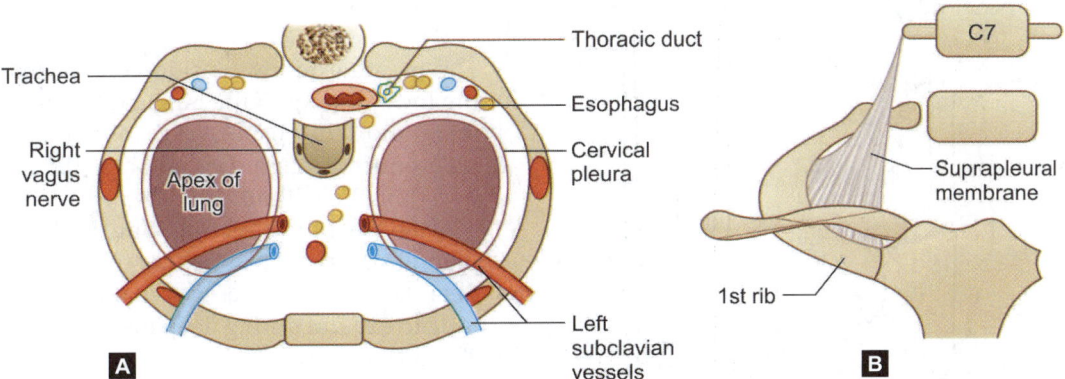

Figs. 11A and B: Cervical pleura.

Costal Pleura Reflexion

- **In front (Fig. 12A)**
  - Behind sternum, it is continuous with the mediastinal pleura along costo-mediastinal line of reflexion which is slightly different on two sides
  - On both sides, the lines extend downwards and medially from the sternoclavicular joints to the middle of the sternal angle, then descend vertically upto the fourth costal cartilge after which the reflexion differs on two sides
  - On the right side, the line passes vertically downward behind the xiphisternal joint, then turns laterally across the right costoxiphoid angle, follows the 7th costal cartilage and is continuous with the costodiaphragmatic line of pleural reflexion
  - On the left side, the line deviates laterally from the sternum and then descends close to the sternum upto the 6th costal cartilage; thereafter it turns laterally as the costodiaphragmatic line of reflexion.
- **Behind (Fig. 12B)**
  - Costal pleura is continuous with mediastinal pleura by the side of the vertebral column along a line known as costovertebral reflexions
  - It extends from a point 2.5 cm lateral to the 7th cervical spine to a point 2.5 cm lateral to the 12th thoracic spine.

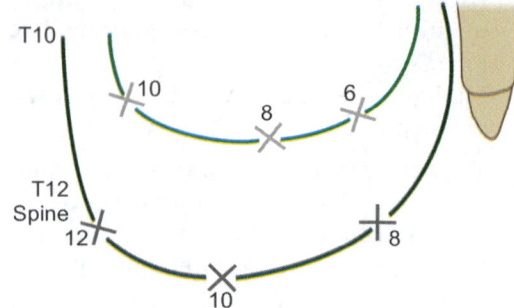

Fig. 13: Costodiaphragmatic recess.

- **Above:** Costal pleura is continuous with the cervical pleura along the inner border of 1st rib.
- **Below:** It is continuous with the diaphragmatic pleura along a line known as costodiaphragmatic reflexions which slightly differs on two sides
  - **On the right side**, the line of reflexions can be drawn by joining the following points:
    - Xiphisternal joint
    - 8th costal cartilage in the mid-clavicular line
    - 10th rib in the mid-axillary line
    - A point 2.5 cm lateral to the 12th thoracic spine.
  - **On the left side**, point (a) on the left 6th sternocostal joint; other points are same as on the right side. Left pleural sac is slightly lower in midaxillary line than the right sac.

Recesses

- The pleura extends considerably beyond the lower border of the lung, and in quiet inspiration the costal and diaphragmatic pleurae of the lung are in contact separated by a thin film of fluid
- The space between the lung and the pleural sac is called as pleural recess
- Recesses is used as reserve spaces for the lung to expand during deep inspiration
- The recesses are:
  - Costomediastinal recess
  - Costodiaphragmatic recess.

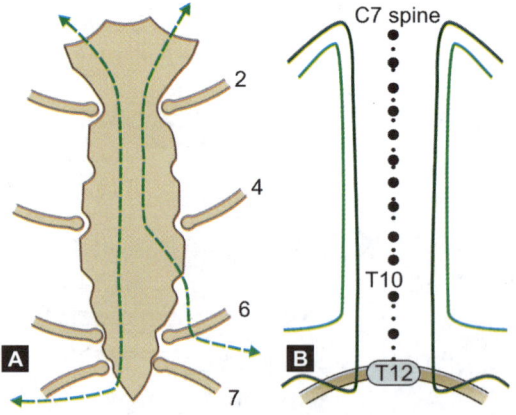

Figs. 12A and B: Reflexion of costal pleura.

Costodiaphragmatic Recess

It is also called as **phrenicocostal sinus**.
- **Shape:** Wedge/crescent shaped
- **Extent:** Lies inferiorly between costal and diaphragmatic pleura
  - The lung lower border corresponds to 6th, 8th, 10th ribs, whereas the lower limit of pleura corresponds to 8th, 10th, 12th ribs in midlavicular, midaxillary, and scapular lines respectively
  - Vertically measures about 5 cm in the midaxillary line.
- **Relations (Figs. 14A and B)**
  - **Right side:** Right lobe of liver, upper part of posterior surface of right kidney
  - **Left side:** Spleen, fundus of stomach, upper part of posterior surface of left kidney.

Costomediastinal Recess

The costomediastinal recess is present behind the sternum and costal cartilages on left side in relation to the anterior border of the left lung and the pleura.

Functions

- Allows expansion of lung in full inspiration
- Most dependent part of the pleural sac, if fluid appears in the pleural sac, it first collects in the costodiaphragmatic recess and obliterates the costodiaphragmatic angle.

Nerve Supply, Blood Supply and Lymphatic Drainage

Nerve Supply

- **Visceral pleura** is supplied by autonomic nerves, through branchial vessels and insensitive to pain
- The **parietal pleura** is supplied by spinal nerve; and sensitive to pain
- The costal pleura and peripheral part of diaphragmatic pleura are supplied by the lower intercostal nerves. Mediastinal and centre of diaphragmatic pleura are by the phrenic nerve.

Blood Supply

Arterial Supply

- The parietal pleura is supplied by internal thoracic, intercostal and musculophrenic arteries
- The visceral pleura by the bronchial arteries.

Venous Drainage

- Parietal pleura by internal thoracic, intercostal and musculophrenic veins
- Visceral pleura drain into bronchial veins.

Lymphatic Drainage

- The parietal pleura drain intercostal and diaphragmatic nodes

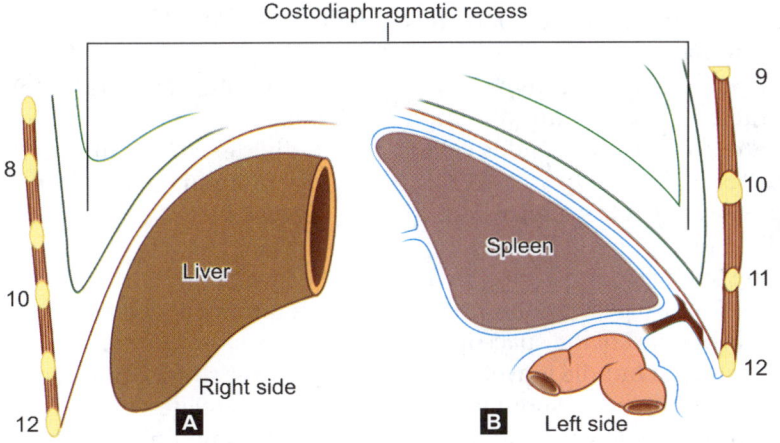

Figs. 14A and B: Relations of costodiaphragmatic recess.

- Visceral pleura drain into nodes at the hilum of lung.

Surface Markings

- A point 2.5 cm above the junction of medial and middle third of clavicle
- The medial end of the line is behind the sternoclavicular joint
- From sternoclavicular joint the line runs downwards and medially, reaches the midline at the sternal angle on both side
- On the right side the line from sternal angle runs downwards in the midline up to the xiphisternal joint
- On the left side the line from sternal angle to the fourth costal cartilage
- It then passes inferolaterally to reach the sixth costal cartilage about 3 cm away from the midline forming the cardiac notch
- From the lower end of this line, the inferior border is marked by joining the points along the 8th rib in the midclavicular line, 10th rib in midaxillary line, 12th rib in scapular line and the side of the body of 12th thoracic vertebra.

Applied Anatomy

- Inflammation of the pleura is referred to as pleurisy
- The pleural cavity is filled with air it is called pneumothorax
- If is filled with serous fluid is referred to as pleural effusion
- The pleural cavity is filled with blood it is called hemothorax
- Presence of pus is called empyema
- If the thoracic cavity is injured, lymph may enter the pleural cavity and is called as chylothorax
- **Paracentesis thoracis:** Aspiration of fluid from the pleural cavity by passing a needle in the 8th intercostal space, in the mid axillary line. By passing the needle through the lower part of the space injury to the neurovascular bundle is avoided
- **Referred pain** to the tip of shoulder and lower part of neck is felt in irritation of diaphragmatic pleura
- The inferior border of right costodiaphragmatic recess is an important consideration in the surgical posterior approach to the kidney.

4. **Describe the temporomandibular joint under the following headings. Articular surfaces, ligaments, relations, movements and muscles producing the movements and applied anatomy.**

Type

Synovial, bicondylar joint.

Articular Surfaces

- **Mandibular/glenoid fossa of temporal bone**
  - The mandibular fossa is restricted in front by the articular eminence of the zygomatic process
  - Mandibular fossa of temporal bone has an articular and nonarticular part separated by squamotympanic fissure
  - The anterior articular part is, formed by the squamous part
  - The posterior nonarticular area, formed by the tympanic part.
- **Condyle of mandible**
  - Is ovoid in shape
  - The transverse dimension is more than the anteroposterior.

Ligaments

1. Articular Disc (Fig. 15)

- Oval in **shape**
- It is **made** of dense fibrous connective tissue
- It divides the joint cavity into two—superior and inferior articular cavities.
- **Surfaces**
  - Upper surface appears concavo-convex, to fit into the convex articular eminence and the concave articular fossa
  - Lower surface has a central depression that is related to the articular surface of the mandibular condyle.
- The **thickness** of the disc varies.

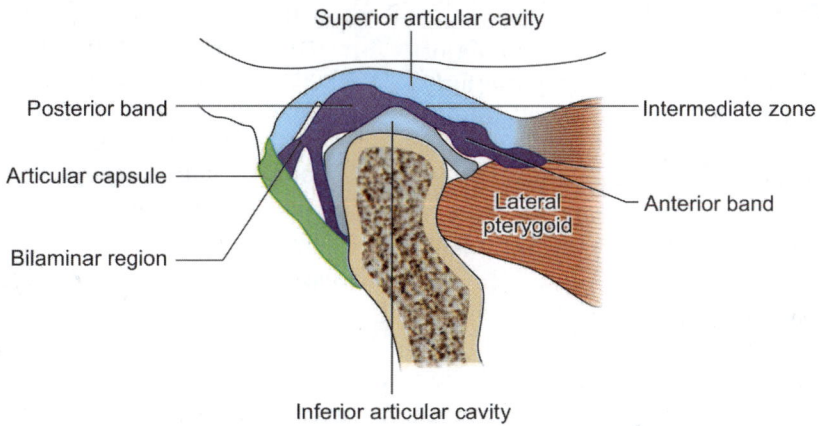

Fig. 15: Articular disc.

- **Parts**
  - The disc has a thin **intermediate zone** and thickened **anterior and posterior bands**, posterior **bilaminar region** which splits into two laminae
  - The upper lamina is made of fibrous tissue with elastic fibers, the lower lamina contains only fibrous tissue, and elastic fibers are absent.
- **Attachment**
  - Posteriorly the upper lamina is attached to the squamotympanic fissure, and the lower lamina, is attached to the back of the condyle. In between the two laminae venous plexus is present
  - Anteriorly attached to the tendon of lateral pterygoid
  - It is **attached** all around to the fibrous capsule.
- **Vascularity**
  - The central part of the disc is avascular, peripherally less vascular
  - No **nerve** supply the disc
  - The disc degenerates as age advances and gets thinned out.
- **Functions of disc are**
  - Stabilizes the condyles within the joint
  - Chondroitin sulphate secreted by the cells in the disc, gives compressive strength
  - As the joint cavity is divided, the sliding movement and rotation occur in different compartments of the joint. The wear due to frictional force on the condyle and the articular eminence is thereby reduced
  - Helps in lubrication of the joint.

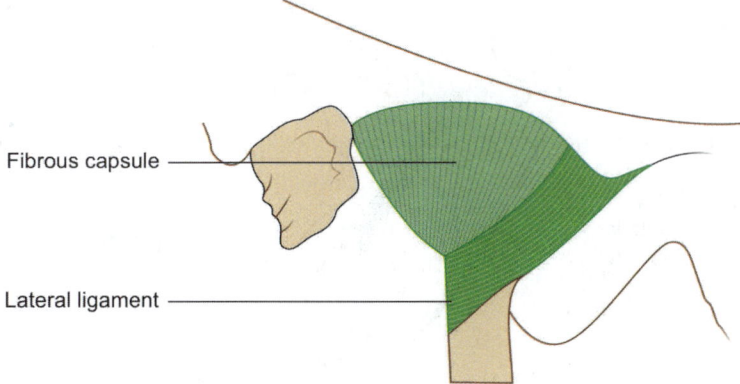

Fig. 16: Fibrous capsule.

2. Fibrous Capsule (Fig. 16)

- The capsule is attached above to the anterior edge of the articular eminence, posteriorly to the squamotympanic fissure, all around to the margins of the articular fossa, and below to the neck of the mandible
- The upper part of the joint is lax, surrounded by loose fibers and lower part by tight fibers.

3. Lateral (Temporomandibular) Ligament (Fig. 16)

- It is attached above to the articular tubercle of the zygomatic process of the temporal bone
- It is directed downwards and backwards
- Attached below to the lateral surface and posterior border of the neck of the mandible.

4. Sphenomandibular Ligament (Fig. 17)

- **Attachment:** Extends from the spine of the sphenoid to the lingula of the mandibular foramen
- It is stretched when the jaw is about half open
- **Development**: It is remnant of fibrous sheath of Meckel's cartilage
- Relations
  - **Lateral:** Lateral pterygoid, the auriculotemporal nerve, and neck and ramus of the mandible
  - The maxillary artery intervenes between the sphenomandibular ligament and the neck of the mandible
  - The ramus of the mandible is separated from the ligament by the inferior alveolar vessels and nerve and parotid
  - **Medial:** In the upper part the chorda tympani nerve and inferomedially medial pterygoid muscle.
- Structure **piercing the ligament**—the vessels and nerve to mylohyoid.

5. Stylomandibular Ligament (Fig. 17)

- The stylomandibular ligament is formed by the thickening of deep cervical fascia
- Extends from the apex and adjacent anterior aspect of the styloid process to the angle and posterior border of the mandible
- Relations
  - Superiorly—middle cranial fossa
  - Medially—middle meningeal artery, maxillary artery
  - Laterally—parotid gland, facial nerve branches.

Movements and Muscles Producing Depression (Fig. 18A)

- Is done to open the mouth
- Occurs in stages
- **Initial stage in opening the mouth:** The condyle rotates within the inferior joint space while the disc remains stationary
- **Middle stage of the opening:** The condyle and disc moves forward together
- **End stage (maximum opening):** The head of condyle moves further forward than the disc so the summit of the condyle,

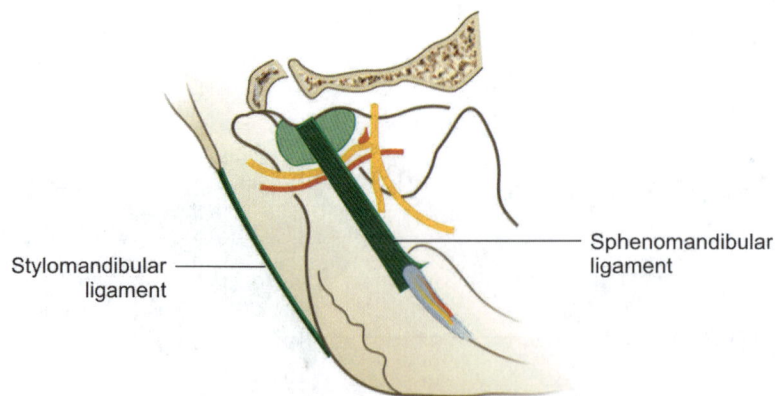

Fig. 17: Sphenomandibular and stylomandibular ligaments.

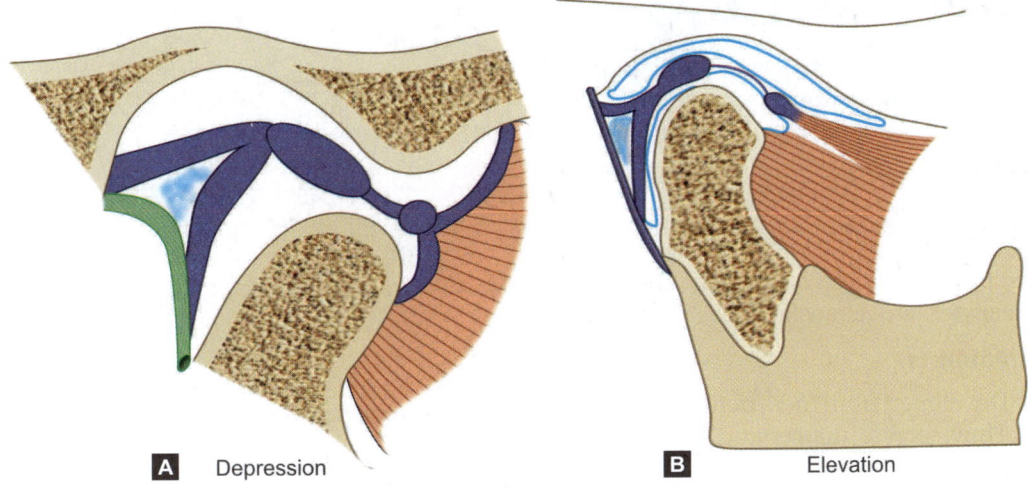

Figs. 18A and B: Movements of TM joint.

will be related above to the anterior band of the articular disc
- The normal range of maximum mouth opening is 35 – 50 mm (between the tips of upper and lower incisor)
- **Muscle producing**: Lateral pterygoid.

Elevation (Fig. 18B)
- This movement is to close the mouth.
- Depressed mandible is elevated.
- The condyle rest back to the mandibular fossa
- The articular disc placed on the head of condyle
- The summit of the condyle will be related above to posterior band
- **Muscle producing**: Masseter, temporalis, medial pterygoid.

Protraction
- Forward movement of mandible
- **Muscles producing:** Lateral and medial pterygoid and masseter.

Retraction
- Protruded mandible is brought back to mandibular fossa
- **Muscle producing**—posterior fibers of temporalis.

Side to Side Movement
- Helps in chewing food
- This movement is produced by the alternating activity both side muscles
- When the medial and lateral pterygoids of right side act together, the mandible of right side is rotated forwards and to the opposite side, with the left mandibular head as a vertical axis and vice versa
- **Muscles producing**: Both side medial and lateral pterygoid muscles act.

Applied Anatomy
- In wide yawning the head of mandible gets dislocated anteriorly. The jaw gets locked and patient cannot close the mouth. It is due to excessive contraction of lateral pterygoid muscle
- Arthritis of the joint—joint gets inflamed from degenerative arthritis
- Injury to the articular branch of auriculotemporal nerve supplying the articular capsule of the joint along with traumatic dislocation and injury to ligaments of the joint leads to laxity and instability of the joint
- Dislocation of joint may also accompany fracture of mandible
- Posterior dislocation is uncommon.

II. SHORT NOTES

1. Microscopic structure of bone in transverse section.

It consists of cells and ground substance (matrix).

CELLS

The **bone cells** are of 3 types: Osteoblasts, osteocytes and osteoclasts.

Osteoblasts

- Developed from mesenchyme
- They secrete matrix and type I collagen fibers
- They have centrally placed nucleus
- The osteoblasts secrete osteocalcin and alkaline phosphatase which release calcium and phosphate radicals from substances
- They help in mineralization
- Osteoblasts are the precursor cells of osteocytes.

Osteocytes

- Once an osteoblast becomes surrounded by matrix, it becomes an osteocyte
- The cells lie in spaces called lacunae
- The cytoplasmic processes of these cells communicate with each other by gap junctions
- They do not undergo mitosis
- They maintain calcification.

Osteoclasts

- They are large cells with multiple nuclei and are macrophages of bone tissue
- They help in resorption of bone and play a role in remodeling of bone
- They lie in depressions called Howship's lacunae
- They do not undergo mitosis.

GROUND SUBSTANCE

It consists of proteoglycans, glycoproteins, minerals and water and type I collagen fibers. The ground substance gets mineralized.

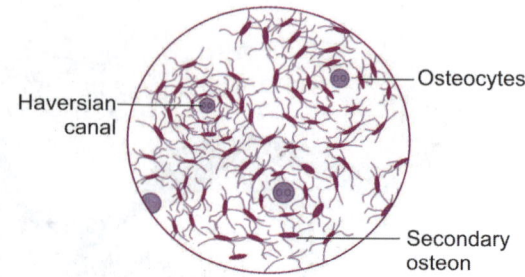

Fig. 19: Transverse section of bone.

Structure of Compact Bone (Transverse Section) (Fig. 19)

- Made up of lamellae
- The lamellae are arranged circumferentially around the Haversian canal
- The Haversian canal encloses the neurovascular bundle
- The Haversian canal along with the surrounding lamellae is called as a **Haversian system** or **secondary osteon**
- The lacunae are present in between the lamellae in which the osteocytes are lodged
- The cytoplasmic processes of the osteocytes pass through the canaliculi and communicate with that of the other cells
- Many such haversian system/secondary osteons are present
- Between the osteons **interstitial lamellae** are present
- Near the surface of the bone the lamellae are arranged parallel to the surface and are named as **circumferential lamellae/ primary osteon**
- In **longitudinal section**, the haversian canals are along the length of the bone
- The **Volkmann's canals** are seen as oblique canals connecting the Haversian canals of adjacent osteons with each other and also with the endosteum and periosteum, through which the blood vessels pass.

2. Intraembryonic mesoderm.

- The intraembryonic mesoderm extends over whole of the embryonic area except

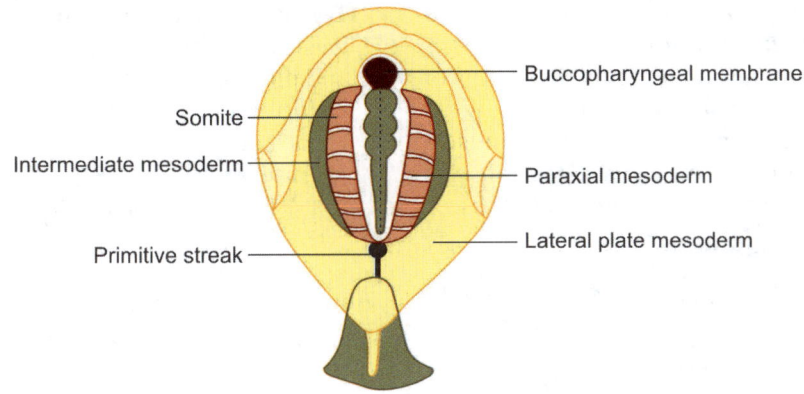

Fig. 20: Intraembryonic mesoderm.

in midline, the prochordal plate and caudal to primitive streak **(Fig. 20)**
- The mesoderm is divided by longitudinal groove into three parts.
    1. Paraxial mesoderm—on each side of notochord and developing neural tube
    2. Intermediate mesoderm—floor of longitudinal groove
    3. Lateral plate mesoderm—extends up to periphery.

Paraxial Mesoderm (Fig. 21)

- It extends from prochordal plate to primitive streak
- It passes on either side of hind brain, close to otic vesicle
- The post otic part of paraxial mesoderm forms bilateral solid cords on either side of notochord
- The paraxial mesoderm undergoes **segmentation** to form somites or metameres
- The process of segmentation extends **craniocaudally**
- Somites appear between **20th to 30th day**. By end of 30 days there will be 44 pairs of somites. Hence 4th week of development is called **somite period**
- Cranial most somites are called **occipital somites**. Situated on either side of hind brain. They give rise to formation of skull
- **Preotic somites** give rise to the base of skull and muscles of head
- Each somite divides into a ventromedial **sclerotome** and dorsolateral **dermomyotome**
- Sclerotome cells become polymorphous and migrate ventromedially around the notochord and neural tube to form primitive vertebrae and ribs

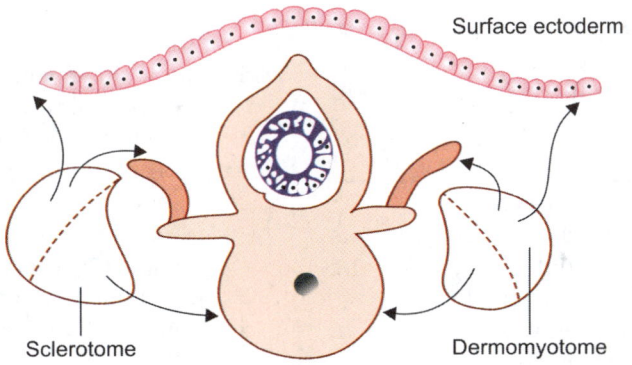

Fig. 21: Paraxial mesoderm.

- The dermomyotome is divided into dermal plate and muscle plate
- The cells of **dermal plate** forms dermis of skin and subcutaneous tissue
- The **myotome** gives rise to skeletal muscle
- The myotome forms the striated muscles of trunk, tongue, diaphragm and limbs.

Intermediate Mesoderm

Gives rise to development of kidneys and gonads.

Lateral Plate Mesoderm

- It is in the peripheral margin of embryonic area
- It is continuous with pericardial bar which encloses a cavity called pericardial sac
- Spaces appear in the lateral plate mesoderm, which join together to form **intraembryonic coelom**
- The intraembryonic coelom forms the pleural, pericardial and peritoneal cavities
- Cephalic end of it forms septum transversum from which the diaphragm is developed
- The coelomic cavity divides the lateral plate into two layers—**somatic and splanchnic**
- The somatic layer with the overlying ectoderm is called as **somatopleure**
- The splanchnic layer with underlying endoderm forms the **splanchnopleure**
- The **somatopleure** gives rise to parietal layer of pericardial, peritoneal and pleural sacs
- It also forms the dermis, subcutaneous tissue of body wall
- The **splanchnopleure** gives rise to the visceral layers of the serous sacs, musculature, connective tissue of gut, respiratory tract, and heart.

3. Brachial artery.

- It is the main artery of the arm
- **Commencement:** The axillary artery is continued as brachial artery from the lower border of teres major
- **Course:** It runs downwards in front of humerus and reaches the cubital fossa
- **Termination:** In the cubital fossa, at the level of neck of radius, it divides into radial and ulnar arteries
- **Relations:** Artery is accompanied by venae comitantes
    - **Anterior**
        - It is superficial covered by skin and fasciae
        - Bicipital aponeurosis
        - Median cubital vein
        - Median nerve crosses from lateral to medial.
    - **Posterior**
        - Medial head of triceps
        - Coracobrachialis
        - Brachialis muscle.
    - **Lateral**
        - Median nerve in upper part
        - Coracobrachialis
        - Biceps tendon.
    - **Medial**
        - Medial cutaneous nerve of forearm
        - Ulnar nerve
        - Median nerve in the lower part.
- **Branches (Fig. 22):**
  1. Profunda brachii artery
     - Large branch
     - Accompanies radial nerve
     - Enters the spiral groove through upper triangular space
     - Supplies muscles, nutrient artery to humerus, and divides into middle and radial collateral branches.
  2. Nutrient branch to humerus
     - Given at the mid-level of arm.
  3. Muscular branches
     - To coracobrachialis, biceps, brachialis.
  4. Superior ulnar collateral artery
     - Arises below the middle of arm
     - Accompanies ulnar nerve
     - Pierces medial intermuscular septum
     - Anastomose with posterior ulnar recurrent artery.
  5. Inferior ulnar collateral artery
     - Arises about 5 cm above elbow
     - Pierces medial intermuscular septum

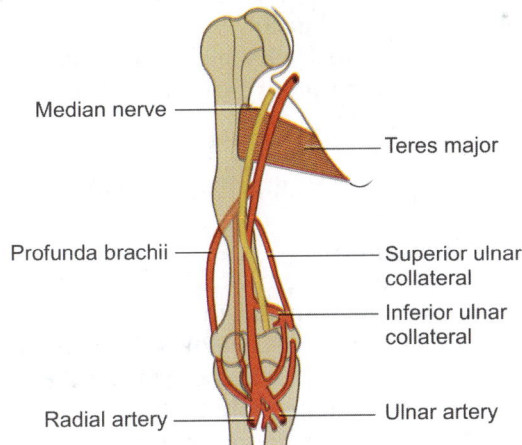

Fig. 22: Brachial artery.

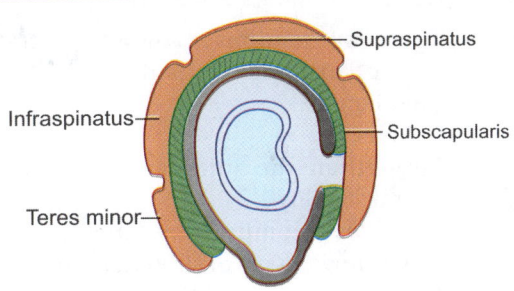

Fig. 23: Rotator cuff.

- Winds around the humerus
- Anastomose with middle collateral artery
- A branch from it descends in front of medial epicondyle and anastomose with anterior ulnar recurrent artery.
- Radial artery—terminal branch
- Ulnar artery—terminal branch.
- Variations:
  - Sometimes higher division into radial and ulnar arteries
  - Artery can sometimes be congenitally compressed by ligament of Struther.

Applied Anatomy

- Ligation is done to prevent blood loss in distal injuries
- Palpation is done by pressing it against the humerus
- For recording the blood pressure, this artery is utilized
- Fracture distal part of humerus may be displaced, anteriorly or posteriorly. The brachial artery may be injured by the displaced bone fragment.

4. Muscles of rotator cuff shoulder.

- The shoulder joint is covered by articular capsule and is strengthened by tendons of muscles around the joint
- The muscles fuse with the capsule of the shoulder joint are called as musculotendinous cuff/rotator cuff of Codmann
- When the humerus is abducted, flexed and internally rotated, the cuff usually impinches against the coracoacromial arch. This position is known as the impingement position
- Components of rotator cuff (**Fig. 23**):
  – **Anteriorly:** Subscapularis
  – **Superiorly:** Supraspinatus
  – **Posteriorly:**
   - Infraspinatus
   - Teres minor.
  These tendons fuse with lateral part of articular capsule to form the cuff.
- **Position of tendons** of muscles in rotator cuff:
  – The posterior surface of tendon of subscapularis gets inserted to lesser trochanter and anterior part of articular capsule
  – Tendon of supraspinatus crosses the shoulder joint and is inserted to the upper facet of greater tubercle and blends with superior part of articular capsule and helps to retain the head of humerus in the glenoid fossa
  – Tendon of infraspinatus passes across the posterior aspect of shoulder joint and is inserted to middle facet of greater tubercle and posterior part of articular capsule. Sometimes a bursa may be present separating the tendon from articular capsule
  – Tendon of teres minor is inserted to the lower facet of greater tubercle and blends with lower part of posterior surface of articular capsule

- These four tendons along with lateral part of articular capsule form the rotator cuff.
- **Functions**:
  - Strengthen the joint and provides lateral stability
  - Produces a compressive force during active movements of shoulder joint
  - Keeps the head of the humerus in contact with the glenoid fossa, and prevents dislocations.

Applied Anatomy

Rotator Cuff Disease
- Is a painful condition in which severe or chronic collision of the rotator cuff tendons on the undersurface of the coracoacromial arch
- The cuff normally presses against the coracoacromial arch
- The supraspinatus tendon is anatomically the most affected by the impact
- Severe impingement can be caused by (a) thickening of the coracoacromial arch, (b) by inflammation of the cuff as in rheumatoid arthritis, (c) due to prolonged overuse, e.g. in cleaning windows.

5. Tibial collateral ligament.

- **Attachment (Fig. 24)**:
  - **Above:** To the medial condyle of the femur just below the adductor tubercle
  - **Below:** It divides into superficial and deep parts.

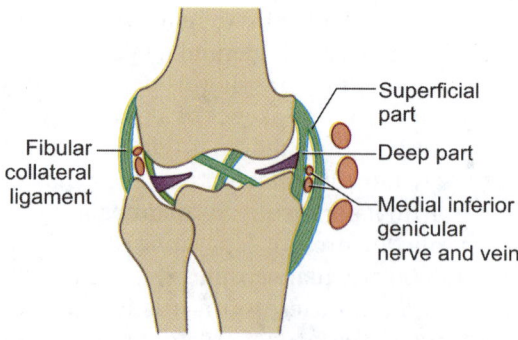

Fig. 24: Tibial collateral ligament.

- **Superficial part:**
  - Attached below to the medial border and posterior part of medial surface of shaft of tibia
  - It is crossed by 3 tendons namely sartorius, gracilis and semitendinosus.
- **Deep part:**
  - Short, blends with the capsule and with the medial meniscus
  - It is attached below to the medial condyle of tibia above the groove for the semimembranosus.
- **Morphology:** Represents the degenerated tendon of the adductor magnus muscle
- **Function:** Stability in extension and strengthens the medial part of capsule.

6. Rectus sheath.

- The rectus abdominis is covered by the aponeurotic sheath
- It has two walls complete anterior and an incomplete posterior, formed by the flat muscles of the anterior abdominal wall
- **Extent:**
  - Above—xiphoid process.
  - Below—pubic symphysis.
- **Features:**
  - **Anterior wall:** Complete, firmly adherent to the tendinous intersections of the rectus abdominis muscle. The thickness varies at different levels
  - **Posterior wall:** Incomplete; deficient above the costal margin and below the midpoint between umbilicus and pubic symphysis (the arcuate line). It is free from the rectus abdominis.
- **Formation: Three levels**
  1. Above the costal margin **(Fig. 25)**:
     - Anterior wall is thin and formed by external oblique aponeurosis
     - Posterior wall deficient, the rectus rests on 5th, 6th and 7th costal cartilages.
  2. Between the costal margin and the arcuate line **(Fig. 26)**:
     - Anterior wall is thicker and formed by the external oblique aponeurosis

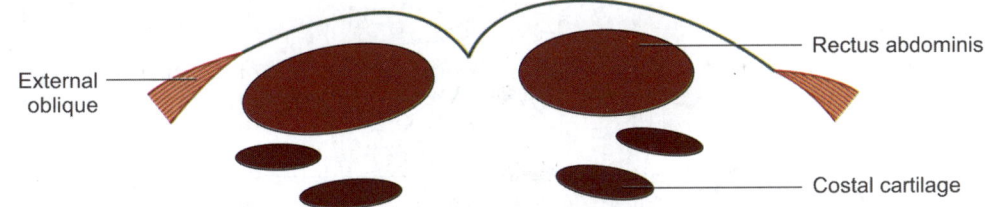

Fig. 25: Rectus sheath above the costal margin.

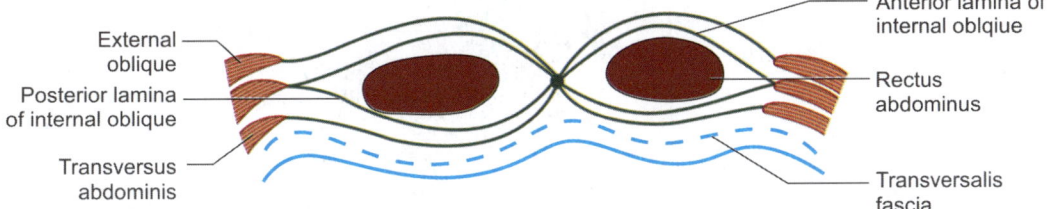

Fig. 26: Between costal margin and arcuate line.

and anterior lamina of aponeurosis of internal oblique
- Posterior wall by the posterior lamina of the aponeurosis of the internal oblique and the aponeurosis of the transversus abdominis muscle.
3. Below the arcuate line (linear semicircular fold of Douglas lies midway between umbilicus and the pubic symphysis) **(Fig. 27)**:
    - Anterior wall is thickest and formed by fusion of the aponeurosis of all the three flat muscles of the abdomen
    - Posterior wall is deficient, the rectus rests on the fascia transversals which is thickened to form iliopubic tract or Thompson's ligament
- Lateral border **(Fig. 28)**: Linea semilunaris extends from tip of 9th costal cartilage to pubic tubercle. The lower six thoracic nerves enter the sheath by piercing this border
- Medial border: Linea alba produced by decussation of aponeurosis of the three anterior abdominal wall muscles.
- **Contents:**
    – Two muscles:
        1. Rectus abdominis
        2. Pyramidalis.
    – Two vessels:
        1. Superior epigastric vessels
        2. Inferior epigastric vessels.

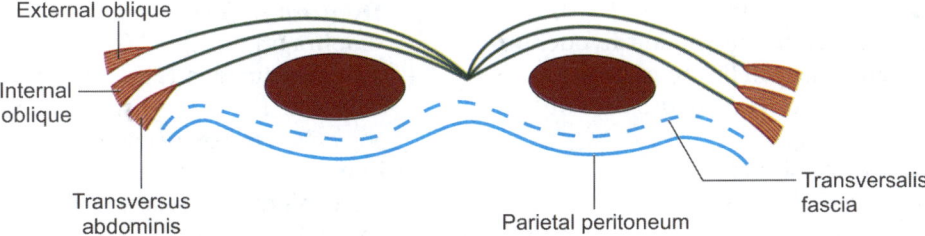

Fig. 27: Below arcuate line.

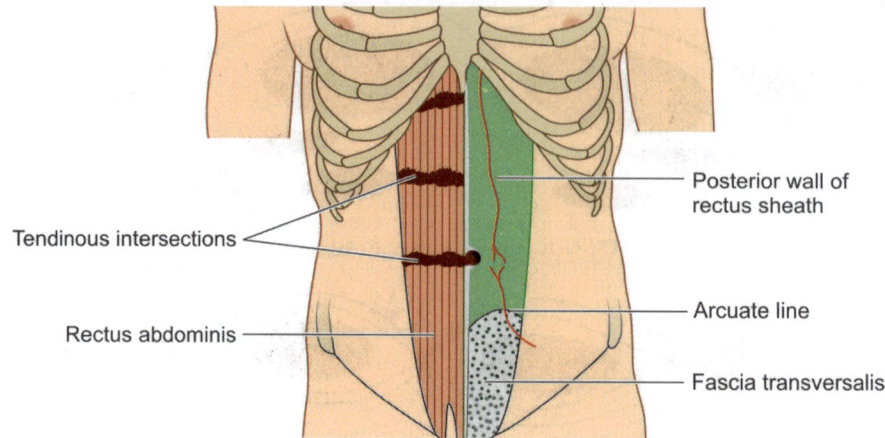

Fig. 28: Rectus sheath.

- Two nerves:
    1. Terminal part of lower 5 thoracic nerves
    2. Subcostal nerve.
- **Functions:**
    - Checks bowing of rectus muscle
    - Maintains the strength of anterior abdominal wall
    - Prevents injury to the midline structures by acting as a shock absorber.
- **Applied anatomy:** Divarification of recti— due to weakness of anterior abdominal muscles usually in multiparous women. Rectus sheath is stretched during coughing, straining and the abdominal viscera protrudes forwards in between the two recti muscles.

7. Spleen.

A wedge-shaped lymphatic organ belonging to reticuloendothelial system.
- **Shape:** Tetrahedral in shape
- **Situation:** Mainly in the left hypochondrium and partly in the epigastrium
- **Measurement:** Harris dictum of odd numbers
    - Thickness—1 inch
    - Breadth—3 inches
    - Length—5 inches
    - Weight—7 ounces
    - Rib level—9 to 11 ribs
- **Axis:**
    - The long axis is along the tenth rib.
    - Directed downwards, forwards and laterally.
- **Features:** It has 2 ends, 3 borders, 2 surfaces.
- **Ends:**
    - **Anterior end:** Expanded at midaxillary line
    - **Posterior end:** Rounded, related to the upper pole of left kidney.
- **Borders:**
    - **Superior border:** Separates diaphragmatic surface from gastric area. Notch present in this border represents the lobulated form of spleen in fetal life
    - **Inferior border:** Separates renal impression from diaphragmatic surface. It is blunt and rounded
    - **Intermediate border.**
- **Surfaces:**
    - **Diaphragmatic surface**—related to diaphragm
    - **Visceral surface (Fig. 29)**—related to stomach, left kidney, splenic flexure of the colon, tail of the pancreas.
- **Hilum:**
    - The splenic vessels and nerves pass through it
    - Gives attachment to gastrosplenic and lienorenal ligaments.

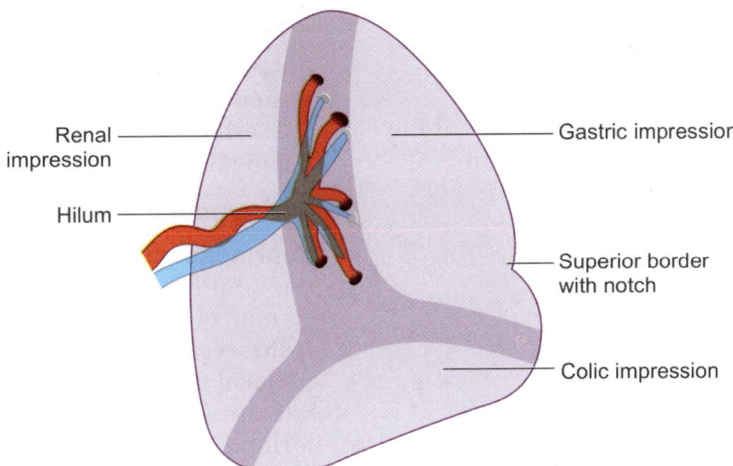

Fig. 29: Viceral surface of spleen.

- **Sustentaculum lienis** for the spleen is phrenicocolic ligament
- **Suspensory ligament**—is lienophrenic (phrenicosplenic) ligament; it is an extension of lienorenal ligament. It extends from spleen to diaphragm **(Fig. 30)**.
- **Blood supply:**
  - Splenic artery is from the coeliac artery and is an end artery. It divides into 5 branches to the segments of the spleen
  - Splenic vein drains into the portal vein.
- **Lymphatic drainage:** The capsular lymphatics drain into pancreaticosplenic nodes. There is no lymphatic drainage for the splenic tissue
- **Nerve supply:** Sympathetic fibers from the coeliac plexus
- **Development:** From mesenchymal nodules—fuse to form spleen (causes splenic notch).
- **Applied anatomy:**
  - Any increase of pressure in the portal system leads to enlargement of spleen
  - Splenomegaly can be palpated deep to left costal margin. It occurs in many hematological and infective conditions.

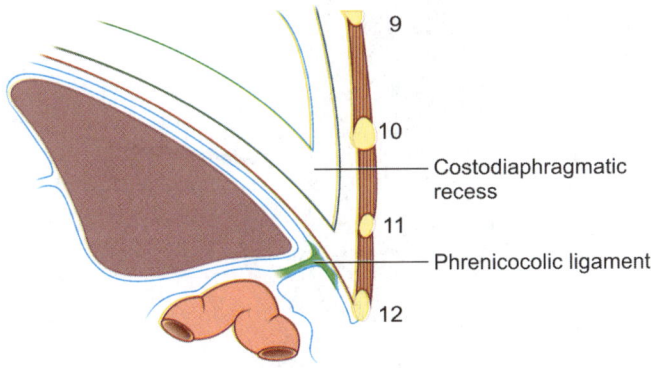

Fig. 30: Relations of diaphragmatic surface.

8. Ischiorectal fossa.

Situation
A wedge-shaped space on each side of the anal canal below the pelvic diaphragm.

Dimensions
- Length – 5 cm
- Width – 2.5 cm
- Depth – 5 cm.

Boundaries
- **Base:** By skin and superficial fascia.
- **Apex:** Formed by the fusion of obturator fascia and anal fascia
- **Anterior boundary:** By the posterior border of the perineal membrane and transverse perineii superficialis and profundus
- **Posterior boundary:** Lower border of gluteus maximus, sacrotuberous ligament
- **Lateral wall:** Obturator internus with fascia, medial surface of ischial tuberosity. Pudendal (Alcock's) canal is present along this wall containing the pudendal nerve, internal pudendal artery and nerve to obturator internus. It is covered by obturator fascia and lunate fascia. The pudendal nerve terminates within the canal
- **Medial wall:** External anal sphincter with fascia, levator ani with anal fascia.

Recesses
- Anterior recess
- Posterior recess
- Horseshoe recess: Connects the two fossae behind the anal canal.

Subdivisions of the Fossa
- **Suprategmental space:** Lies above the tegmentum, which is formed by the summit of lunate fascia
- **Ischiorectal space:** Between lunate and perianal fascia. The perianal fascia is the lateral most septum of conjoint tendon formed by longitudinal muscular coat of rectum and pubo rectalis fibers. This space contains fat
- **Perianal space:** Between the skin and perianal fascia. It contains loculated fat.

Contents
- Internal pudendal vessels in the pudendal canal
- Pudendal nerve divides into dorsal nerve of penis and perineal nerve
- Inferior rectal nerve and vessels crosses the fossa from lateral to medial wall
- Posterior scrotal or labial nerves and vessels
- Perineal nerve of S_4
- Perforating cutaneous branches of nerves S_2, S_3
- Ischiorectal pad of fat.

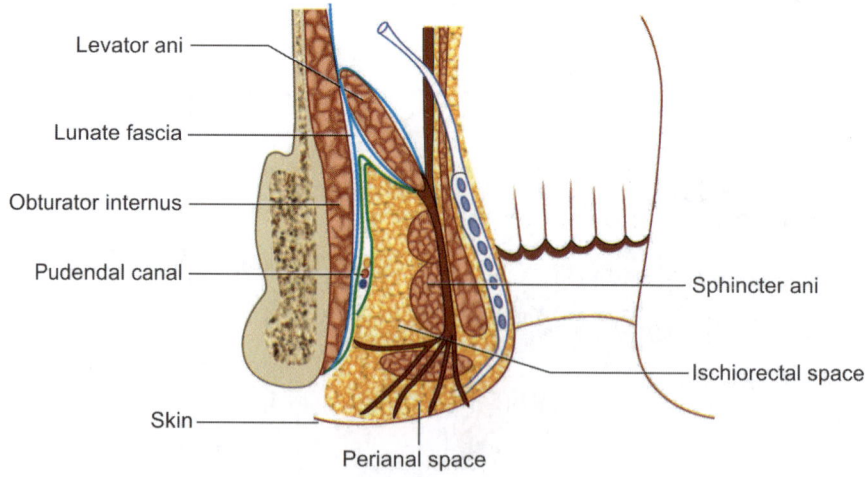

Fig. 31: Ischiorectal fossa.

Function

Space allows distension of anal canal during defecation.

Applied Anatomy

- Ischiorectal abscesses are common and painful because of the nerves crossing it
- Pelvic contents may herniate into this via hiatus of Schwalbe (defect in the pelvic diaphragm) at the apex of the fossa
- Fistula-in-ano if the abscess opens into the anal canal.

9. Development of testis.

- Testis is developed retroperitoneally in the abdominal region
- Initially gonads appear as longitudinal ridge on either side called **genital or gonadal ridges**
- The proliferation of the epithelium with the underlying mesenchyme form these ridges
- The underlying mesenchyme is penetrated by the proliferated epithelial cells of the ridges
- They form the **primitive sex cords** which are irregular shaped cords
- The genital ridge is divided into an outer cortex and inner medulla
- The **primodial germ cells** from the epiblast migrate and reach the endodermal cells of yolk sac
- In the fourth week, these cells travel through the dorsal mesentery of hind gut
- Reaches the genital ridge by 6th week.
- The testis developed from medulla of the undifferentiated genital ridge and the cortex atrophies
- The solid irregular primitive sex cords developed in the ridge are known as **testis/medullary cords**
- Close to the blind end of mesonephric duct and towards hilum of the gland they form a plexus called **rete cords**
- Loose mesenchymal cells intervene between the testis cords
- The **tunica albuginea** is formed by the dense layer of connective tissue, that separates the testis cords from surface epithelium
- The **testis cord is composed** of male germ cells and the supporting Sustentacular cells of Sertoli
- The surface epithelium of the gland **forms the Sustentacular cells**
- The **interstitial cells of Leydig** are derived from mesenchyme of the genital ridge
- The Leydig cells secrete testosterone
- Testis cords remain solid until puberty
- The testis is formed in the abdominal region
- The peritoneum of the abdominal cavity forms an evagination called the **processus vaginalis**
- There is a fibromuscular band called **gubernaculum testis**
- The upper end of the gubernaculum divides and is attached to lower pole of testis, processus vaginalis, mesonephric duct

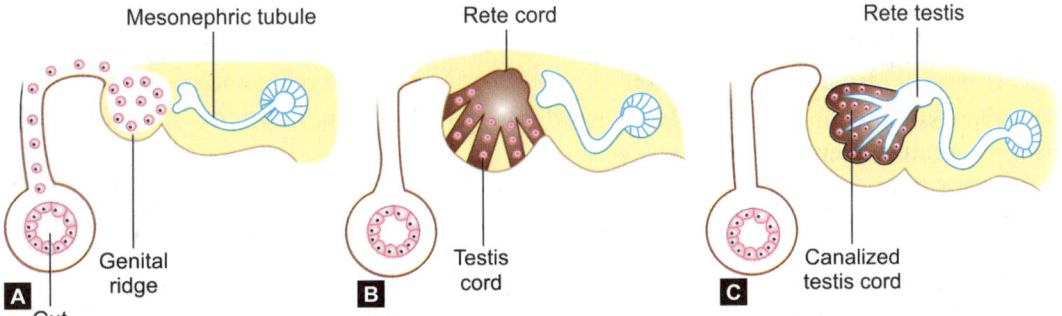

Figs. 32A to C: Development of testis.

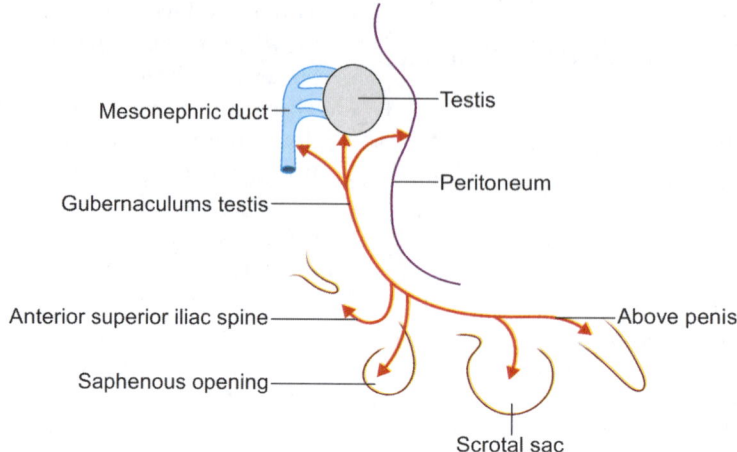

Fig. 33: Descent of testis—tail of Lockwood.

- Lower end initially it extends up to inguinal region
- The lower end of the gubernaculum splits into many fibrous bands called **tail of Lockwood (Fig. 33)**
- When the testis begins to descend the gubernaculum grows towards the scrotal swelling
- The processus vaginalis follows the gubernaculum into the scrotal swellings
- The **factors for descent** of testis are:
  - Gubernaculum testis
  - Increased intra-abdominal pressure
  - Intra-abdominal temperature
  - Contraction of arching fibers of internal oblique muscle
  - Uncurling of fetus
  - Testicular hormone.
- The testis reach inguinal region by 12 weeks, passes through inguinal canal by 28 weeks, and reach the scrotum by 33 weeks.

10. Microscopic structure of pancreas.

Glandular tissue of pancreas is made of two types—exocrine and endocrine parts

1. **Exocrine part**
   - **Cells:** Formed by branched tubular acini.
     - The **acinar cells** are serous acini
       * The cells are pyramidal in shape
       * Cells are provided with basal round nuclei
       * The infranuclear part contains abundant roughened endoplasmic reticulum, and zymogen granules in the apical region
       * Supranuclearly golgi complex and membrane bound granules containing pancreatic secretion
   - **Centroacinar cells** are seen between duct and acinus lined by flattened or cuboidal cells
   - **Pancreatic stellate cells** (PaSCs) are similar to myofibroblast, and situated in the periacinar space with processes in contact with acini.
   - **Ducts:** (a) Sections of **intercalated** and (b) **Intralobular ducts** lined by cuboidal epithelium are present. (c) The **interlobular ducts** lined by columnar cells are present.

2. **Endocrine part**
   - It consists of **islets of Langerhans**
   - Arranged in cords and clumps, between which the connective tissue and extensive capillary network are found
   - Thin connective tissue capsule is present separating the islets from acinar cells
   - Found numerous at the tail part
   - The islet is a group of polyhedral cells with fenestrated capillaries and nerve endings

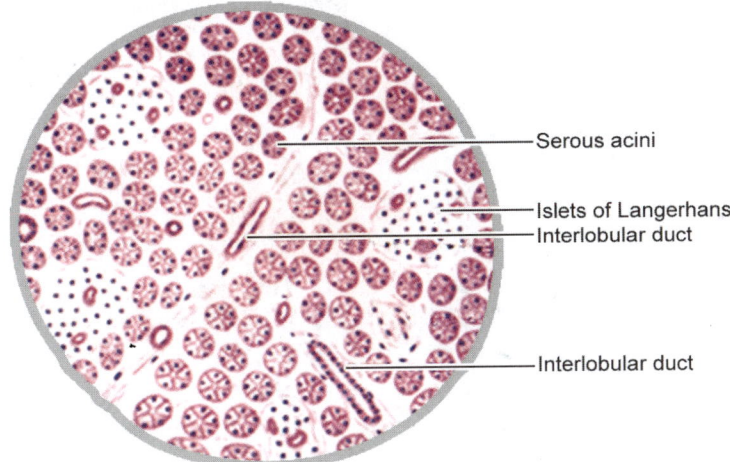

Fig. 34: Histology of pancreas.

- Alpha (A) cells—20 percentage of cell population; Occupy periphery of islet, secretes glucagon
- Beta (B) cells—70 percentage of cell population. Seen in the center of islet and secrete insulin
- Delta (D) cells—seen in the periphery. Produce gastrin and somatostatin
- F cells secrete pancreatic polypeptide (PP)
- D1 cells secrete vasoactive intestinal polypeptide (VIP).

The islet is divided into outer cortex and inner medulla. The beta cells form the medulla and is homotypical and the other cells are at periphery forming the cortex and is heterotypical.

11. Superior vena cava.

- Superior vena cava is a large venous channel which **collects** blood from the upper half of the body and drains into the right atrium.
- It has no valve.
- **Situation**:
  - Extrapericardial part: In superior mediastinum
  - Intrapericardial part: In middle mediastinum.
- **Measurements:**
  - Length—7 cm
  - Width—2 cm
- **Formation:** The right and the left brachiocephalic veins unite behind the lower border of the first right costal cartilage close to the sternum.
- **Course:**
  - Begins behind the lower border of sternal end of the first right costal cartilage
  - Opposite the second right costal cartilage pierces the pericardium
- **Termination:** Opens into the upper part of sinus venarum part of right atrium behind the third right costal cartilage.
- **Relations:**
  - Anterior
    - Chest wall
    - Internal thoracic vessels
    - Anterior margin of right lung and pleura
    - Pericardium in its lower half.
  - Posterior
    - Trachea and right vagus
    - Root of right lung.
  - To the left
    - Ascending aorta
    - Brachiocephalic artery.
  - To the right
    - Phrenic nerve with accompanying vessels
    - Right lung and pleura.

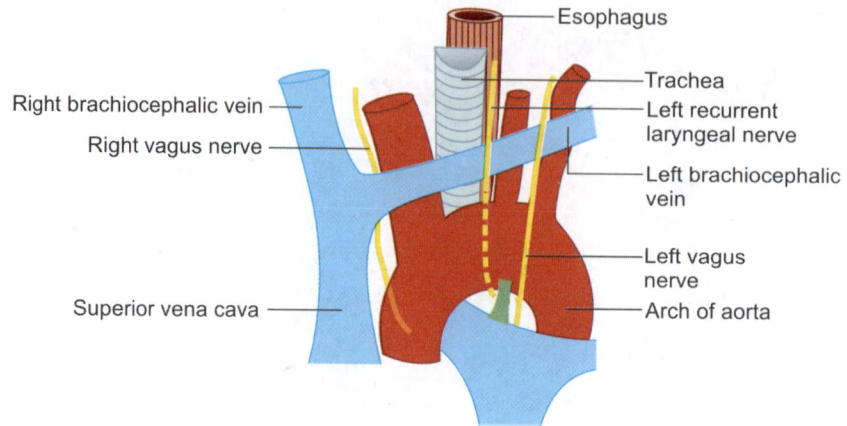

Fig. 35: Formation of superior vena cava.

- **Tributaries**:
  - Right and left brachiocephalic veins.
  - Azygos vein
  - Small mediastinal veins
  - Pericardial veins.
- **Development**:
  - Intrapericardial part from common cardinal vein (duct of Cuvier)
  - Extrapericardial part from anterior cardinal vein below oblique anastomoses.
- **Applied Anatomy:**
  - Superior vena cava may be obstructed above or below the termination of the azygos vein
  - If obstructed above, collateral circulation may be established through the tributaries of internal thoracic vein and lateral thoracic vein
  - When obstructed below, collateral circulation follows the azygos vein, superior and inferior epigastric veins, lateral thoracic and thoracoepigastric veins, hence to inferior vena cava and finally into the right atrium
  - Important channel through which blood from lower half of the body drains in obstruction of inferior vena cava through the azygos vein.

12. Third ventricle of the brain.

- It is a cavity of diencephalon
- It is like a slit
- **Developmentally** from primitive forebrain vesicle
- **Situated** between the two thalami
- **Communication**: With lateral ventricles through interventricular foramen (foramen of Monro) and with fourth ventricle through cerebral aqueduct
- **Boundaries:** It has a roof, floor, anterior, posterior, and lateral walls **(Fig. 36)**
  - **Roof:** Ependymal layer bridging between the two thalami
  - **Floor:** By the hypothalamic structures – infundibulum of pituitary, tuber cinerium, mammillary body, crus cerebri
  - **Anterior wall**: Lamina terminalis, anterior commissure, anterior columns of fornix
  - **Posterior wall:** Pineal gland, posterior commissure, cerebral aqueduct.
  - **Lateral wall**:
    - Upper part by two-third of the medial surface of the thalamus and lower part by the hypothalamus and subthalamus
    - The lateral wall is limited by stria medullaris thalami
    - A sulcus extends from interventricular foramen to the cerebral aqueduct called hypothalamic sulcus
    - The sulcus divides the thalamus and hypothalamus

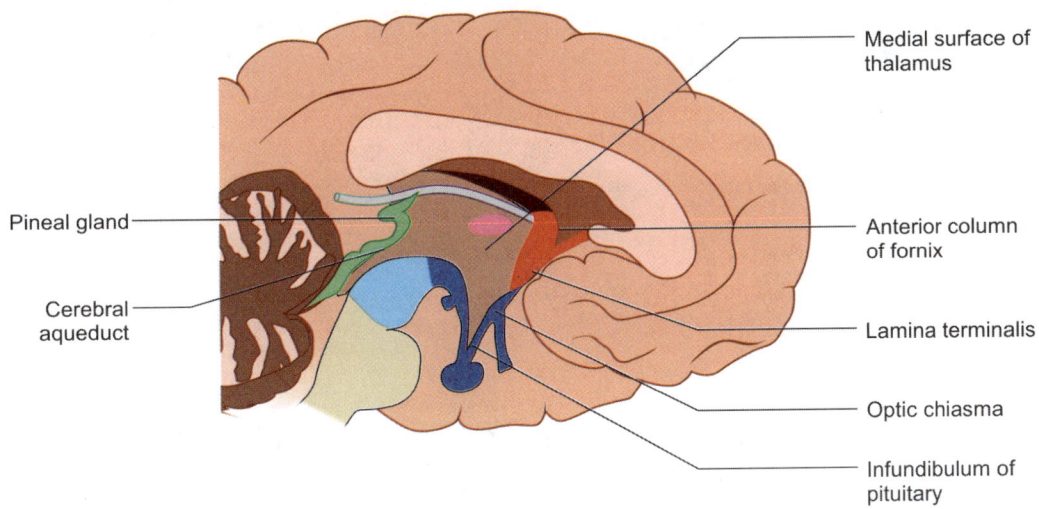

Fig. 36: Boundaries of third ventricle.

- Just behind the interventricular foramen a strip of gray matter extends from the medial wall of one thalamus to other, crossing the ventricle called interthalamic adhesion.
- **Recesses:**
  - Infundibular recess
  - Suprapineal recess
  - Pineal recess.
- **Applied anatomy:**
  - The anterior communicating artery is in the cistern of lamina terminalis. Any aneurysm formation can cause intraventricular bleed through lamina terminalis
  - The anterior and posterior commissures are used as markers in radiological landmarks
  - Any tumor in the ventricle can compress hypothalamus and also blocks the cerebral aqueduct resulting in hydrocephalus.

13. Metathalamus.

MGB for **M**usic—hearing (auditory pathway).
LGB for **L**ight—vision (visual pathway).
- The metathalamus includes medial and lateral geniculate bodies.
- They are collection of gray matter
- They form one of the component of dorsal part of diencephalon.

- **Situation:**
  - Below the pulvinar of thalamus
  - Lateral to the superior colliculus.
- **Medial geniculate body (Fig. 37)**
  - It is a relay station for auditory pathway.
  - Afferent fibers:
    - Receives fibers from lateral lemniscus
    - Few fibers through inferior brachium after relay in inferior colliculus.
  - Efferent: Fibers project to the primary auditory area 41, 42 situated in the Heschl's gyrus (transverse temporal gyrus).
- **Lateral geniculate body (Fig. 37)**
  - It is a relay station for visual pathway
  - **Afferent**: It receives fibers from.
    - Ipsilateral temporal retina
    - Contralateral nasal retina
      It contains third order of neurons in the visual pathway
    - Fibers from nuclei of reticular formation in the brainstem
    - Fibers from pulvinar of thalamus.
  - **Structure (Fig. 38):**
    - It is made up of six layers
    - Layer 1, 4, and 6 receive contralateral fibers
    - Layer 2, 3 and 5 receive ipsilateral fibers

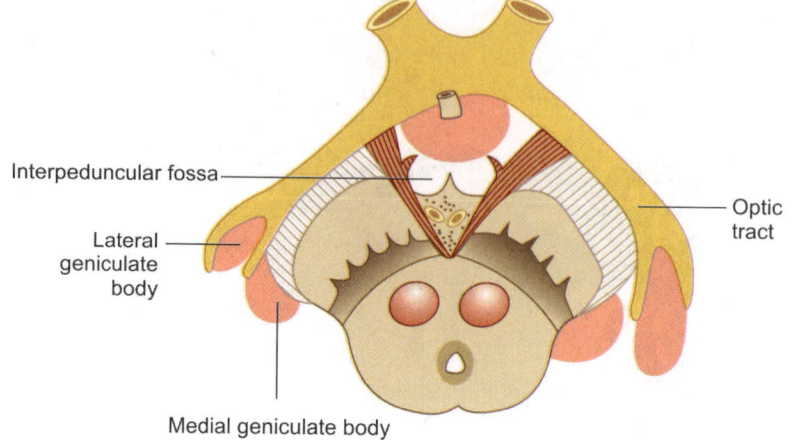

Fig. 37: Medial and lateral geniculate bodies.

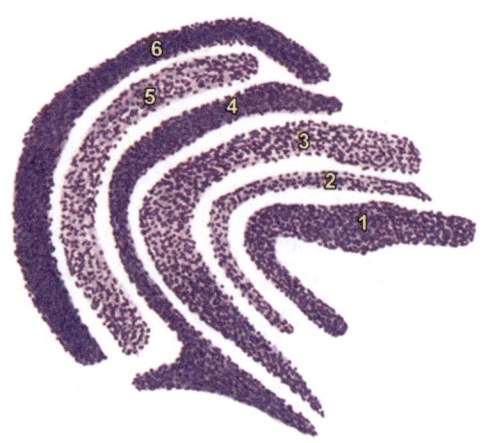

Fig. 38: Structure of lateral geniculate body.

- **Efferent:**
  - The fibers from medial geniculate body form the optic radiation (geniculocalcarine tract)
  The optic radiation ends in primary visual area 17 in the calcarine sulcus of occipital lobe
  - The retinotectal fibers responsible for visual reflex leave the MGB to the pretectal nucleus and superior colliculus.
- **Blood supply**: Posterior choroidal and posterior cerebral arteries supply.

14. Submandibular salivary gland.

Location and Part

- Large salivary gland situated on the anterior part of the digastric triangle. It is a seromucous type of gland
- J-shaped; mylohyoid muscle divides it into large **superficial** and small **deep** parts (Fig. 39A).

Relations

- **Superficial part (Fig. 39B):**
  - **Extent:**
    - **Anteriorly:** Anterior belly of digastric
    - **Posteriorly:** The stylomandibular ligament. The ligament seperates the submandibular and parotid gland
    - **Above:** Passes medial to the body of the mandible
    - **Below:** Covers the intermediate tendon of digastric and the insertion of stylohyoid
  - **Parts**: It has 3 surfaces—inferior, lateral, medial
  - **Inferior surface is related to:**
    - Skin, superficial fascia
    - Platysma
    - Investing layer of deep fascia
    - Submandibular lymph nodes

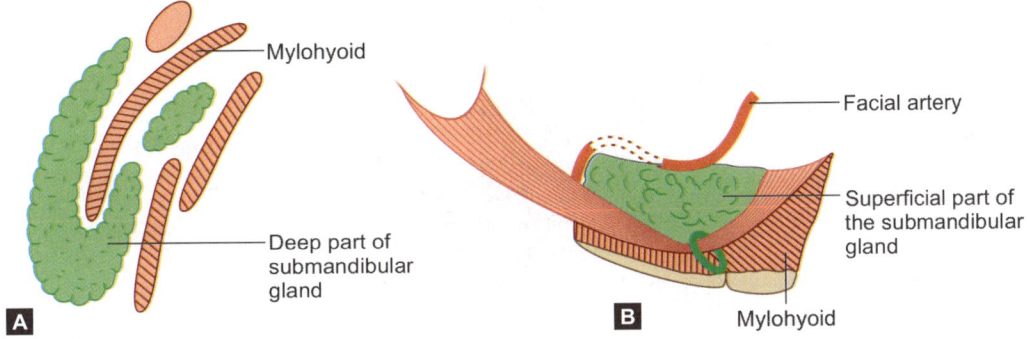

Figs. 39A and B: Submandibular salivary gland: (A) Superficial and deep parts; (B) Relations of superficial part.

- Crossed by common facial vein and cervical branch of facial nerve.
- **Lateral surface is related to:**
  - Submandibular fossa of mandible
  - Medial pterygoid muscle
  - Facial artery loops between the muscle and bone **(Fig. 40)**.
- **Medial surface is related to:**
  Anterior part
  - Mylohyoid muscle and nerve and vessels
  - Submental branch of facial artery.

  Intermediate part
  - Hyoglossus
  - Lingual nerve
  - Submandibular ganglion
  - Hypoglossal nerve.

  Posterior part
  - Styloglossus
  - Stylohyoid ligament
  - Glossopharyngeal nerve.
- **Deep part:**
  - Lies on hyoglossus muscle
  - Extends up to the posterior end of the sublingual gland.
  - Relations:
    - Laterally—mylohyoid
    - Medially—hyoglossus and styloglossus
    - Above—lingual nerve and submandibular ganglion
    - Below—hypoglossal nerve and deep lingual vein.

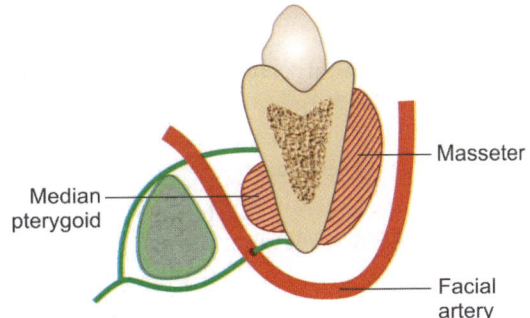

Fig. 40: Relation of facial artery.

- **Submandibular duct/Wharton's duct (Fig. 41):**
  - The submandibular duct is usually 5 cm long
  - It formed by many tributaries in the superficial part of the gland
  - From the medial surface of superficial part, passes through the deep part of the gland
  - It receives the smaller ducts of deep part
  - It runs forwards between mylohyoid and hyoglossus
  - Then passes between the sublingual gland and genioglossus
  - It opens in the floor of the mouth on the summit of the sublingual papilla on either side of the frenulum of the tongue
  - On hyoglossus it lies between the lingual and hypoglossal nerves but, at

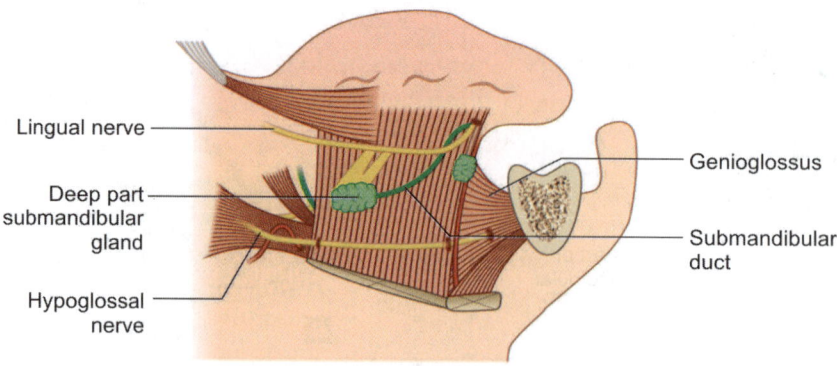

Fig. 41: Submandibular duct.

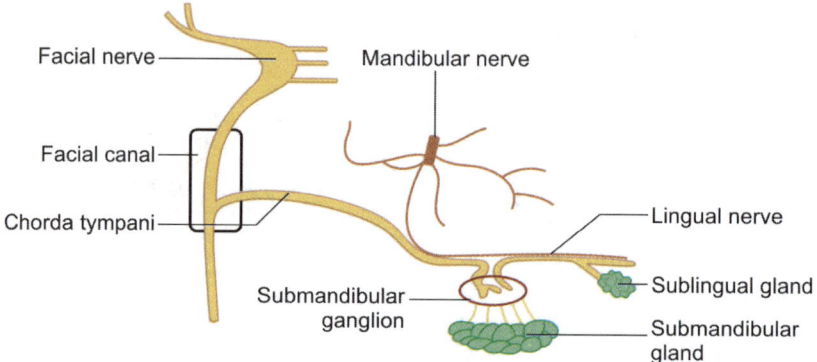

Fig. 42: Nerve supply of the gland.

the anterior border of the muscle, it has triple relation with the lingual nerve- lateral, inferior and medial.

- **Blood supply:**
  - Facial artery
  - Lingual artery
  - Veins drain into common facial or lingual vein.
- **Nerve supply (Fig. 42):**
  - Secreto motor (parasympathetic) Superior salivatory nucleus---------- facial nerve ---------- chorda tympani ----Joins------ Lingual nerve ------- submandibular ganglion Postganglionic fibers ------------------- -------------- gland
  - Sympathetic Postganglionic fibers from superior cervical ganglion ---------- plexus around facial artery ---------------- gland

- **Lymphatic drainage:** Lymph passes to jugulo-omohyoid nodes interrupted by submandibular nodes.

15. Facial nerve.

- Facial nerve is the nerve of the second branchial arch
- It is the seventh cranial nerve
- It is a mixed type of nerve.

Structures Supplied

- **Motor fibers:**
  - **Branchiomotor**—to the muscles developed from 2nd branchial arch
  - Secretomotor fibers—to submandibular, sublingual, lacrimal glands and mucous glands of nose, pharynx and palate.
- **Sensory fibers:**
  - Special sensory fibers—carry taste sensation from anterior two-third of tongue
  - General sensation from skin of auricle.

Origin and Termination

Nuclei

- **Motor nucleus**: Located at the level of facial colliculus in the lower pons
- **Lacrimatory nucleus**: Is a parasympathetic nucleus situated in pons close to motor nucleus
- **Superior salivatory nucleus**: Parasympathetic nucleus situated in lower pons. Send fibers into the sensory root of the facial nerve
- **Nucleus tractus solitarius** in the medulla oblongata concerned with taste fibers
- **Spinal nucleus of trigeminal** in the medulla for general sensation from auricle.

Termination

Enters the face through posteromedial surface of parotid gland. Within the gland terminates by dividing into five branches— temporal, zygomatic, buccal, mandibular and cervical.

Course and Relations

- **Intracranial course (Fig. 43)**
  - **Motor root:** The motor fibers incline dorsally and medially, below the abducent nucleus, and ascend medial to it. Then forms a loop around the abducent nucleus and descend through the reticular formation ventrolaterally
  - **Sensory root:** The sensory root is called as **nervus intermedius**, contains

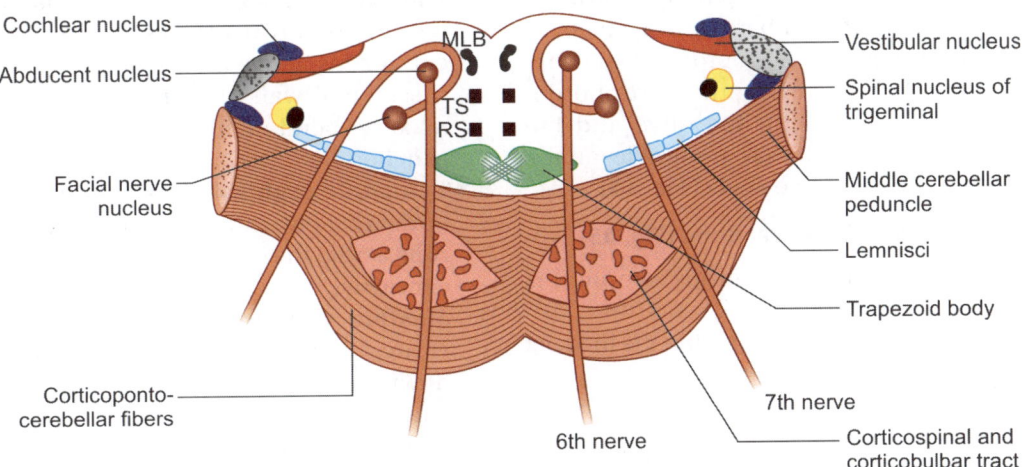

Fig. 43: Lower pons showing facial nucleus and the facial nerve.

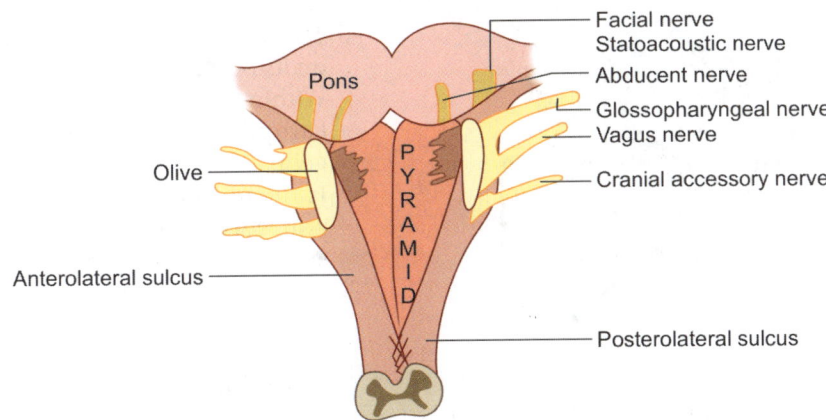

Fig. 44: Emergence of facial nerve.

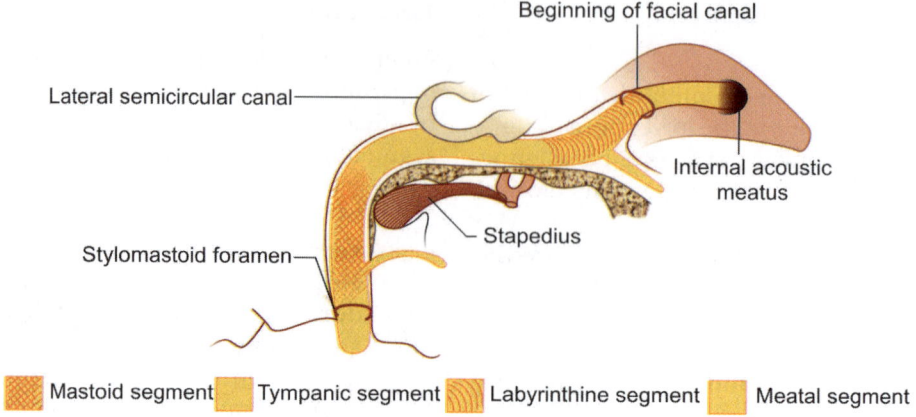

Fig. 45: Course of facial nerve within the petrous temporal bone.

taste fibers and parasympathetic (secretomotor) fibers to the glands
- **Emergence:** The motor and sensory roots emerge along the lower border of pons between the olive and the inferior cerebellar peduncle at the cerebellopontine angle **(Fig. 44)**.

Within Petrous Temporal Bone (Fig. 45)

The course within the petrous temporal is divided into four segments:
1. **Meatal segment** as it is within the internal acoustic meatus **(Fig. 46)**.

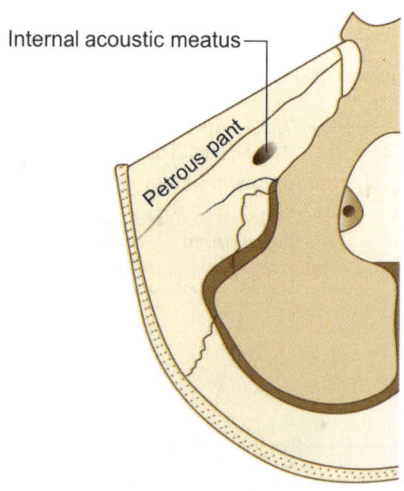

Fig. 46: Internal acoustic meatus.

2. **Labyrinthine segment:** It extends from formation of trunk to vestibule of inner ear. It runs above the vestibule to reach the medial wall of middle ear. Here it makes a bend and bears the geniculate ganglion.
3. **Tympanic segment:** It is related to the horizontal part of facial canal. The canal runs across the medial wall of the middle ear cavity.
4. **Mastoid segment:** It is related to the vertical part of facial canal. Then runs downwards in the posterior wall of the tympanic cavity to reach the stylomastoid foramen.

- **Extracranial course (Fig. 47):**
  - The facial nerve crosses the base of styloid process laterally
  - The nerve then enters the parotid gland on its posteromedial surface
  - Within the gland it crosses the external carotid artery and retromandibular vein
  - It terminates into temporofacial and cervicofacial trunks within the substance of the gland
  - The trunks branch further to form five branches: temporal, zygomatic, buccal, marginal mandibular, and cervical
  - The branches form a parotid plexus called **pes anserinus**.

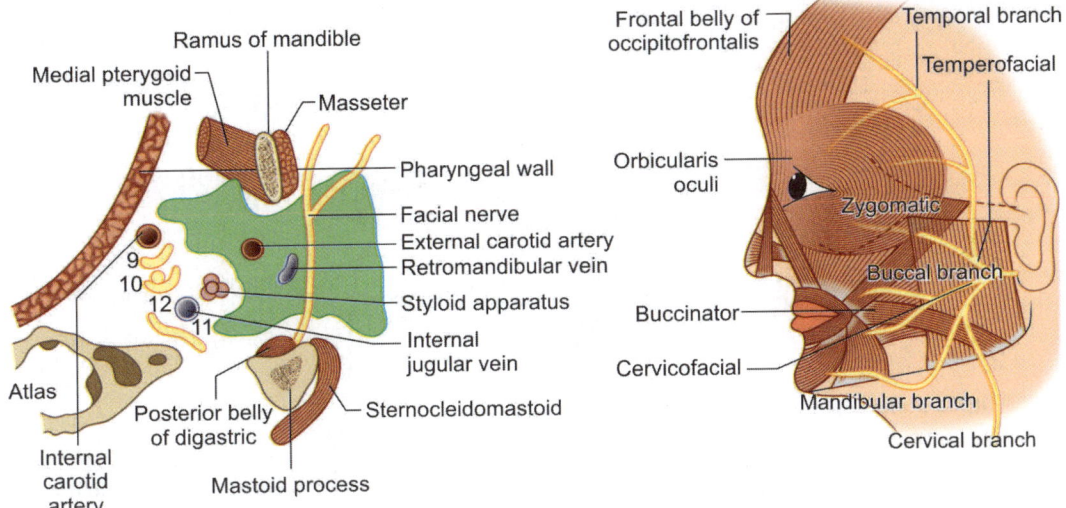

Fig. 47: Extracranial course within parotid gland and on face.

Branches

Branches are classified as communicating and distributing branches.

Communicating Branches (Fig. 48)

The facial nerve communicates with other nerves at various levels.

- **Intracranial part:**
  - Within cranial cavity—with vestibulocochlear nerve
  - Geniculate ganglion three branches arise from this ganglion:
    i. Greater petrosal nerve to communicate with pterygopalatine ganglion
    ii. To communicate with otic ganglion
    iii. External petrosal nerve to communicate with sympathetic plexus around middle meningeal artery
  - Facial canal—with auricular branch of vagus.
- **Extracranial part**
  - At stylomastoid foramen—with glossopharyngeal, vagus, auriculotemporal
  - Behind the ear—with lesser occipital nerve
  - On face—with trigeminal nerve
  - In the neck—with transverse cutaneous nerve of neck.

Distributing Branches (Fig. 49)

Distributing branches are given at various levels

- **Intracranial part**
  - Facial canal
    - Nerve to stapedius muscle
    - Chorda tympani which carries secretomotor fibers for submandibular and sublingual gland and taste fibers from anterior two-third of tongue.
- **Extracranial part**
  - At stylomastoid foramen
    - Posterior auricular branch to supply occipital belly of occipitofrontalis and auricular muscles
    - Nerve to posterior belly of digastric
    - Nerve to stylohyoid muscle.
  - Face
    - The facial nerve terminates by dividing into temporofacial and cervicofacial
    - Temporofacial in turn divides into temporal and zygomatic branches
    - Cervicofacial terminates by dividing into buccal, marginal mandibular, cervical.

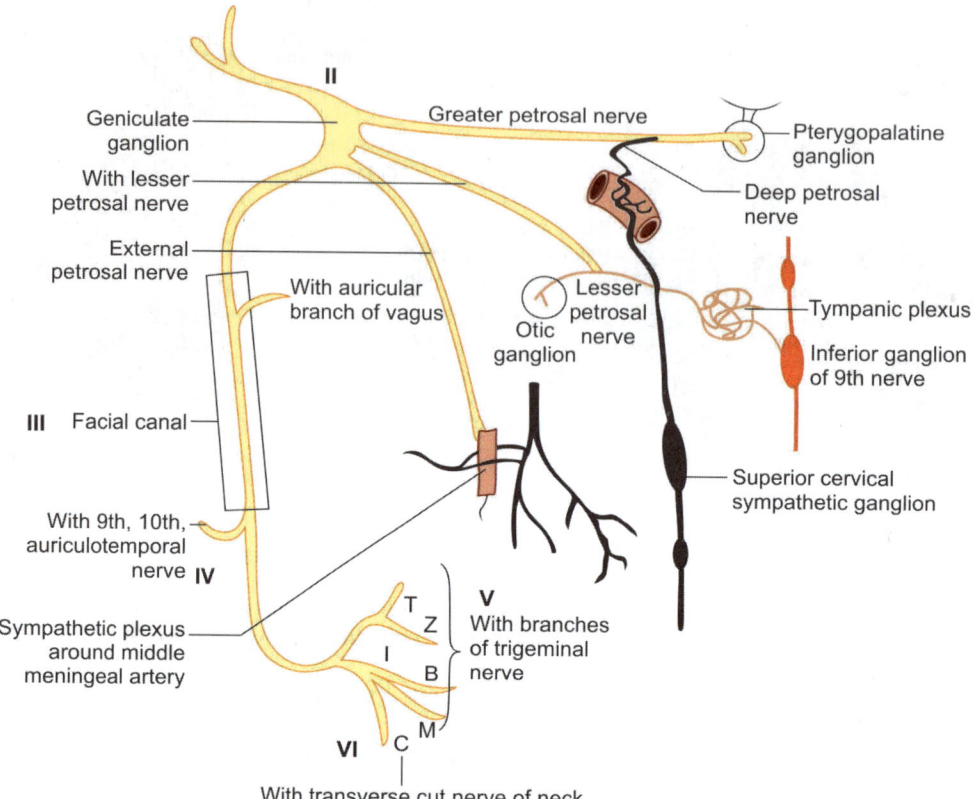

Fig. 48: Communicating branches.

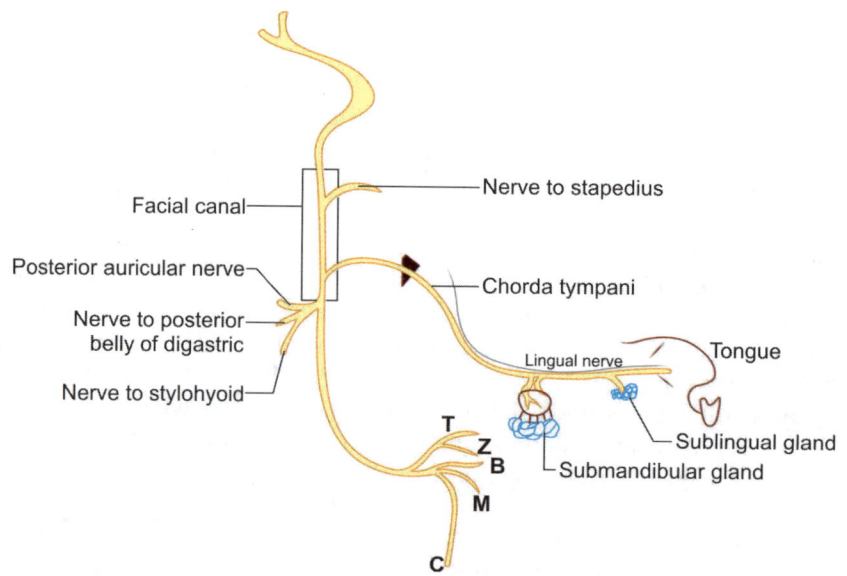

Fig. 49: Distributing branches.

Applied Anatomy

- **Facial paralysis due to an**
  - **Upper motor neuron lesion** paralysis of the lower half of face on the contralateral side when frontalis is partially spared due to the bilateral innervation of the muscle of the upper part of the face
  - **Lower motor neuron lesion** paralysis of muscles of one half of face on the ipsilateral side called Bell's palsy
  - **Bell's palsy:** Bell's palsy is due to paralysis of one side muscles of facial expression
  - **Crocodile tears syndrome:** Lacrimation during eating occurs due to aberrant regeneration after trauma.

16. Esophagus.

Level of Origin

It is continuation of pharynx from the level of lower border of cricoid cartilage corresponding to C6 vertebra.

Parts and Relations

Parts

- Cervical part
- Thoracic part
- Abdominal part.

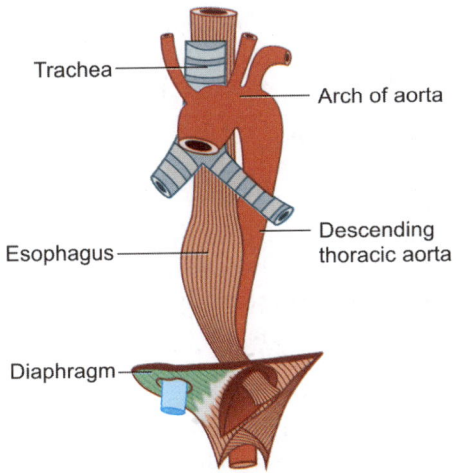

Fig. 50: Esophagus.

Course

- **In the superior mediastinum:**
  - It is situated to the left of midline
  - Passes between the trachea in front and the vertebral column behind
  - As esophagus descends first the aortic arch is anterior and then to the left.
- **In the posterior mediastinum:**
  - The esophagus is first along right side, then crosses in front and lies to the left of descending thoracic aorta
  - Enters the abdomen through the oesophageal orifice of the diaphragm at the level T_{10}.

Relations

- **Cervical part**
  - *Anterior:* Trachea, recurrent laryngeal nerves in tracheo oesophageal groove
  - *Posterior:* T5 – T12 vertebrae, longus colli, prevertebral fascia
  - *Lateral:* Common carotid arteries, lateral lobe of thyroid gland.
- **Thoracic part**
  In the superior mediastinum (Fig. 51)
  - *Anterior:* Trachea, Right pulmonary artery, Left main bronchus
  - *Posterior:* T1 – T4 vertebrae, longus colli
  - *Left lateral:* The terminal part of the aortic arch, left subclavian artery, thoracic duct, left pleura, left recurrent laryngeal nerve.

  In the posterior mediastinum (Figs. 52A to C)
  - *Anterior:*
    - Pericardium (separating it from the left atrium)
    - The diaphragm
  - *Posterior:*
    - Vertebral column, longus colli, right posterior intercostal arteries, thoracic duct, azygos vein, terminal parts of the hemiazygos and accessory hemiazygos veins
    - Aorta—near the diaphragm.
  - *Left lateral:* The descending thoracic aorta.
    - Left pleura

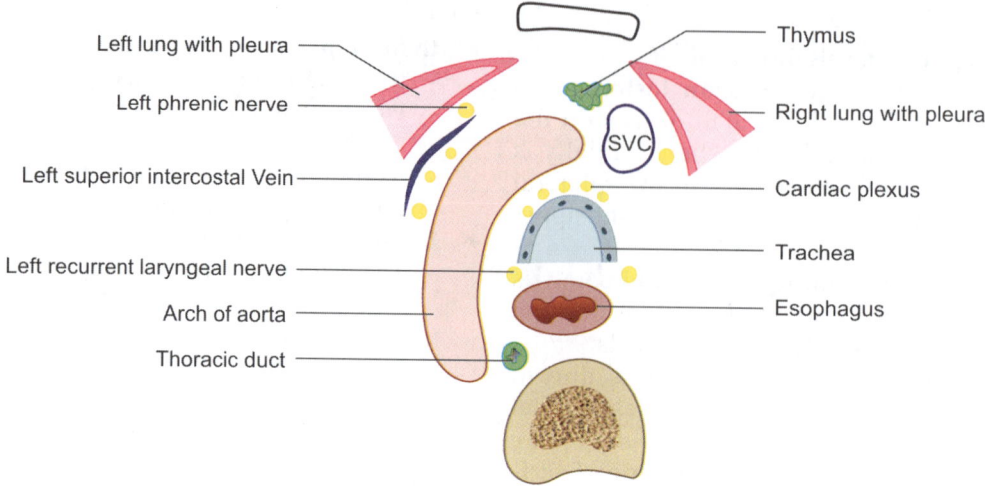

Fig. 51: Relations in superior mediastinum.

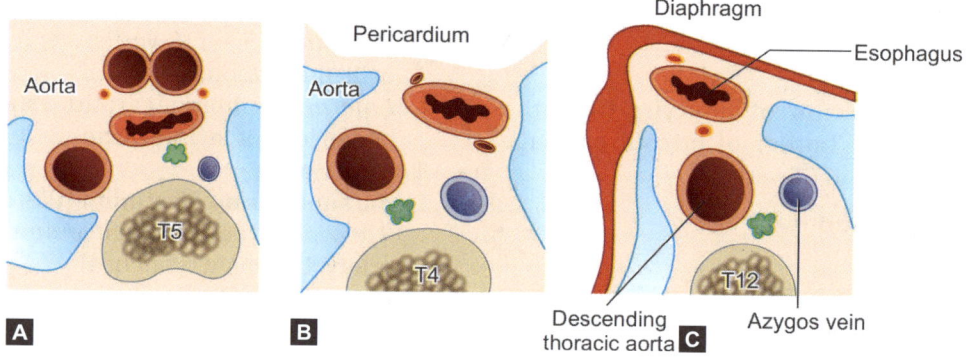

Figs. 52A to C: Relations in posterior mediastinum.

- Right lateral
- Right pleura
- Arch of azygos.
- **Abdominal part:**
  - It is about 1 – 2.5 cm in length.
  - It is connected to diaphragm by the thickening of transversalis fascia called inferior phrenoesophageal ligament
  - It lies posterior to left lobe of the liver.

Levels of Constriction
- Pharyngoesophageal junction (15 cm from the incisor teeth)
- Crossing of the aortic arch (22.5 cm from the incisor teeth)
  - Crossed by the left principal bronchus (27.5 cm from the incisors)
  - As it passes through the esophageal orifice of diaphragm (40 cm from the incisors).

17. Nasal septum.

- The septum of the nose divides the nasal cavity into two
- It forms the medial wall of each nasal cavity
- It is made of a sheet of bone (posteriorly) and cartilage (anteriorly)
- It extends between the roof and floor of the cavity
- **Bony component**
  - **Major contribution**:
    - The posterosuperior part—the vomer, which is attached above to the body of the sphenoid and below to the hard palate.

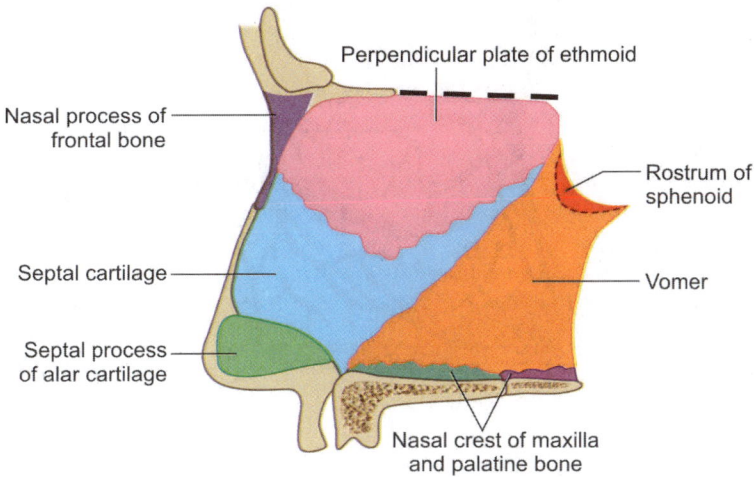

Fig. 53: Bony components of nasal septum.

- The anterosuperior part—the perpendicular plate of the ethmoid.
- **Minor contributions**
  - Anterosuperiorly—nasal bones and the nasal spine of the frontal bones
  - Posterosuperiorly—the rostrum of the sphenoid
  - Inferiorly—the nasal crests of the maxilla and nasal crests of palatine bones.
- **Cartilaginous part**
  - The septal cartilage is quadrilateral and prolongs behind between the vomer and the perpendicular plate of the ethmoid
  - Septal process of major alar cartilage
  - The cartilage is absent in the anteroinferior part of the nasal septum between the two nostril and hence called the **membranous septum**. It is continuous with the columella anteriorly
  - A blind pouch called vomeronasal organ situated close to base of septum and is vestigial in human.
- **Nerve supply (Fig. 54B)**
  - Nasopalatine nerve supplying posterior three-fourth and anterior ethmoidal nerve supplying anterosuperior, and anterior superior alveolar nerves supplying anteroinferior part of septum.
- **Blood supply (Fig. 54A)**
  - **Arterial supply**
    - Anterior ethmoidal artery branch of ophthalmic
    - Sphenopalatine artery and
    - Greater palatine branches of maxillary
    - Septal branch of superior labial of facial artery
    - There is arteriovenous anastomosis between these arteries in the anteroinferior part of septum. This area is called **Little's area (Kisselbach's plexus)** which is the commonest site of epistaxis.
  - **Venous drainage:** From posterior part to pterygoid venous plexus, from anterior part to ophthalmic or facial veins
- **Lining epithelium**
  - Close to roof—olfactory epithelium
  - Near the nostrils lined by skin
  - Rest of the region—pseudostratified ciliated columnar epithelium.
- **Applied anatomy**
  - Deviation of nasal septum causes nasal block, sinusitis
  - Most common site of epistaxis—anteroinferior part of nasal septum.

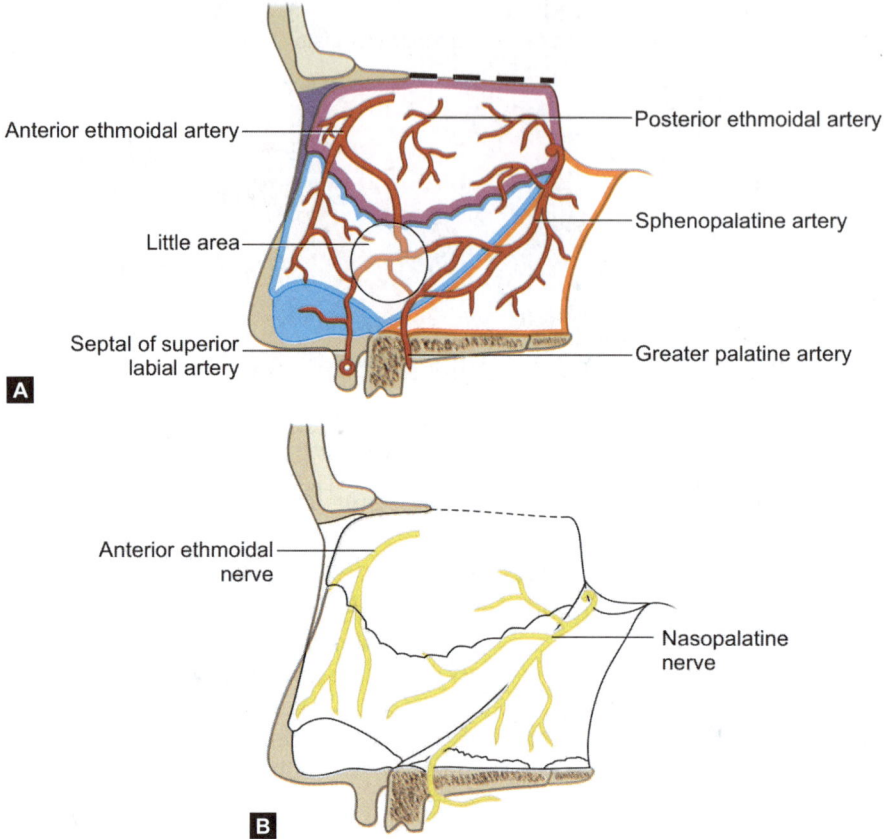

Figs. 54A and B: Blood supply and nerve supply of septum.

18. Microscopic structure of cerebral cortex.

The cells of the cerebral cortex are pyramidal cells, horizontal cells, Martinoti cells, granular/stellate cells, basket cells **(Fig. 55)**.

- **Pyramidal cell**:
  - Are more in number
  - Are triangular in shape, apex facing upwards
  - The axon arises from base of the cell, and dendrites from the angles
  - The dendrite from apex is large and extend to the entire thickness of cortex
  - The size of the pyramidal cells varies. The larger cell is known as Betz cells.
- **Granular cell**:
  - Small and multipolar
  - They form one-third of total neuronal population
  - The axon ramifies within the gray matter
  - The dendrites are many and radiate from cell body
  - The cerebral cortex is made of six layers **(Fig. 56)**
  - **Outer molecular layer**: Consists of horizontal cells of Cajal, axons of stellate cells, Martinoti cells, dendrites of pyramidal cells
  - **Outer granular layer**: This layer is packed with granule cells and less number of small pyramidal cells
  - **Outer pyramidal layer**: Small and medium sized pyramidal cells and less number of granule cells
  - **Inner granular layer**: Densely packed with stellate neurons, less number

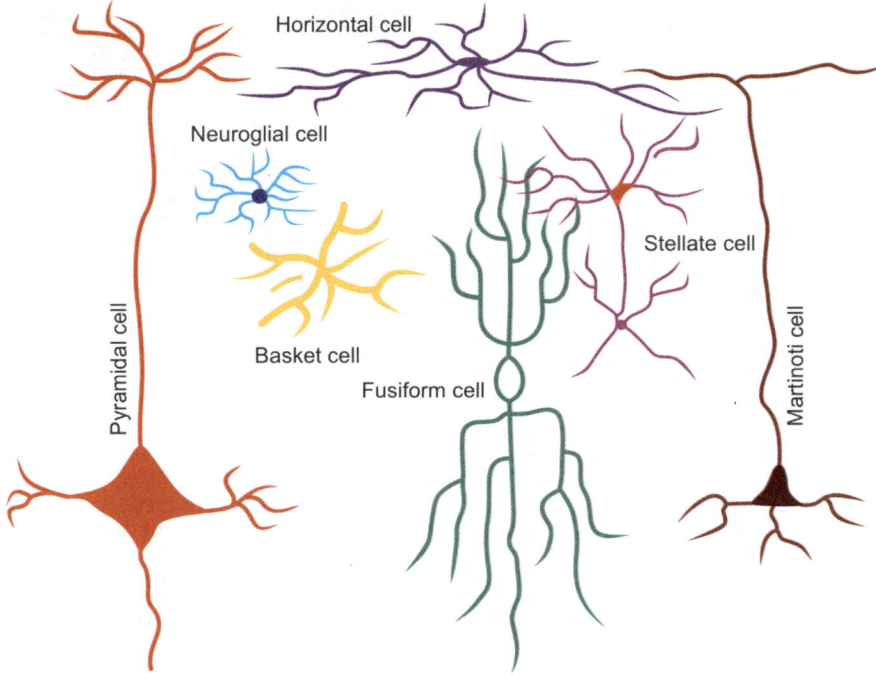

Fig. 55: Neurons of cerebellum.

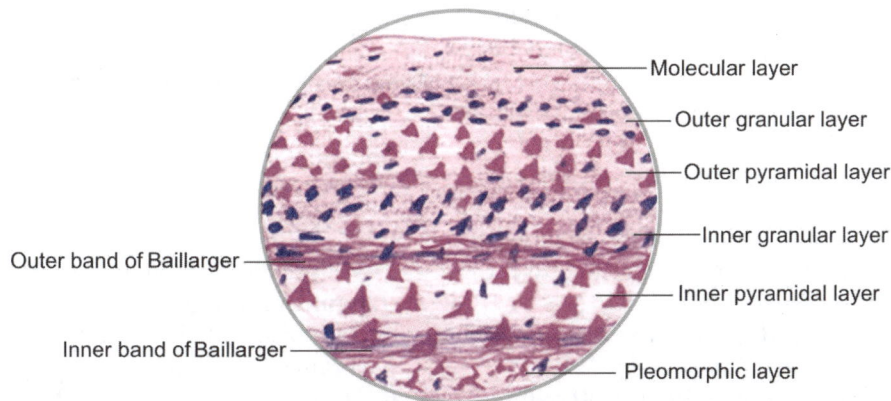

Fig. 56: Histology of cerebellum.

of medium sized pyramidal cells. Lower part of this layer is traversed by association fibers forming **outer band of Baillarger**
- **Inner pyramidal layer:** Large pyramidal neurons called Betz cells are present. **Inner band of Baillarger** is seen in the lower part of the layer
- **Pleomorphic layer:** Contains multipolar neurons, which are modified pyramidal cells. Cells of Martinoti are more in this layer.

19. Development of palate.

- The palate is developed by 8th week of intrauterine life
- The palate is developed from three sources
  - Primitive palate
  - Two palatine processes of maxillary process

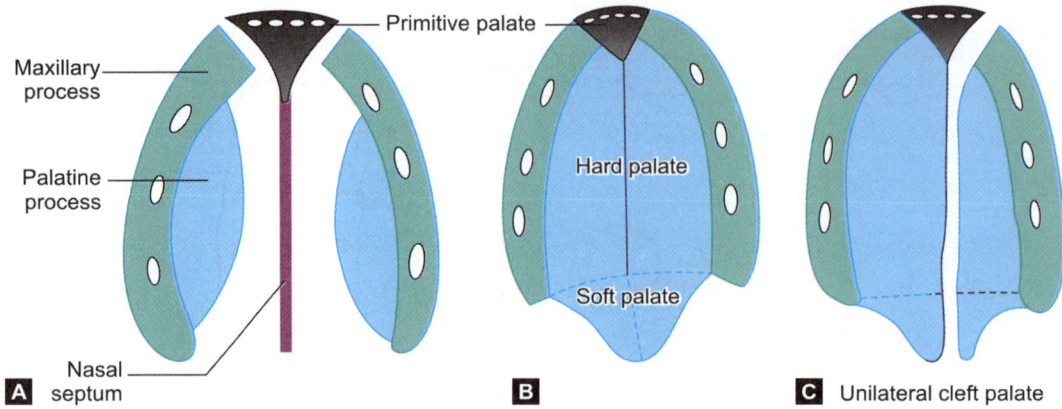

Figs. 57A to C: Development of palate.

- **The primitive palate**
  - Is triangular in shape bearing sockets for incisors
  - Protrudes below and between the nasal cavities
  - Derived from median nasal process
  - Posteriorly the nasal septum is attached to it.
- **Palatine process of maxillary process**
  - Is shelf like projection from maxillary process
  - The three processes join in the form of letter "Y"
  - The union starts from anterior to posterior
  - The portion of the palate attached to the nasal septum gets ossified to form hard palate
  - The posterior part remains unossified to form soft palate.
- **Congenital abnormality** is **cleft palate**
  - The cleft can be classified as complete and incomplete
  - **Complete cleft** in turn is divided into unilateral and bilateral cleft.
    - **Unilateral cleft** is failure of fusion of one of the palatine process with other palatine process and premaxilla
    - **Bilateral cleft** is both the palatine processes fail to fuse with each other and with premaxilla
  - In **incomplete cleft** the soft palate will be divided or bifid uvula.

20. Development of tongue.

- The tongue appears by 4th week of intrauterine life
- Development of tongue is studied under two headings **(Fig. 58)**:
  i. Development of mucous membrane
  ii. Development of muscles

Development of Mucous Membrane

- Development of anterior two-third of tongue
- Development of posterior one-third of tongue.

Development of Anterior Two-third

- **Lingual swellings**
  - It is seen at the ventral ends of 1st branchial arches
  - The underlying mesoderm at the ventral ends proliferate to form the enlargement.
- **Tuberculum impar**
  - Behind this swelling between first and the second arch another enlargement is seen in midline called **tuberculum impar**
    - Behind the tuberculum impar is the median thyroid rudiment which grow downwards to form thyroglossal duct

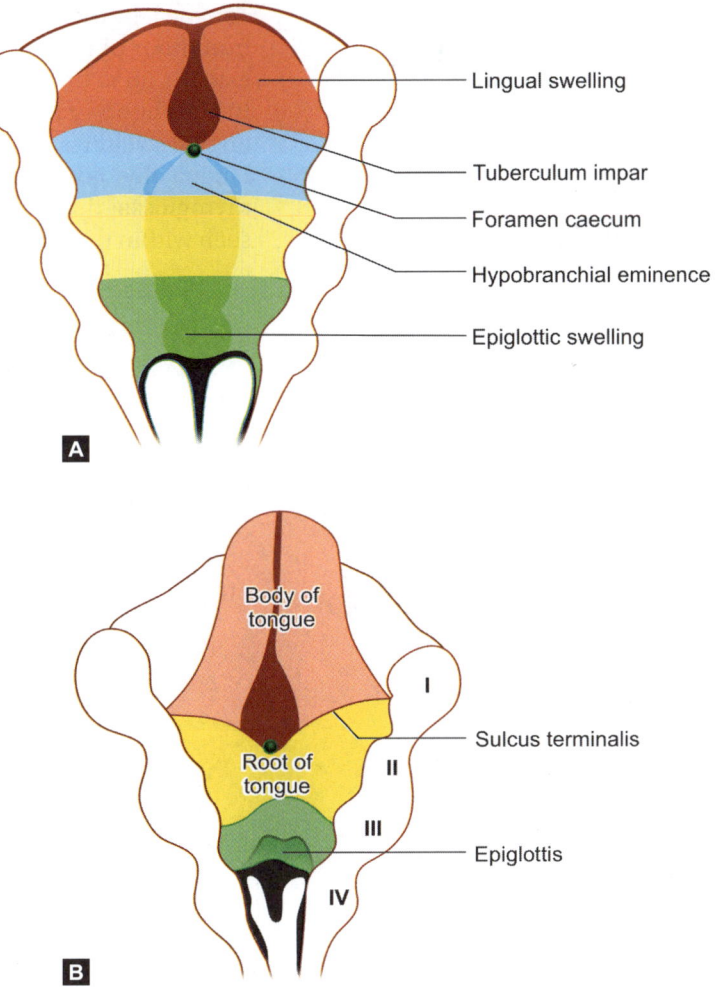

Figs. 58A and B: Development of tongue.

- The duct disappears
- The upper end is represented as **foramen cecum** and lower end forms thyroid gland.
- **The two lingual swellings and tuberculum impar fuse to form mucous membrane of the anterior two-third of tongue**
- An alveolingual groove appears laterally and anteriorly
- The groove separates the tongue from floor of oral cavity and alveolar processes.

Development of Posterior One-third of Tongue

- From **hypobranchial eminence/copula**
- It is an enlargement produced by cells of ventral ends of 2, 3, and 4th arches
- This in turn divides into a ventral and caudal part
- The caudal part develops into epiglottis derived from 4th arch
- The ventral part is formed by the 2nd and 3rd arch
- The cells of the 3rd arch overgrow the 2nd arch cells and form mucous membrane of posterior one-third of tongue

- The fusion between the anterior and posterior parts is in a form of "V" represents the **sulcus terminalis.**

Development of Muscles

- From occipital myotome
- Congenital anomalies
  - Agenesis of tongue
  - Tongue tie—the tongue is not separated from floor of mouth and the frenulum extends up to tip
  - Bifid tongue—failure of fusion of the lingual swellings
  - Lingual thyroid—failure of formation of thyroglossal duct and thyroid gland is seen within the tongue.

MBBS Examination 2004

ANSWER ALL QUESTIONS

I. Essay questions   **(15/10 Marks each)**

1. Describe the hip joint under the following headings: Articular surfaces, ligaments, movements and muscles producing the movements, and applied anatomy.
2. Describe the uterus under the following headings: Normal position, external features, supports, peritoneal and visceral relations, and applied anatomy.
3. Describe the lungs under the following headings: External features, fissures and lobes, bronchopulmonary segments and applied anatomy.
4. Describe the parotid gland under the following heading: External features and relations, structures lying within the gland, nerve supply, and applied anatomy.

II. Short notes: **(2 Marks each)**

1. Microscopic structure of mixed salivary gland.
2. Yolk sac.
3. Ulnar nerve in the hand.
4. Structures under cover of deltoid muscle.
5. Inguinal lymph nodes.
6. Portal vein.
7. Ureter.
8. Perineal body.
9. Microscopic structure of duodenum.
10. Development of kidney.
11. Arch of aorta.
12. Corpus striatum.
13. Labeled diagram of section of pons at the level of facial colliculus.
14. Oculomotor nerve.
15. Hyoglossus muscle.
16. Lateral wall of nasal cavity.
17. Thyroid gland.
18. Microscopic structure of cerebellum.
19. Derivatives of 3rd and 4th pharyngeal pouches.
20. Development of neural tube.

I. ESSAY QUESTIONS

1. Describe the hip joint under the following headings: Articular surfaces, ligaments, movements and muscles producing the movements, and applied anatomy.

Type of Joint

- It is a multi-axial, synovial joint of ball and socket variety.

Articular Surfaces (Fig. 1)

- **Acetabulum**
  - The articular surface is horse-shoe shaped called **lunate surface**
  - It is deficient inferiorly at the acetabular notch
  - The articular surface is contributed by all three parts of hip bone—ilium, ischium, and pubis
  - The floor of the acetabulum is non-articular forming the acetabular fossa containing fat (Haversian pad of fat).
- **Head of the femur**
  - It is spheroid with flattening of its upper surface
  - The fovea present in the head gives attachment for ligamentum teres

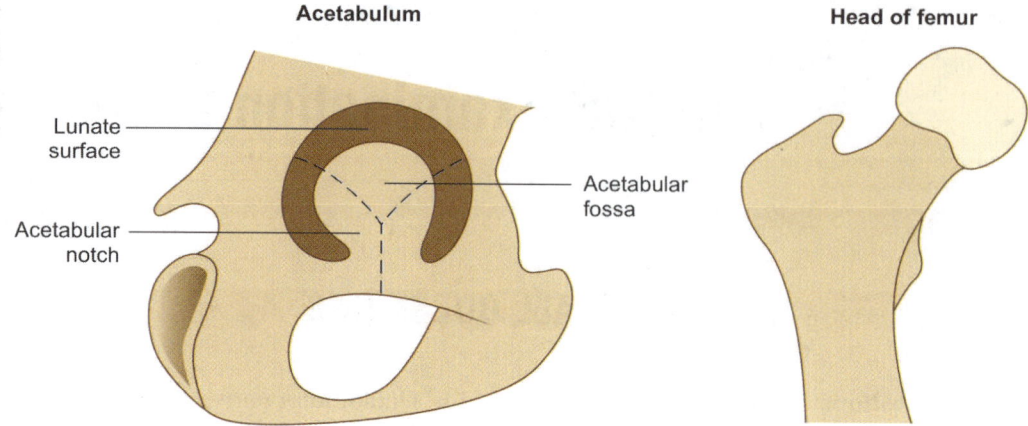

Fig. 1: Articular surfaces.

- Both the articular surfaces are covered with hyaline cartilage.

Ligaments

- **Fibrous capsule (Fig. 2)**
  - Proximally attached close to the acetabular margin and transverse acetabular ligament below
  - Distally to inter trochanteric line and crest
  - From inter trochanteric line, a few fibers of the capsule are reflected upward and medially along the neck and beneath the synovial membrane as **retinacular fibers**. These fibers carry blood vessels to neck and the head of femur
  - The deep fibers of the capsule are circularly arranged and form **zona orbicularis**
  - The inner surface of the capsule is covered by synovial membrane.
- **Acetabular labrum**
  - It is a fibro cartilaginous structure attached to the acetabular margin
  - It deepens the socket
  - It also holds the head tightly and retains the head in position.

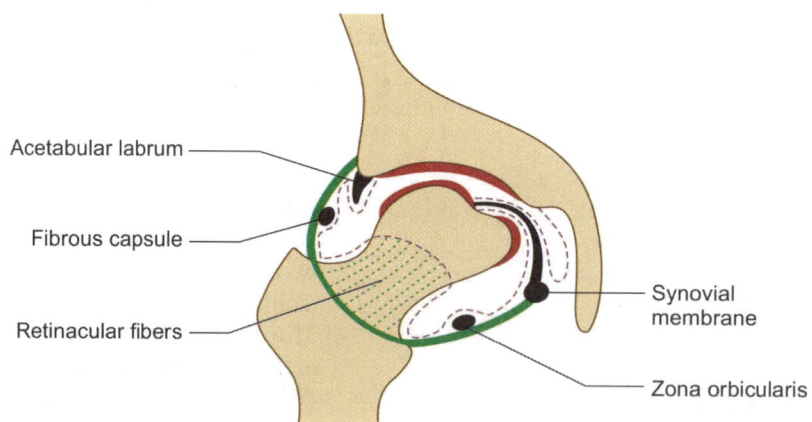

Fig. 2: Fibrous capsule.

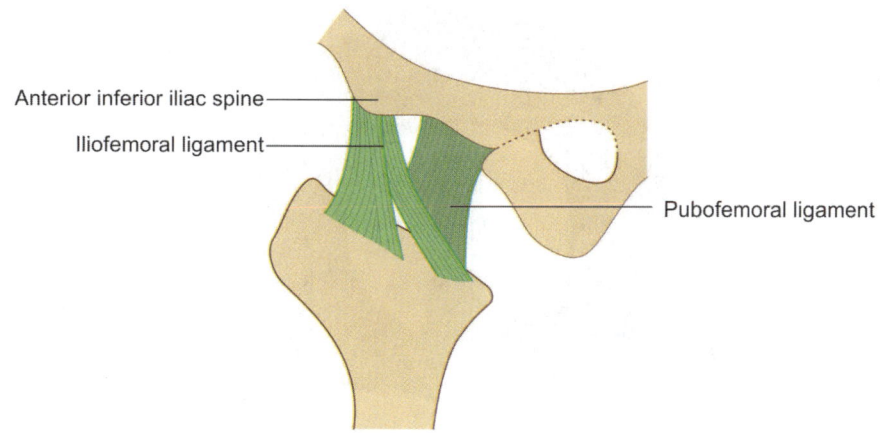

Fig. 3: Ligaments of hip joint.

- **Iliofemoral ligament (ligament of Bigelow) (Fig. 3)**
  - It is a strong inverted Y-shaped ligament
  - One of the strongest ligaments in the body
  - Its base is attached to anterior inferior iliac spine
  - The two limbs of Y are attached to the upper and lower parts of the inter trochanteric line.
- **Pubofemoral ligament**
  - Triangular in shape
  - Attached to iliopubic ramus, obturator crest, superior pubic ramus and below to the capsule of the joint
  - Fibers pass deep to iliofemoral ligament
- **Ischiofemoral ligament (Fig. 4)**
  - It is spiral in shape
  - It is attached to the body of ischium near the margin of acetabulum
  - The fibers are continuous with zona orbicularis.
- **Transverse acetabular ligament (Fig. 5):**
  - It is attached to the margins of the acetabular notch
  - It converts the notch into a foramen for the passage of blood vessels and nerves to the joint.
- **Ligament of head of femur** (ligamentum teres femoris/round ligament of head of femur):

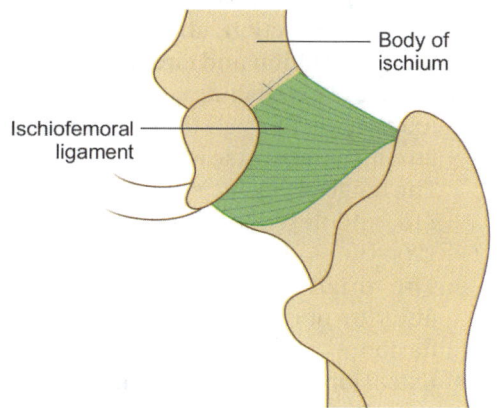

Fig. 4: Ischiofemoral ligament.

  - It is also called as round ligament
  - It is triangular in shape
  - Its apex is attached to the fovea on head of femur and base to ends of acetabular notch and transverse acetabular ligament
  - It is an intracapsular ligament and is covered by synovial membrane
  - It conveys blood vessels to the head of femur.

Movements and Muscles Producing

- Stability and strength are important for this joint
- Movements are limited

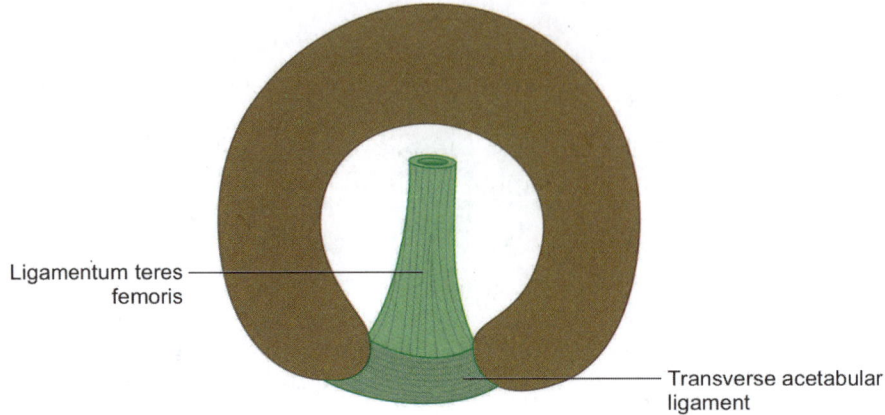

Fig. 5: Acetabulum with transverse ligament.

- Movements permitted are flexion, extension, adduction, abduction, medial and lateral rotation and circumduction.
- **Flexion and extension**
  - Axis passes through the neck of femur around a transverse axis
  - The range of flexion is in extended knee 110° and flexed knee it is increased to 120°
  - The thigh comes in contact with anterior abdominal wall with spinal flexion
  - Extension is, the limb and the trunk are in the same vertical plane.
  - Muscles producing are:
    - **Flexion:** Iliopsoas and rectus femoris
    - **Extension:** Gluteus maximus and hamstrings.
- **Abduction and adduction**
  - Axis passes through head of femur around anteroposteriorly
  - The range of abduction is 60°
  - Adduction is when both thighs come in contact with each other
  - Is increased as in cross kicking
  - Muscles producing are
    - **Abduction:** Gluteus medius, gluteus minimus and tensor fascia lata
    - **Adduction:** Adductor longus, brevis, magnus and gracilis.
- **Medial and lateral rotation**
  - Occurs around vertical axis passing through the center of head of femur
  - Muscles producing are **medial rotation,** anterior fibers of gluteus medius and minimus
  - **Lateral rotation:** Gluteus maximus, piriformis, obturator externus, obturator internus and two gemelli.
- **Circumduction:** Combination of all these movements in sequence.

Applied Anatomy

- Congenital dislocation is more common in the hip than in any other joint of the body
- Perthes's disease or Pseudocoxalgia: In this disease there is destruction and flattening of the head of the femur, and can be identified in X-ray by an increase in joint space
- Coxa vara is a condition in which the neck shaft angle is reduced from the normal angle of about 150° in a child and 127° in an adult
- In arthritis of hip joint, the position of joint is partially flexed, abducted and laterally rotated
- **Shenton's line**: The upper border of obturator foramen and the lower border of the neck of the femur is seen as a continuous curve in the X-ray known as

Shenton's line. In case of fracture neck of femur this line is disturbed
- **Nelaton's line:** The tip of greater trochanter, the ischial tuberosity and the anterior superior iliac spine lie in a line known as Nelaton's line. In fracture neck of femur, or dislocation of hip, the greater trochanter lies above the line.

2. **Describe the uterus under the following headings: Normal position, external features, supports, peritoneal and visceral relations, and applied anatomy.**

Normal Position

- Anteversion **(Fig. 6A)**
  - Normally, in majority of women, long axis of the cervix is bent forward on the long axis of the vagina forming an angle of 90°
  - This position is referred to as anteversion of the uterus
  - The uterus corresponds to the axis of pelvic inlet and vagina to the axis of pelvic outlet.
- Anteflexion **(Fig. 6B)**
  - The axis of the body of uterus is bent forward with the long axis of the cervix forming an angle at about 125°
  - This position is called anteflexion of the uterus
  - The mobile part tilts forward than the fixed part by its own weight.

External Features: Parts of Uterus (Fig. 7)

- (i) Fundus, (ii) Body, (iii) Cervix
- The **fundus** is the part of the uterus that lies above the entrance of the uterine tubes
- The **body** lies below the entrance of the uterine tubes and becomes narrow to become continuous with the cervix. The shape of the cavity of the body of uterus in coronal section is triangular and in sagittal section merely a slit
- The **cervix** pierces the anterior wall of the vagina and is divided into supravaginal and vaginal parts. The cervical canal is spindle shaped and communicates with the cavity of the body via the internal os and with the vagina via the external os.

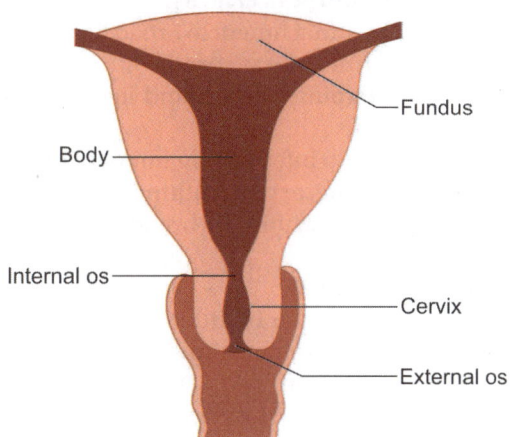

Fig. 7: Parts of uterus.

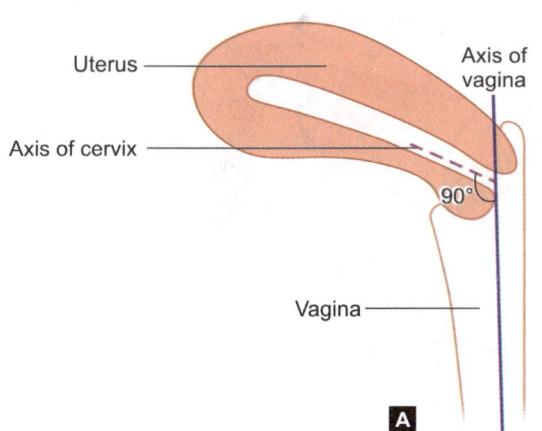

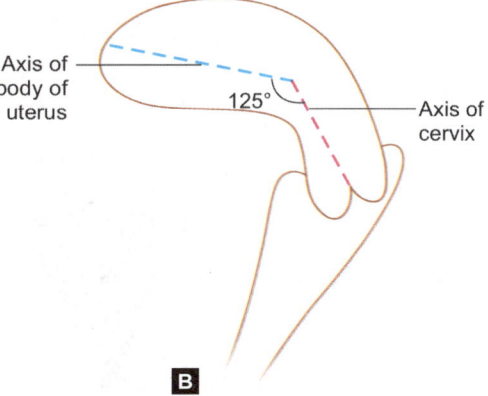

Figs. 6A and B: Normal position: (A) Anteversion; (B) Anteflexion.

Peritoneal and Visceral Relations (Fig. 8)

- **Fundus:** Covered with peritoneum, related to coils of small intestine
- **Body:**
    - **Anterior surface:**
        - Covered with peritoneum, extends up to internal os
        - Urinary bladder separated by uterovesical pouch.
    - **Posterior surface:**
        - Covered with peritoneum
        - The peritoneum is reflected to rectum forming rectouterine pouch (pouch of Douglas) from posterior wall of vagina
        - Related to coils of terminal ileum and sigmoid colon.
    - **Lateral borders (Fig. 9):**
        - Gives attachment to broad ligament, uterine tube at cornua
        - Anteroinferiorly round ligament of uterus
        - Postero inferiorly ligament of ovary
        - Uterine artery related to lateral surface within the broad ligament.
- **Cervix:**
    - **Supravaginal:**
        - **Anteriorly:** Bladder, separated by loose parametrium. Not covered by peritoneum
        - **Posteriorly:** Covered by peritoneum forming rectouterine pouch with coils of intestine, sigmoid colon
        - **On each side:** Ureter and uterine artery, attachment of Mackenrodt's ligament.
    - **Vaginal part:**
        - It is surrounded by vaginal canal
        - The tip presents the external os through which the cervix communicates with vagina.

Supports

- The uterus is a mobile organ
- It undergoes changes in size during reproductive period
- The uterus is supported by muscles, ligaments, and viscera

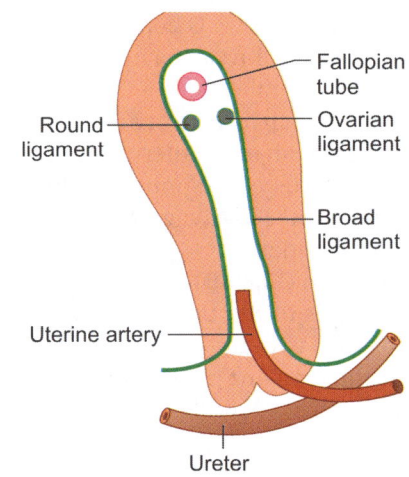

Fig. 9: Relations of lateral border.

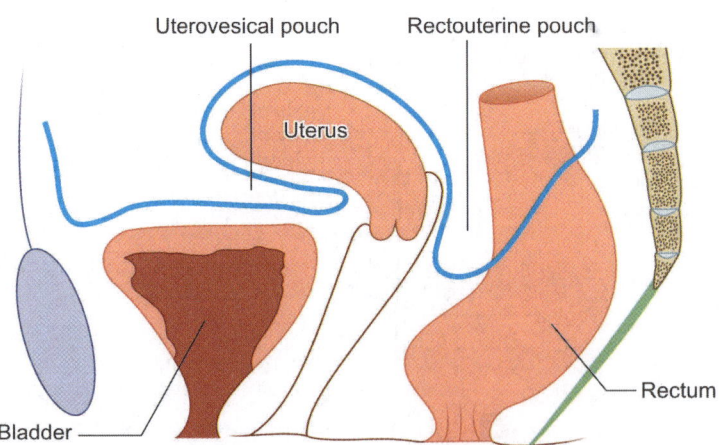

Fig. 8: Peritoneal relations.

- These supports prevent the uterus from sagging down.

Muscles (Fig. 10)
The muscles form the **primary supports**
1. **Levator ani muscle**
   - The **pubovaginalis** part forms a sling around posterior wall of the vagina and converges towards perineal body. It has a hammock action and narrows the urogenital opening preventing descent of uterus
   - **The puborectal** sling wraps around the anorectal junction and maintains the anorectal flexure. This supports the posterior wall of vagina
   - **Pubococcygeus part** is inserted to the perineal body and form a sphincter for the vagina and supports the uterus and bladder indirectly.
2. **Perineal body** called central tendon of perineum/gynecological perineum (Fig. 11): Formed by aggregation of fibromuscular tissue.
   - **Muscular contribution**
     - Posteriorly—fibers from the middle part of the external anal sphincter and the conjoint longitudinal coat
     - Superiorly—the rectoprostatic or rectovaginal septum, including

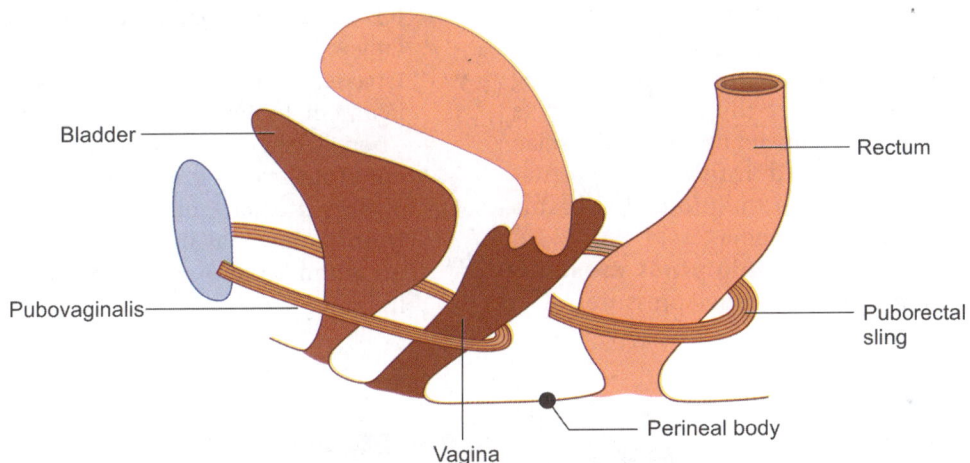

Fig. 10: Muscular supports.

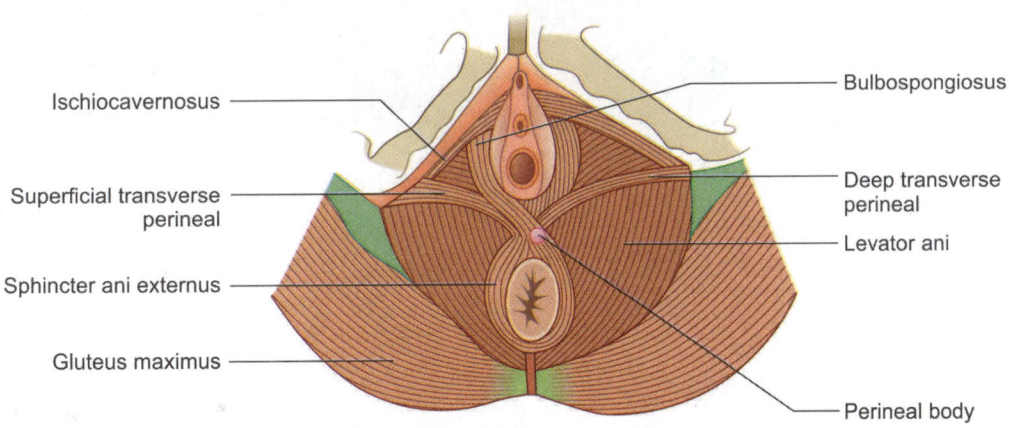

Fig. 11: Perineal body.

fibres from levator ani (puborectalis or pubovaginalis)
- Anteriorly—contribution from the deep transverse perineal, the superficial transverse perineal and bulbospongiosus.
- **Fascial contribution**
  - The perineal membrane and the superficial perineal fascia are connected with perineal body
  - It is attached to the skin of perineum through the superficial perineal fascia
  - **Function**: Through the muscles attached to it, it helps to maintain the integrity of the pelvic floor and keeps rectum and vagina in position
3. **Urogenital diaphragm**: Muscles forming the diaphragm are the deep transverse perineal and sphincter urethra and fasciae are superior and inferior urogenital membranes, close the urogenital hiatus and constrict the vagina
4. **Muscle tone of abdominal muscles**: Maintain intra-abdominal pressure.

Ligaments (Fig. 12)
The ligaments form the **mechanical supports**. The ligaments are divided as true and false.

True Ligaments
- **Mackenrodt's ligament**
  - It is also called as cardinal/transverse cervical ligament
  - It extends from lateral surface of cervix and lateral fornix of vagina to fascia covering levator ani muscle
  - It prevents downward displacement of uterus.
- **Round ligament (Fig. 13)**
  - It extends from anteroinferior to lateral cornua of uterus to labium majus
  - It is a fibromuscular band about 10 – 12 cm long
  - It passes between the two layers of broad ligament, to the lateral wall of pelvis
  - Then it traverses the inguinal canal entering through the deep inguinal ring
  - It splits into many bands after emerging from superficial inguinal ring to be attached to mons pubis and labia majora.

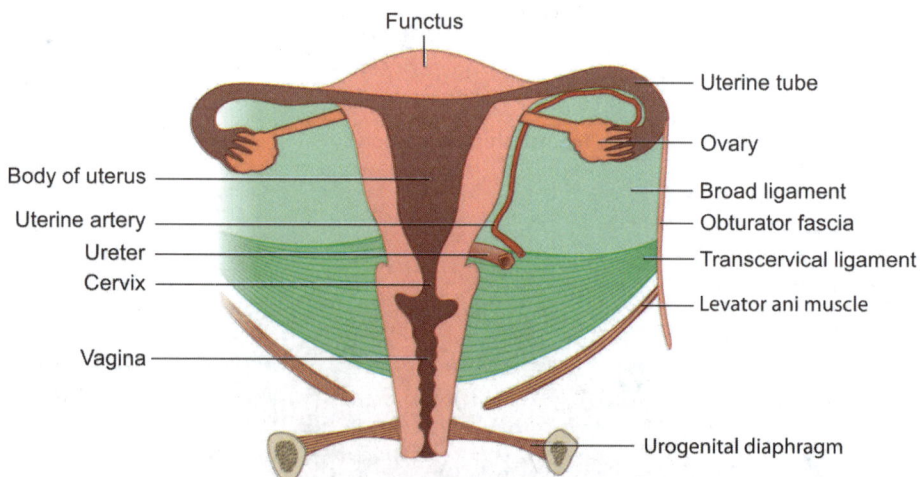

Fig. 12: Supports of uterus.

- **Uterosacral ligament (Fig. 13)**
  - It is formed by condensation of the endopelvic fascia
  - It extends from cervix to 3rd sacral vertebra
  - It keeps the cervix in position against the forward pull of the round ligament.
- Round ligament and uterosacral ligament maintain the anteversion and anteflexion of uterus
- **Pubocervical ligament**: From cervix to posterior surface of pubic bones. Prevents excessive traction on cervix.

False Ligaments
- **False ligaments** formed by the peritoneal reflexions and form the **secondary supports**
- **Uterovesical fold**—fold of peritoneum reflected from bladder to the uterus at the level of junction of body of uterus and cervix (internal os)
- **Rectovaginal fold**—peritoneum from posterior vaginal fornix to the anterior surface of rectum
- **Broad ligament**—fold of peritoneum from lateral surface of uterus to the lateral wall of pelvis. It contains uterine vessels, ovarian vessels, round ligament of uterus, suspensory ligament of ovary, epoophoron and paroophoron. It is divided into mesoovarium, mesosalpinx, and mesometrium. The uterine tube lies along the free upper border.

Viscera
- **Anorectal flexure** supports the obliquity of the posterior wall of vagina
- **Upper surface of urinary bladder** acts as support upon which the body of anteverted uterus rests.

Functional Supports
- **Peritoneal folds**—acts as sling and prevents descent
- **Parametric tissue** fills the space between pelvic peritoneum and pelvic floor. Around the cervix it is thickened and acts as anchorage to the uterus.

Applied Anatomy
- **Fibroid uterus:** Common benign tumor affecting the muscles. According to position they may be intramural, submucosal, subserous
- **Endometriosis:** Proliferation of endometrial tissue outside uterine cavity
- **Prolapsed uterus:** During parturition or any damage to the supports of uterus results in descent of uterus into the vagina. Complete protrusion of uterus outside the vaginal orifice is called procidentia
- Lacerations of the perineal body sustained during childbirth results in damage to

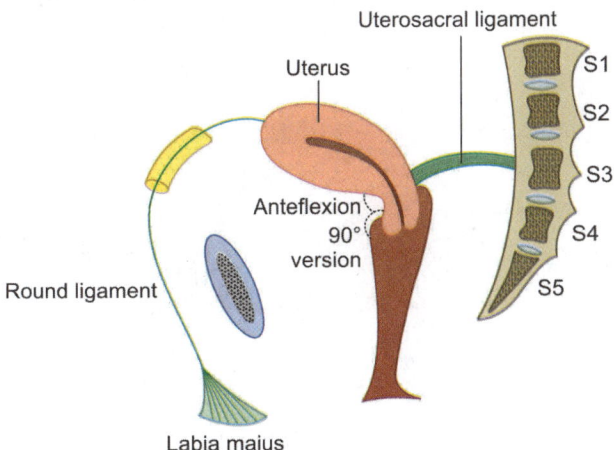

Fig. 13: Round and uterosacral ligaments.

the anterior fibers of the sphincter ani externus
- **Episiotomy:** It is division of perineum to facilitate delivery. The division should be angled laterally to avoid injuries of the perineal body.

3. **Describe the lungs under the following headings: External features, fissures and lobes, bronchopulmonary segments and applied anatomy.**

External Features

- Presenting parts:
  - Apex
  - Base
  - Surfaces: Costal and medial
  - Borders: Anterior, posterior, inferior.

Apex (Fig. 14)

- Tip 2.5 cm above the clavicle and 4 cm above the 1st rib
- Covered externally by cervical pleura and suprapleural membrane
- **Relation of apex of lung**
  - *Right lung*
    - Right brachiocephalic vein
    - Brachiocephalic trunk
    - Trachea with right vagus.
  - *Left lung*
    - Brachiocephalic vein
    - Subclavian artery
    - Esophagus
    - Thoracic duct.

Base
- Related to diaphragm
- Below diaphragm
- Right side liver, and left side left lobe of liver, stomach, spleen.

Surfaces
- **Costal surface**—related to ribs and endothoracic fascia
- **Medial surface** is divided into:
  - **Vertebral surface** – 1 to 10 thoracic vertebrae, sympathetic chain, splanchnic nerves
  - **Mediastinal surface**.

Right Lung (Fig. 15)

- Cardiac impression: Formed by the right atrium and its auricle and by the right ventricle
- Posterosuperior to cardiac impression is the hilum of the lung
- The pleura extends down below the hilum and behind cardiac impression as pulmonary ligament
- Arched groove above and behind the hilum—by arch of azygos vein
- Deep groove anterior to hilum extending upwards is for superior vena cava and terminal part of brachiocephalic vein
- Behind the hilum and pulmonary ligament is a vertical groove for esophagus
- Posteroinferior part of cardiac impression short groove for inferior vena cava

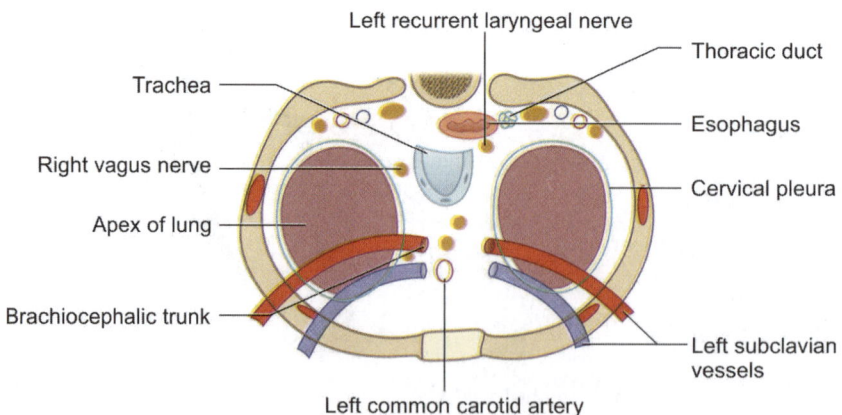

Fig. 14: Apex of lung.

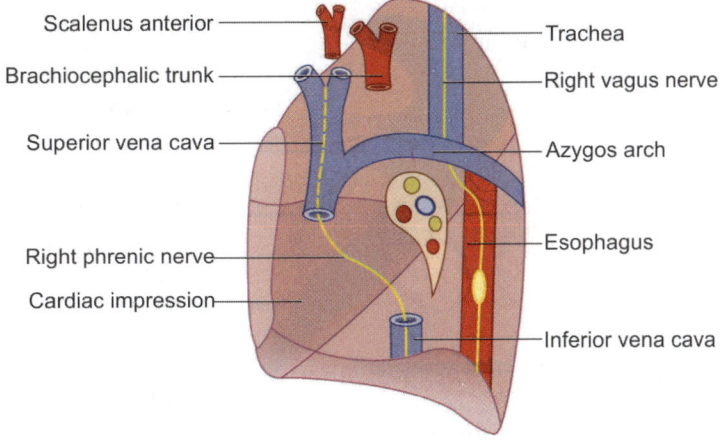

Fig. 15: Mediastinal surface of right lung.

- Between apex and azygos groove the trachea, right vagus are related
- Right phrenic nerve: In contact with the groove for right brachiocephalic vein, groove for superior vena cava, cardiac impression and the groove for inferior vena cava.

Left lung (Fig. 16)

- **Cardiac impression:** Related to anterior and left surfaces of the left ventricle and left auricle; part of anterior surface of right ventricle
- A groove for pulmonary trunk passes upwards in front of the hilum from the upper part of the cardiac impression
- Arch of aorta lies in a groove above the hilum
- A vertical groove for descending thoracic aorta runs behind the hilum and pulmonary ligament as a continuation of the arched groove
- Left subclavian artery is related to the groove above the groove for arch of aorta, which extends towards the apex
- The left lung comes in contact with the left edge of esophagus and thoracic duct above the aortic arch and behind the left subclavian artery
- Left edge of esophagus forms a shallow groove between the descending thoracic aorta and left pulmonary ligament

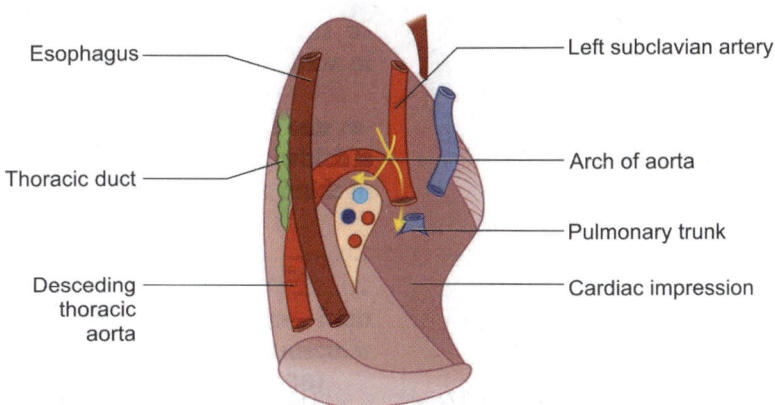

Fig. 16: Mediastinal surface of left lung.

- Left phrenic and left vagus nerves run between the arch of aorta and the lung.

Hilum of lungs

- The heart and trachea are connected to the medial surface of the lung by the pulmonary root
- Is formed by structures related to the hilum, covered by a sleeve of pleura.

Right lung (Fig. 17)

- **Contents:**
  - The eparterial and hyparterial bronchus
  - One pulmonary artery
  - Two pulmonary veins—superior and inferior
  - One bronchial artery
  - Bronchial veins
  - Pulmonary autonomic plexus
  - Lymph vessels
  - Bronchopulmonary lymph nodes
  - Loose connective tissue.
- **Relations:**
  - Anterior relations
    - The phrenic nerve, pericardiacophrenic artery and vein, and anterior pulmonary plexus, superior vena cava and right atrium
    - Posterior relations
    - Vagus nerve and posterior pulmonary plexus, terminal part of the azygos vein
    - Inferior relation
    - The pulmonary ligament.
- **Arrangement of structures**
  - Anterior to posterior
    - Superior pulmonary vein
    - Pulmonary artery
    - Principal bronchus
    - Bronchial vessels.
- **Above downwards**
  - Eparterial bronchus
    - Pulmonary artery
    - Hyparterial (principal) bronchus
    - Inferior pulmonary vein.

Left Lung (Fig. 18)

- **Contents:**
  - The principal bronchus
  - One pulmonary artery
  - Two pulmonary veins—superior and inferior
  - Two bronchial arteries
  - Bronchial veins
  - Pulmonary autonomic plexus
  - Lymph vessels
  - Bronchopulmonary lymph nodes
  - Loose connective tissue.
- **Arrangement of structures:**
  - **From above downward:**
    - Left pulmonary artery
    - Left principal bronchus
    - Lower pulmonary vein.

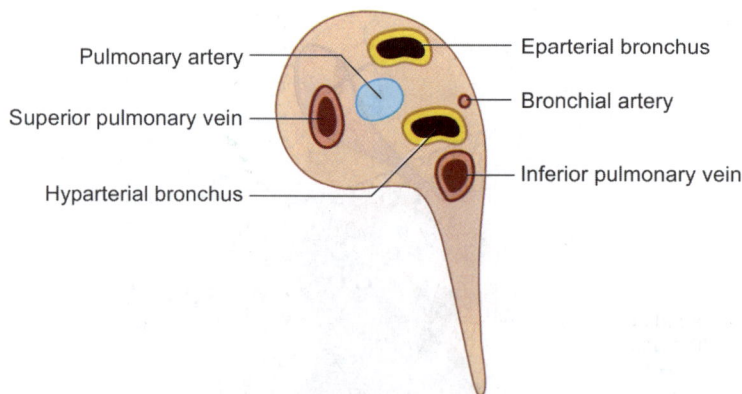

Fig. 17: Hilum of right lung.

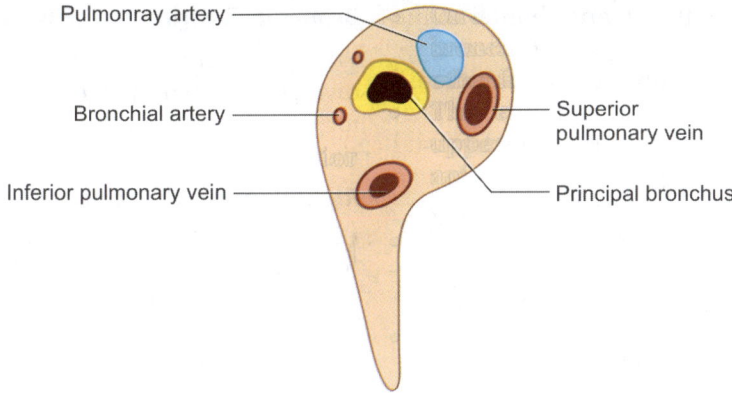

Fig. 18: Hilum of left lung.

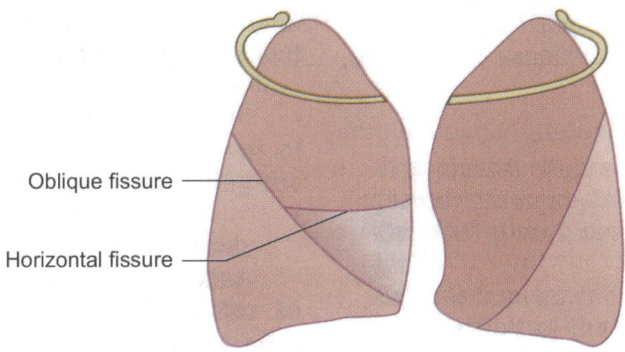

Fig. 19: Fissures and lobes.

- **From before backward:**
  - Superior pulmonary vein
  - Left pulmonary artery
  - Bronchus
  - Bronchial vessels.

Borders
- **Anterior**: Thin and shorter than the posterior border. Separates the costal surface from the mediastinal surface. Cardiac notch is present in the anterior border of left lung below the level of the fourth costal cartilage
- **Posterior**: Thick and ill-defined. It is related to thoracic vertebrae, heads of the ribs. Extends from the level of the seventh cervical spine to the tenth thoracic spine
- **Inferior:** The costal and medial surfaces are separated from the base by this border. Related to costodiaphragmatic recess.

Fissures and Lobes (Fig. 19)

- Right lung is divided into 3 (upper, middle, lower) lobes by 2 (oblique, horizontal) fissures
- **Oblique fissure**
  - It separates the lower lobe from upper and middle lobes
  - Extends deep into the whole thickness of the lung except at the hilum
  - Passes obliquely downwards and forwards
  - Crosses the posterior border about 6 cm below the apex at the level of spine of T4 descends across 5th intercostal space and along 6th rib to sixth costochondral junction.
- **Horizontal fissure**
  - Separates superior lobe from middle
  - Only in the right lung

- It runs from the anterior border to the oblique fissure
- Extends from oblique fissure in mid axillary line to anterior border at the sternal end of the fourth costal cartilage.
- **Lobes**
  - Right lung—3 lobes
  - Upper, middle and inferior lobes
  - Left lung—2 lobes.

Bronchopulmonary Segments

Definition (Fig. 20)

- A structurally separate, independent functional unit of lung tissue is called a broncho pulmonary segment
- It is a part of lung aerated by one tertiary bronchus
- Each segment is wedge shaped with the base directed to the surface
- Each segment is a separate respiratory unit, separated by connective tissue septa, which extends from the visceral pleura
- Tributaries of pulmonary vein are inter segmental, lie in the septa
- Branches of pulmonary artery are segmental
- A segmental bronchus, and its divisions along with associated arteries occupy a central position in each segment.

Bronchial Distribution (Fig. 21)

Within the lung each principal bronchus divides into secondary or lobar bronchi, one for each lobe; 2 in the left lung and 3 in the right lung.

Right Principal Bronchus

- The right principal bronchus divides into eparterial and hyparterial bronchi before entering the hilum of the right lung
- The eparterial bronchus enters the upper lobe and divides into **three** apical, anterior and posterior tertiary or segmental bronchi
- The hyparterial bronchus on entering the lung divides into two lobar bronchi, one for the middle lobe and the other for the lower lobe
- The middle lobar bronchus divides into **two** medial and lateral segmental bronchi
- The lower lobar bronchus divides into **five** apical of lower lobe, medial basal, lateral basal, anterior basal and posterior basal segmental bronchi.

Left Principal Bronchus

- In the left lung, the principal bronchus on entering the hilum divides into the upper and lower lobar bronchi.
- The upper lobar bronchus subdivides into upper and lower divisions. The

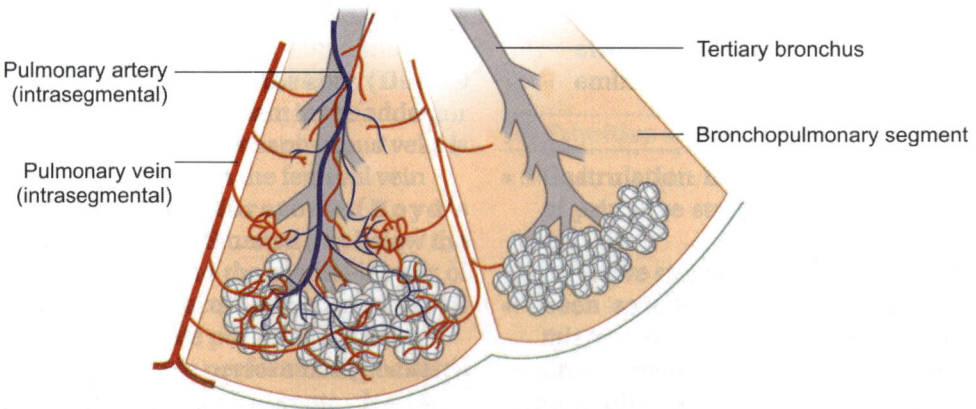

Fig. 20: Bronchopulmonary segment.

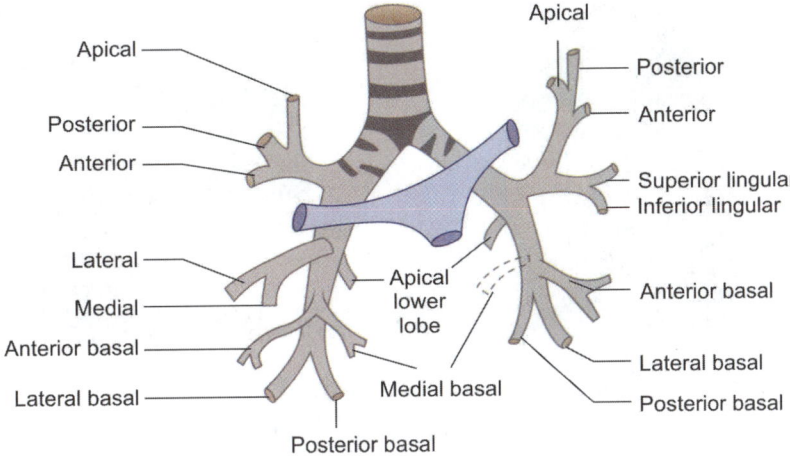

Fig. 21: Bronchial distribution.

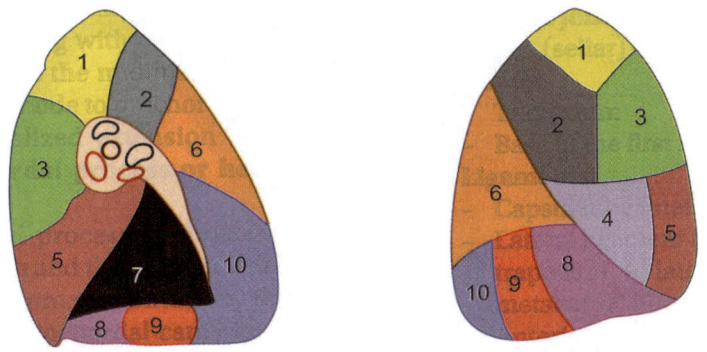

Upper lobe: 1 – Apical segment of upper lobe, 2 – Posterior, 3 – Anterior
Middle lobe: 4 – Lateral, 5 – Medial
Lower lobe: 6 – Apical segment of lower lobe, 7 – Medial basal,
8 – Anterior basal, 9 – Lateral basal, 10 – Posterior basal

Fig. 22: Bronchopulmonary segments of right lung.

upper division divides into **two** anterior segmental bronchi, and apicoposterior bronchus which in turn divides into apical and posterior segmental bronchi. The lower division gives of superior lingular and Inferior lingular segmental bronchi
- The lower lobar bronchus subdivides into **four or five** apical segment of lower lobe, medial basal, lateral basal, anterior basal and posterior basal segmental bronchi. Of these, the medial basal segment is usually suppressed/absent.

Segments of Right Lung (Fig. 22)
- **Upper:** Apical, anterior, posterior, medial, lateral
- **Middle:** Lateral, medial
- **Lower:** Apical, anterior basal, medial basal, posterior basal, lateral basal.

Segments of Left Lung (Fig. 23)
- **Upper:** Apical, anterior, posterior, superior lingular, inferior lingular
- **Lower:** Apical, anterior basal, medial basal, posterior basal, lateral basal.

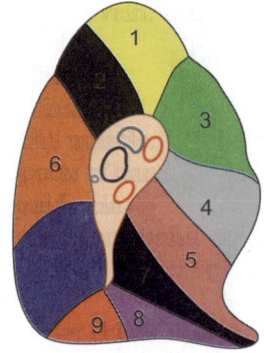 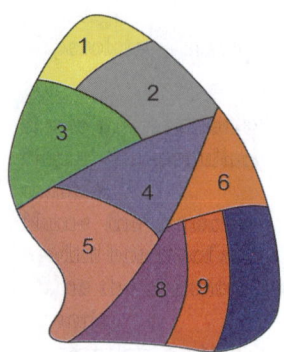

Upper lobe: 1 – Apical segment of upper lobe, 2 – Posterior, 3 – Anterior
4 – Superior lingula 5 – Inferior lingula
Lower lobe: 6 – Apical segment of lower lobe, 7 – Medial basal occasional),
8 – Anterior basal, 9 – Lateral basal, 10 – Posterior basal

Fig. 23: Bronchopulmonary segments of left lung.

Applied Anatomy

- Fibrous septa prevent spread of infection by acting as natural barriers. Hence segmental resection can be done
- Carcinoma and tuberculosis of the lung, however, break through the barrier and spreads widely
- Apical segment of lower lobe and posterior segment of upper lobe are common sites of lung abscess due to aspiration of infected material. They are the most dependent segments in the supine position
- Aspiration pneumonia involves most frequently the apical segment of lower lobe.

---

4. **Describe the parotid gland under the following heading. External features and relations, structures lying within the gland, nerve supply, and applied anatomy.**

Parotid gland is the largest of salivary glands, serous type and lies in the parotid region.

External Features and Relations

Location and Parts

- Situation: Parotid bed is formed by the of masseter muscle, below the zygomatic arch, in front of the external acoustic meatus, and overlaps the sternocleidomastoid, posteroinferior to angle of mandible.
- Parts:
    - Shape: Inverted pyramid and has a base, apex, and superficial, anteromedial and posteromedial surfaces.

Coverings Capsule (Fig. 24)

- Inner true capsule: Condensation of the connective tissue
- Outer false capsule:
    - It is the parotid sheath
    - Formed by the splitting of investing layer of deep cervical fascia
    - Superficial layer—thick and adherent to gland, blends with epimysium of masseter muscle to form—**parotido-masseteric fascia**
    - It is attached above to zygomatic arch.
- Deep layer: Thin, after covering the gland attached to tympanic plate and styloid process
- The part of fascia from styloid process to angle of mandible it is thickened to form—**stylomandibular ligament**
- The ligament separates the parotid from submandibular gland.

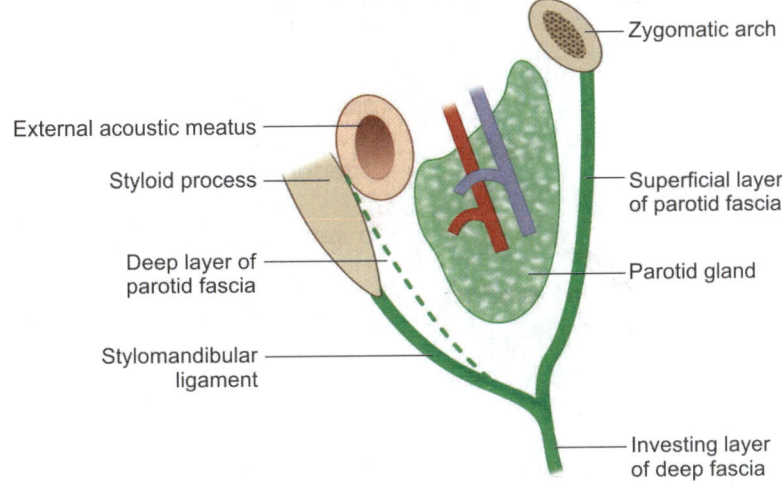

Fig. 24: Parotid fascia.

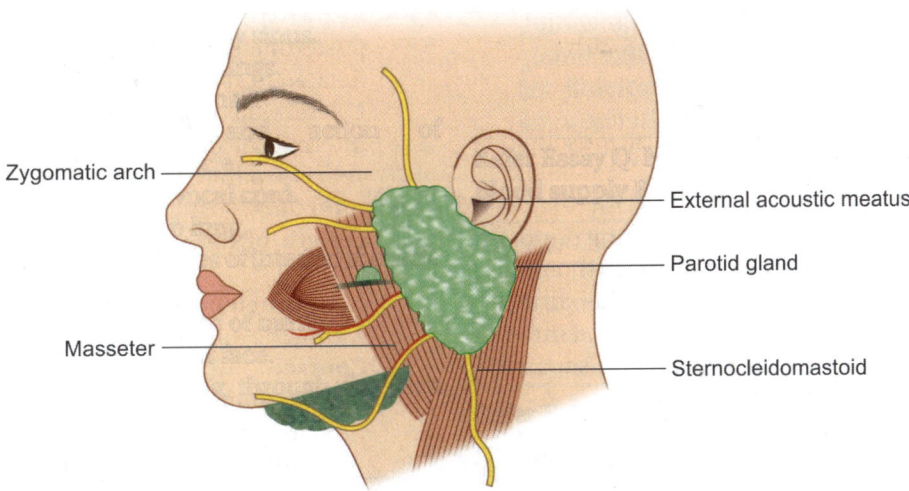

Fig. 25: Relations of parotid gland.

Relations (Fig. 25)

- **Apex:**
  - Directed below
  - Overlaps posterior belly of digastric muscle
  - Cervical branch of facial nerve and 2 divisions of retromandibular vein emerge.
- **Base (superior surface):**
  - Directed above
  - Related to: External acoustic meatus and posterior surface of temporomandibular joint
  - Structures emerging: Superficial temporal vessels, auriculotemporal nerve and temporal branch of facial nerve.
- **Superficial or lateral surface:**
  - Covered by skin, superficial fascia with platysma and parotid-masseteric fascia
  - Related to branches of greater auricular nerve and parotid lymph nodes.
- **Anteromedial surface (Fig. 26):**
  - Posterior border of ramus of mandible
  - Temporomandibular joint

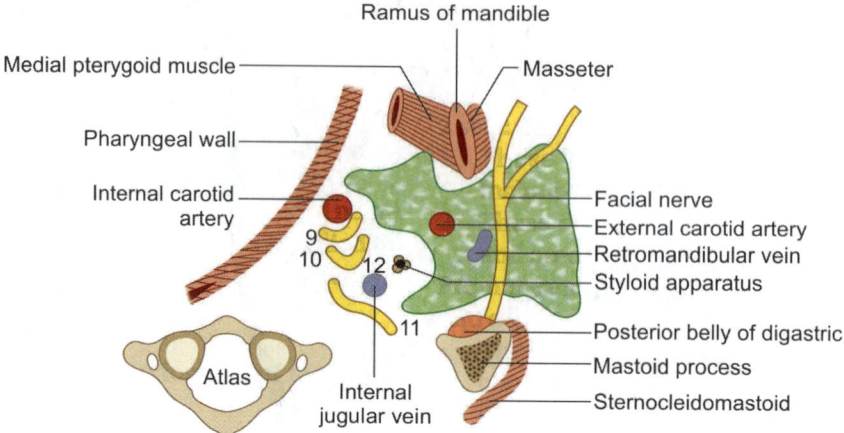

Fig. 26: Anteromedial and posteromedial surfaces.

- Masseter
- Medial pterygoid muscles.
- **Posteromedial surface (Fig. 26):**
  - Mastoid process
  - Sternocleidomastoid
  - Posterior belly of digastric muscle
  - Styloid apparatus
  - This surface is grooved by external carotid artery before entering the gland
  - Facial nerve enters the gland piercing through the upper part of this surface
  - The internal carotid artery and internal jugular vein are medial and separated by the styloid apparatus.
- **Anterior border:**
  - Separates anteromedial and lateral surfaces
  - Structures emerging (from above downwards):
    - Zygomatic branch of facial nerve
    - Transverse facial artery
    - Upper buccal branch of facial nerve
    - Parotid duct
    - Lower buccal branch of facial nerve
    - Marginal mandibular branch of facial nerve.
- **Posterior border:**
  - Separates lateral and postero medial surfaces
  - Related to sternomastiod muscle
  - Posterior auricular nerve and pass upwards beneath this border.

- **Medial border:**
  - Separates anteromedial and posteromedial surfaces
  - Related to styloid apparatus
  - Lateral wall of pharynx
  - Internal carotid artery, internal jugular vein is separated by the styloid process.
- **Parotid duct:**
  - **Length** of the parotid duct are 5 cm long.
  - It is **formed** by the union of tributaries within the anterior part of the gland
  - **Course:**
    - The duct emerges from the upper part of the gland, along the anterior border
    - Runs horizontally, crosses masseter, approximately midway between the angle of the mouth and the zygomatic arch
    - Reaching the anterior border of masseter it turns at right angle medially
    - It pierces the buccal fat pad, buccopharyngeal membrane and buccinator opposite the upper third molar tooth
    - For a short distance runs forwards between buccinator and the oral mucous membrane obliquely
    - The oblique course of the duct acts as a valve preventing entry of air into

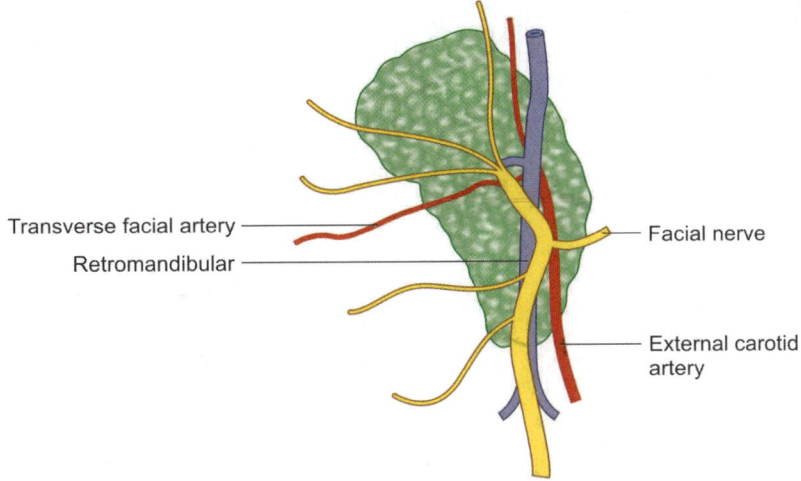

Fig. 27: Structures within the gland.

the gland whenever there is raise in intraoral pressures.
- **Termination:** It opens into the vestibule opposite the upper second molar.
- **Relations:**
  - Below: Upper buccal branch of the facial nerve
  - Above: The accessory part of the gland, the transverse facial artery and lower buccal branch of the facial nerve.

Structures Lying within the Gland

From deep to superficial (Fig. 27)
- **External carotid artery:**
  - Enters the gland through its posteromedial surface
  - Terminates inside the gland behind the level of neck of mandible into its two branches: superficial temporal and maxillary arteries.
- **Retromandibular vein:**
  - Superficial temporal and maxillary vein unite within the gland to form retromandibular vein
  - The vein divides into anterior and posterior divisions.
- **Facial nerve:**
  - Divides into:
    - Temporofacial division (temporal and zygomatic)
    - Cervicofacial division (buccal, marginal mandibular and cervical).

Nerve Supply (Fig. 28)

- **Secretomotor (parasympathetic) root**
  Inferior salivatory nucleus ----- Tympanic branch of IX nerve ----- Tympanic plexus ----- Lesser petrosal nerve ---- Otic ganglion ---- Auriculotemporal nerve ---- Parotid gland
- **Sympathetic supply**
  Post ganglionic fibers from superior cervical ganglion -----------through plexus around middle meningeal artery------ to otic ganglion ----------- auriculotemporal nerve---------gland
- **Sensory root**
  Sensations from parotid—Auriculotemporal nerve
  Sensations from parotid fascia—Greater auricular nerve.

Applied Anatomy

- **Parotid swellings:** Mumps, parotid abscess, pleomorphic adenoma, malignancy
- **Sialolithiasis and Sialography:** Dye injected into the parotid gland through its duct to visualize its ductal pattern and for any stones obstructing it
- **Acute sialadenitis:** Acute inflammation of the parotid gland results in severe pain in

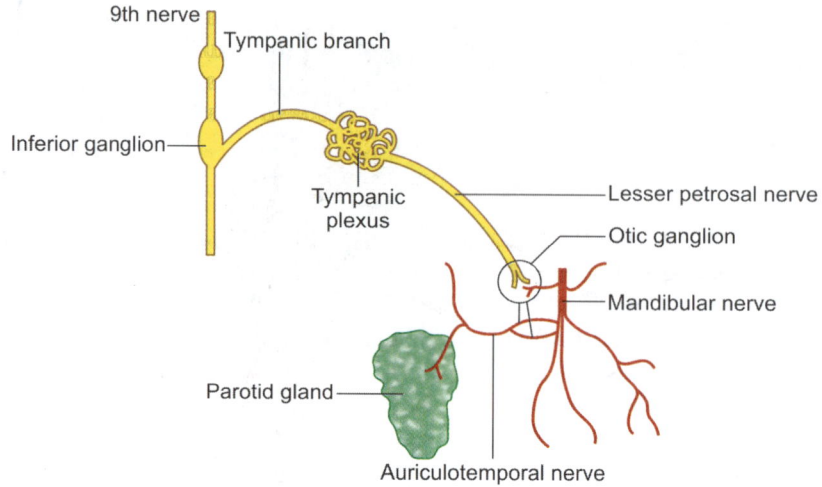

Fig. 28: Nerve supply of gland.

the preauricular region as the capsule of the parotid gland is stretched and the great auricular nerve is stimulated
- **Frey's or auriculotemporal syndrome**: The patient presents with sweating warmth and redness of the face by the smell or taste of the food after parotid surgery. This is due to the aberrant innervations of sweat glands by the regenerating secretomotor fibers. This leads to sweating of the skin over the parotid every time the patient attempts to eat
- **Patey's plane**: It is a fasciovenous plane. The parotid gland is divided into a larger superficial part and small deep part. Both the parts are connected by an isthmus, so the gland appears H – shaped. The plane between the two parts in which nerves and the veins lie is called as Patey's fasciovenous plane. The surgeons use this plane to remove tumor without damaging the nerve.

II. SHORT NOTES

1. **Microscopic structure of mixed salivary gland.**

- The submandibular gland is a mixed type of salivary gland
- The gland consists of both serous and mucous acini.
- It is covered by capsule
- Connective tissue septae extends and divides the gland into many lobules.
- **Acini:**
    - **Serous acini**
        - Is pyramidal in shape
        - The spherical nucleus situated in the center
        - The cytoplasm is filled by zymogen granules supranuclearly
        - Kallikrein, lactoferrin and lysozyme are secreted by serous cells.
    - **Mucous cells**
        - Are cylindrical in shape
        - The nucleus is flattened, and situated towards base
        - Large, and electron-translucent secretory droplets occupy the cytoplasm above nucleus.
    - **Demilunes**
        - Semilunar shaped serous demilunes are attached to the mucous acini
        - The ducts of the demilunes open along with mucous acini
        - The serous demilunes secrete an antibacterial enzyme.
- **Ducts**
    - **Intercalated ducts**: The lining cells are flat close to the secretory end piece, but become cuboidal.

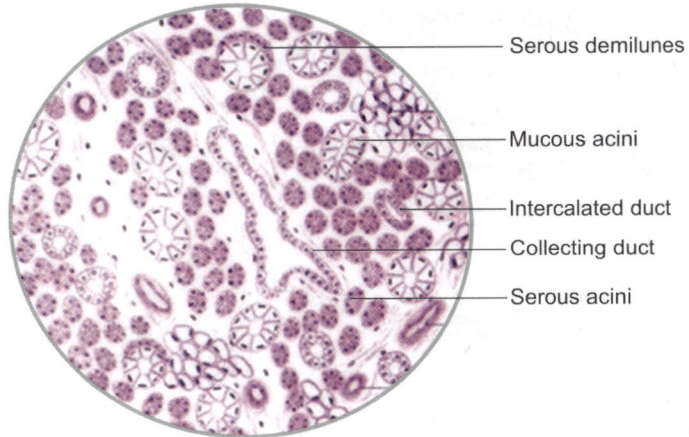

Fig. 29: Histology of mixed salivary gland.

- **Striated ducts:**
  - Are lined by a low columnar epithelium
  - Basal striations are present in the cells and hence are called as striated cells
  - The infoldings of the basal cell membrane produce the striation
  - Between the folds mitochondria are situated
  - The nuclei are apically situated
  - The function of the cells are to carry potassium and bicarbonate into saliva
  - They reabsorb sodium and chloride ions in excess of water and produce a hypotonic saliva
  - Striated ducts modify electrolyte composition
  - Secrete IgA, lysozyme and kallikrein.
- **Collecting ducts**
  - The lining epithelium varies
  - It may be pseudostratified columnar, stratified cuboidal or columnar
  - Near termination it becomes a stratified squamous epithelium.
- **Myoepithelial cells**
  - Also called as basket cells
  - Present between the basement membrane and the acinar cells
  - Help to empty the secretions from the acinus.

2. **Yolk sac.**
- The embryoblast differentiates into two layers on 8th day
- On 9th day, flattened mesothelial cells appear on the inner surface of cytotrophoblast at abembryonic pole to form Heuser's membrane
- The Heuser's membrane along with primary endoderm forms a cavity known as **primary yolk sac or exocoelomic cavity**
- On 13th day the cells of the hypoblast proliferate and form a new cavity within the primary yolk sac called secondary **yolk sac** or definitive yolk sac
- The secondary yolk sac is small
- Large part of yolk sac is pinched off and so the size is reduced
- The pinched off part is known as **exocoelomic cyst**, in the extraembryonic coelomic cavity
- After the formation of the secondary yolk sac, a diverticulum appears, the **allantois**, towards the connecting stalk
- During 4th week the lateral body wall folds are formed
- The endoderm also folds and form the gut tube
- The gut is connected with yolk sac by vitellointestinal duct or yolk sac duct
- The yolk sac becomes coated with extraembryonic mesenchyme, which forms mesenchymal and mesothelial layers.

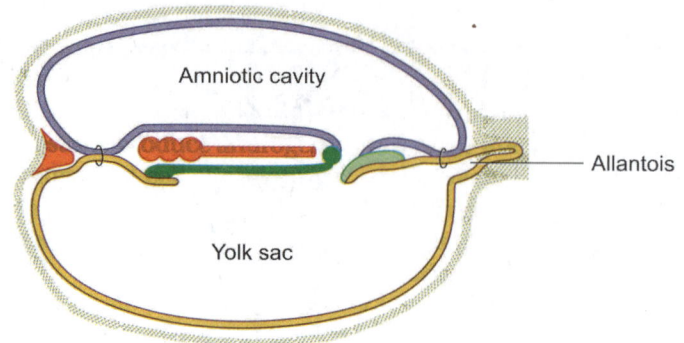

Fig. 30: Yolk sac.

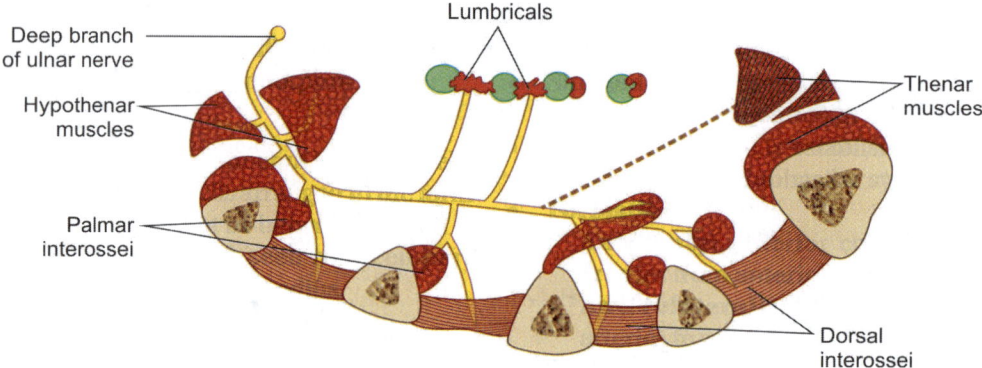

Fig. 31: Deep branch of ulnar nerve.

3. **Ulnar nerve in the hand.**

- The ulnar nerve supplies the intrinsic muscles of hand which are responsible for finer movements
- Hence it is called as **musician's nerve**
- The ulnar nerve passes superficial to the flexor retinaculum along with ulnar artery through Guyon's canal (ulnar tunnel) and enters the palm
- It divides into superficial and deep branches.

Distribution

- **Terminal branches**
  - **Superficial branch**
    - Supplies palmaris brevis
    - Two palmar digital branches to supply medial one and a half digits.
      1. One to medial side of little finger
      2. One common palmar digital nerve divides to supply adjacent sides of ring and little fingers
      3. It also supplies the nail beds of medial one and fingers.
  - **Deep branch of ulnar nerve:** Supplies most of the intrinsic muscles of the hand.
  - **Course and relation:**
    - It is accompanied by the deep branch of ulnar artery
    - It passes in between abductor digiti minimi and flexor digiti minimi
    - Pierces the opponens digiti minimi
    - It curves along the deep palmar arch
    - It lies deep to the flexor tendons
    - It terminates by supplying adductor pollicis.
  - **Structures supplied**:
    - Three hypothenar muscles namely flexor digiti minimi, abductor digiti minimi, opponens digiti minimi.

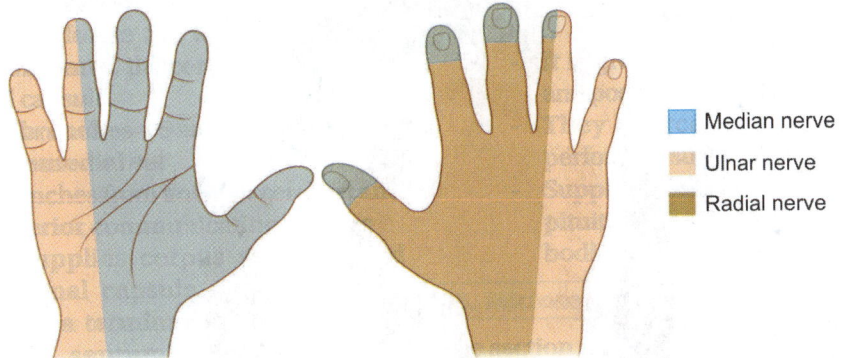

Fig. 32: Cutaneous innervation of palmar and dorsal surfaces of hand.

- 4th and 3rd lumbricals
- All dorsal interossei
- All palmar interossei
- Adductor pollicis
- Occasionally, branch to the deep head of flexor pollicis brevis.
- **Palmar cutaneous branch of ulnar nerve**
  - It is given in the middle of forearm.
  - It passes superficial to flexor retinaculum
  - Supplies the skin of medial half of palm.
- **Dorsal branch**
  - Arises 5 cm above the wrist
  - Passes dorsally deep to flexor carpi ulnaris
  - Divides into two dorsal digital branches:
    1. One branch supplies the medial side of little finger
    2. The other branch supply the adjacent sides of little and ring fingers.
  - In the little finger the dorsal branch supplies up to base of distal phalanx and ring finger up to base of middle phalanx.

Applied Anatomy

- Ulnar tunnel syndrome:
  - The nerve may be compressed by (i) trauma, (ii) ganglion, (iii) by accessory muscles as it passes deep to Guyon's canal
  - The patient complains of pain and sensory loss over medial one and a half digits
  - There will be weakness and wasting of intrinsic muscles of hand supplied by the ulnar nerve
  - Loss of hypothenar eminence
  - It produces ulnar claw hand—Marked clawing of 4th and 5th digits.
    - If ulnar nerve is injured, there is partial **claw-hand**.
  - Manifests in the form of partial claw hand of the medial two fingers
  - This results in flexion of interphalangeal joints and extension of metacarpophalangeal joints of the little and ring fingers of the hand. This occurs due to paralysis of interossei and medial two lumbricals
- If ulnar nerve is **injured at the wrist**, the clawing of the fingers is more as the nerve supply to flexor digitorum profundus is intact and flexes the digits more called as **ulnar paradox**.

4. **Structures under cover of deltoid muscle.**

- **Bones:** Lesser and greater tubercles of the humerus, intertubercular sulcus, upper part of shaft and surgical neck of humerus, coracoid process of scapula.
- **Muscles**
  - Insertions of:
    - Pectoralis minor to coracoid process
    - Supraspinatus, infraspinatus, and teres minor inserted to greater tubercle.

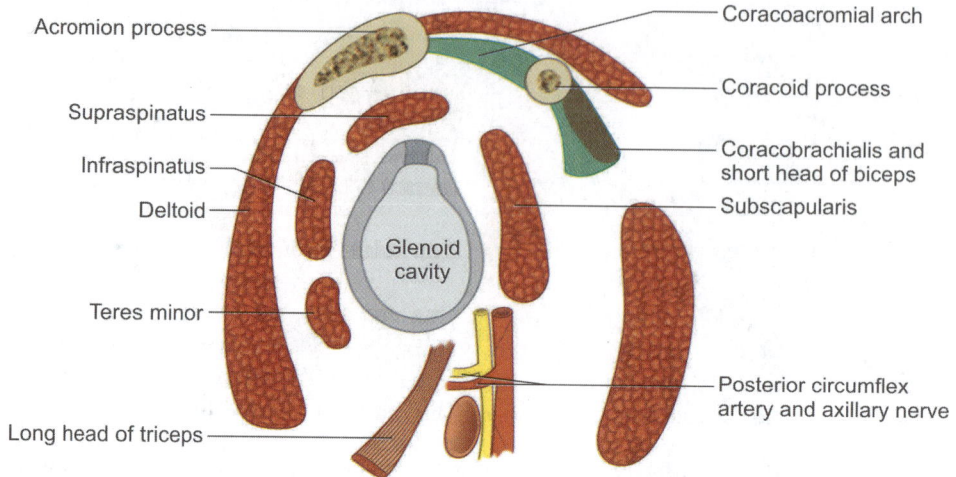

Fig. 33: Structures deep to deltoid muscle.

- Pectoralis major, teres major and latissimus dorsi on the intertubercular sulcus
- Subscapularis inserted to lesser tubercle.
- Origins of:
  - Coracobrachialis and short head of biceps brachii from the coracoid process
  - Long head of the biceps brachii from the supraglenoid tubercle
  - Long head of the triceps brachii from the infraglenoid tubercle
  - The lateral head of the triceps brachii from the upper end of the humerus.
- **Vessels:** Anterior circumflex humeral and posterior circumflex humeral vessels
- **Nerve:**
  - Axillary nerve
- **Joints and ligaments:**
  - Shoulder joint, coracoacromial ligament.
- **Bursae:** All bursae around the shoulder joint
- **Spaces:** Quadrangular lower and upper triangular spaces.

5. Inguinal lymph nodes.

- **Superficial inguinal lymph nodes:**
  - The superficial inguinal lymph nodes are variable in their number and size
  - Their arrangement is T-shaped, and grouped as a vertical group and an upper horizontal group
  - The **upper horizontal nodes** can be subdivided into the upper lateral and upper medial groups
  - The lymph nodes lie parallel to and below the inguinal ligament
  - **Upper lateral group** drains lymph from infraumbilical part of anterior abdominal wall and gluteal region
  - **Upper medial group** drains lymph from anterior abdominal wall below umbilicus, external genital the terminal part of the urethra, lower part of anal canal, and in female the lower part of vagina, and cornua of uterus
  - **Vertical group** drains lymph from most of the lower limb except areas drained by popliteal nodes
  - The nodes are situated along the terminal part of great saphenous vein.
- **Deep inguinal lymph nodes:**
  - Lie deep to the deep fascia
  - Situated medial to the upper part of the femoral vein
  - One to three in number
  - One at the junction of great saphenous and femoral veins

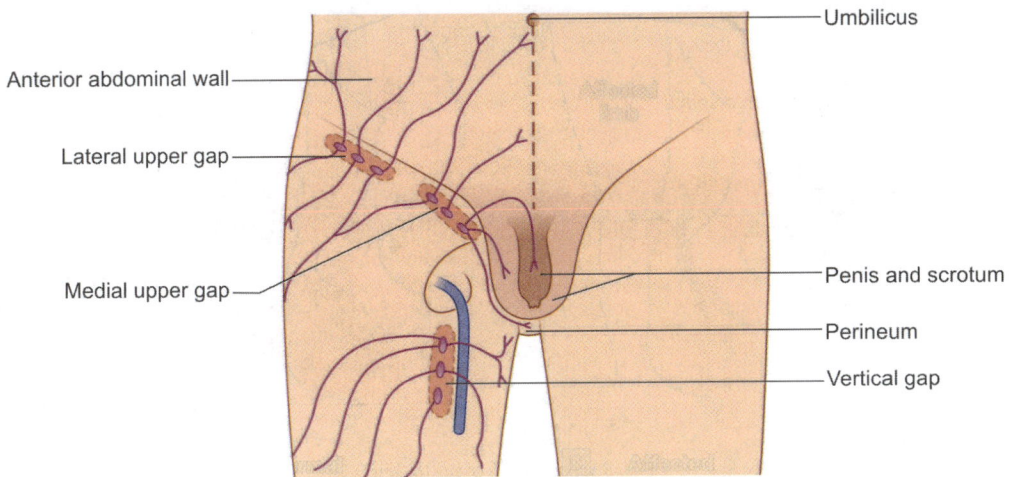

Fig. 34: Superficial inguinal lymph nodes.

- Another in the femoral canal (gland of Cloquet or Rosenmuller)
- The third in the lateral part of femoral ring
- Receive lymph from superficial inguinal lymph nodes, from glans penis or clitoris and deep lymphatics of lower limb.

- **Applied anatomy:**
  - Various groups of lymph nodes may be enlarged due to spread of infection or malignant growth extending from the areas drained by these nodes
  - The lesions of prepuce, penis, labia majora, lower part of vagina and anal canal, cornua of uterus, cause enlargement of horizontal group of superficial inguinal nodes
  - Infection in gluteal region results in enlargement of upper lateral horizontal group of superficial inguinal nodes.

6. Portal vein.

Portal vein is a large vein which collects blood from abdominal part of GIT except lower part of anal canal, from abdominal part of esophagus, gallbladder, pancreas, and spleen.
- **Length:** It is about 8 cm long

- **Formation (Fig. 35):**
  - Formed by the union of the superior mesenteric and splenic veins
  - Behind the neck of the pancreas
  - At the level of second lumbar vertebra
  - Splenic vein receives the inferior mesenteric vein.
- **Peculiarities:**
  - Portal vein starts as capillaries and ends as capillaries
  - It carries digested nutritive materials
  - Valves are present in foetal life and absent in adult
  - Two streams of blood circulate in the portal vein. The blood from superior mesenteric vein passes through right branch and blood from splenic vein is carried by left branch
  - 65–75% blood supply to liver is provided by the portal vein and the rest by the hepatic artery.
- **Course:**
  - It runs upwards and a little to the right first behind the neck of the pancreas
  - Behind the first part of the duodenum
  - In the right free margin of the lesser omentum

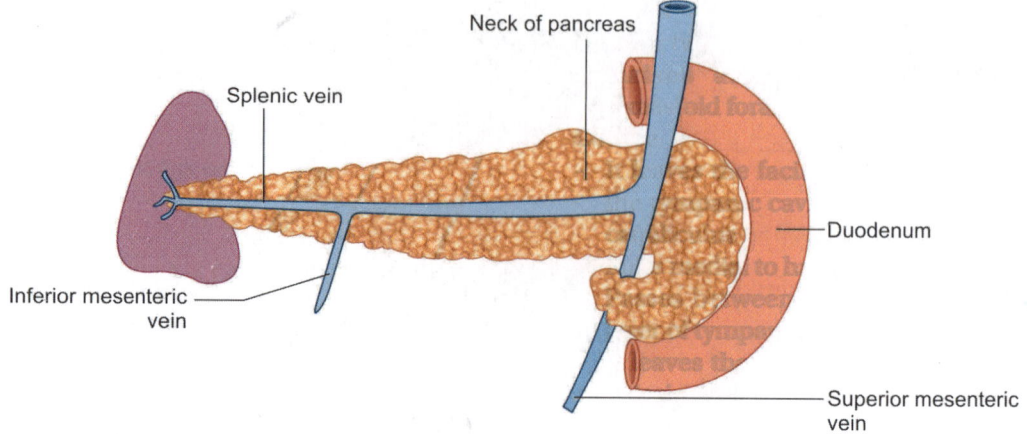

Fig. 35: Formation of portal vein.

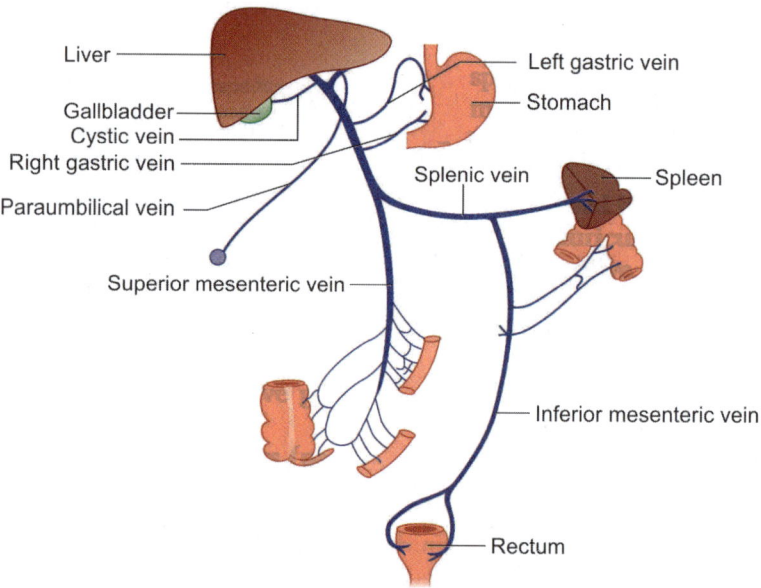

Fig. 36: Tributaries of portal vein.

- The vein ends at the right end of the porta hepatis by dividing into right and left branches and enter the liver.
- **Tributaries** portal vein receives the following veins **(Fig. 36)**:
  - **Formative tributaries**:
    - Splenic vein
    - Superior mesenteric vein
  - **Direct tributaries to portal vein**:
    - Left gastric vein
    - Right gastric vein
  - **Tributary to right branch**: Cystic vein
  - **Tributary to left branch**: Paraumbilical veins.
- **Portosystemic anastomoses:** These communications form important routes of collateral circulation in portal obstruction. The portal vein obstruction is seen in alcoholic cirrhosis of liver, carcinoma head of pancreas, congestive cardiac failure. In these cases, there is enlargement of these anastomotic areas.

Important sites of portosystemic communications (Fig. 37)

S. No.	Sites of porto-systemic (caval) anastomosis	Systemic veins	Portal veins	Surgical anatomy
1	Abdominal part of esophagus	Esophageal veins of azygos system	Esophageal veins of left gastric vein	In portal obstruction, there is esophageal varices leading to hematemesis
2	Anal canal	Middle rectal and inferior rectal veins	Superior rectal vein	In portal obstruction, there is enlargement of these veins resulting in hemorrhoids/piles and bleeding per rectum.
3	Umbilicus	The superior epigastric, lateral thoracic, posterior intercostal, inferior epigastric, superficial epigastric veins	Paraumbilical vein	In portal obstruction, there is enlargement of these veins seen resembling spokes of a wheel called caput medusae.
4	Bare area of the liver	Diaphragmatic vein	Portal vein tributaries	—
5	Posterior abdominal wall	Renal vein, the lumbar veins	Veins of spleen and colon (veins of Retzius)	
6	Falciform ligament	Diaphragmatic veins	Paraumbilical vein	
7	Patent ductus venosus	Inferior vena cava.	Left branch of portal vein	

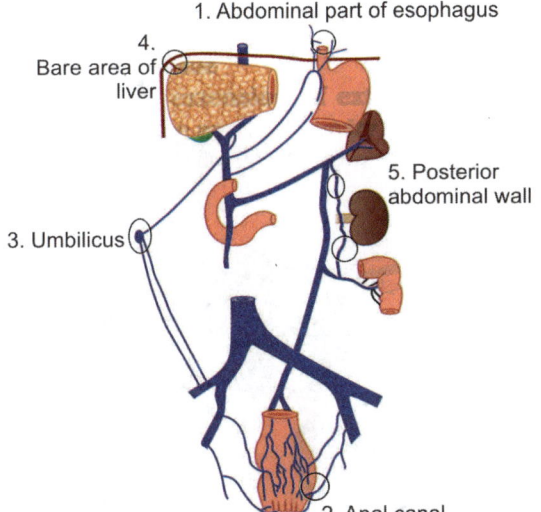

Fig. 37: Portocaval anastomosis.

7. Ureter.

- The ureter is a muscular tube
- Extends from the lower end of the renal pelvis to the urinary bladder
- It is about 25 cm long.
- **Course:**
  - From renal pelvis it runs downwards and medially
  - The abdominal part passes beneath the peritoneum of the posterior abdominal wall
  - At the brim of the pelvis, the upper end of the external iliac artery is crossed by the ureter, and reach the lateral wall of the pelvis
  - In the lateral wall of pelvis runs along the anterior margin of greater sciatic notch.

- It leaves the pelvic wall and turns medially and forwards at the level of ischial spine to reach the posterolateral part of the urinary bladder
- It passes within the wall of the bladder to open at the lateral angle of trigone.
- **Relations (Fig. 38):** Abdominal part of ureter:
  - **Anteriorly:**

On the right side	On the left side
• Peritoneum	• Peritoneum
• 2nd part of duodenum	• Gonadal artery
• Gonadal vessels	• Left colic vessels
• Right colic vessels	• Sigmoid colon
• Ileocolic vessels	• Sigmoid mesocolon
• Root of the mesentery	
• Terminal part of the ileum.	

  - **Posteriorly:**
    - Psoas major
    - Tips of transverse processes of lumbar vertebrae
    - Genitofemoral nerve.
  - **Medially:**
    - On the right side—inferior vena cava
    - Left side—left gonadal vein, inferior mesenteric vein.

- **Pelvic part of the ureter**
  - **Posteriorly:**
    - Internal iliac vessels
    - Lumbosacral trunk
    - Sacroiliac joint.
  - **Laterally:**
    - Fascia covering the obturator internus
    - Obturator nerve and vessels
    - Inferior vesical artery
    - Middle rectal artery.
  - In male—the ureter hooks the vas deferens
  - In female—in the lateral wall form posterior boundary of ovarian fossa, and the uterine artery is anterosuperior to the ureter and crosses the ureter from lateral to medial.
- **Constrictions:** 3 constrictions
  1. Pelviureteric junction
  2. Pelvic brim
  3. At the site of piercing the bladder wall.
- **Blood supply:**
  - Renal, gonadal, lumbar, perineal, common and internal iliac, inferior vesical arteries
  - In female uterine and vaginal arteries
  - These arteries form longitudinal anastomosis by dividing into ascending and descending branches.

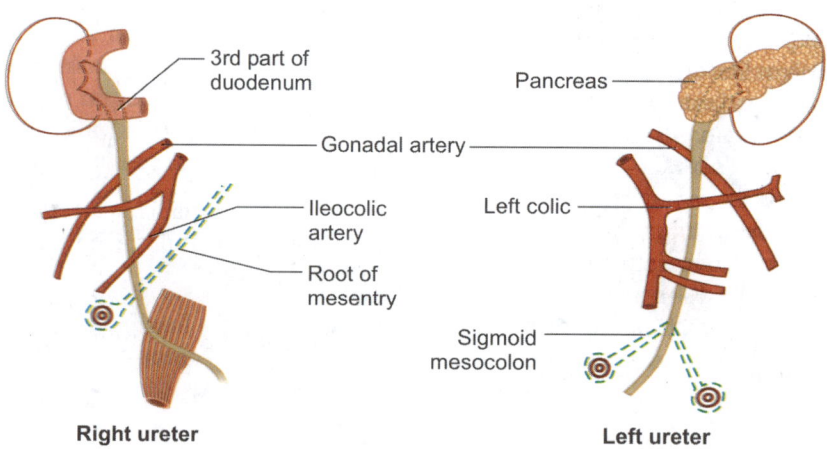

Fig. 38: Relations of ureter.

- **Development:** Ureteric bud, a diverticulum from mesonephric duct.
- **Applied anatomy**
  - Ureteric colic: Pain due spasm of the muscle produced by the ureteric stones radiates from loin to groin, scrotum or labium major
  - Impaction of the ureteric calculi is seen at the levels of constrictions as they are the narrowest points of ureter.

8. Perineal body.

- The perineal body (or) **central tendon of the perineum** is **formed** by aggregation of fibromuscular tissue
- It is also called as **gynecological perineum**
- **Situation:**
  - In the median plane at the junction of the anal and urogenital triangles
  - In male it separates the anal canal from the membranous urethra and the bulb of the penis. It is continuous with the raphe in the scrotal skin
  - In female it separates anal canal from the vagina. It is attached to the posterior commissure of labia majora.
- **Structures contributing**
  Ref Essay 2 perineal body
- **Development:** At the end of 7th week the urorectal septum comes in contact with the cloacal membrane and divides it into urogenital and anal membranes. The tip of the septum meets the cloacal membrane forms the future perineal body.
- **Applied anatomy:**
  - Damage to the perineal body during child-birth can weaken the perineum and may lead to prolapse of pelvic organs
  - Lacerations of the perineal body sustained during childbirth results in damage to the anterior fibers of the external anal sphincter
  - Perineal body is used for positioning the radiological marker to evaluate the dysfunction of floor of pelvis
  - Episiotomy: It is division of perineum to facilitate delivery. The division is angled laterally to avoid traumatic tear of the perineal body.

9. Microscopic structure of duodenum.

- The duodenum is proximal part of small intestine
- The small intestine is lined by four layers—mucous, submucous, muscular, and serous layers
- The mucous layer has permanent circular folds called plica circularis or valve of Kerkring
- The mucous layer has finger like, highly vascular, projections visible to naked eye called villi. These villi are broad and leaf like in duodenum. They increase the surface area and helps for absorption

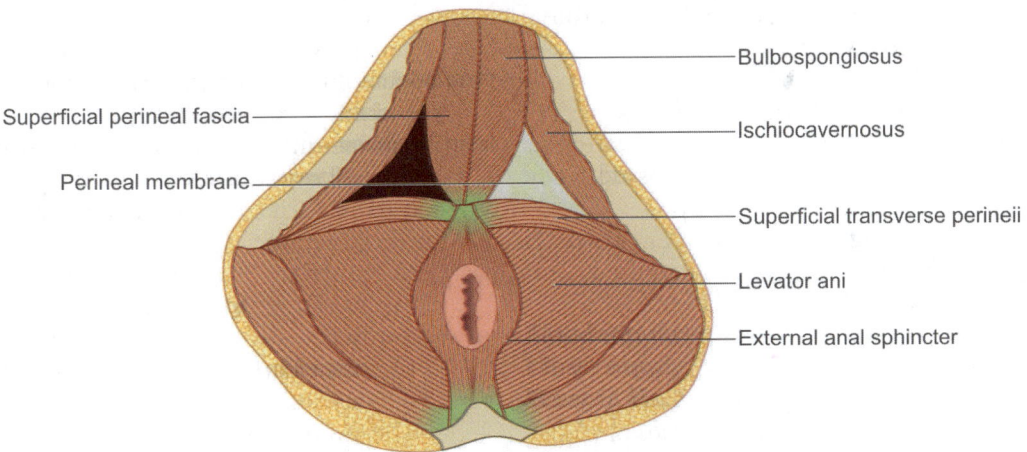

Fig. 39: Perineal body.

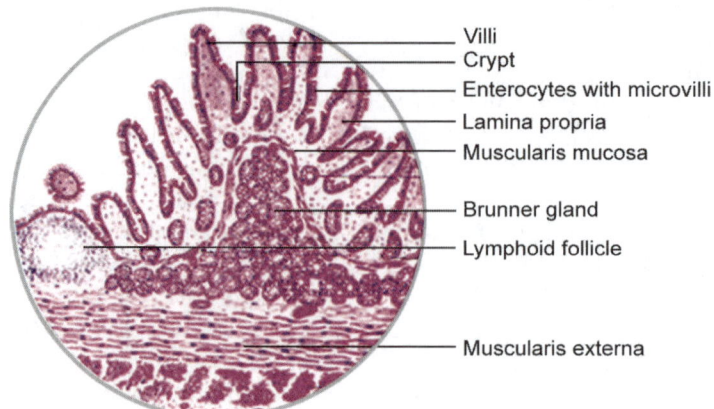

Fig. 40: Histology of duodenum.

- Duodenum is provided with from outer to inner are.
  - **Serous/adventitial layer**: Outermost – incomplete and formed by connective tissue
  - **Muscularis externa**: Outer longitudinal and inner circular smooth muscle fibers
  - **Submucosa**: Full of mucus secreting Brunner's glands. They are branched tubuloacinar type of glands. They secrete alkaline to neutralize the stomach chyme
  - **Mucous layer**: Lined by single layer epithelium which covers the villi and the intestinal glands. The villi are long and numerous. Invaginations in the form of crypts of Lieberkühn (intestinal glands) are seen.

  Epithelium: Lined by columnar cells with microvilli and goblet cells
    - The columnar cells are called as **enterocytes** and are absorptive in function
    - The goblet cells secretion is protective against microorganisms and help for lubrication
    - M cells are present over the lymph nodules
    - **Intestinal glands** open into the lumen between the bases of villi.
  - **Lamina propria**: Supports the epithelium. Contains connective tissue, intestinal glands (crypts of Lieberkühn), fibroblast, lymphocytes, vascular plexus, smooth muscle fibers. The cells present in the glands are: (i) Enterocytes—dilutes the chyme, (ii) Paneth cells secrete lysozyme, (iii) Mucous cells, (iv) Stem cells, (v) Neuroendocrine cells
    - **Muscularis mucosa**—Inner circular and outer longitudinal smooth muscle fibers.

10. Development of kidney.

The kidney develops from two different sources.
- The excretory tubules (nephrons) are derived from the lowest part of the nephrogenic cord. This part is the metanephros, the cells of which form the metanephric blastema in the lumbosacral region
- The collecting part of the kidney is derived from a diverticulum called the ureteric bud which arises from the lower part of the mesonephric duct.
- **Collecting part (Fig. 42):**
  - 5th week, the ureteric bud grows cranially towards the metanephric blastema, and its growing end becomes dilated
  - The dilated part divides repeatedly. It undergoes 13 or more successive divisions

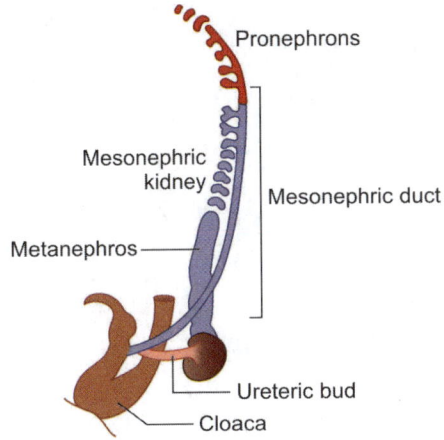

Fig. 41: Development of kidney.

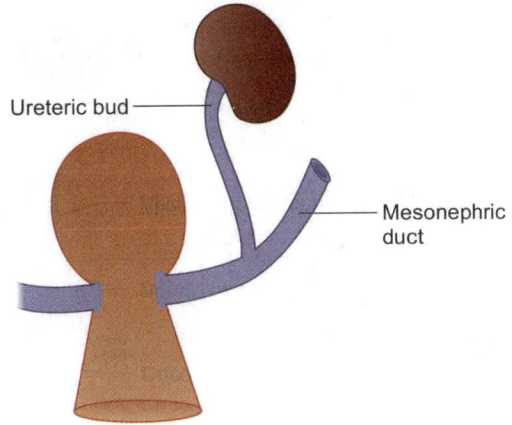

Fig. 42: Collecting part.

- The dilated end forms the pelvis and 1st division the major calyces
- The 2nd to 4th generations form the minor calyces
- While further divisions form the collecting tubules
- The stalk of the ureteric bud forms the ureter.

- **Excretory part (Fig. 43):**
  - Each division of the ureteric bud is capped with metanephric blastema, made of bilaminar cells
  - Some of the blastema cells separate and lie along the sides of subdivisions of ureteric bud
  - They enlarge to form hollow renal vesicle
  - One end of vesicle is dilated and another end narrow
  - Into the dilated part the internal glomerulus invaginates, and thereby converting vesicle into Bowman's capsule, together forming the nephron
  - The narrow end becomes an 'S' shaped tube which later forms the proximal convoluted tubule (PCT), Henle's loop, distal convoluted tubule (DCT)
  - Later a communication is established between collecting and secretory part
  - The kidney lies in pelvic cavity, receives blood from median sacral artery

- Later it ascends to reach iliac fossa, undersurface of diaphragm
- Further ascent is arrested by the supra renal gland
- During ascent, the kidney undergoes rotation so that the hilum faces medially.
- Congenital anomalies:
  - Agenesis of kidney
  - Pelvic kidney—failure to ascend
  - Horse shoe kidney—lower pole of both kidneys are connected and pass in front of aorta and inferior vena cava (IVC)
  - Polycystic kidney—failure of fusion between the collecting and excretory parts.

11. Arch of aorta.

- **Formation:** Continuation of ascending aorta, behind right 2nd sterno costal joint
- **Termination:** Continues as descending aorta, at the 2nd left sterno costal joint (T4)
- **Extent:** From 2nd right costal cartilage to 2nd left costal cartilage
- **Curvatures:** Presents two curvatures.
  - One is convex above
  - Other is convex in front and to the left
  - Summit of the upper curve is situated at the middle of the manubrium sterni.

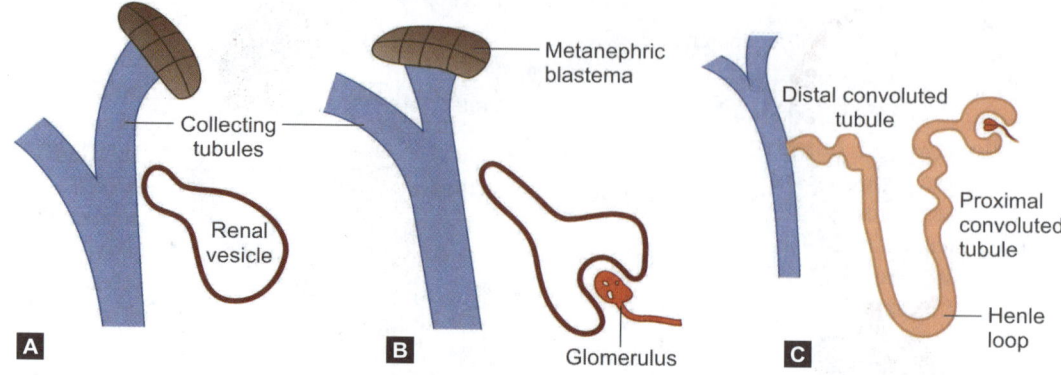

Figs. 43A to C: Excretory part.

- **Relations (Fig. 44):**
  - **Below**
    - Left principal bronchus
    - Bifurcation of pulmonary trunk
    - Left recurrent laryngeal nerve
    - Ligamentum arteriosum
    - Superficial cardiac plexus.
  - **Above**
    - Origin of brachiocephalic trunk, left common carotid artery, left subclavian artery
    - Left brachiocephalic vein
    - Crossing of left phrenic nerve over left vagus nerve.
  - **Posterior and to the right**
    - Trachea
    - Esophagus
    - Left recurrent laryngeal nerve
    - Thoracic duct
    - Deep cardiac plexus
    - Vertebra.
- **Anterior and to the left**
  - Left mediastinal pleura
  - Left phrenic nerve
  - Inferior cervical cardiac branch of left vagus
  - Superior cervical cardiac branch of left sympathetic trunk
  - Left vagus nerve
  - Left superior intercostal vein.
- **Branches from arch of aorta:**
  - Brachiocephalic trunk
  - Left common carotid artery
  - Left subclavian artery

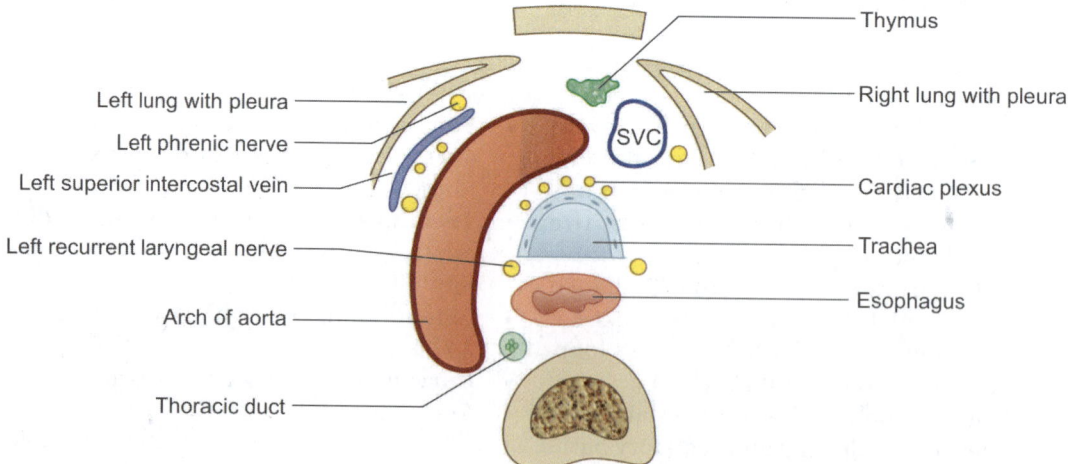

Fig. 44: Relations of arch of aorta.

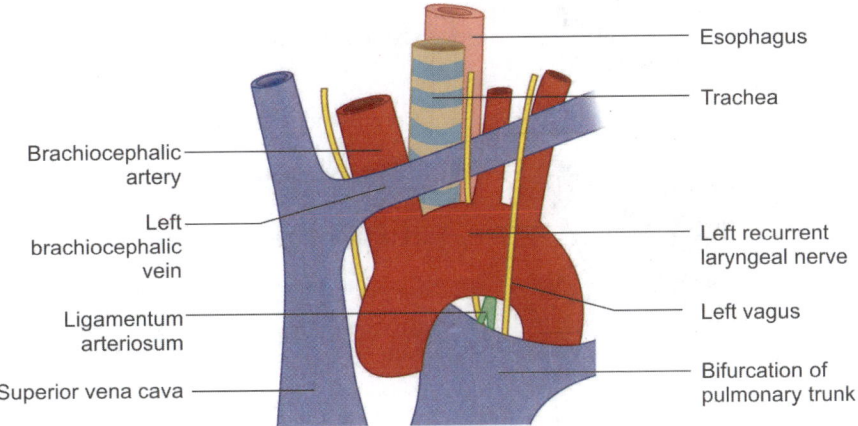

Fig. 45: Branches of arch of aorta.

- Occasional branches—thyroidea ima, vertebral artery, right subclavian.

12. Corpus striatum.

- Basal nuclei are gray masses forming major part of motor system
- They help to maintain normal voluntary movements and regulate coordinated voluntary movements
- The basal ganglia include caudate nucleus, lentiform nucleus, subthalamic nucleus, substantia nigra.
  - **Corpus striatum** includes the caudate nucleus and putamen of lentiform nucleus
  - Caudate nucleus is divided into head, body and tail.
- The putamen is larger and lateral part of lentiform nucleus.
- **Connections:**
  - **Afferent:**
    - From cerebral cortex—cortico striate fibers from motor and premotor areas
    - From thalamus—thalamo striate fibers from intralaminar nuclei of thalamus to striatum and are excitatory
    - From substantia nigra—nigrostriate fibers carry dopamine from substantia nigra to putamen.
  - **Efferent:**
    - To globus pallidus—striopallidal fibers from putamen and caudate nucleus to globus pallidus.
    - To substantia nigra—strionigral fibers from putamen to substantia nigra.
- **Functions:**
  - Programming of voluntary movements
  - Regulation of muscle tone
  - Control involuntary movements of skeletal muscles
  - Has a role in mood, and behavioral response.
- **Applied anatomy:**
  - Parkinsonism:
    - The disease is due to reduction of secretion of dopamine leads to degeneration of neurons of substantia nigra or nigrostriate fibers.
    - **Effect of lesion:**
      * Increased muscle tone leading to rigidity, tremors, abnormal movements
      * Akinesia—slow movement
      * Cogwheel or lead pipe rigidity
      * Pill rolling movement
      * Mask-like face
      * Shuffling gait
      * Stopped posture.

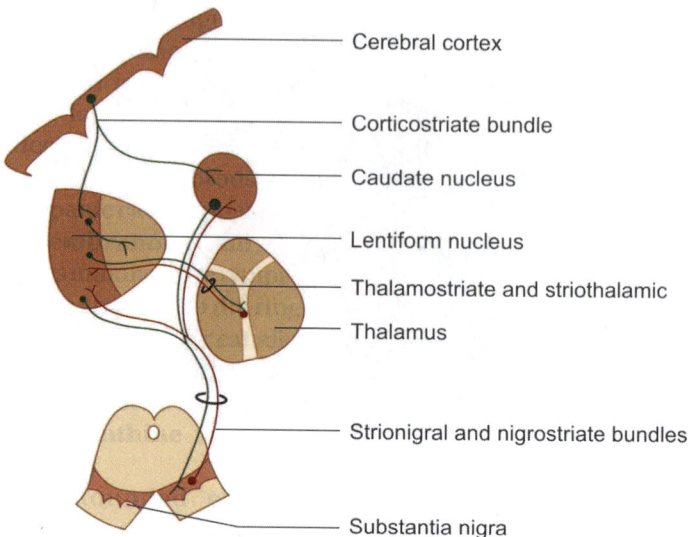

Fig. 46: Connections of corpus striatum.

13. Labeled diagram of section of pons at the level of facial colliculus.

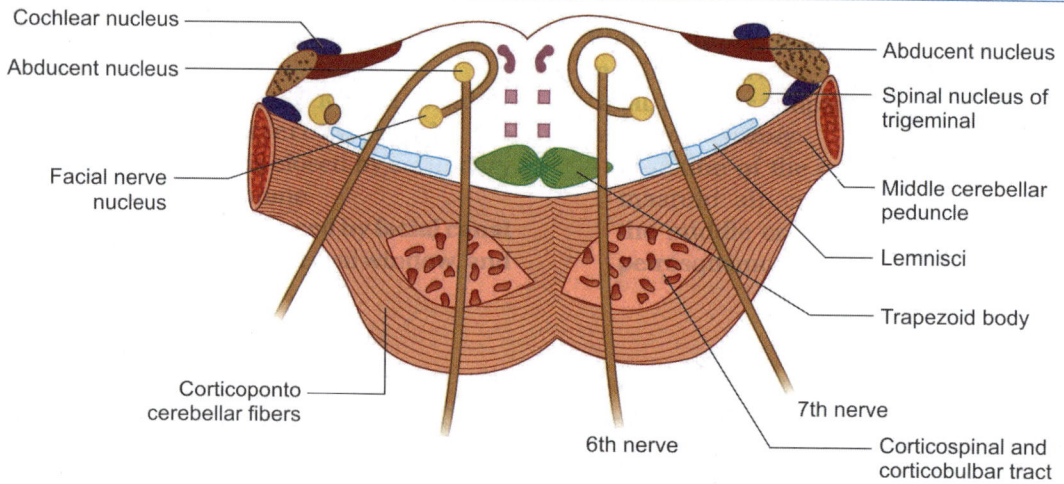

Fig. 47: Pons-facial colliculus level.

14. Oculomotor nerve.

- It is the third cranial nerve
- Purely motor
- Supplies the extraocular muscles which are developed from somitomere 1 and 2
- **Structures supplied**
  - The nerve supplies
    - The extraocular muscles except lateral rectus and superior oblique muscle
    - The intraocular muscles—sphincter papillae and ciliaris.
- **Functional component**
  - Somatic efferent—supplying the extraocular muscles which are developed from head somitomeres
  - General visceral efferent: Parasympathetic fibers for sphincter papillae and ciliaris.

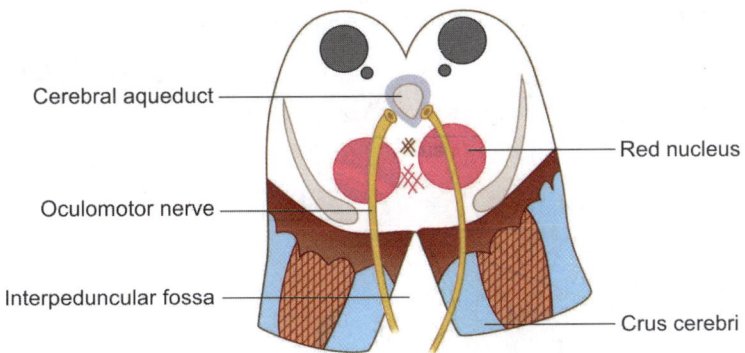

Fig. 48: Midbrain—superior colliculus.

- **Nucleus of origin (Fig. 48)**
  - Oculomotor nucleus situated in the periaqueductal gray matter in the midbrain at the level of superior colliculus
  - The nucleus is divides into **motor nuclei** supplying extraocular muscles
  - A preganglionic **parasympathetic the Edinger – Westphal nucleus** which supply the intraocular muscles, sphincter papillae and ciliaris.
- **Course**
  - **Within midbrain:** The nerve fibers pass through red nucleus, crus cerebri and emerge medial to the crus cerebri.
  - **Interpeduncular fossa:**
    - It becomes a content of interpeduncular fossa
    - Situated between the posterior cerebral and superior cerebellar arteries
    - The nerve is lateral to the posterior communicating artery.
  - **Intracranial:**
    - It runs forward related to the roof of cavernous sinus
    - It pierces the duramater between attached and free border of tentorium cerebelli (oculomotor triangle) to reach the lateral wall of cavernous sinus.
  - **Lateral wall of cavernous sinus (Fig. 49)**
    - In the **lateral wall of cavernous sinus,** it terminates by dividing into superior and inferior divisions

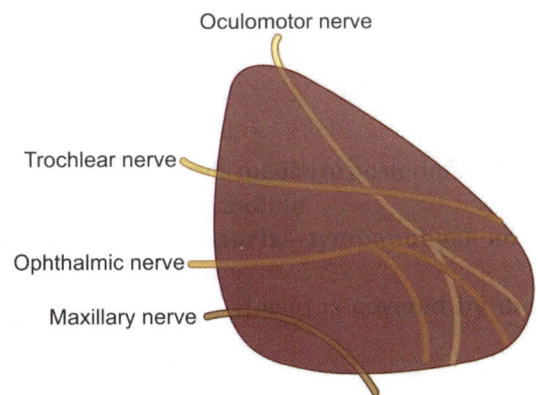

Fig. 49: Lateral wall of cavernous sinus.

  - It is related below to the trochlear, ophthalmic and maxillary nerves.
  - **Superior orbital fissure (Fig. 50)**
    - The two divisions enter the orbit through the **superior orbital fissure**
    - It passes within the common tendinous ring (oculomotor foramen)
    - It is related to the abducent and nasociliary nerves.
  - **In the orbit**:
    - The superior division passes above the optic nerve
    - The inferior division passes below the optic nerve and terminates into three branches.
- **Distribution (Fig. 51)**
  - Superior division—supplies superior rectus and levator palpabrae superioris

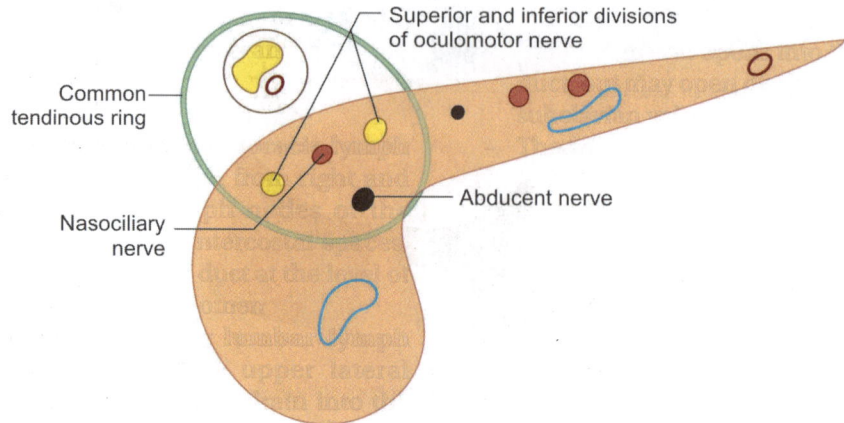

Fig. 50: Superior orbital fissure.

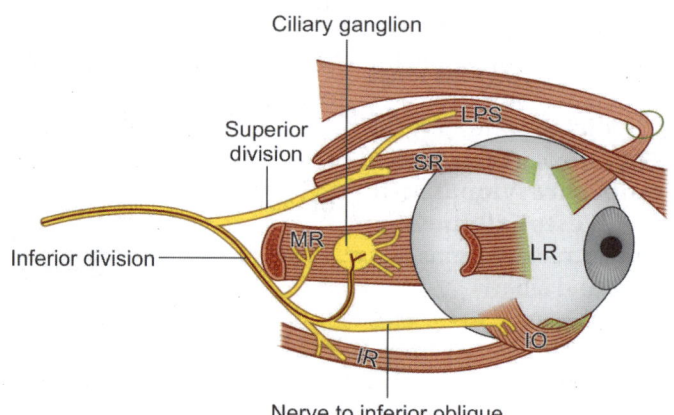

Fig. 51: Distribution of oculomotor nerve.

- Inferior division—supply inferior rectus, medial rectus and inferior oblique muscles
- The branch to inferior oblique gives a communicating branch to ciliary ganglion which contains the parasympathetic fibers. Through this branch, it supplies intraocular muscles sphincter pupillae and the ciliary muscle.
- **Connections:**
  - Cerebral cortex through corticobulbar fibers
  - To visual cortex
  - To pretectal nucleus
  - Through medial longitudinal fasciculus the nerve is connected to 4th, 6th, and 8th nerve for coordinated movement of the eyeball.
- **Communications:**
  - With sympathetic plexus around internal carotid artery
  - With ophthalmic nerve.
- **Applied anatomy**
  - **Oculomotor syndrome**—injury to oculomotor nerve results in:
    - Ptosis—due to paralysis of levator palpabrae superioris
    - Lateral squint—due to unopposed action of lateral rectus
    - Dilated pupil—due to paralysis of sphincter pupillae
    - Enophthalmos—as most of the extraocular muscles are paralyzed

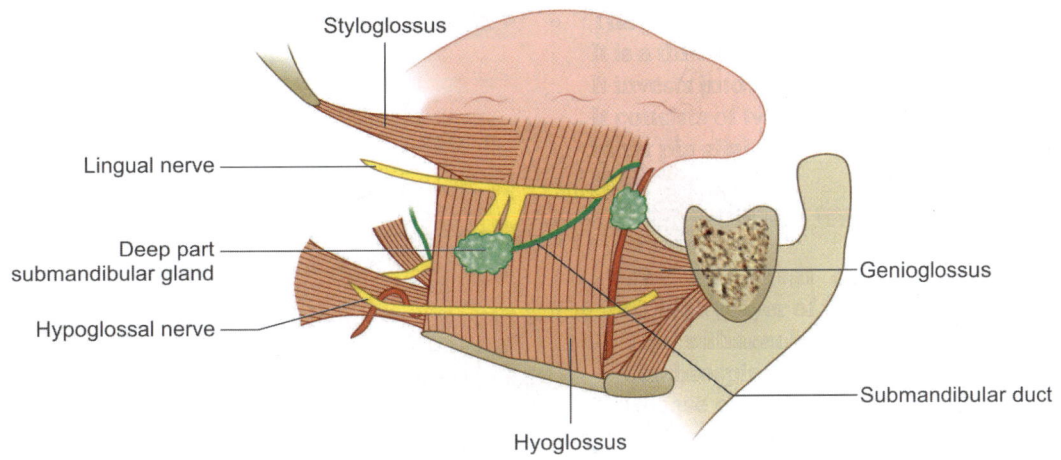

Fig. 52: Relations of hyoglossus.

- Loss of accommodation—due to paralysis of ciliaris.
- **Weber's syndrome:** Due vascular lesion affecting mid brain the oculomotor nerve fiber, corticospinal tract will be affected resulting in oculomotor syndrome and contralateral hemiplegia.

15. Hyoglossus muscle.

- It is an extrinsic muscle of tongue
- It is a quadrilateral muscle
- **Origin:** From whole length of the upper border of greater horn and part of body of hyoid bone
- **Insertion:** Side of tongue lateral to geniohyoid muscle
- **Nerve supply:** Hypoglossal nerve
- **Action:** Depresses the tongue
- **Relations (Fig. 52):**
  - **Superficial:** Tendon of digastric muscle, styloglossus, mylohyoid, lingual nerve, deep part of submandibular gland and its duct, sublingual gland, submandibular ganglion, hypoglossal nerve and deep lingual veins
  - **Deep:** Stylohyoid ligament, lingual artery, middle constrictor, genioglossus, glossopharyngeal nerve
  - **Posterior border:** Glossopharyngeal nerve, stylohyoid ligament, lingual artery.

16. Lateral wall of nasal cavity.

Skeleton of Lateral Wall (Fig. 53)

- The lateral wall of nasal cavity is formed by bones and cartilages
- Bony component
  - Body and the frontal process of maxilla
  - Labyrinth of ethmoid bone
  - Inferior concha
  - Perpendicular plate of palatine bone
  - Lacrimal bone
  - Nasal process of frontal bone
  - Medial pterygoid plate
  - Nasal bone.
- Cartilage
  - Major alar cartilage
  - Minor alar cartilage
  - Lateral process of septal cartilage.

Features

Vestibule

Seen close to the anterior nasal orifice. It is bounded above by a ridge called limen nasi and is lined by stratified squamous epithelium.

Conchae and Meatuses

Three projections are seen curving inferomedially called **conchae**. Depressions/ grooves seen below these conchae are called **meatuses**.

- Conchae
  - **Superior concha** is smallest and is from ethmoid bone

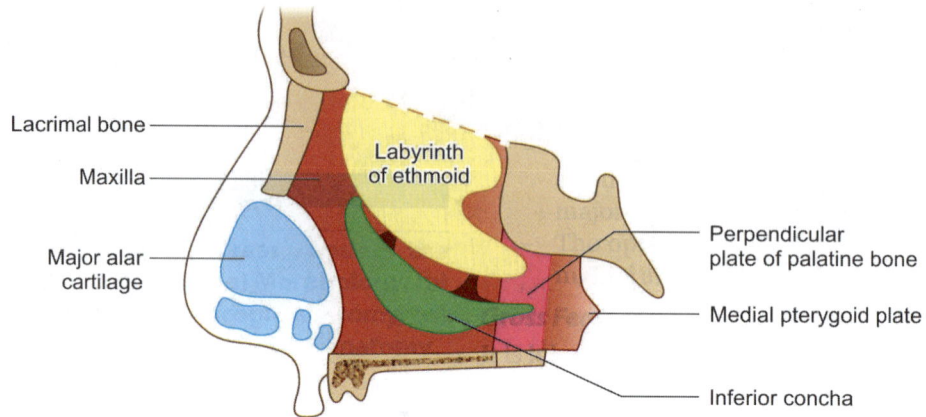

Fig. 53: Skeleton of lateral wall.

- The **middle concha** is from labyrinth of ethmoid bone. It articulates with perpendicular plate of palatine bone posteriorly
- The **inferior concha** is an individual bone and articulates with body of maxilla and perpendicular plate of palatine bone
- Sometimes a fourth concha is seen and if present seen above the superior concha and is called as **supreme/highest concha**.
- **Meatuses (Fig. 54)**
  - **Superior meatus**:
    - The posterior ethmoidal sinus opens into it
  - The depression above superior concha is called **sphenoethmoidal recess**. Into this space the sphenoidal sinus opens.
  - **Middle meatus**:
    - Lies below and lateral to the middle concha
    - There is a rounded bulge in the center known as **bulla ethmoidalis** produced by middle ethmoidal air cells.
  - **Hiatus semilunaris**:
    - Curved cleft below bulla formed by the edge of uncinate process
    - Expands anteriorly as a slit like space called **ethmoid infundibulum**

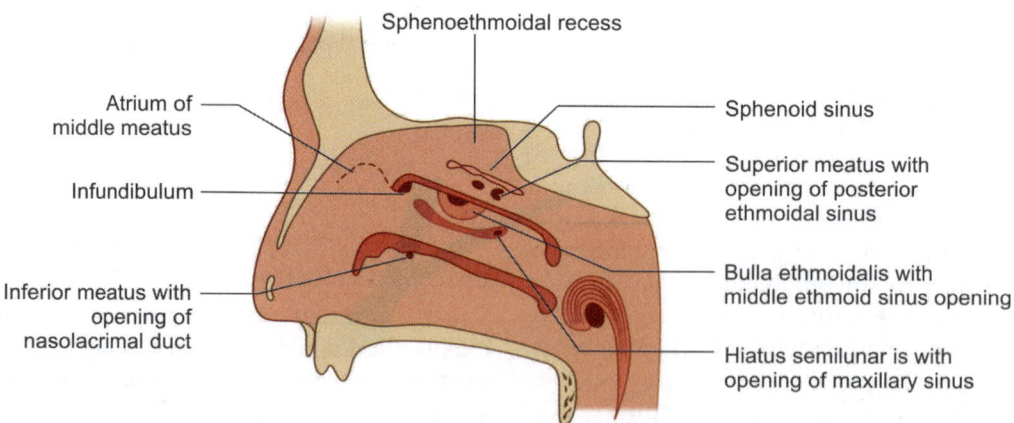

Fig. 54: Meatuses.

- In front of middle meatus is a depression—**atrium**
- It is bounded above by a ridge—**agger nasi.**
- **Sinuses opening** into it are:
  - Maxillary sinus into the hiatus semilunaris
  - Anterior ethmoidal air sinuses into the infundibulum
  - Middle ethmoidal sinus on top of bulla
  - Frontal air sinus opens into middle meatus.
- **Inferior meatus**
  - It is the largest meatus
  - The nasolacrimal duct opens into it
  - The opening is at the junction of anterior one-third and posterior two-third of the meatus
  - The opening is guarded by a mucous fold called **lacrimal fold**/Hasner's valve.
- **Nerve supply (Fig. 55)**
  - Anterosuperiorly—anterior ethmoidal nerve branch of ophthalmic nerve
  - Anteroinferiorly—anterior superior alveolar nerve branch of maxillary nerve
  - Posterosuperiorly—posterior superior lateral nasal branches from pterygopalatine ganglion
  - Posteroinferiorly—posterior inferior lateral nasal branches of greater palatine nerve from pterygopalatine ganglion.
- **Blood supply**
  - **Arterial supply**
    - Anterosuperiorly—anterior ethmoidal artery of branch ophthalmic artery
    - Anteroinferiorly—greater palatine and facial arteries
    - Posterosuperiorly—sphenopalatine artery branch of maxillary artery
    - Posteroinferiorly—greater palatine branch of maxillary artery
  - **Venous drainage:** Drains into pterygoid venous plexus, facial and ophthalmic veins
  - **Applied anatomy:** Deviation of the nasal septum can cause unilateral nasal obstruction.

17. Thyroid gland

Parts

- 2 lateral lobes and an isthmus
- Lateral lobes—roughly pyramidal shape; has an apex, base, anterolateral, medial and posterolateral surfaces, anterior and posterior borders
- Isthmus—quadrilateral with 2 borders and 2 surfaces.

Apex (Fig. 56)

- Extends up to oblique line of thyroid cartilage
- Covered by the sternothyroid attached to oblique line, which prevents upward extension
- Related to superior thyroid artery and external laryngeal nerve.

Base

- Extends up to 4th or 5th ring of trachea
- Related to loop of inferior thyroid artery and recurrent laryngeal nerve.

Superficial Surface (Fig. 57)

Overlapped by sternothyroid, sternohyoid, superior belly of omohyoid and sternocleidomastoid muscles.

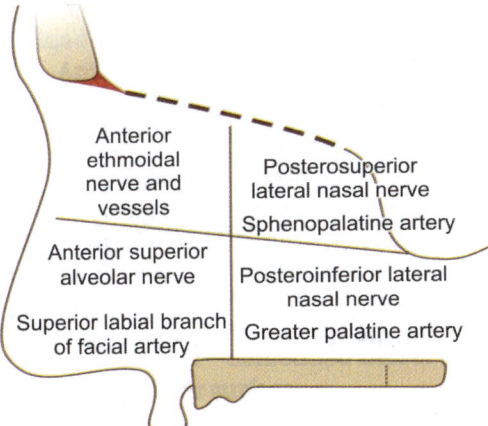

Fig. 55: Nerve and arterial supply of lateral wall.

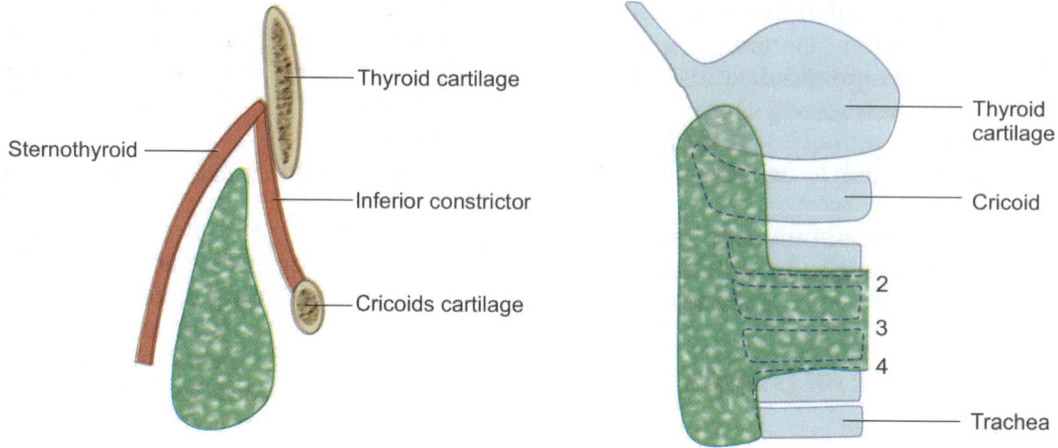

Fig. 56: Extent of thyroid gland.

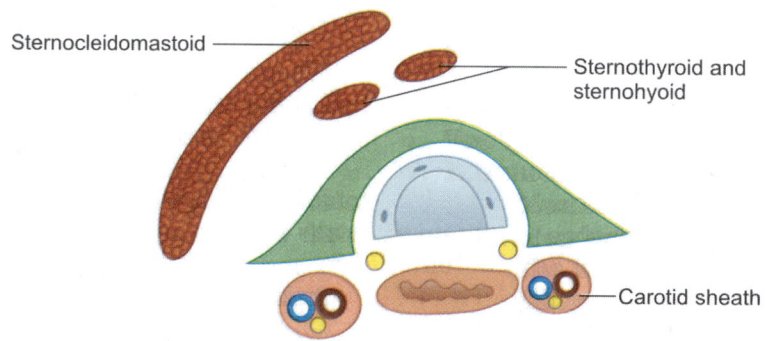

Fig. 57: Relations of lateral lobe.

Posterolateral Surface

Related to carotid sheath and its contents common carotid artery, internal jugular vein, vagus.

Medial Surface (Fig. 58)

- 2 tubes: Esophagus and trachea
- 2 muscles: Inferior constrictor muscle and cricothyroid muscle
- 2 nerves: External and recurrent laryngeal nerves
- 2 cartilages: Thyroid and cricoid cartilages.

Anterior Border

- Separates anterolateral and medial surfaces
- Related to anterior branch of superior thyroid artery.

Posterior Border

- Separates posterolateral and medial surfaces
- Anastomosis between superior and inferior thyroid arteries
- Parathyroid glands are situated.

Isthmus (Fig. 59)

- Lies across midline
- Connects the two lateral lobes
- **Anterior surface**—covered by sternothyroid, sternohyoid, investing layer of deep cervical fascia, anterior jugular veins
- **Posterior surface**—related to 2nd to 4th tracheal rings
- **Upper border**
  - Anastomosis between the superior thyroid arteries

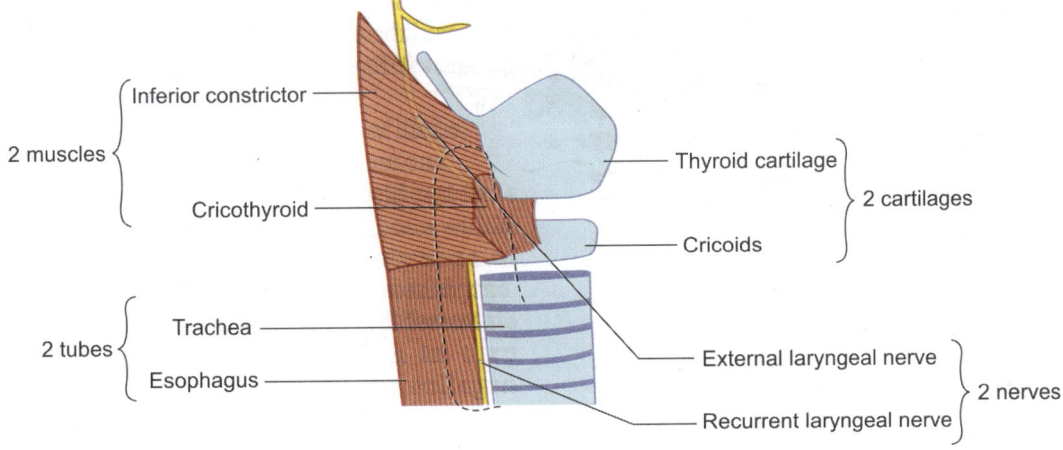

Fig. 58: Medial relations of lateral lobe.

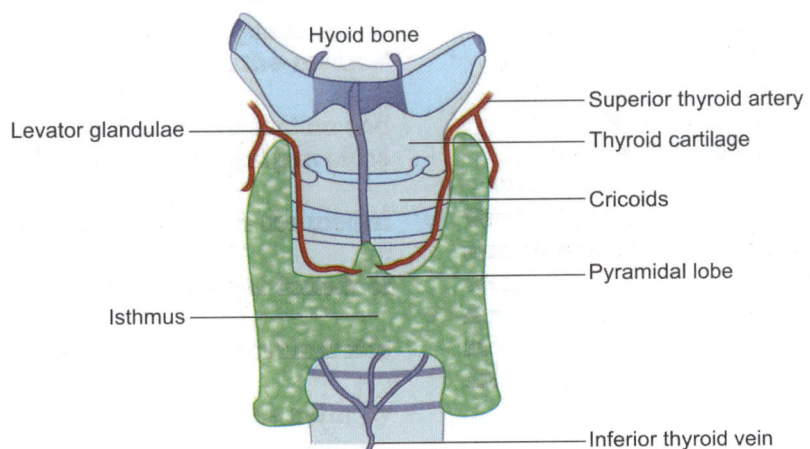

Fig. 59: Relations of isthmus.

- Pyramidal lobe – projection from upper border of isthmus towards hyoid bone. Sometimes it will be attached to hyoid bone by a fibromuscular strand called levator glandulae thyroidea.
- **Lower border**
  - Inferior thyroid veins emerge from lower border
  - Arteria thyroidea ima.
- **Blood supply**
  - Arterial supply by superior thyroid artery from external carotid artery, inferior thyroid artery from thyrocervical trunk, and thyroidea ima
  - Venous drainage—superior and middle thyroid veins end in internal jugular vein. Inferior thyroid vein to brachiocephalic vein.

18. Microscopic structure of cerebellum.

- The surface of cerebellum is more folded and thin called folia
- It has outer gray matter and inner white matter
- The **gray matter** is made of three layers —outer molecular, middle purkinje, and inner granular layers
- The neurons in the cerebellar cortex are Purkinje cell, golgi cell, granule cell, horizontal cell, basket cell and neuroglial cells
- **Stellate cell** present in molecular layer. Dendrites synapse with parallel fibers of

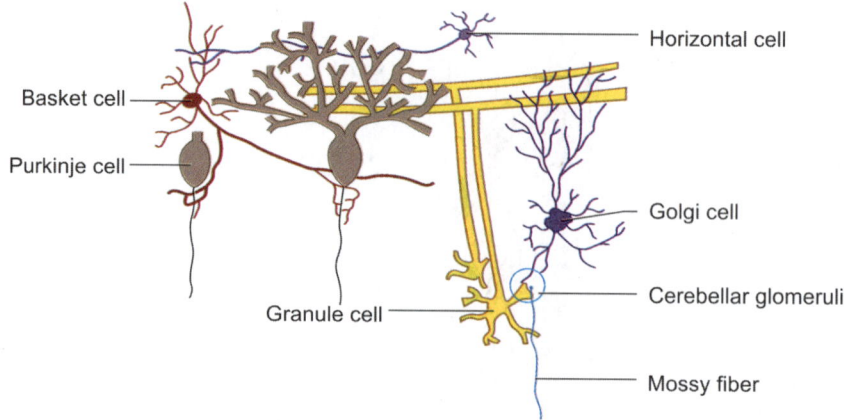

Fig. 60: Cells of cerebellum.

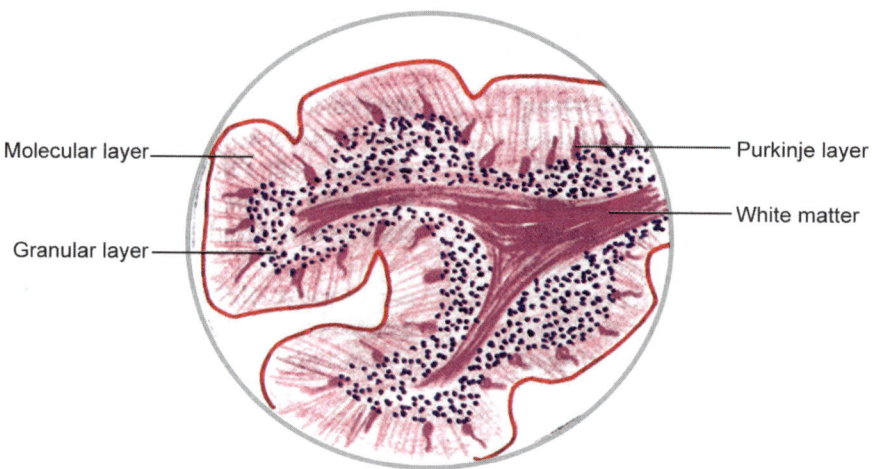

Fig. 61: Histology of cerebellum.

granule cell and axon with dendrites of the Purkinje cells
- **Basket cell** present in molecular layer. The axon synapse with pre axon part of Purkinje and dendrites with dendrites of Purkinje, mossy and climbing fibers
- **Purkinje cells** are flask shaped. The dendritic tree arises from the cell neck and pass on to molecular layer. The axon passes through the granular layer and it forms the only efferent fibers. They are inhibitory
- **Granular cells** situated in the granule layer. The axon passes to the molecular layer and divide into the form of letter T, the fibers run parallel to each other. The dendrites of the granule cells have processes which take part in glomeruli
- **Golgi cell** present in granular layer. The dendrite enters the molecular layer. The axon take part in glomeruli
- The **molecular layer** contains—(i) dendritic tree of purkinje cells, (ii) soma, axon and dendrites of horizontal cell, (iii) soma, axon and dendrites of basket cells, (iv) axons of granule cells which divides as T branches, (v) dendrites of golgi cells (vi) climbing fibers (vii) neuroglial cells
- **Purkinje layer** contains the soma of Purkinje cells

- **Granular layer** contains—soma, axon, and basal dendrites of golgi cells, soma and dendrites of granule cells, axons of purkinje cells, neuroglial cells, cerebellar glomeruli, mossy and climbing fibers
- The **white matter** is made of **afferent and efferent fibers**:
  - **Afferent** is formed by mossy and climbing fibers
  - The **climbing fiber** is from olivocerebellar fibers and end in purkinje cells.
  - All the other fibers entering form the **mossy fibers**
  - They are vestibule, ponto, spino cerebellar fibers
  - The only **efferent** is formed by axons of purkinje cells.

19. Derivatives of 3rd and 4th pharyngeal pouches.

- Pharyngeal pouches are endodermal derivatives
- Initially there are five pouches
- As the fifth pharyngeal arch disappears the fifth become rudimentary or disappears
- The endoderm of the pouches thickens and evaginates into mesenchymal condensations and the neural crest enter into the condensation
- The second, third and fourth pouches are prolonged to form dorsal and ventral wings.

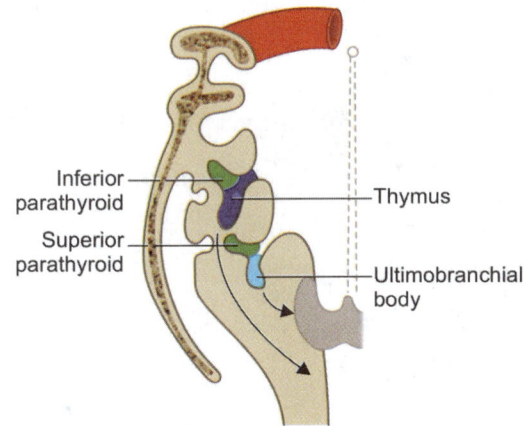

Fig. 62: Pharyngeal pouches.

Derivatives of third pouch
- Ventral wing gives rise to **thymus** and dorsal wing **parathyroid III/inferior parathyroid**
- Thymus grow caudally into the surrounding cardiac mesenchyme
- Ventral to the aortic sac the two thymic rudiments are united by connective tissue
- As the neck is fully developed the heart descends and the thymus is also pulled to the anterior mediastinum
- The connection with the third pouch is soon lost
- The connection between the parathyroid III and the thymic rudiments persists for some time
- When the thymus descends the parathyroid III is also pulled and it becomes the inferior parathyroid gland.

Derivatives of fourth pouch:
- Fourth pouch divides into dorsal wing and ventral wing
- The superior parathyroid gland (**parathyroid IV**) develops from the dorsal wing
- The ventral portion of the fourth pouch, form **ultimobranchial body**
- The ultimobranchial body gives rise to **parafollicular/C cells** of thyroid gland.

20. Development of neural tube.

- The neuroectodermal cells become thickened to form medullary/neural plate
- During somite period, a depression appears known as **neural groove (Fig. 63)**
- The tips of the groove are lined by specialized cells called **neural crest** cells
- The neural groove extends in midline from Henson's node to buccopharyngeal membrane
- The neural groove gradually fuses to form neural tube and the process is called **neurulation**
- The fusion starts from cervical region extending caudally with appearance of two pores
- The cephalic and caudal pores are called anterior and posterior neural pores
- The amniotic fluid circulates through neuropores

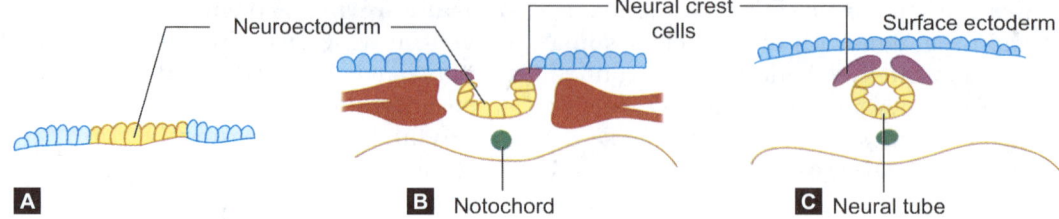

Figs. 63A to C: Development of neural tube.

- The anterior pore closes by middle of 4th week and the posterior pore by end of 4th week
- The position of anterior pore is represented as lamina terminalis
- The neural tube gets detached dorsally from surface ectoderm
- The neural tube is lined by pseudostratified neuroepithelial cells
- Continued proliferation of the neuroepithelial cells forms three layers in the walls of neural tube—inner ependymal, intermediate mantle and outer marginal zones
- The cells lining the neural tube form **ependymal zone** and are non-migratory lining the ventricles of brain
- After closure of the neural tube the neuroepithelial cells migrate outwards to give rise to **neuroblast and spongioblast cells**. The neuroblast differentiate into neurons. The spongioblast form glial cells
- These cells form **mantle zone** around the neuroepithelial layer **(Fig. 64)**
- They form the **gray matter in the spinal cord**
- The processes (nerve fibers) of the neuroblast cells form the marginal zone
- They are myelinated and form the **white matter of spinal cord**
- The neural crest cells are seen dorsal to the neural tube between the surface ectoderm and neural tube. It extends from midbrain vesicle to the caudal end of neural tube
- The cephalic part of tube enlarges to form 3 vesicles—fore, mid and hind brain vesicles
- Forebrain vesicle gives rise to—telen and diencephalon, midbrain—mesencephalon, hindbrain—myelin and metencephalon
- The rest of the tube forms the spinal cord.
- **Congenital anomaly**:
  – Anencephaly—the failure of closure of neural tube in the cranial region results in this condition
  – Spina bifida—if the neural tube fails to close anywhere from cervical region to caudal part **(Figs. 65A to C)**
  – Types of spina bifida are due to failure of development of the vertebral laminae.

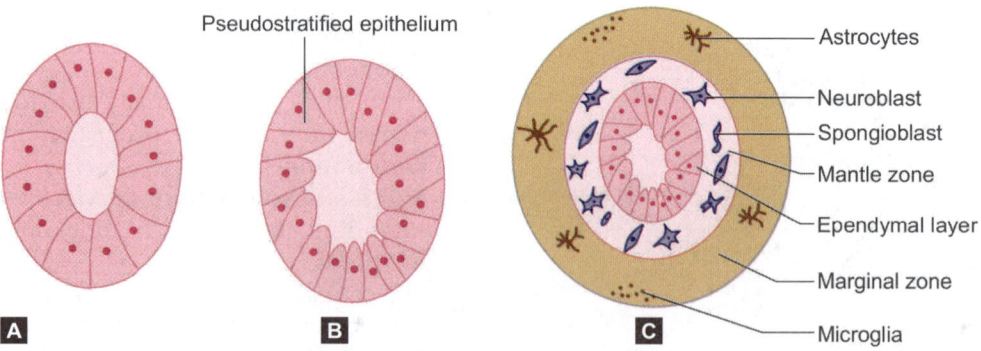

Figs. 64A to C: Cellular differentiation of neural tube.

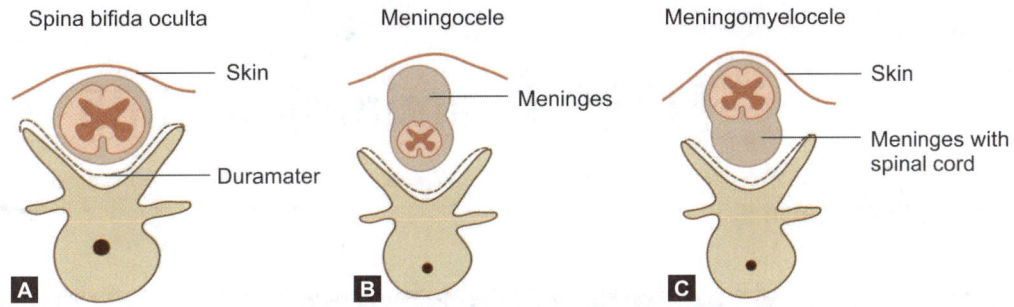

Figs. 65A to C: Spina bifida.

- Spina bifida oculta—where the overlying skin and muscles are present
- Meningocele—the meninges protrude through the defect
- Meningomyelocele—the meninges and spinal cord lies within the meninges protruded.

MBBS Examination 2005

ANSWER ALL QUESTIONS

I. Essay questions (15/10 Marks)

1. Describe the arches of the foot under following headings: Name of arches and their constitution factors maintain them applied aspects.
2. Describe the extrahepatic biliary apparatus parts, position, peritoneal and visceral relations, blood supply and applied anatomy.
3. Write about brachial plexus under the following headings: Formation, relations, branches and its clinical significance.
4. Describe the anal canal parts positions, interior relations, blood supply, lymphatic drainage and applied aspects.
5. Write about coronary circulation. Mention the origin, course, distribution, branches, termination, anastomosis and clinical importance.
6. Describe extraocular muscles—enumerate. Give an account of their attachments, nerve supply, actions and applied anatomy.
7. Describe the parts, relations, constituent fibers, blood supply and applied anatomy of internal capsule.
8. Describe the thoracic diaphragm under the following headings: Parts, attachments, major and minor openings, blood supply, nerve supply, actions, and applied anatomy.

II. Short notes (5/3/2 Marks)

1. Corpus luteum.
2. Midgut rotation.
3. Microscopic structure of spleen.
4. Femoral sheath.
5. Trigone of the bladder.
6. Development of pancreas.
7. Pronation and supination.
8. Cutaneous nerve supply of the foot.
9. Perineal membrane.
10. Lesser sac.
11. Microscopic structure of appendix.
12. Meckel's diverticulum.
13. Inferior mesenteric artery.
14. Great saphenous vein.
15. Primitive streak.
16. First carpometacarpal joint.
17. Microscopic structure of bone.
18. Pelvic diaphragm.
19. Lymphatic drainage of the mammary gland.
20. Radial nerve in spiral groove.
21. Nasal septum.
22. Down's syndrome.
23. Histology of hypophysis cerebri or Pituitary gland.
24. Circle of Willis.
25. Microscopic structure of the lung.
26. Tympanic membrane.
27. Second branchial arch.
28. Chorda tympani.
29. Amnion.
30. Lateral pterygoid muscle.
31. Muscles of tongue.
32. Microscopic structure of trachea.
33. Vocal cords.
34. Microscopic structure and development of palatine tonsil.
35. Hilum of lungs.
36. Dentate nucleus.
37. Boundaries of tympanic cavity.
38. Styloid process.
39. Klinefelter's syndrome.
40. Pleural recesses.

I. ESSAY QUESTIONS

1. **Describe the arches of the foot under following headings: Name of arches and their constitution factors maintain them applied aspects.**

Refer essay Q. No. 1 – 2003

2. **Describe the extrahepatic biliary apparatus parts, position, peritoneal and visceral relations, blood supply and applied anatomy.**

The extra biliary apparatus collects the bile from the liver, stores it in the gallbladder and drains to the second part of duodenum.

Parts of Extrahepatic Biliary Apparatus (Fig. 1)

- Right and left hepatic ducts
- Common hepatic duct
- Gallbladder
- Cystic duct
- Bile duct
- Ampulla of Vater

Peritoneal and Visceral Relations

- **Hepatic ducts**
  - The right and left hepatic ducts from corresponding lobes of liver emerge at the porta hepatis
  - At porta hepatis, the arrangement from behind forwards is—right and left branches of portal vein, hepatic artery and hepatic ducts.

- **Common hepatic duct**
  - Near the right end of porta hepatis the right and left hepatic ducts unite to form common hepatic duct
  - It runs downwards for about 3 cm
  - The cystic duct joins at an acute angle with it, to form the bile duct.

- **Gallbladder**
  - It is a flask shaped hollow organ
  - Situated in the fossa on the inferior surface of right lobe of liver separated by loose areolar tissue
  - It is connected to the common bile duct by the cystic duct
  - Length: 7 – 10 cm long
  - Capacity: 50 mL

  Parts of gallbladder
  - Fundus
  - Body
  - Neck.

  - **Relations – visceral and peritoneal (Fig. 2A)**
    - **Fundus**
      * Entirely surrounded by peritoneum
      * Projects beyond the inferior border of the liver
      * It is along the transpyloric plane in the angle between the right lateral border of the rectus abdominis and the 9th costal cartilage
      * **Relations:** In front—anterior abdominal wall
      * Posteriorly—the transverse colon.

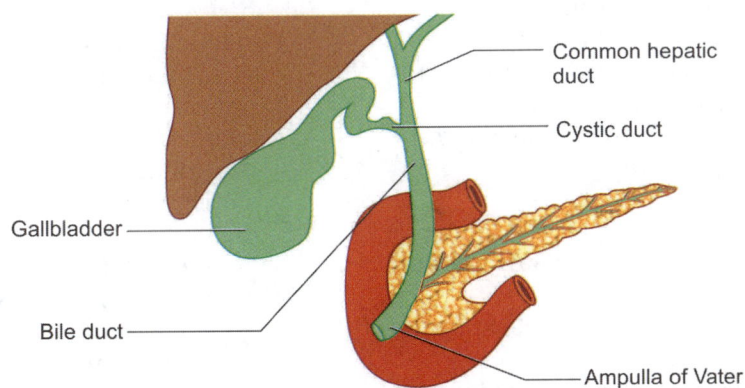

Fig. 1: Extrahepatic biliary apparatus.

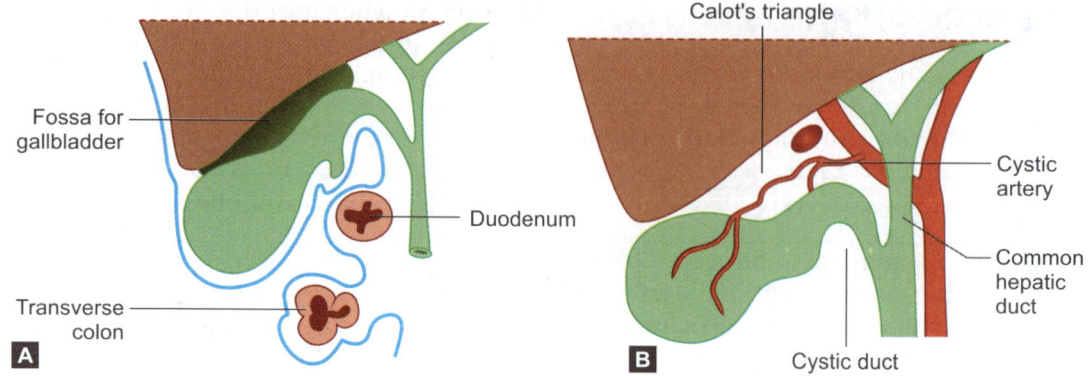

Figs. 2A and B: (A) Relations of gallbladder; (B) Cystic duct.

- **Body**
  * Superior surface devoid of peritoneum and attached to liver by areolar tissue
  * The inferior surface is covered with peritoneum
  * Situated in the fossa for gallbladder on the liver
  * Above it is continuous with the neck
  * **Relations:** Inferior surface—the transverse colon and the 1st and 2nd parts of duodenum.
- **Neck**
  * Above not covered with peritoneum
  * It is S shaped
  * Extends from the body and is continued as cystic duct
  * Sometimes a diverticulum arises from the neck called Hartmann's pouch
  * **Relations:** Above—non peritoneal, to liver
  * Below—1st part of duodenum.
- **Cystic duct (Fig. 2B)**
  - 3 – 4 cm long
  - Begins at the neck of the gallbladder
  - Descends downwards, backwards and to the left
  - Unites with the common hepatic duct to form the bile duct
  - Its mucous membrane is provided with a **spiral valve of Heister (Fig. 3)**.

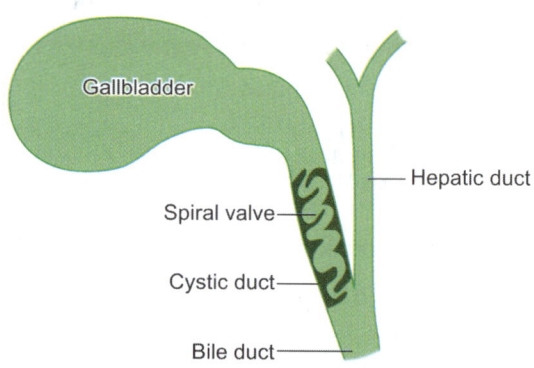

Fig. 3: Valve of cystic duct.

- Boundaries of Calot's triangle:
  - Below and laterally—cystic duct
  - Above and laterally—liver
  - Medially—common hepatic duct
  - Contents—cystic artery and cystic lymph node of Lund.
- **Bile duct**
  - Formation: By the union of the cystic duct and the common hepatic duct
  - Length: 8 cm long
  - Course:
    - Runs downwards and backwards along the free border of lesser omentum
    - Behind 1st part of duodenum and head of pancreas
    - It comes into contact with the pancreatic duct
    - Then runs through the wall of the second part of the duodenum obliquely

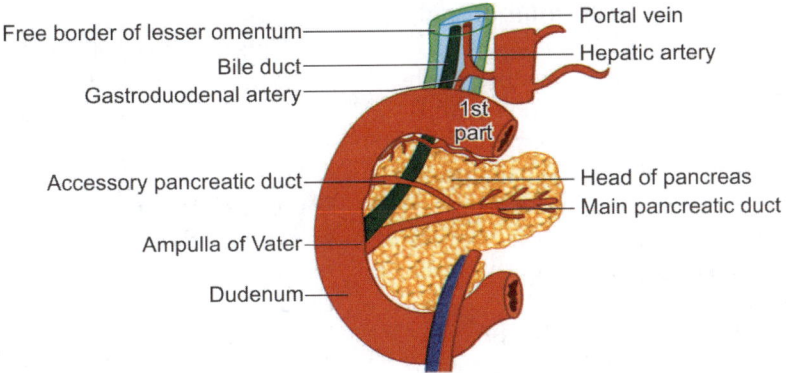

Fig. 4: Bile duct.

- Here it forms the hepatopancreatic duct or ampulla of Vater
- Opens on the summit of the major duodenal papilla about 8 – 10 cm distal to the pylorus.
- **Relations (Fig. 4)**
  - Supraduodenal part (along free border of lesser omentum):
    * Posterior—portal vein and epiploic foramen
    * Left—hepatic artery.
  - Retroduodenal part:
    * Anterior—1st part of duodenum
    * Posterior—inferior vena cava
    * Left—gastroduodenal artery.
  - Infraduodenal part:
    * Anterior—Head of pancreas
    * Posterior—inferior vena cava.
- **Sphincters (Fig. 5)**
  - Sphincter choledochus—surrounds the terminal part of bile duct

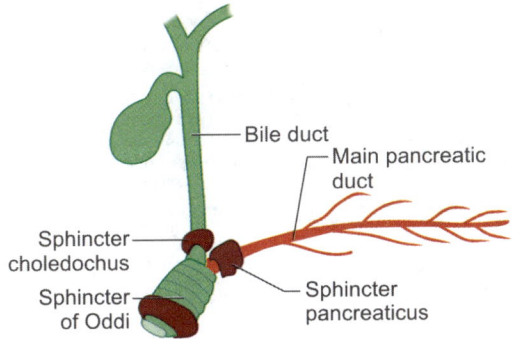

Fig. 5: Sphincters.

  - Sphincter pancreaticus—at the end of the pancreatic duct
  - Sphincter of Oddi—around the hepatopancreatic ampulla.

Blood Supply

- **Arterial supply**
  - Cystic artery: Main artery to the gallbladder, the cystic duct, the hepatic ducts and the upper part of the bile duct
  - Posterosuperior pancreaticoduodenal artery—supplies the lower part of the bile duct
  - Right hepatic branch—supplies the middle part of the bile duct.
- **Venous drainage**
  - Cystic vein drains the gallbladder and in turn drains into the right branch of portal vein
  - Veins of bile duct drain into portal vein.

Applied Anatomy

- **Cholecystitis:** Inflammation of gallbladder
- **Gallstones:** May be formed in the gallbladder, this condition called as cholelithiasis may produce spasmodic pain called biliary colic. The gallstones are more commonly found in (Four Fs) Forty years, Female, Fertile, and Fatty
- **Cholecystectomy:** Removal of gallbladder
- **Referred pain:** Pain of stretch of common bile duct or gallbladder is referred to the epigastrium or even to the right shoulder and inferior angle of right scapula

- **Phrygian cap:** Folded fundus of gallbladder
- **Courvoisier's law:** The patients with jaundice due to gallstones have non-distensible gallbladder but patient with jaundice due to malignant obstruction have a distensible gallbladder. This proves that the dilatation of gallbladder occurs due to compression by extrinsic structures than the intrinsic
- **Endoscopic retrograde cholangio-pancreatography (ERCP):** Catheter is inserted to hepatopancreatic duct and radio-opaque contrast medium is injected to visualize the bile and pancreatic ducts.

3. **Write about brachial plexus under the following headings: Formation, relations, branches and its clinical significance.**

Formation (Fig. 6)

Anterior primary rami of spinal nerves C5, C6, C7, C8 and T1, with contribution from the anterior primary rami of C4 and T2.

Mode of Formation

Five stages are in the formation of brachial plexus namely—root, trunk, division, cord and branches.
- **Roots:** The anterior primary rami of C5, C6, C7, C8 and T1.
- **Trunks:**
  - Roots C5 and C6 join to form the upper trunk
  - Root C7 forms the middle trunk
  - Roots C8 and T1 join to form the lower trunk.
- **Divisions:** Each trunk divides into ventral and dorsal divisions. These divisions join to form cords as follows.
- **Cords:**
  - **Lateral cord**—formed by the union of ventral divisions of the upper and middle trunks
  - **Medial cord**—formed by the ventral division of the lower trunk
  - **Posterior cord**—formed by the union of the dorsal divisions of all the three trunks.
- **Branches:** Cords divide into **branches**.

Types of Formation

- **Pre fixed:** When the anterior primary rami of C4 joins; C5 is large, T1 is reduced and T2 is absent
- **Post fixed:** The anterior primary rami of T2 joins; T1 is large, C4 is absent and C5 is reduced.

Relations

- **Roots** lie between scalenus medius and anterior muscles in the posterior triangle of neck

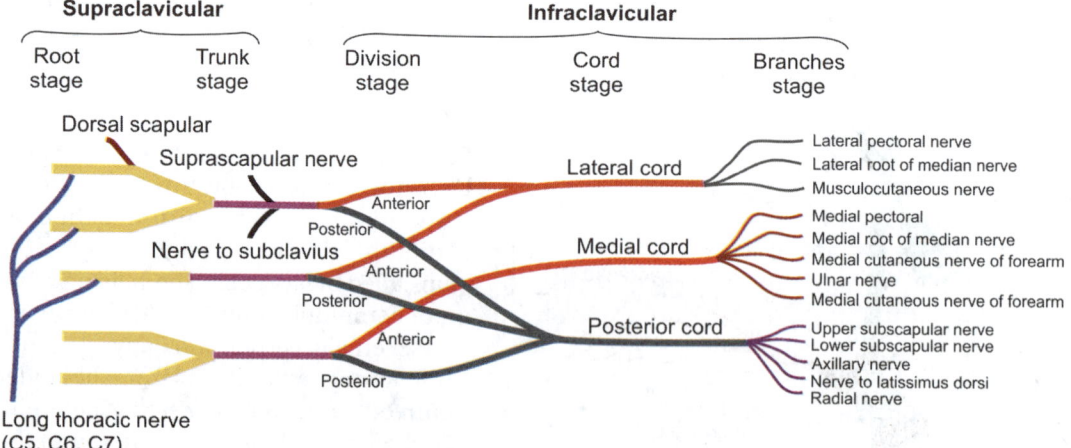

Fig. 6: Formation of brachial plexus.

- **Trunks** lie in the posterior triangle of neck
- **Divisions** situated behind the clavicle
- **Cords** formed in the axilla and are related to the 1st and 2nd parts of axillary artery
- **First part of axillary artery (Fig. 7A)**
  - Lateral and posterior cords are lateral
  - Medial cord posterior.
- **Second part of axillary artery (Fig. 7B):** Cords are related to the corresponding side, medial cord medially, lateral cord laterally, posterior cord posteriorly
- **Branches** are related to the 3rd part of axillary artery correspondingly **(Fig. 8)**.

Branches

They are grouped as supraclavicular and infraclavicular branches.

Supraclavicular Branches

These arise from the roots and trunks.

- **Branches of the roots:**
  - Nerve to serratus anterior (long thoracic nerve) (C5, C6, C7)
  - Nerve to rhomboids (dorsal scapular nerve) (C5)
  - Branch to join phrenic nerve (C5)
  - Nerve to prevertebral muscles.
- **Branches of the trunks:** Arises from the upper trunk in relation to Erb's point where six nerves meet (VR of C5, C6, anterior and posterior divisions of upper trunk and the branches from upper trunk)
  - Suprascapular nerve (C5, C6)
  - Nerve to subclavius (C5, C6).

Infraclavicular Branches

These arise from the cords.

Branches of the cords:

- **Branches of lateral cords**
  - Lateral pectoral nerve (C5, C6, C7): It pierces the clavipectoral fascia and supplies pectoralis major and minor muscles
  - Musculocutaneous nerve (C5, C6, C7): It pierces the coracobrachialis

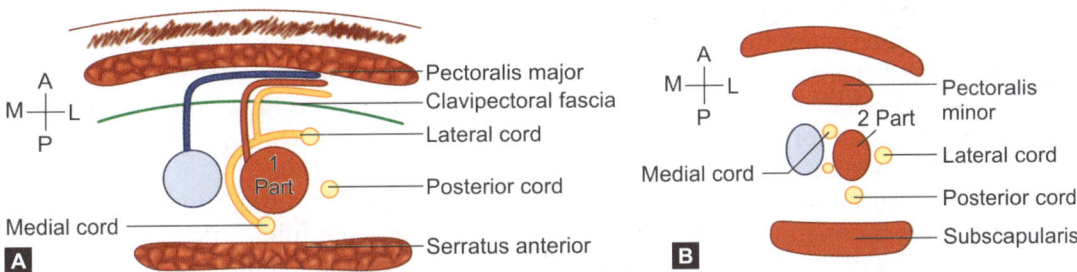

Figs. 7A and B: Relations of cord stage: (A) First part of axillary artery; (B) Second part of axillary artery.

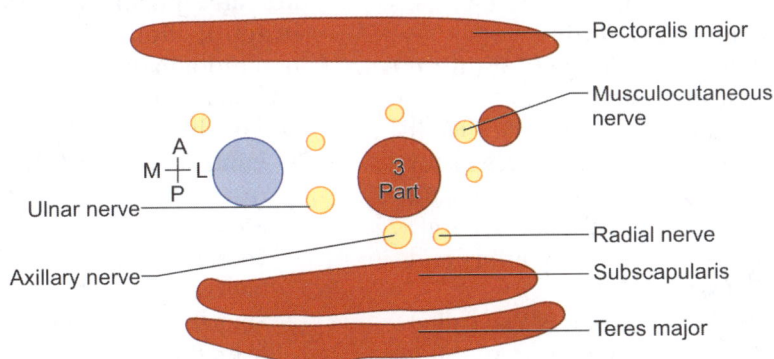

Fig. 8: Relations of branches. Third part of axillary artery.

and supplies biceps brachii, coracobrachialis, brachialis. It is continued as lateral cutaneous nerve of forearm
- Lateral root of median nerve (C5, C6, C7): It joins with the medial root, after crossing the axillary artery.
- **Branches of medial cord:**
  - Medial pectoral nerve (C8, T1): The nerve passes between axillary artery and vein. It pierces the pectoralis minor and supplies pectoralis minor and major
  - Medial cutaneous nerve of forearm (C8, T1): Passes in between the axillary artery and the vein. Then passes medial to the brachial artery. In the middle of the arm pierces the deep fascia along with basilica vein. It supplies the skin along the anteromedial side of forearm upto wrist
  - Medial cutaneous nerve of arm (C8, T1): It is related to the medial side of axillary vein. It receives a communication from the intercosto brachial nerve. It supplies the skin of the medial side of distal third of arm
  - Ulnar nerve (C7, C8, T1): It receives an additional contribution from C7 through median nerve, and supply flexor carpi ulnaris in the forearm. It descends between axillary artery and vein. It mainly supplies the intrinsic muscles of hand
  - Medial root of median nerve (C8, T1): Joins with medial root.
- **Branches of posterior cord:**
  - Upper subscapular nerve (C5, C6): It supplies subscapularis
  - Lower subscapular nerve (C5, C6): It supplies subscapularis and teres major
  - Nerve to latissimus dorsi (C6, C7, C8): It is also known as thoracodorsal nerve. It accompanies subscapular artery and supplies latissimus dorsi
  - Axillary nerve (C5, C6): It is also called as circumflex nerve. Winds around the surgical neck of humerus along with posterior circumflex humeral artery. It supplies deltoid and teres minor muscles. It is continued as upper lateral cutaneous nerve of arm
  - Radial nerve (C5-C8, T1): It passes behind the arm and enters the spiral groove by passing through the lower triangular space. It is nerve of extensor compartments of arm and forearm.

Applied Anatomy

Lesion of Root Stage

Injury to the nerve to serratus anterior:
- **Causes:** Sudden pressure on the shoulder from above, carrying heavy loads on the shoulder
- **Deformity**
  - Loss of pushing and punching actions. When patient tries to push, **winging of the scapula** occurs
  - Arm cannot be raised beyond 90°, i.e. overhead abduction is not possible.

Lesion of Trunk Stage

Upper trunk injury
- **Erb's Paralysis:**
  - **Site of injury**: Erb's point in the upper trunk of brachial plexus (six nerves meet here) **(Fig. 9)**
  - **Causes of injury**: Birth injury, fall on the shoulder, during anesthesia, excessive stretching
  - **Nerve roots involved**: Mainly C5 and partly C6
  - **Muscles paralyzed**: Mainly biceps brachii, deltoid, brachialis and brachioradialis. Partly supraspinatus, infraspinatus and supinator.
  - **Deformity**:
    - Limb hangs by the side
    - Arm adducted
    - Medially rotated
    - Forearm pronated, and palm facing backwards
    - Sensations is lost over a small area over the lateral part of the upper arm.

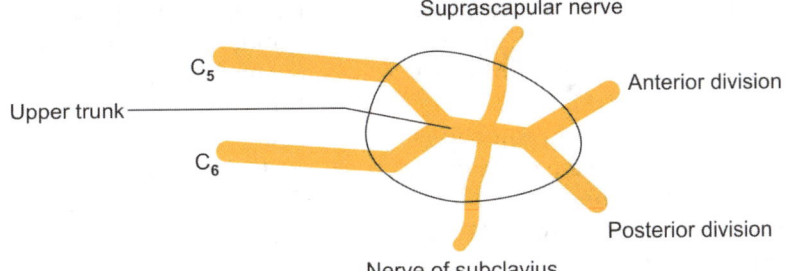

Fig. 9: Erb's point.

- **Reasoning:**
  - Adducted due to supraspinatus and deltoid
  - Medially rotated due to teres minor and infraspinatus
  - Extended forearm due to biceps, brachialis and brachioradialis
  - Pronated forearm due to biceps and supinator
  - The deformity is known as **Policeman's tip position or Porter's tip position.**

Lower trunk injury
- **Klumpke's paralysis:**
  - **Site of injury:** Lower trunk of the brachial plexus
  - **Cause of injury:** Upward traction of arm as in birth injury—breech delivery
  - **Nerve roots involved:** Mainly T1
  - **Muscles paralysed:** Intrinsic muscles of the hand
  - **Deformity: Claw hand** due to injury to intrinsic muscles of hand.

Lesion of Cord Stage
- **Hyper abduction syndrome:**
  - **Cause of injury:** Prolonged hyper abduction
  - **Deformity:** Pain radiating down the arm, tingling, and erythema of skin (due to capillary vasodilatation) and weakness of hand. Associated with compression of axillary vessels.

Brachial Plexus Block
Anesthetic blockade of brachial plexus through supraclavicular route. The site of injection is 2 cm above the midclavicular point, or axillary approach around the axillary artery.

4. Describe the anal canal parts positions, interior relations, blood supply, lymphatic drainage and applied aspects.

Position
- Extends from anorectal junction to the anus
- The anus is the external opening of the anal canal
- It is about 4 cm below and in front of the tip of the coccyx
- **Direction:** Directed downwards and backwards
- **Parts:** Three parts
  1. Upper mucous part—15 mm long
  2. Middle part or transitional zone—15 mm long
  3. Lower cutaneous part—8 mm long.

Interior (Fig. 10)
Upper mucous part: Covered by mucous membrane lined by columnar cells. The cells are secretory and absorptive in function.
- This part is endodermal in origin, developed from primitive rectum of hind gut
- The subepithelial area is rich with submucosal arterial and venous plexus
- 6 – 10 mucous vertical folds—called **anal columns** of Morgagni
- Terminal part of superior rectal artery lies deep to each column
- **Anal valves** connect the lower ends of anal columns

- Depression above each valve is called **anal sinus**
- The ducts of **anal glands** open into the floor of the sinuses **(Fig. 11)**
- In the anal valves epithelial projections called **anal papillae** which are remnant of embryonic anal membrane.
- Anal valves together form a transverse line called the **pectinate line**
  - **Pectinate line**
  - Is also known as **Dentate line**
  - Situated at the middle of internal anal sphincter
  - It forms the mucocutaneous junction of the anal canal
  - Developmentally it is the junction of the ectodermal (anal pit) and endodermal (cloaca) parts
  - It corresponds to the position of the anal valves
  - It divides the anal canal into upper and lower parts which are different in nerve supply, blood supply, development, lymphatic drainage and lining epithelium.

Middle part or pecten: Covered by mucous membrane.

- Mucosa—bluish due to underlying venous plexus

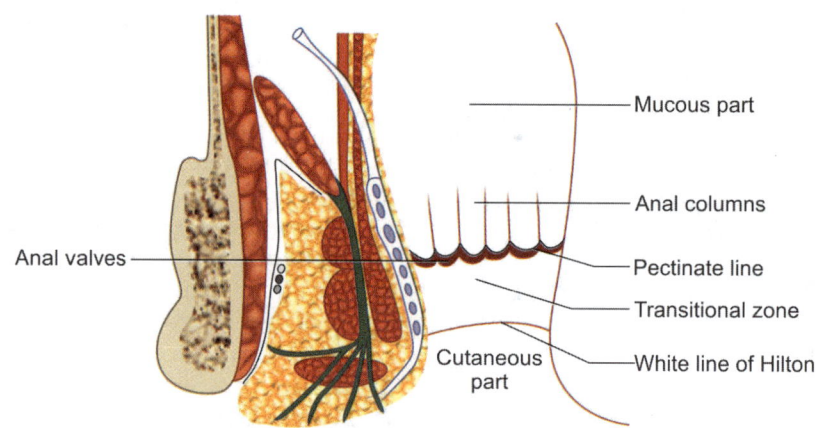

Fig. 10: Interior of anal canal.

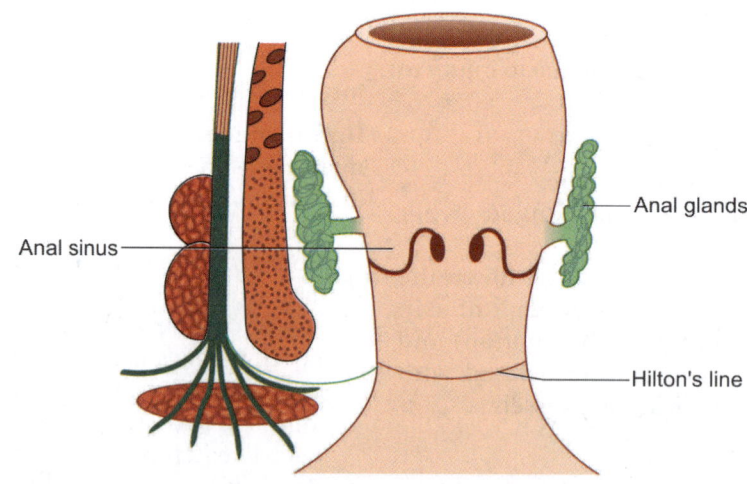

Fig. 11: Anal glands.

- Lined with non-keratinized stratified squamous epithelium. The sweat, sebaceous glands and hair follicles are absent
- This part is transitional zone
- Numerous nerve endings are present
- The lower limit of the pecten is white in color—called **white line of Hilton**
- The white line is the inter sphincteric groove—the interval between the subcutaneous part of external anal sphincter and the lower part of internal anal sphincter.

Lower cutaneous part: Lined by skin
- Keratinized stratified squamous epithelium and the sweat and sebaceous glands are present in this region
- It is continuous with perianal skin
- More arterial and venous plexus are present in the submucosa
- Number of radiating skin folds converge which are produced by the fibroelastic septa of the conjoint tendon.

Sphincters of the anal canal (Fig. 12): Sphincters are external and internal sphincters.

External sphincter:
- It is made up of skeletal muscle and voluntary in function
- Surrounds the entire anal canal
- It is divided into 3 parts—subcutaneous, superficial and deep parts

- **Subcutaneous part** is around anus separated from skin by venous plexus
- **Superficial part** arises from tip of coccyx and anococcygeal raphe and is inserted to perineal body
- **Deep part** surrounds anorectal junction. No bony attachment. Inserted to perineal body.

Internal sphincter:
- It is made up of smooth muscle and involuntary in function
- It is formed by thickening of circular muscle fibers
- It surrounds the upper three-fourth of anal canal— up to white line of Hilton
- It is separated from mucous membrane by internal venous plexus
- It is separated from external sphincter by conjoint sheath.

Blood Supply

- **Arterial supply (Fig. 13A)**
  - The part above the pectinate line is supplied by the superior rectal artery which is continuation of inferior mesenteric artery
  - Below the line—supplied by inferior rectal artery branch of pudendal artery.
- **Venous drainage (Fig. 13B)**
  - Internal rectal venous plexus— communicates with external venous plexus and drains into the superior rectal vein

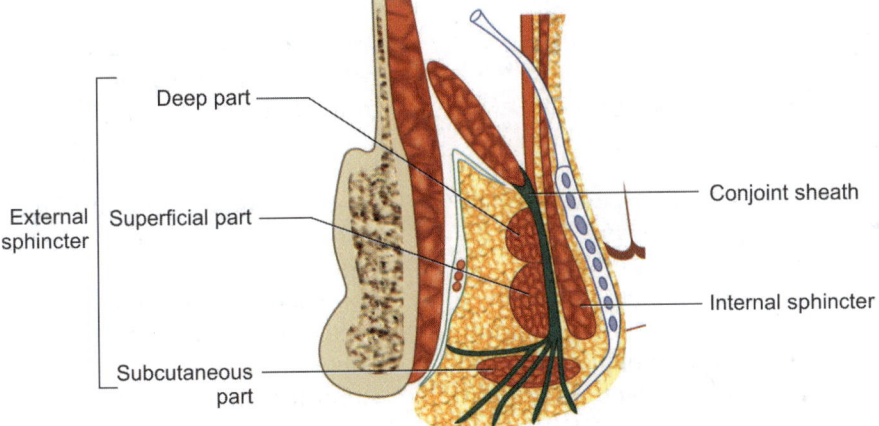

Fig. 12: Sphincters—external and internal.

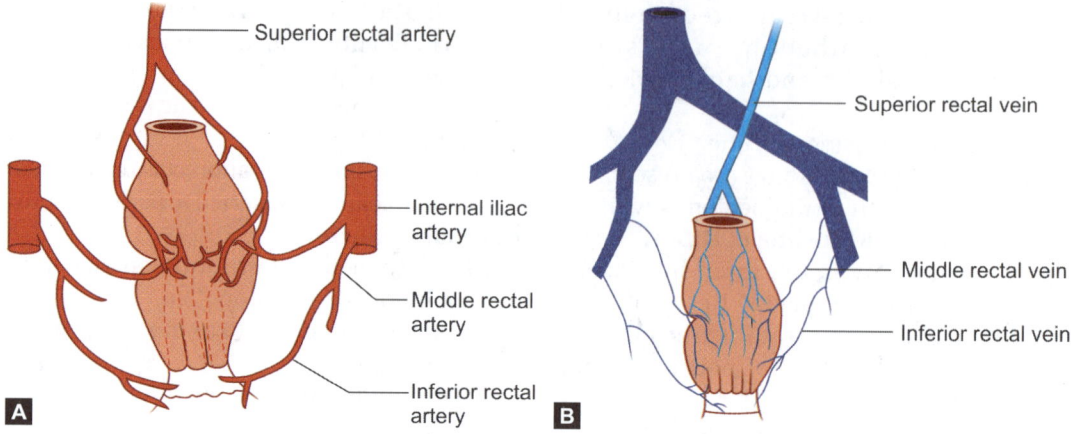

Figs. 13A and B: Blood supply: (A) Arterial supply; (B) Venous drainage.

- Veins present in 3 anal columns at 3, 7 and 11'o clock positions are large sites for primary internal piles
- **The external rectal venous plexus** lies outside the muscular coat, communicates with internal venous plexus—is drained by inferior rectal vein
- **Anal veins** placed radially around the anal margin communicate with internal rectal venous plexus and inferior rectal veins.

Lymphatic Drainage (Fig. 14)

- Above pectinate line—into internal iliac nodes
- Below pectinate line—into superficial inguinal nodes.

Applied Anatomy

- **Digital examination per rectum**—many structures can be palpated:
  - Anteriorly:
    - In male prostate, seminal vesicles, terminal part of ureters, bulb of penis, and spongy urethra
    - In female—the uterus and vagina
  - Posteriorly—coccyx and sacrum, enlarged sacral lymph nodes
  - Laterally—ischiorectal fossae and ischial spines, appendix (tenderness

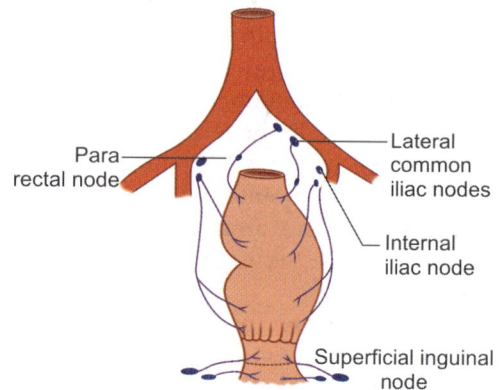

Fig. 14: Lymphatic drainage.

  felt in appendicitis), enlarged pelvic nodes, and in female the ovary and uterine tube.
- **Anal fistula**—fibrous tract communication between skin and anorectal mucosa and formed due to abscess. The abscess may spread circumferentially producing horse shoe abscess
- **Hemorrhoids**—internal hemorrhoid is distended varicose veins above pectinate line
- External hemorrhoids are below the pectinate line. Straining during defecation may rupture the anal veins resulting in subcutaneous perianal hematoma or external piles.

5. **Write about coronary circulation. Mention the origin, course, distribution, branches, termination, anastomosis and clinical importance.**

- The myocardium is supplied by the two coronary arteries—the right and the left
- They anastomose with each other
- But they function as end arteries
- **Origin**: Arise from the aortic sinuses of the ascending aorta.

Right Coronary Artery

- **Origin:** From anterior aortic sinus of the ascending aorta.
- **Course:**
  - Runs forwards and to the right between the pulmonary trunk and the right auricle
  - Then runs downwards in the right along the anterior coronary sulcus to the right border of the heart
  - It winds around the border to reach the posterior coronary sulcus
  - The artery reaches the crux
  - To the left of the crux it terminates by anastomosing with the circumflex branch of left coronary artery
  - From origin to the inferior border is called as 1st/anterior segment
  - From inferior border to the termination is 2nd/posterior segment.

- **Branches:**
  - **From anterior segment**
    - Right conus artery—it anastomoses with the conus branch of anterior inter ventricular artery around the infundibulum to form **annulus of Vieussens.** Sometimes it arises directly from aortic sinus and it is named as **third coronary artery**
    - Right atrial branches—to supply right atrium. One of the branch called **SA nodal branch** to supply the SA node situated along the base of superior vena cava
    - Right ventricular branches—to supply right ventricle. One of the branch is large runs parallel to the inferior border called **marginal branch**.
  - **From posterior segment**
    - Right atrial branches
    - Right ventricular branches
    - Posterior inter ventricular artery—to supply right and left ventricles. This branch determines the dominance of coronary artery. It also gives septal branches to supply posterior one-third of interventricular septum
    - AV nodal artery—to supply the AV node.

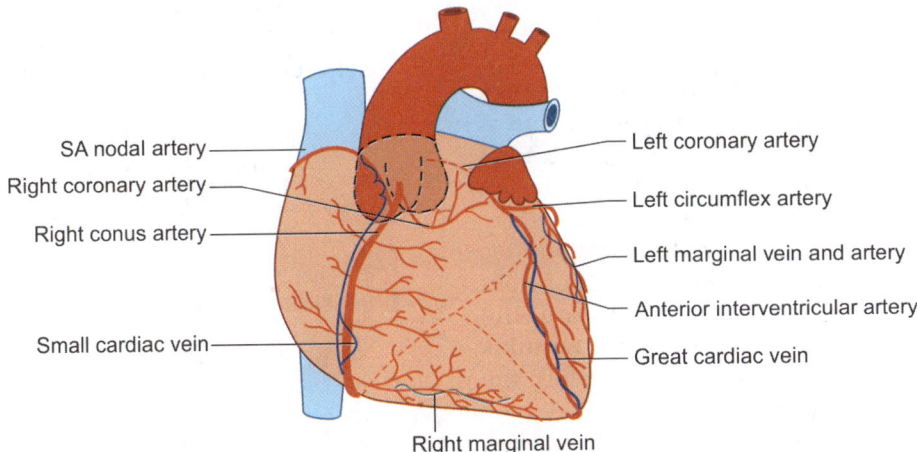

Fig. 15: Coronary arteries.

- Area of distribution
  - Right atrium
  - Greater part of right ventricle except the part along the anterior inter ventricular groove
  - Smaller part of left ventricle along the posterior inter ventricular groove
  - Posterior one-third of interventricular septum
  - Whole of conducting system of heart except a part of the left branch of AV bundle.

Left Coronary Artery

- **Origin**: Arises from the left posterior aortic sinus of ascending aorta.
- **Course:**
  - Runs forwards and to the left
  - Emerges between the pulmonary trunk and the left auricle
  - Terminates by dividing into anterior interventricular and circumflex arteries
  - The portion from origin to termination is called the **stem** of the artery
  - No branch arises from the stem.
- **Branches:**
  - **Anterior interventricular artery**
    - Descends in the anterior interventricular sulcus accompanied by great cardiac vein
    - It terminates by anastomosing with posterior interventricular branch of right coronary in the lower one-third of posterior interventricular groove
    - Branches:
      * Ventricular branches to supply right and left ventricles; One of these branches is large called diagonal **artery** to supply the left ventricle
      * Left conus branch anastomoses with the conus branch of right coronary artery around the infundibulum to form **annulus of Vieussens.** It supplies the infundibulum
      * Septal branches supply anterior two-third of interventricular septum.
  - **Circumflex artery**
    - Winds around the left margin of the heart and runs along the posterior interventricular sulcus
    - It anastomoses with right coronary artery to the left of crux
    - Branches:
      * Diaphragmatic surface of left ventricle
      * Left atrial branches
      * Left marginal branch.
    - Occasional branches are (i) SA nodal artery in about 40% (ii) Posterior interventricular branch (10 to 20%), (iii) Kugel's artery/arteria anastomotica auricularis magna (left atrial branch).

Area of Distribution of Left Coronary

- Left atrium
- Greater part of left ventricle except the region along the posterior inter ventricular groove
- Smaller part of right ventricle along the anterior interventricular groove
- Anterior 2/3 of interventricular septum
- A part of left branch of AV bundle.

Venous Drainage (Fig. 17)

- Coronary sinus
- Anterior cardiac veins
- Venae cordis minimi
- **Coronary sinus**:
  - Large vein draining the heart
  - Lies in the posterior coronary sulcus between left atrium and ventricle

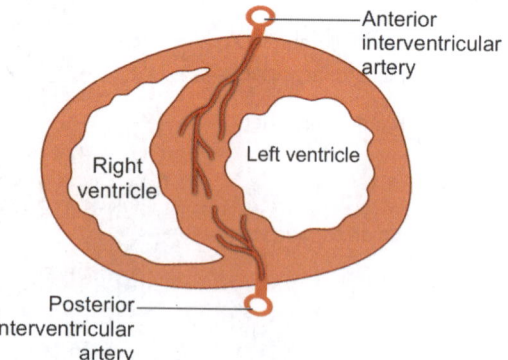

Fig. 16: Blood supply to interventricular septum.

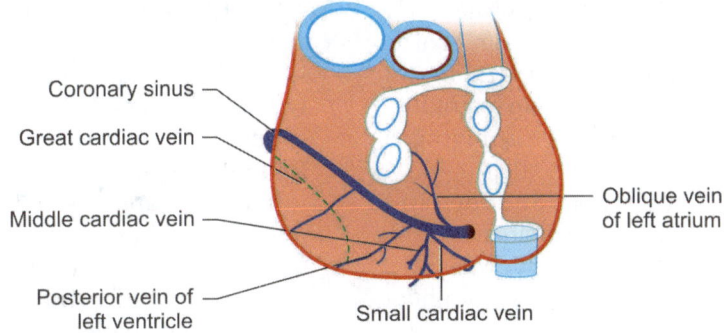

Fig. 17: Venous drainage of heart.

- 3 cm long
- Runs downwards and to the right
- Terminates into the sinus venarum part of right atrium between IVC and right atrioventricular orifice
- The opening is guarded by the Thebesian valve.
- Tributaries:
  - **Great cardiac vein**: Starts at the apex of heart and lies in anterior inter ventricular sulcus accompanied by anterior interventricular artery and ends in the coronary sinus at the level of origin
  - **Middle cardiac vein**: Starts at apex and lies in posterior interventricular sulcus accompanied by posterior interventricular artery; ends in coronary sinus
  - **Small cardiac vein**: Accompanies the right coronary artery in the right posterior coronary sulcus and ends in coronary sinus. It also receives the right marginal vein
  - **Posterior vein of left ventricle**: Lies on diaphragmatic surface, ends in the middle of coronary sinus to the left of middle cardiac vein
  - **Oblique vein of Marshall**: Small vein on the posterior surface of left atrium; ends in coronary sinus.
- **Anterior cardiac veins:** 3 or 4, lie on the anterior wall of right ventricle and open into right atrium

- **Venae cordis Minimi (Thebesian veins)**
  - Very small veins, numerous, open directly into all chambers of the heart
  - More numerous on the right side of the heart, hence infarcts are common on the left side.

Coronary Dominance in Man

- Most people have right coronary dominance (60%), where the posterior interventricular artery arises from the right coronary artery
- Few people have left coronary dominance (40%), where the posterior interventricular artery arises from the circumflex branch of left coronary artery.

Anastomosis (Myocardial Circulation)

- **Interarterial anastomosis:** Anastomosis exists between the branches of the coronary arteries. So the coronary arteries are not typical end arteries, but function like end arteries
- **Arteriovenous anastomosis:** Anastomosis between coronary arteries and cavities establishing myocardial sinusoids. These help to supply the myocardium, by backflow from the coronary sinus
- **Arterioluminal:** Some branches of the coronary artery directly open into the lumen of the heart.

Applied Anatomy

- **Angina pectoris:** Incomplete and spasmodic obstruction of the coronary

arteries leads to intense precordial pain which is referred along the left upper arm
- **Myocardial ischemia:** Lack of blood supply to the myocardium due to gradual obstruction of an artery supplying a particular region
- **Myocardial infarction:** Sudden and complete obstruction of the branches of the coronary artery leading to sudden death
- **Coronary angiography:** Radiological procedure using contrast for localization of block in the artery
- **Coronary artery by-pass graft:** The great saphenous vein, internal thoracic artery and radial artery are used as graft to connect the aorta and the part of the occluded artery distal to the block
- Left anterior descending artery is commonly prone for atherosclerotic changes causing fatal myocardial infarction
- PTCA (percutaneous transluminal coronary angioplasty) and CABG (coronary artery bypass graft) are the procedures used for restoration of normal blood flow in the blocked arteries.

6. **Describe extraocular muscles enumerate. Give an account of their attachments, nerve supply, actions and applied anatomy.**

- The extraocular muscles are situated within the orbit
- They are seven in number
- They help in the movement of eyeball in all directions and elevation of the upper eyelid
- They are levator palpabrae superioris, four recti and two oblique muscles (**LR6 SO4**).

Recti Muscles

- They are four in number—superior, inferior, medial, and lateral recti. They are strap muscles
- **Origin:**
  - Four recti arise from common tendinous ring
  - Superior rectus from upper part above and lateral to optic canal
  - Inferior rectus—lower part below optic canal
  - Medial rectus—from medial part
  - Lateral rectus—lateral part and from the spine of greater wing of the sphenoid.
- **Insertion (Fig. 18A):**
  - The recti are inserted into the sclera in front of equator, a little posterior to limbus. The insertion is in oblique manner called **spiral line of Tilloux**
  - The distance between the insertion of the tendons and limbus are
    - Medial rectus – 5.5 mm
    - Inferior rectus – 6.6 mm
    - Lateral rectus – 7 mm
    - Superior rectus – 7.5 mm.
- **Nerve supply (Fig. 18B):**
  - Superior rectus- oculomotor nerve
  - Inferior rectus - oculomotor nerve
  - Medial rectus - oculomotor nerve
  - Lateral rectus - abducent nerve.
- **Actions (Fig. 19)**
  - Medial rectus - adduction
  - Lateral rectus - abduction
  - Superior rectus - elevation, adduction, intorsion
  - Inferior rectus - depression, adduction, extorsion.

Oblique Muscles (Fig. 20)

Superior Oblique

- **Origin:** From the body of the sphenoid above and medial to optic canal
- **Course:** It runs along the medial wall of the orbit and ends in a tendon. The tendon is attached to the trochlear fossa of frontal bone by a fascial sling. From here the muscle is directed backwards and superiorly. From origin to tendon is called **straight part** and from tendon to insertion is known as **reflected part**
- **Insertion:** To the sclera behind the equator, between the superior and lateral recti, in the posterior quadrant superolaterally
- **Nerve supply:** It is supplied by the trochlear nerve
- **Action:** Abduction, depression and intorsion.

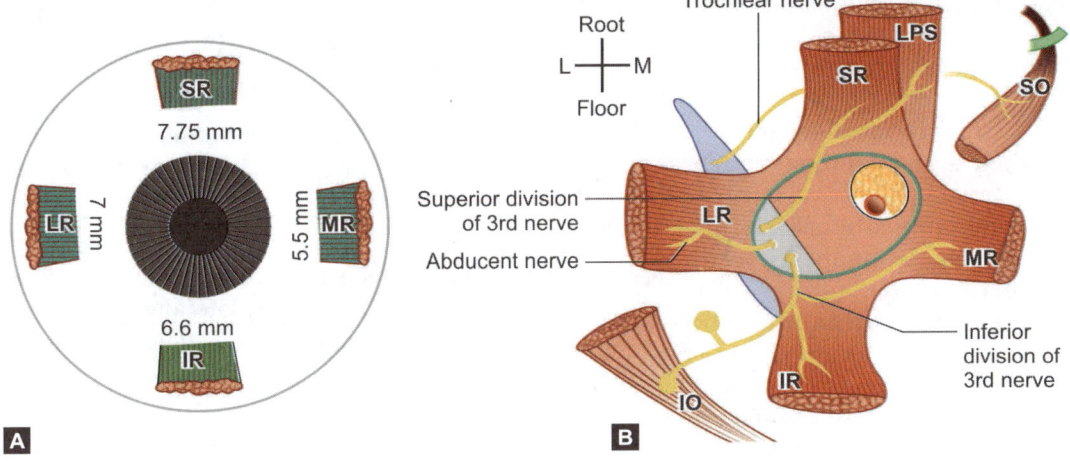

Figs. 18A and B: Recti muscles: (A) Insertion of recti; (B) Nerve supply.

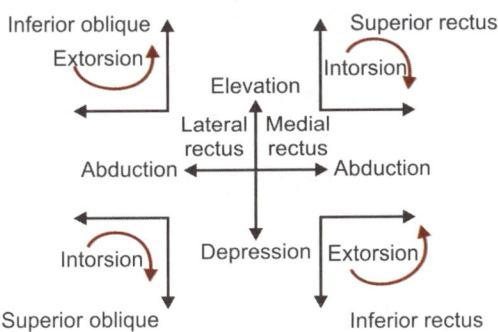

Fig. 19: Action of extraocular muscles.

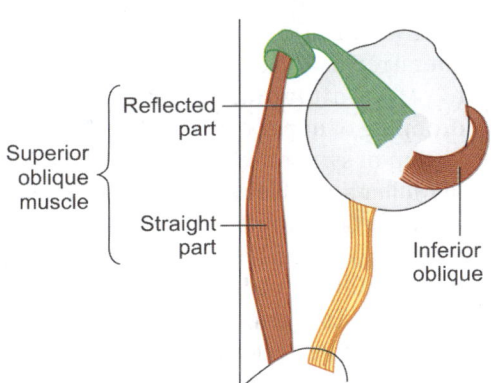

Fig. 20: Oblique muscles.

Inferior Oblique

- **Origin:** Arises from the floor of orbit – from the orbital surface of the maxilla
- **Course:** Directed upwards and backwards. It lies parallel to the reflected part of superior oblique muscle
- **Insertion:** It is inserted into the sclera behind the equator, between the inferior and lateral recti in the inferolateral part of posterior quadrant
- **Nerve supply:** It is supplied by the inferior division of oculomotor nerve
- **Action:** Abduction, elevation, extorsion.

Levator Palpabrae Superioris (Fig. 21)

- **Origin:** Arises from the orbital surface of the lesser wing of the sphenoid bone above and in front of optic canal

- **Insertion:** The muscle divides into superior and inferior laminae.
    - **Superior lamina**
        - Superior lamina expands into a wide aponeurosis
        - It divides the lacrimal gland into two.
        - It is inserted:
            * Medially to medial palpebral ligament
            * Laterally to Whitnall's tubercle
            * Middle part passes through orbicularis oculi fibers and is inserted to the skin of upper eyelid
            * Few fibers to the anterior surface of tarsal plate.

- **Inferior lamina** is replaced by smooth muscle fibers called **Muller's muscle** and is inserted to upper border of superior tarsal plate. It is also known as **superior tarsal muscle**.
- There is an **additional attachment** to the superior conjunctival fornix by a conjoint tendon formed by fusion of fibers of levator palpabrae with superior rectus.
- **Nerve supply:**
  - Levator palpabrae superioris is supplied by oculomotor nerve
  - Muller's muscle by sympathetic nerves.
- **Action:** Elevation of upper eyelid.

Applied Anatomy

- Injury to oculomotor nerve results in paralysis of all extraocular muscles except lateral rectus and superior oblique leading to **4Ds**—diplopia, divergent squint, drooping of upper eyelid, dilated pupil
- Lesion of sympathetic results in paralysis of Muller's muscle results in partial ptosis as in Horner's syndrome
- Paralysis of lateral rectus due to injury to 6th nerve results in medial/convergent squint
- Paralysis of superior oblique due to injury to 4th nerve results in diplopia when patient looks upward
- Retrobulbar anesthesia is given for cataract surgery to immobilize the extraocular muscles.

7. **Describe the parts, relations, constituent fibers, blood supply and applied anatomy of internal capsule.**

- Internal capsule is a bent white band
- It is collection of bundles of projection fibers with convexity laterally
- It contains afferent and efferent fibers.

Boundaries (Relations)

- Laterally—lentiform nucleus
- Medially—thalamus and head of caudate nucleus
- Above—continuous with corona radiate
- Below—continuous with crus cerebri.

Parts/divisions (Fig. 22A)

- Anterior limb—between head of caudate nucleus and lentiform nucleus
- Posterior limb—between thalamus and lentiform nucleus
- Genu—bent part between thalamus and caudate nucleus
- Retrolentiform
- Sublentiform.

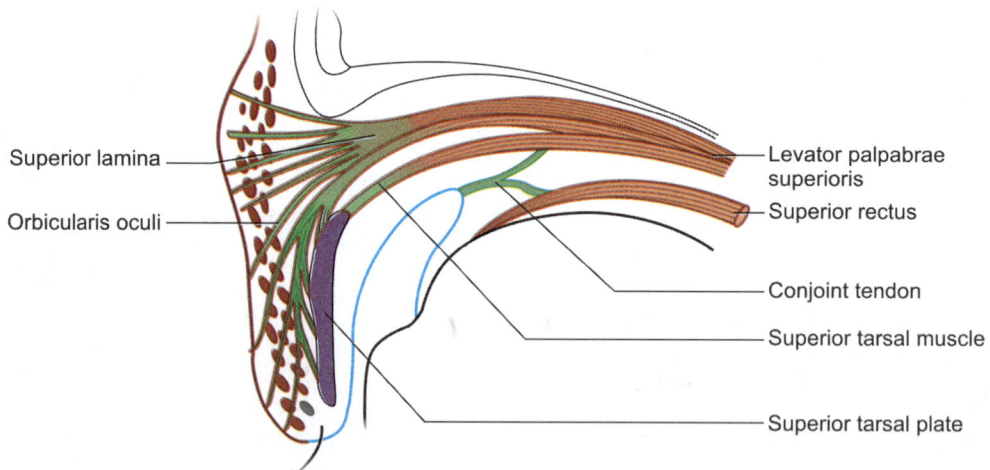

Fig. 21: Levator palpabrae superioris.

Constituent Fibers (Fig. 22B)

- **Anterior limb**
  - Frontopontine fibers—from frontal lobe to pontine nuclei and reach opposite cerebellar hemisphere
  - Anterior thalamic radiation—from medial and anterior thalamic nuclei to frontal lobe of cerebrum.
- **Genu**
  - Corticonuclear/corticobulbar fibers—from area 4, 6 (precentral gyrus) and to the contralateral motor nuclei of cranial nerves
  - Superior thalamic radiation, extension from posterior limb.
- **Posterior limb**
  - Corticospinal fibers—fibers from motor area to opposite side of body. The fibers for upper limb are anterior. The fibers for trunk and lower limb are posteriorly placed
  - Frontopontine fibers from area 4 and 6 to pontine nuclei
  - Corticorubral fibers from frontal lobe (area 4, 6) to red nucleus
  - Superior thalamic radiation from ventral nucleus of thalamus to post central gyrus.
- **Retrolentiform part**
  - Parieto and occipitopontine fibers—from parietal and occipital lobes to pontine nuclei
  - Optic radiation—from lateral geniculate body to visual area
  - Posterior thalamic radiation—from pulvinar of thalamus to occipital lobe.
- **Sublentiform part**
  - Temperopontine fibers—from temporal lobe to pontine nuclei
  - Auditory radiation—from medial geniculate body to superior temporal and transverse temporal gyrus (areas 41, 42)
  - Inferior thalamic radiation – from thalamus to temporal lobe and insula.

Blood Supply (Figs. 23A and B)

- Anterior limb—branches from anterior cerebral, recurrent artery of Heubner, middle cerebral artery
- Genu—direct branches from the internal carotid artery and from posterior communicating artery and middle cerebral artery
- Posterior limb—branches from anterior choroidal artery posterior communicating and middle cerebral artery

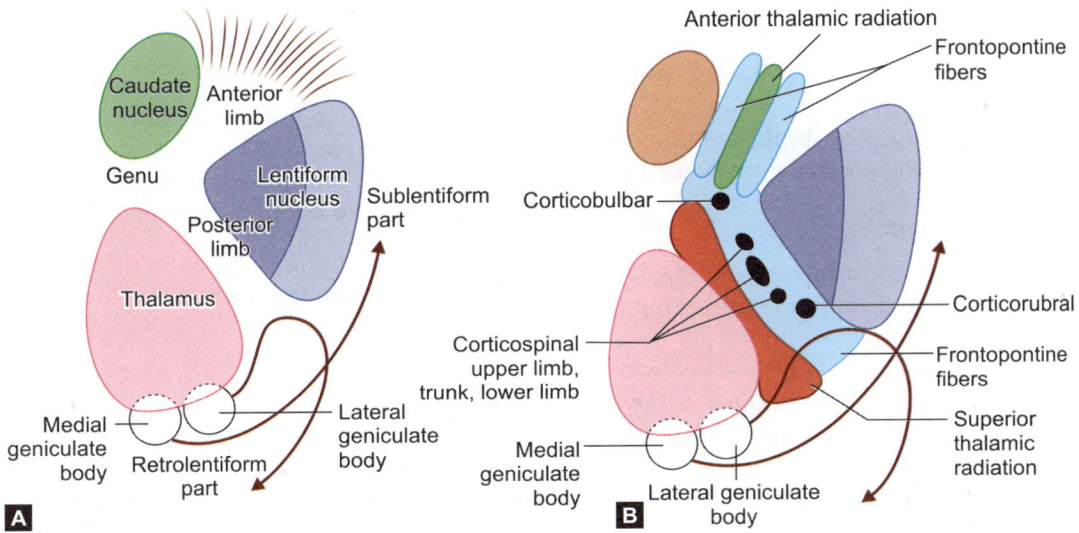

Figs. 22A and B: (A) Parts of internal capsule; (B) Constituent fibers.

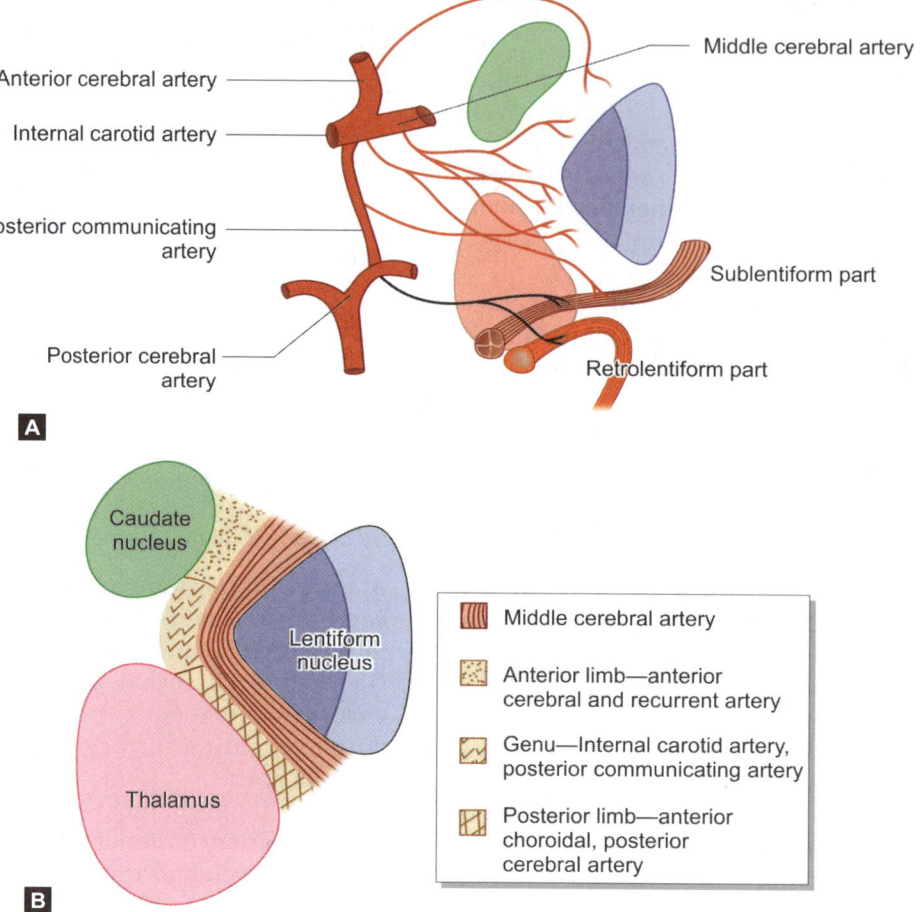

Figs. 23A and B: Blood supply.

- Retrolentiform part—by the posterior cerebral artery
- Sublentiform part—by the anterior choroidal artery and posterior cerebral artery.

Applied Anatomy

- Hemiplegia—paralysis of one half of body due to thrombosis or rupture of the one of the lateral/lenticulo striate artery (Charcot's artery of cerebral hemorrhage)
  - Lesions of genu produce paralysis of face and monoplegia of the upper limb of opposite side
  - Lesions of posterior limb produce paralysis of the opposite side and loss of sensation in the opposite side.

8. Describe the thoracic diaphragm under the following headings: Parts, attachments, major and minor openings, blood supply, nerve supply, actions, and applied anatomy.

It is a dome-shaped musculoaponeurotic partition which intervenes between the thorax and the abdomen.

Parts

- Thoracic surface is convex on the right and left sides and is depressed in the middle
- The convexities are known as the **cupola**
- The right cupola is slightly higher than the left due to the presence of liver

- The peripheral part of the diaphragm is muscular and the central part is tendinous which is occupied by the central tendon.

Attachments (Fig. 24)

- **Origin:** It has three parts namely sternal, costal and vertebral (lumbar) parts:
    - **Sternal origin:** As two fleshy slips from the posterior surface of xiphoid process
    - **Costal origin:** From the inner surfaces of the cartilages and the adjacent parts of the lower six ribs on each side
    - **Lumbar origin:** It has 3 parts—crura, from medial and lateral arcuate ligaments (lumbocostal arches)
        - **The right crus** from the sides of bodies and intervertebral discs of upper three lumbar vertebrae
        - **The left crus** arise from the sides of bodies and intervertebral discs of upper two lumbar vertebrae
        - **Median arcuate ligament** is a tendinous arch connecting the medial margins of the two crura
        - **Medial arcuate ligament:** It is formed by thickening of the psoas fascia extending between the side of body of L1 vertebra and transverse process of L1 vertebra
        - **Lateral arcuate ligament:** Thickening of anterior layer of thoracolumbar fascia covering the upper part of quadratus lumborum muscle extending between the transverse process of L1 vertebra and lower border of 12th rib.
- **Insertion:** Into the central tendon of diaphragm.
    - **The central tendon:**
        - The central tendon is aponeurotic
        - Receives the insertion of all parts of diaphragm.
        - It is more anterior
        - It has 3 parts:
            1. Central portion which is triangular in shape
            2. The right leaflet is broader and short. At the junction of right leaflet and central portion is the opening of inferior vena cava (IVC)
            3. The left leaflet is narrower and longer than the right. To the left of IVC orifice, four diagonal fibers decussate in the central tendon.

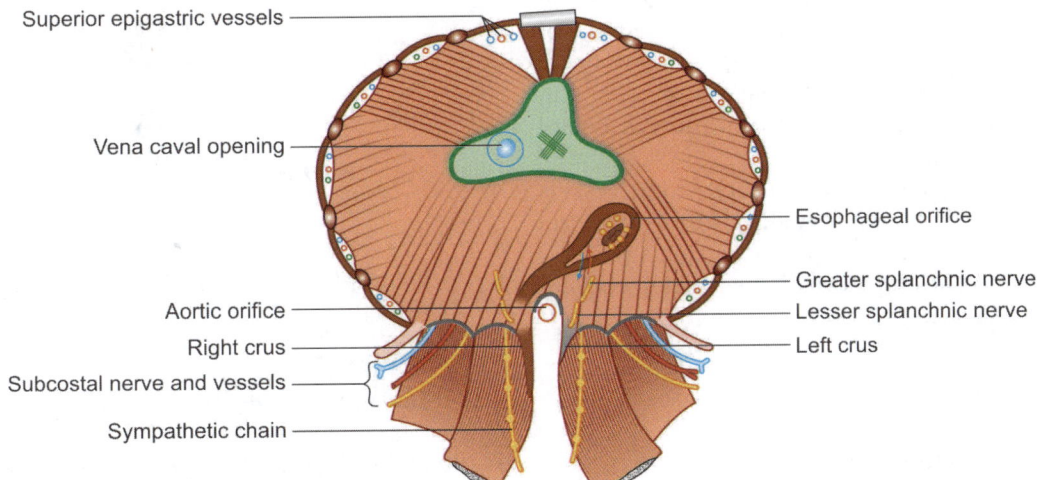

Fig. 24: Attachment of diaphragm.

Major and Minor Openings

Major Openings (Fig. 25)

Name of the orifice	Position and formation	Vertebra level	Shape of orifice	Nature of orifice	Structures passing	Function
Vena caval orifice	To the right of midline. In the central tendon at the junction of right leaflet and central part	T_8	Quadrilateral	Aponeurotic	IVC, right phrenic nerve, lymphatics from liver	Dilates the opening and increases venous return.
Esophageal orifice	To the left of midline. Formed by the right crus of diaphragm	T_{10}	Elliptical	Muscular	Esophagus, right and left vagal trunks, esophageal branch of left gastric artery, lymphatics from liver.	Constricts the orifice and prevents regurgitation.
Aortic orifice	In midline. Formed deep to median arcuate ligament	T_{12}	Round	Osseoaponeurotic	Abdominal aorta, thoracic duct, azygos sometimes	No change

Minor Openings

- Each crus of the diaphragm is pierced by the greater and lesser splanchnic nerves
- Subcostal nerve and vessels pass behind the lateral arcuate ligament
- Sympathetic trunk and least splanchnic nerve passes behind the medial arcuate ligament.
- The superior epigastric vessels and some lymphatics pass between the xiphoid process and costal origins of the diaphragm through a gap called **space of Larrey**
- Musculophrenic vessels pierce the diaphragm between 7th and 8th costal cartilages
- Lower five intercostal nerve and vessels pass between the slips from lower six costal cartilages
- Left phrenic nerve pierces the left cupola.

Blood Supply

- **Arteries**
  - Musculophrenic artery
  - Superior phrenic artery
  - Inferior phrenic artery
  - Subcostal artery
  - Lower intercostal arteries.

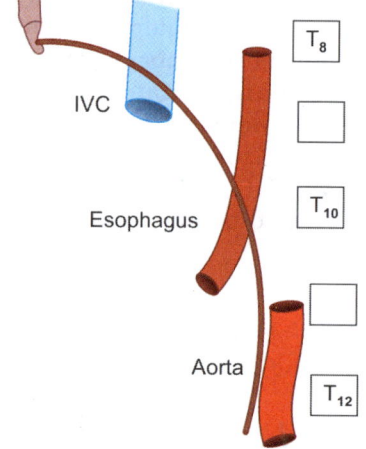

Fig. 25: Major openings.

- **Veins**: Corresponding veins drain the diaphragm.

Nerve Supply

- **Motor supply:** By the right and left phrenic nerves (root value C3, C4, C5).
- **Sensory supply:** By phrenic nerve from central part and lower six intercostal nerves from periphery.

Actions

- It is the principal muscle of inspiration
- It helps in all expulsive acts like sneezing, coughing, laughing, crying, vomiting, micturition, defecation and parturition.

Applied Anatomy

- **Foramen of Morgagni**: Gap due to failure of sternal origin of the diaphragm, through which the abdominal viscera may herniate into the thorax (**Morgagni's hernia**)
- **Bockdalek's triangle**: Triangular gap in the posterior part of the diaphragm due to failure of the diaphragm to take origin from the lateral arcuate ligament. Congenital herniation of the abdominal viscera through this gap is called **Bockdalek's hernia**
- **Hiatus hernia**: Herniation of the upper part of the stomach through the dilated esophageal opening.

II. SHORT NOTES

1. Corpus luteum.

- Graafian follicle contains ovum, surrounded by cumulus ovaricus and the membrane granulose cells surrounding the antrum folliculi
- The maturing graafian follicle moves towards the surface of ovary
- During ovulation there is rupture of the graffian follicle and the ovum is expelled out
- The granulose cells and the theca interna cells proliferate and fill up the intrafollicular cavity and are vascularized by the surrounding capillaries
- This solid cellular mass formed within the graffian follicle form the **corpus luteum**
- There are **two types of cells** seen in the corpus luteum
    1. **Granulose lutein cells**: The enlarged granulose cells forms the bulk of corpus luteum. The cytoplasm of the cell contains yellow carotinoid pigment
    2. **Para lutein cells**: The cells of tunica interna lie in the periphery and in between the lutein cells.

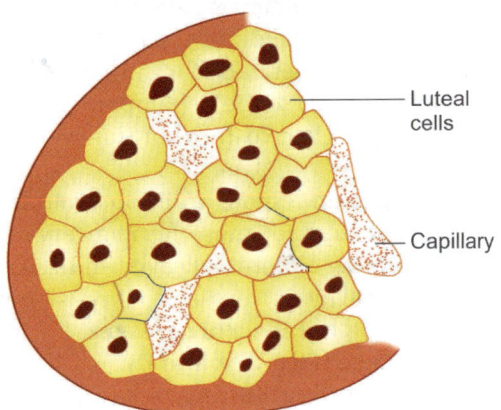

Fig. 26: Corpus luteum.

- **Functions:**
    - Progesterone is secreted by it which is important for the continuance of pregnancy
    - It stimulates the changes in uterus, mammary gland, thyroid
    - It suppresses the formation of FSH from anterior pituitary, so that the maturation of the follicle is suppressed.
- **Fate of corpus luteum**:
    - The fate depends on fertilization
    - If the fertilization takes place then it is called **corpus luteum of pregnancy**
    - It enlarges in size, and longevity is increased
    - The role of corpus luteum will continue up to 16 weeks
    - If there is no fertilization then it is called **corpus luteum of menstruation**
    - It is small and short span of life—12 to 14 days
    - The corpus luteum is later replaced by fibrous tissue called **corpus albicans**.

2. Midgut rotation.

- The midgut extends from anterior intestinal pore to posterior intestinal pores
- It is suspended by dorsal mesentery from posterior wall
- The superior mesenteric artery is found in the center of the mesentery
- By the artery the midgut is divided into pre-arterial and post-arterial segments

- The apex of the midgut is connected to the yolk sac by the vitellointestinal duct
- The structures derived from midgut are duodenum distal to the hepatopancreatic duct to the right two-third of transverse colon
- The midgut undergoes rotation around the axis of superior mesenteric artery— 90° outside the abdominal cavity and 180° inside the cavity.
- **The rotation is under three stages**.
  - **First stage (Figs. 27A and B)**:
    - The midgut elongates and so temporarily the midgut herniates outside into the extraembryonic coelomic cavity
    - The herniation is called as **physiological umbilical herniation**
    - The **herniation is due** to: (1) The large size of the liver; (2) The abdominal cavity is small to accommodate the midgut and (3) Mesonephric kidneys in the lumbar region
    - The herniation is **during** 5th week
    - The midgut undergoes **90° rotation**, anticlockwise to the right
    - The **rotation is due** to the pressure exerted by the liver
    - By this rotation the prearterial segment become right limb and the post arterial left limb.
  - **Second stage (Fig. 27C)**:
    - The period of physiological hernia is 5 weeks (5th to 10th wk)
    - **During 10th week** the herniated mass reenters the abdominal cavity
    - **Return** is due to: (1) Reduction in size of liver; (2) Increase in the abdominal cavity and (3) Regression of mesonephric kidneys
    - The return is not all together, but in stages
    - The pre-arterial segment increases in length to form the coils of jejunum and ileum
    - The cecal bud appears in the post-arterial segment
    - The coils of jejunum and ileum (pre-arterial segment) return to the abdominal cavity first
    - The coils of jejunum and ileum occupy the posterior, right and left part of the abdominal cavity
    - Finally, the post-arterial segment of the midgut loop returns to the abdominal cavity
    - Initially it reaches the left side of abdomen
    - As the dorsal part of abdomen is filled with coils of intestine, the cecum undergoes a search for fixation to dorsal wall
    - It rotates upwards and to the right anterior to superior mesenteric artery and small gut
    - At the end of this stage, the cecum lies just below the liver.
  - **Third stage (Fig. 27D)**:
    - Gradually, the cecum descends to the iliac fossa and the ascending, transverse and descending parts of the colon become distinct
    - The appendix is a diverticulum from cecal bud
    - The total range of rotation is 270° in anticlockwise
    - The first 90° is within umbilical hernia, and 180° within abdomen.
- **Congenital anomalies**:
  - Abnormal rotation of the intestinal loop results in volvulus
  - Reverse rotation occurs in the initial 90° rotation and the transverse colon passes deep to the duodenum and superior mesenteric artery.

3. Microscopic structure of spleen.

- Spleen is a lymphoid organ
- Spleen is covered by a capsule made of connective tissue
- Numerous fibrous septa extend from the capsule into the substance of spleen
- The septae are continuous with the reticular network
- The substance of the spleen has red pulp and white pulp

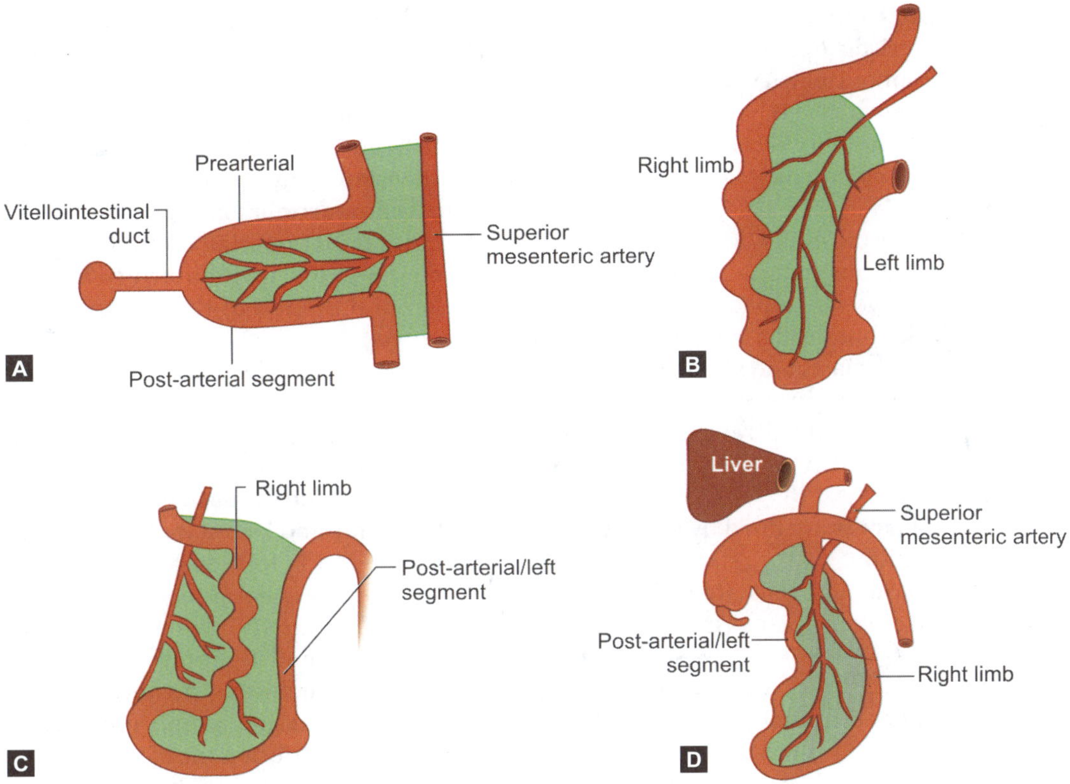

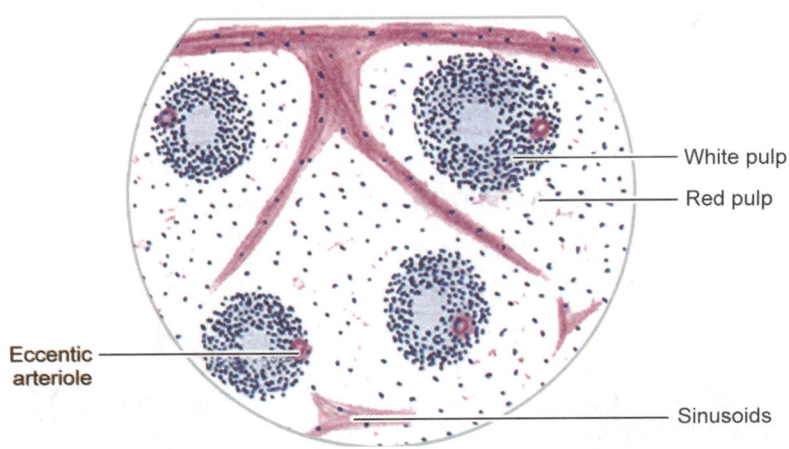

Figs. 27A to D: Midgut rotation.

Fig. 28: Histology of spleen.

- **White pulp**:
  - The branches of splenic artery enter through the trabeculae, and form arterioles. The adventitia is replaced by peri-arteriolar lymphatic sheath (PALS) by the T lymphocytes
  - In some places the sheath is surrounded by B lymphocytes to form lymphoid follicles
  - The white pulp also contains the terminal parts of the arterioles and the arteriole is located eccentrically.

Eccentric arteriole, which is a characteristic feature of the spleen
- The lymphoid follicles contain germinal center with active B lymphocytes
- The lymphoid follicles are reduced or absent in elderly people.
- **Red pulp:**
  - This forms the bulk (75%) of the spleen
  - Has numerous venous sinusoids
  - The sinusoids are separated by reticular network containing collagen type III fibers, fibroblasts and macrophages
  - In between the sinusoids, the lymphocytes are arranged as cords or strips known as **Splenic cords of Billroth**
  - The **sinusoids** are lined by incomplete endothelium
  - The endothelial cells are called **stave cells** resembling planks in a barrel.

4. Femoral sheath.

- It is a flattened funnel shaped sleeve of fascia
- Encloses the upper 3 or 4 cm of the femoral vessels.
- It is wider above and narrows in the lower part
- Merges with tunica adventitia of the vessels
- In new born the sheath is shorter
- Formation:
  - Anterior wall by fascia transversalis
  - Posterior wall by the fascia iliaca.
- Lateral wall of sheath—vertical
- Medial wall—oblique and slopes downwards and laterally
- Function of sheath: Allows the vessels to glide freely below the inguinal ligament
- Subdivisions **(Fig. 29A)**: Sheath is divided into **3 compartments:**
  1. Lateral or arterial compartment – contains the femoral artery and the femoral branch of the genitofemoral nerve
  2. Intermediate or venous compartment contains femoral vein
  3. Medial or lymphatic compartment called **femoral canal** about 1.25 cm in length is a dead space. Its medial wall is oblique and lateral wall straight. The upper end is formed by the **femoral ring** which is bounded by the lateral border lacunar ligament medially, the inguinal ligament anteriorly and the pectineus posteriorly. The canal **contains** a lymph node called Cloquet's node or node of Rosenmuller which drains the glans penis/glans clitoris. The canal allows the expansion of femoral vein.
- Structures piercing femoral sheath **(Fig. 29B):**
  - Laterally, femoral branch of genito-femoral nerve
  - In front, the superficial branches of femoral artery
  - Medially, great saphenous vein.

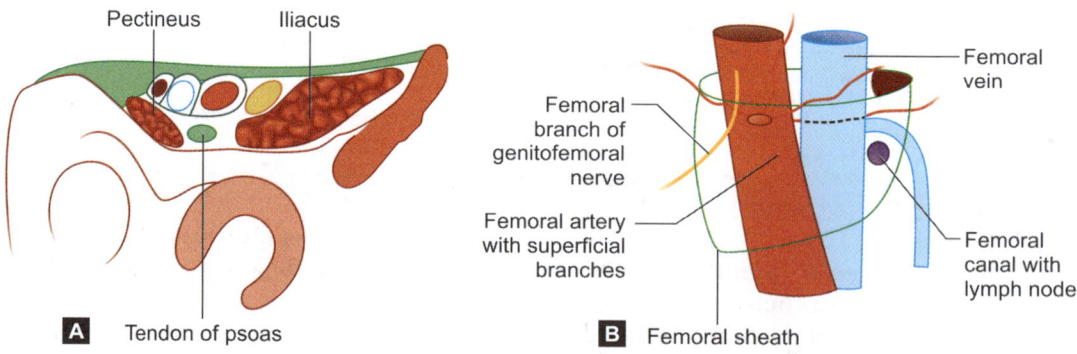

Figs. 29A and B: Femoral sheath.

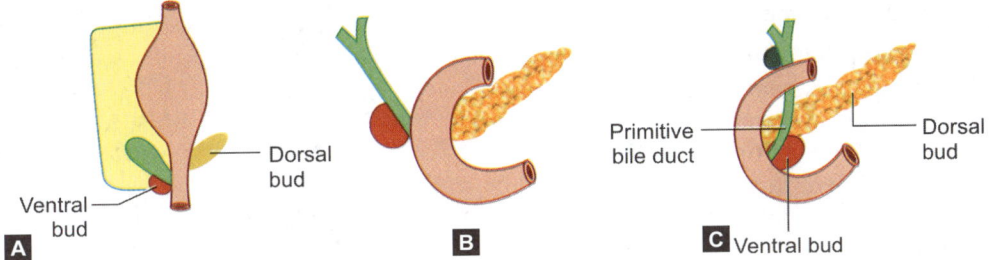

Figs. 30A to C: Development of pancreas.

Applied anatomy: Femoral hernia is common in female because of wider femoral canal. It is below and lateral to the pubic tubercle.

5. Trigone of the bladder.

Refer essay Q. No. 2 – 2003.

6. Development of pancreas.

- Pancreas is endodermal in origin
- It is developed from the lower end of foregut which forms the second part of duodenum
- Developed in 2 parts—dorsal bud and ventral bud
- Dorsal bud—larger; ventral bud—smaller
- Dorsal bud arises from dorsal wall of primitive duodenum. It is proximal to ventral bud
- Ventral bud has two components and is from the bile duct which arises from junction of foregut and midgut. The two components fuse and then undergoes rotation
- The second part of duodenum undergoes axial rotation
- The ventral and dorsal buds unite to form the pancreas
- **Ventral bud** gives rise to uncinate process and inferior part of head of pancreas
- **Dorsal bud** gives rise to part of the head, neck, body and tail of pancreas
- Main pancreatic duct is derived from three sources **(Fig. 31)**:
  1. Distal part of dorsal duct
  2. Oblique communication between the ducts of dorsal and ventral buds
  3. Primitive bile duct.
- Accessory pancreatic duct is from proximal part of dorsal duct.

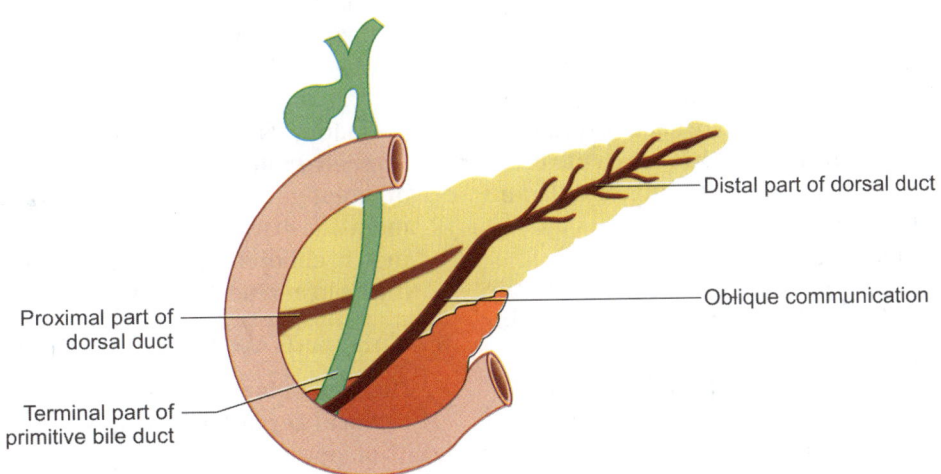

Fig. 31: Development of duct.

Developmental Anomalies

Annular pancreas: The two components of the ventral pancreatic bud sometimes fail to fuse. In such conditions, these two components grow in opposite directions around the duodenum and meet the dorsal pancreatic bud. The annular pancreas thus formed produces duodenal obstruction.

7. Pronation and supination.

These are rotatory movements of the forearm.
- **Supination (Fig. 32A)**:
  - The palm is directed upwards (in front)
  - The radius and ulna lies parallel to each other
  - More powerful
  - It is an antigravity movement
  - Helps in all screwing movements of hand.
- **Pronation (Fig. 32B)**:
  - The head of radius spins around within the annular ligament
  - The lower end of radius carries the hand with it and rotates forwards and medially across the lower end of ulna
  - The interosseous membrane is spiralised during pronation.
- **Axis**: It passes obliquely from the center of the head of the radius to the ulnar attachment of the articular disc below.
- **Range of movement**:
  - In flexed elbow, it is about 140 – 150 degrees
  - In extended elbow, the range of movement is raised to 360 degrees along with rotation of head of humerus.
- **Joint producing this movements**: Radioulnar joints—superior, middle and inferior joints.
- **Movements occurring**:
  - During **pronation,** the head of the radius spins within the annular ligament, and is lateral to ulna
    - The lower end of radius along with the hand rotates forwards and medially
    - The radius crosses the lower end of ulna, lies medial to ulna

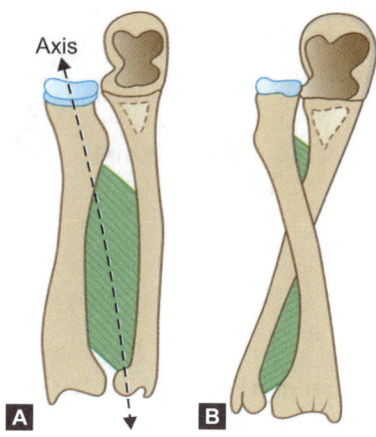

Figs. 32A and B: (A) Supination; (B) Pronation.

  - The interosseous membrane is spiralised
  - The lower end of ulna moves backwards and laterally.
  - **During supination**—the movement is reversed
    - The lower end of radius returns to the lateral position
    - The interosseous membrane is despiralized
    - The lower end of ulna move forwards and medially.
- **Muscles producing**:
  - **Supination:** Biceps brachii, supinator and brachioradialis. Biceps brachii is the most powerful supinator (in semi-flexed elbow). Supinator comes into play when the forearm is extended
  - Pronation: Pronator teres and pronator quadratus.
- **Applied anatomy:** Pulled elbow – the head of radius gets slips out of the annular ligament due to traction on the wrist. It is common in children below 6 years as the size of the head and neck of radius are same.

8. Cutaneous nerve supply of the foot.

- **Dorsum of foot (Fig. 33A)**
  - **Sural nerve:** Supplies the lateral border of foot
  - **Saphenous nerve:** Supplies the medial border of foot up to ball of the great toe

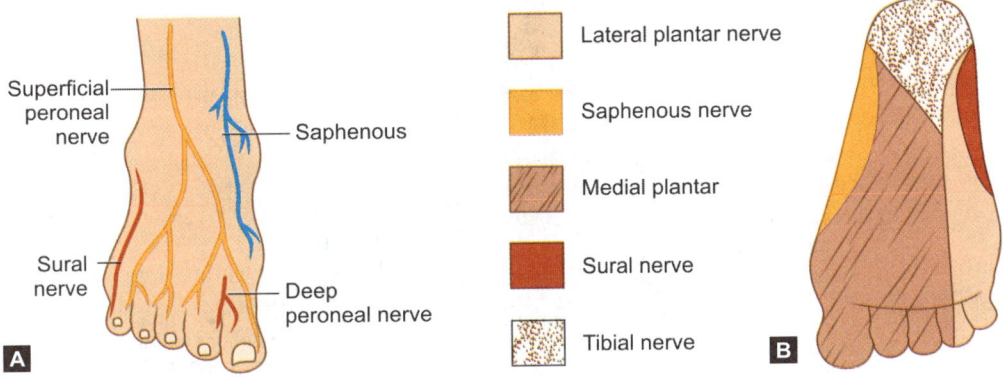

Figs. 33A and B: Cutaneous innervation of foot: (A) Dorsum; (B) Sole.

- **Anterior tibial/deep peroneal nerve:** Inter digital cleft between great toe and second toe
- **Superficial peroneal nerve:** Supplies the entire dorsum of foot except the areas supplied by the above nerves.
- **Sole of foot (Fig. 33B)**
  - Heel – supplied by medial calcanean branches of tibial nerve
  - Lateral 1/3 of sole with lateral one and half toes – by lateral plantar nerve
  - Medial 2/3 of sole with medial three and half toes – by medial plantar nerve.
- **Applied anatomy**
  - Morton's toe – it is a painful condition due to neurofibroma in the digital nerves supplying the adjacent sides of 3rd and 4th toes. The cause may be due to trauma resulting from weight bearing in small or ill fitting shoes
  - Plantar reflex is elicited by stroking the skin of the sole along the lateral border.

9. Perineal membrane.

- It is a triangular membrane present between the superficial and deep perineal pouches
- It is also known as **inferior layer of urogenital diaphragm**
- **Attachments:**
  - Laterally to ischiopubic rami
  - Apex to transverse perineal ligament
  - Posterior border is attached to perineal body
  - Fuses with fascia over the deep transverse perineii.
- Structures piercing it **(Fig. 34)**:
  - **In both sex**
    - Urethra about 2 – 3 cm behind the lower border of pubic symphysis
    - Dorsal artery of penis/clitoris behind pubic arch near the lateral border
    - Deep artery of the penis/clitoris about 2.5 cm behind the pubic arch near lateral border
    - 2 posterior scrotal/labial nerves and vessels close to posterior border.
  - **In male**
    - Duct of bulbourethral gland
    - Artery to bulb of penis posterolateral to urethra.
  - **In female**: Vagina in the center.

10. Lesser sac.

Lesser sac is a diverticulum of greater sac, situated behind the stomach and extends beyond the stomach. It allows expansion of stomach and hence known as **omental bursa**. It is closed on all sides except at the epiploic foramen through which it communicates with the greater sac.

- Shape: Resembles an empty hot water bag with the opening at its lower right margin

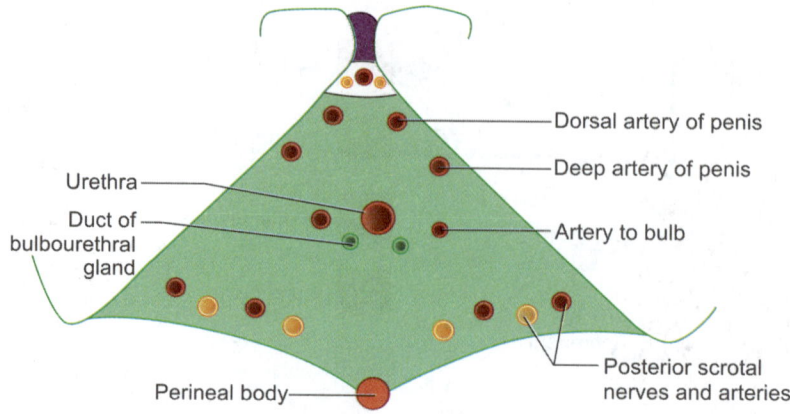

Fig. 34: Perineal membrane.

- Boundaries **(Fig. 35A)**: It has two walls—anterior and posterior and four margins—upper, lower, right and left.
- Anterior wall
  - Peritoneum covering caudate lobe and caudate process of liver
  - Posterior layer of lesser omentum
  - Peritoneum covering the postero-inferior surface of stomach and adjoining part of proximal half of first part of duodenum
  - Second layer of greater omentum
- Posterior wall
  - Third layer of greater omentum
  - Peritoneum covering the anterosuperior surface of transverse colon
  - Upper layer of transverse mesocolon
  - Peritoneum covering the stomach bed structures.
- Upper margin
  - Formed by the reflection of peritoneum from the diaphragm to the upper end of caudate lobe of liver
  - Extends from the groove for inferior vena cava to the cardiac end of stomach.
- Lower margin
  - In new born—lower margin of greater omentum
  - After puberty—second and third layers of greater omentum are fused. Hence does not usually extend below the transverse colon.
- Right margin
  - Below transverse colon: Right free margin of greater omentum
  - Between transverse colon and first part of duodenum: Reflection of peritoneum from the neck of pancreas to the posterior surface of first part of duodenum
  - Between duodenum and liver: Deficient and presents the epiploic foramen through which it communicates with the greater sac.
- Left margin
  - Below transverse colon: Left free margin of greater omentum
  - Between transverse colon and cardiac end of stomach: Inner layer of gastrosplenic and inner layer of lienorenal ligaments.
- Communication **(Fig. 35B)**: Communicates with greater sac through epiploic foramen.
- **Interior of lesser sac:**
  - Two sickle-shaped peritoneal folds are seen known as superior and inferior gastropancreatic folds
  - Superior gastropancreatic fold is produced by left gastric artery
  - Inferior gastropancreatic fold is produced by common hepatic artery.

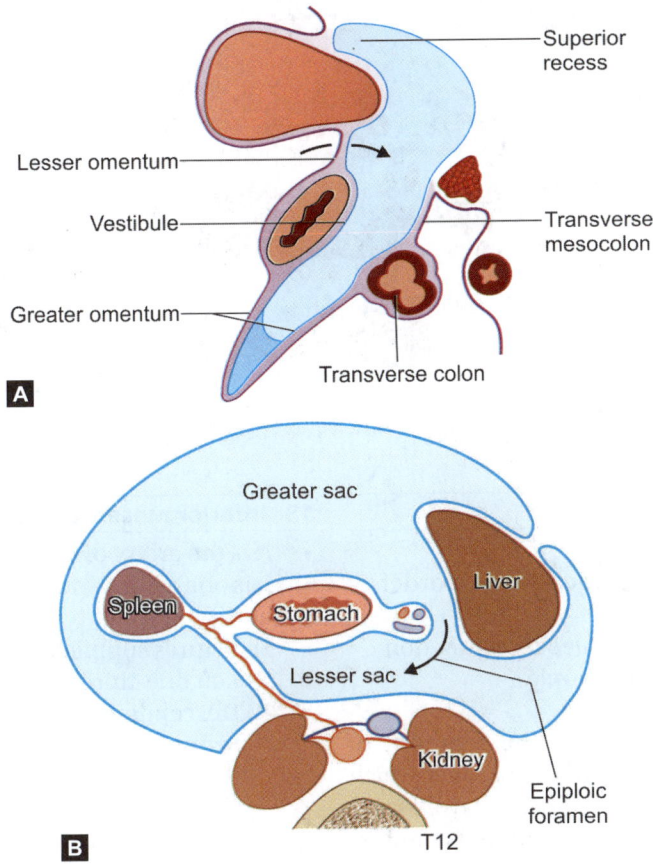

Figs. 35A and B: Lesser sac: (A) Boundaries; (B) Communication.

- **Applied Anatomy:**
  - **Internal hernia:** Herniation of intestines into the lesser sac through the epiploic foramen
  - **Perforation of posterior wall of stomach** can result in accumulation of fluid in the omental bursa
  - **Inflamed or injured pancreas can result in pseudo:** Pancreatic cyst, which is due to collection of pancreatic fluids in the lesser sac.

11. Microscopic structure of appendix.

- Appendix is made up of four layers—from outer to inner are: (i) serous (ii) muscular (iii) submucous (iv) mucous **(Fig. 36)**.
  - Serous layer- is formed by peritoneum.
  - Muscular layer - is complete. Made of inner circular and outer longitudinal layers. At certain sites the muscle fibers are deficient called **hiatus muscularis**
  - Submucous layer: Loose areolar tissue, blood vessels, and numerous lymphatic follicles are present. The lymphatic nodules are formed in lamina propria and extend to submucosa. Hence appendix is known as **abdominal tonsil**
  - Mucous layer: Consists of **epithelium** lined by columnar epithelium with goblet cells, **lamina propria** with intestinal glands (crypts of Lieberkuhn), **muscularis mucosa**. Villi are absent.

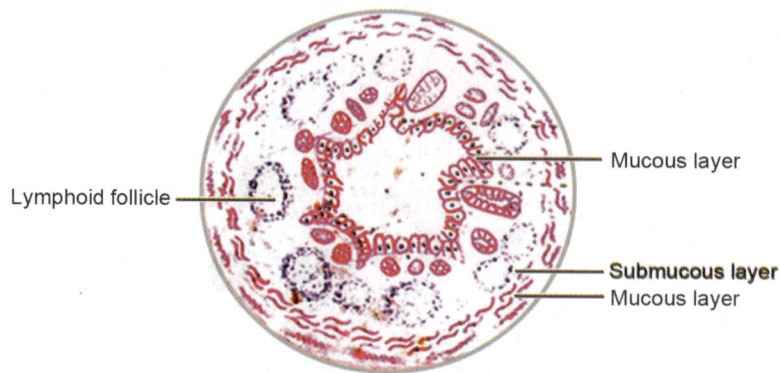

Fig. 36: Histology of appendix.

12. Meckel's diverticulum.

- It is a blind pouch
  - Arises from antimesenteric border of ileum
  - 2 feet proximal to ileocecal junction
  - Present in 2% of people
  - 2 inch in length.
- **Developmentally** it is the remnant of proximal part of vitellointestinal duct, which in fetal life connects midgut with yolk sac
- The caliber of the diverticulum is same as that of ileum
- The tip may be free or attached to umbilicus by a fibrous band
- Oxyntic cells are occasionally present leading on to peptic ulcer.

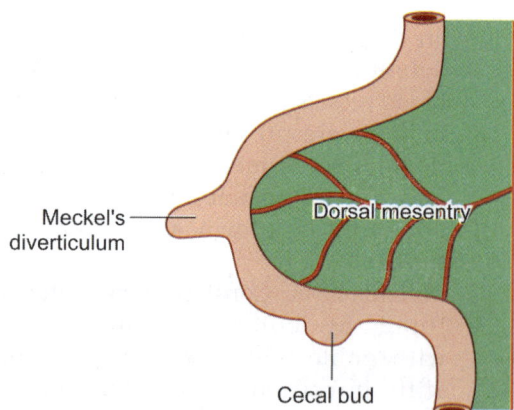

Fig. 37: Meckel's diverticulum.

13 Inferior mesenteric artery

- It is the artery of the hind gut
- It is one of the ventral branch of abdominal aorta
- Structures supplied:
  - Left one-third of transverse colon
  - Descending colon
  - Sigmoid colon
  - Rectum
  - Upper part of the anal canal up to pectinate line.
- Origin:
  - From the abdominal aorta
  - At the **level** of 3rd lumbar vertebra
  - Behind the 3rd part of the duodenum
  - About 3 – 4 cm above the bifurcation of aorta.
- Course:
  - Runs downwards and to the left behind the peritoneum
  - Crosses the origin of left common iliac artery
  - Medial to the left ureter and inferior mesenteric vein.
- Termination: Continues down as the superior rectal artery.
- Branches:
  - Left colic artery:
    - The artery supplies transverse colon and descending colon
    - It divides into ascending and descending branches

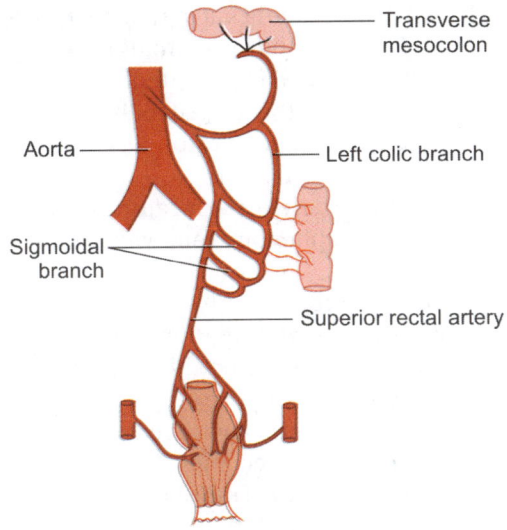

Fig. 38: Inferior mesenteric artery.

- Pierces the wall of rectum and enters the submucosa
- It terminates by anastomosing with branches of inferior rectal artery.

14. Great saphenous vein.

Great saphenous vein is the longest superficial vein of the lower limb.
- Formation and termination
  - **Formation**: Continuation of medial end of dorsal venous arch of foot and united by medial marginal vein
  - **Termination**: It pierces the cribriform fascia and femoral sheath to open into the femoral vein distal to inguinal ligament.
- Course and relations
  - **Course**
    - It starts from the medial end of the dorsal venous arch on the dorsum of the foot
    - Runs upwards 2.5 cm in front of the medial malleolus, crosses the lower part of tibia and reaches the medial side of the leg
    - Then it curves backwards a hand breadth behind the patella to the back of the knee
    - It ascends to reach the saphenous opening, along the medial side of

- The ascending branch anastomose with left branch of middle colic within the transverse mesocolon
- The descending branch anastomose with highest branch of sigmoid artery.
- Sigmoid arteries:
  - Supplies descending colon and sigmoid colon
  - Usually seen as three to five branches
  - They divide and form arterial arcade close to the wall of colon
  - From arches smaller branches arise to supply the sigmoid colon
  - First sigmoid branch anastomoses with left colic artery and supply descending colon
  - The last sigmoid branch anastomoses with superior rectal artery.
- Superior rectal artery:
  - The superior rectal artery is continuation of inferior mesenteric artery
  - It descends into the pelvis and crosses the sacral promontory in midline
  - It terminates into two branches at the level of S3
  - They lie on either side of rectum

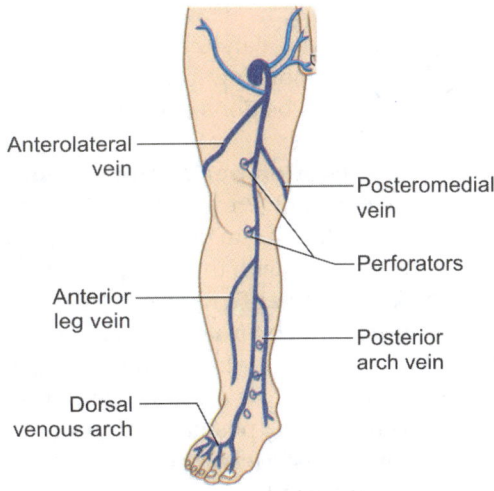

Fig. 39: Great saphenous vein.

thigh. The opening is 3 cm inferior and lateral to the pubic tubercle
- It contains about 10 - 20 valves.
- **Relations:**
  - The vein is posterior to all the structures mentioned in relations
  - In the thigh—branches of medial cutaneous nerve of thigh
  - At the knee—saphenous branch of descending genicular artery
  - In the leg and foot—saphenous nerve.
- **Tributaries and perforators**
  - **Tributaries**
    - Below the knee:
      * Medial marginal vein
      * The anterior vein of the leg
      * The posterior arch vein (vein of Leonardo da Vinci)
      * A vein from the calf through short saphenous vein.
    - In the thigh:
      * Accessory saphenous vein
      * Anterior cutaneous vein.
    - Just before piercing the cribriform fascia:
      * Superficial epigastric vein
      * Superficial circumflex iliac vein
      * Superficial external pudendal vein.
  - **Perforators:** Connect saphenous vein or its tributaries with the deep veins after piercing the deep fascia. They are provided with valves at each end and direct the blood flow from superficial to deep veins. Positions of the perforators are as follows:
    - **Mid-Hunter perforator (Dodd's perforator):** Present in the adductor canal. The great saphenous vein is connected with the femoral vein
    - **Knee perforator (Boyd's perforator):** Situated just below the knee, close to the medial border of tibia. Connects the great saphenous vein with the posterior tibial vein
    - **Three ankle perforators (Cockett's perforator):** Connects the great saphenous vein with the posterior tibial vein at three levels.
      1. Upper one lies at the junction of the middle and lower thirds of tibia
      2. Lower one is situated below and behind the medial malleolus
      3. Middle perforator lies midway between them.
    - Lateral ankle perforator connects short saphenous vein with peroneal vein.
- **Applied Anatomy**
  - **Varicose veins:** Superficial veins of the lower limb are often dilated, tortuous and become varicose
  - **Varicose ulcers:** Over the area of varicosity, the skin becomes pigmented and suffers from lack of nutrition which leads to varicose ulcers that often bleed profusely and require surgical intervention
  - **Coronary by-pass graft:** Great saphenous vein is used for arterial grafting. Due to presence of valves, the vein has to be reversed to replace an arterial obstruction
  - **Venous cut downs:** The great saphenous vein is used just in front of medial malleolus
  - **Trendelenburg's test:** Test to check the patency of saphenofemoral valve. Positive Trendelenburg test indicates treatment by surgery
  - **Deep vein thrombosis (DVT)** is a complication after major surgeries, due to less activity of the legs, there is stasis of venous blood and thrombosis. The thrombi can enter into venous circulation leading to pulmonary embolism.

15. Primitive streak.

- Gastrulation begins with the formation of primitive streak on the surface of the epiblast
- Primitive streak appears by 15th day
- Seen as a narrow median groove with raised lateral margins
- At the cephalic end of the primitive streak, the cells proliferate to form a knob like enlargement called **Henson's/Primitive node**.

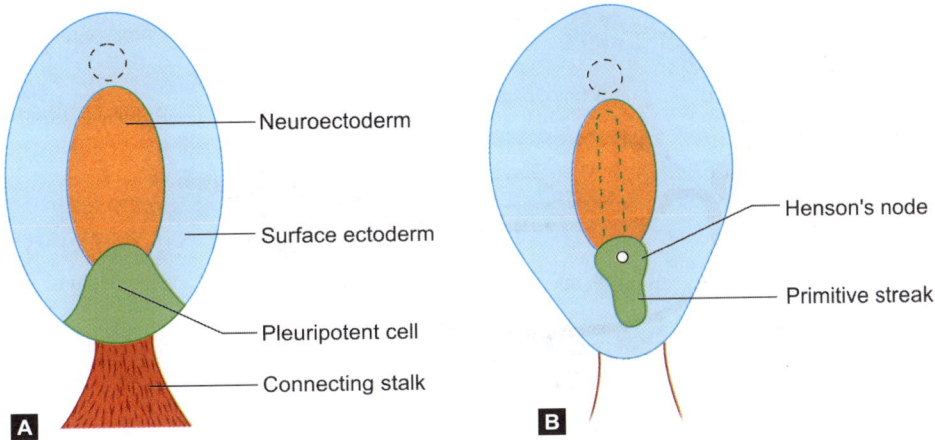

Figs. 40A and B: Primitive streak.

- In the center of Henson's node, a depression appears called **primitive pit**
- The pit along with cord of cells extends forwards in the midline. It extends from Henson's node to prochordal plate
- The canalized extension is called the **notochordal process or head process** (Fig. 41)
- The head process is situated between endoderm and the neuroectoderm
- As development continues, the cells of floor of notochordal canal fuse with the endodermal cells of the roof of yolk sac
- Later both groups of cells disappear and communicate with yolk sac
- A temporary **neuroenteric canal** is formed communicating yolk sac with amniotic cavity to provide nutrition (Fig. 42)
- Later the notochordal plate folds and gradually escalates from the roof of yolk sac
- The endodermal layer is also lined by uninterrupted layer
- The notochordal plate forms solid cord called **definitive notochord**
- Notochord **persists (remnant)** as **nucleus pulposus** in the center of intervertebral disc, and **apical ligament**
- It **induces differentiation** of neural tube from the medullary plate
- It also acts as **forerunner** in development of vertebral column.

16. First carpometacarpal joint.

- **Type of joint:** It is a synovial, multiaxial, saddle (sellar) variety.
- **Bones:**
  – Trapezium
  – Base of the first metacarpal bone.
- **Ligaments:**
  – Capsular ligament
  – Lateral ligament from lateral surface of trapezium to lateral surface of base of metacarpal bone
  – Anterior ligament from palmar surface of trapezium to ulnar side of base of metacarpal bone
  – Posterior ligament from dorsal surface of trapezium to ulnar side of base of metacarpal bone.
- **Blood supply:** Radial artery and first dorsal metacarpal branch
- **Nerve supply:** Posterior interosseous and superficial branch of radial nerve
- **Movements and muscle causing movements:**
  – Flexion and extensions
    - Are parallel with palmar plane
    - The movement is in the interphalangeal or metacarpophalangeal joints
    - In flexion the thumb moves across the palm and it comes in contact with the palm

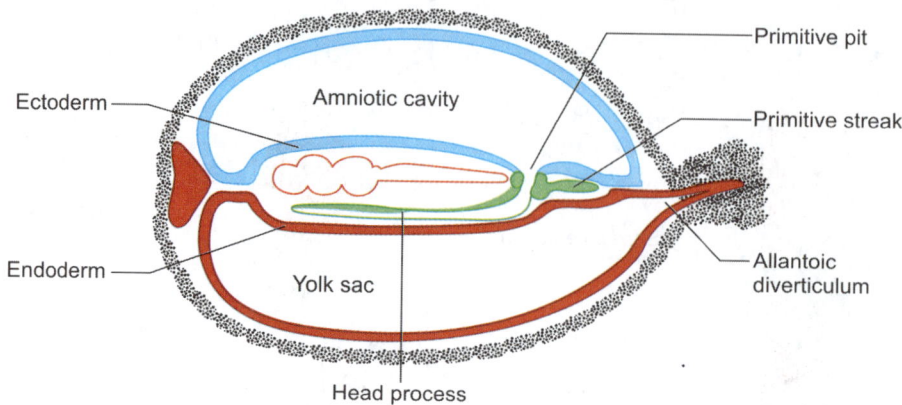

Fig. 41: Notochordal process.

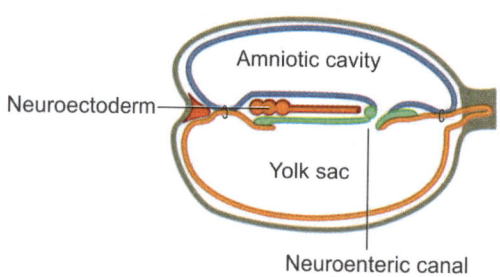

Fig. 42: Neuroenteric canal.

- In extension the thumb moves away from palm and is accompanied by lateral rotation of thumb.
- Muscles producing:
  * Flexion: Flexor pollicis brevis, opponens pollicis
  * Extension: Extensor pollicis longus and brevis and abductor pollicis longus.
- **Abduction and adduction**
  - Are at right angles to flexion and extension
  - In abduction the thumb moves away from the index finger
  - In adduction the thumb comes in front and in contact with the index finger
  - Muscles producing:
    * Abduction: Abductor pollicis longus, Abductor pollicis brevis
    * Adduction: Adductor pollicis.

- **Opposition**
  - The thumb crosses the palm and touches the tips of other fingers
  - The opposition is movement of flexion and medial rotation of abducted thumb
  - Muscles producing opposition: Opponens pollicis, flexor pollicis brevis.
- **Circumduction**
  - Is a rotatory movement
  - Rotation along the long axis of metacarpal shaft
  - Muscles producing circumduction: Extensors, abductors, flexors, and adductors acting in order.

17. Microscopic structure of bone.

Refer short notes 1 – 2003.

18. Pelvic diaphragm.

- Levator ani and coccygeus of both sides together form the pelvic diaphragm
- It separates the pelvis from the perineum
- The pelvic diaphragm is divisible from before backwards into:
  – Pubococcygeus
  – Iliococcygeus
  – Ischiococcygeus
- Pubococcygeus and iliococcygeus together form levator ani
- Ischiococcygeus is called as coccygeus muscle

- **Levator ani:**
  - **Pubococcygeus part:** Arises from anterior half of white line of obturator fascia and body of pubis. It is divided into:
    - **Pubourethralis**—
      * The fibers from body of pubis pass medially close to urethra in both sexes
      * The fibers from both side form part of urethral sphincter
      * Behind the urethra the fibers intersect across midline
      * In male few of these fibers form **levator prostatae** pass lateral and below the prostate.
    - **Pubococcygeus proper:** Most posterior fibers inserted to ano coccygeal raphe and tip of coccyx.
    - **Puborectalis:**
      * The fibers form a sling around the ano rectal junction and is continuous with opposite side muscle
      * Few of these fibers blend with the external sphincter
    - **Puboanalis:**
      * Some fibers decussate and merges with the longitudinal coat of anal canal
      * After merging the fibers are called as **conjoint tendon of anal canal.**
    - **Pubovaginalis:**
      * In female the anterior fibers pass by the side of vagina
      * It forms a loop around the posterior wall of vagina
      * The fibers are inserted to perineal body.
  - **Iliococcygeus part:**
    - Origin:
      * Posterior half of white line of the obturator fascia extending up to obturator canal
      * Pelvic surface of the ischial spine.
    - Insertion:
      * To the tip of sacrum and coccyx
      * The fibers decussate with opposite side to form raphe
      * The raphe is prolonged to the anococcygeal ligament.
- **Ischiococcygeus:**
  - It is a triangular muscle occupying the posterior part
  - The muscle may be absent or tendinous.
  - **Sacrospinous ligament** is the degenerated part of the muscle
  - Origin: Medial surface and tip of ischial spine.

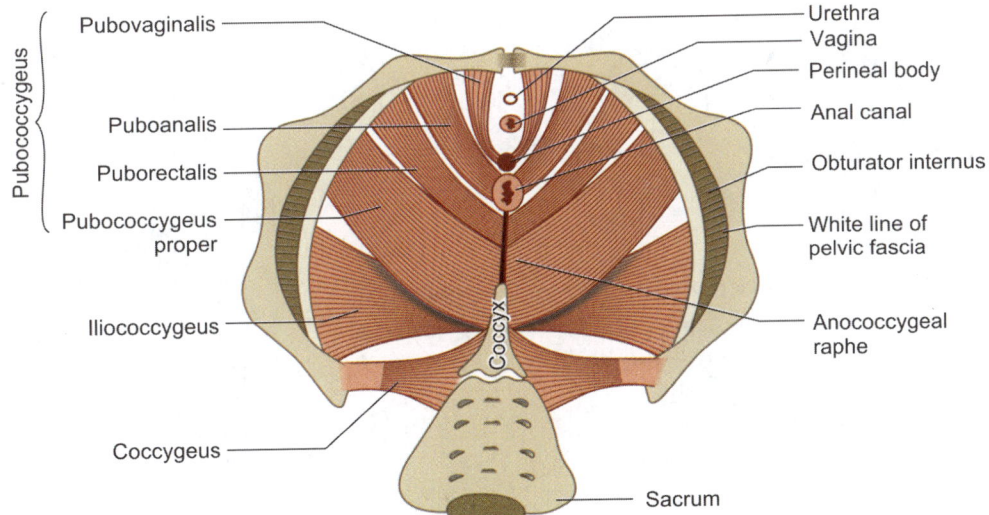

Fig. 43: Pelvic diaphragm.

- Insertion:
  - Lateral margin of coccyx
  - Lateral margin of fifth sacral segment.
- **Nerve supply:**
  - The levator ani is supplied by:
    - Branch from 4th sacral nerve
    - Branch from the inferior rectal nerve.
  - Ischiococcygeus muscle is supplied by
    - Branch from 3rd and 4th sacral nerves.
- **Actions:**
  - Closes the posterior part of the pelvic outlet
  - Supports the pelvic viscera
  - Helps to increase the intra-abdominal pressure
  - Prevents any prolapse through the pelvic floor.
- **Applied anatomy:**
  - Hiatus Schwalbe: Herniation of the pelvic contents into ischiorectal fossa, due to a gap between tendinous origin of levator and obturator fascia. The hernia is known as **ischioanal hernia**
  - The pelvic diaphragm is weakened by the perineal tear during childbirth. The weak pelvic floor can lead to prolapse of uterus.

19. Lymphatic drainage of the mammary gland.

Lymph vessels draining breast are divided as 2 sets:
1. Those draining parenchyma of breast including nipple and areola
2. Those draining the skin excluding nipple and areola.

From parenchyma of breast including nipple and areola (**Fig. 44**)
- The lymph vessels form plexus in the connective tissue and walls of lactiferous ducts
- Subareolar plexus of Sappey collects lymph from the nipple and areola
- Both these vessels join together
- 75% of lymphatic from the gland drain into axillary nodes. They accompany lateral thoracic artery
- 20% of lymphatic drain into parasternal nodes. They accompany internal thoracic artery
- 5% from lateral and posterior part of the gland drain into posterior intercostal nodes. They accompany posterior intercostal arteries.

Lymphatics from skin excluding nipple and areola (**Fig. 45**):

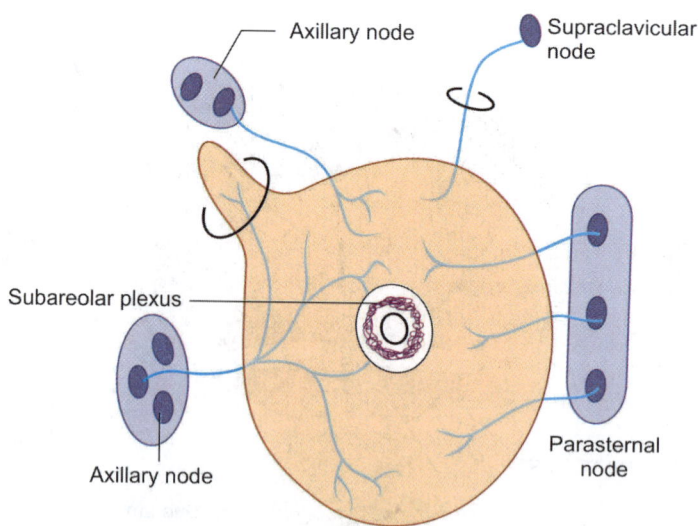

Fig. 44: Lymphatic drainage of parenchyma.

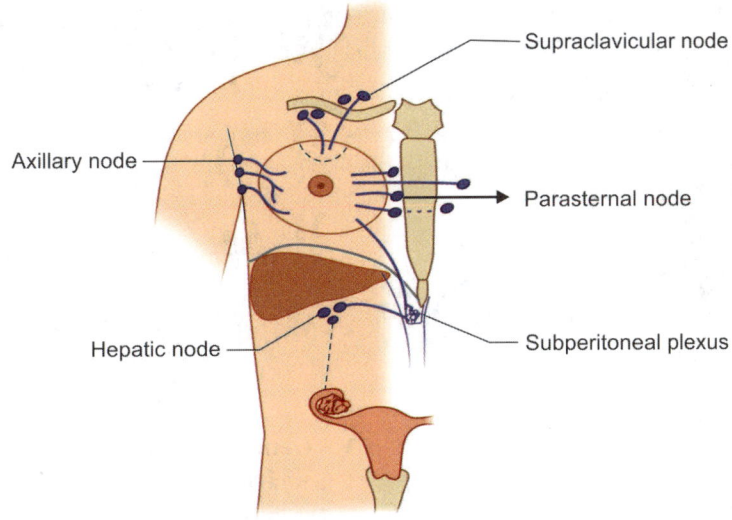

Fig. 45: Lymphatic drainage of skin.

- From outer part—axillary nodes
- From upper part—infra and supra clavicular nodes
- From inner part—parasternal nodes of both sides
- From lower part—communicate with those of rectus sheath and form subperitoneal plexus. They drain into sub diaphragmatic nodes
- Lymphatics of both sides communicate with each other across the midline
- **Applied Anatomy**
  - Cancer cells may infiltrate the suspensory ligaments; hence the breast becomes fixed. Contraction of the ligaments cause retraction of skin
  - Peau d'orange appearance: Infiltration of the cutaneous lymphatic leading to obstruction of lymph vessels of the skin over the breast. Lymphedema of the skin of the breast with intermittent pitting due to retraction of hair follicles resulting in peau d'orange appearance
  - Infiltration of lactiferous ducts—results in retraction of nipple
  - Cancer may spread to the opposite side because of the communications of the superficial lymphatics of the breast across the midline
  - Cancer can spread to the liver; may drop into pelvis—secondaries in the pelvic organs (Krukenberg's tumor)
  - Cancer can spread through veins to vertebrae, humerus and to the brain
  - Mastectomy: Removal of the breast is called mastectomy. Simple mastectomy is removal of axillary nodes along with breast and preserving the pectoral muscles. Radical mastectomy is preferred which is removal of the breast along with lymph nodes and pectoral muscles and the skin overlying the tumour
  - While performing radical mastectomy, the long thoracic nerve should be taken care. If injured results in winging of scapula
  - The mammography is a soft tissue X-ray of the breast, with minimal radiation risk. This method is useful in locating clinically undetected lesions.

20. Radial nerve in spiral groove.

- Radial nerve by passing through the lower triangular space the nerve reaches the radial groove (spiral groove) on the back of the humerus

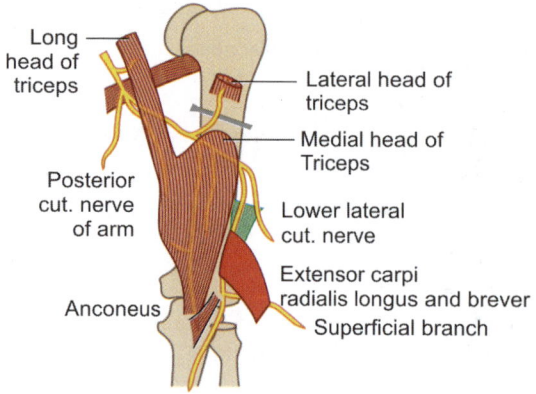

Fig. 46: Radial nerve in spiral groove.

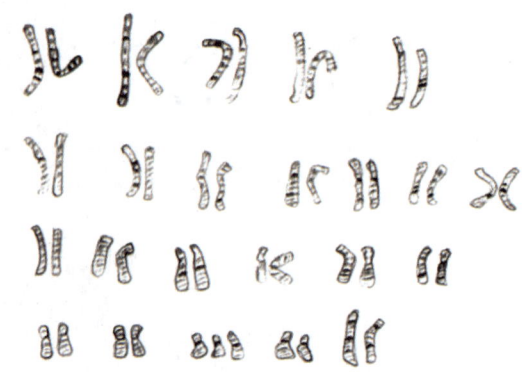

Fig. 47: Trisomy 21.

- In the spiral groove, it runs downwards and laterally
- Pierces the lateral intermuscular septum to enter front of arm.
- Branches:
  - Muscular branches:
    - Branch to lateral head of triceps
    - Branch to medial head of triceps
    - Branch to anconeus given in spiral groove descends within the medial head of triceps and terminate by supplying the muscle.
  - Cutaneous branches:
    - Lower lateral cutaneous nerve of arm supplies the skin of lower half of lateral part of arm
    - Posterior cutaneous nerve of forearm supplies dorsum of forearm.
  - Articular branch: To elbow joint. Nerve to anconeus supplies the elbow joint.

21. Nasal septum.

Refer short notes 17 – 2003.

22. Down's syndrome.

- **Down syndrome** is the most common form of chromosomal disorder in human
- It is rare in young mothers, but increases with maternal age
- It is an extra copy of chromosome 21.
- **Genotype (Fig. 47)**
  - Trisomy 21
    - Due to meiotic nondisjunction of chromosome during oocyte formation
    - Unbalanced translocation between chromosome 21
    - Mosaicism from mitotic non-disjunction.
- **Features in Phenotype**: A child with Down syndrome may have:
  - Growth retardation
  - Intellectual disability
  - Characteristic facial features
    - Upward slant of palpabral fissure
    - Epicanthal folds
    - Low set small ears that folded over slightly at the top
    - Macroglossia: Mouth is small, and large tongue
    - Their nose small, with a flat nasal bridge.
  - Some babies have short necks and small hands with short fingers
  - Has one single crease that goes straight across the palm (Simian crease)
  - The child or adult with Down syndrome often short and has
  - Hypotonia (poor muscle tone and looseness of the joints).
- **Complications:**
  - Leukemia
  - Infections
  - Thyroid dysfunctions
  - Premature ageing.

23. Histology of hypophysis cerebri or pituitary gland.

- Pituitary is divided into anterior and posterior parts
- The anterior is further divided into pars anterior (distalis), pars intermedius, and pars tuberalis
- The posterior is divided as pars nervosa, infundibulum, and median eminence.

Structure and Functions

Anterior Lobe

Pars anterior

- Irregular clusters of epithelial cells arranged as irregular clusters.
- Two types of cells:
  1. **Chromophobes:**
     - 50% of cells of anterior are chromophobic
     - Agranular cytoplasm, considered to be immature precursor cells
     - Under electron microscope few granules are identified.
  2. **Chromophils**:
     - 50% of cells of pars anterior are chromophilic
     - Granular cytoplasm
     - The chromophils are subdivided into acidophils and basophils depending on the stain
  - **Acidophils (alpha cells):** 40% of chromophilic cells are acidophilic. Granules stain with acid stain. They include somatotrophs and mammotrophs
    - **Somatotrophs** secrete growth hormone. It constitutes 50% of the cell population. It is situated in the lateral part of the anterior lobe
    - **Mammotrophs** produce prolactin
    - It constitutes 25% of the cell population
    - It is situated throughout the anterior lobe
  - **Basophils (beta cells):** 10% of cells form basophilic cells. The cells stain poorly with hematoxylin. The basophilic cells include corticotrophs, thyrotrophs, gonadotrophs.
    * **Corticotrophs** produce corticotropic hormone (ACTH): It forms 15 – 20% of the cell population. It occupies the posterior and median part of the anterior lobe. **Thyrotrophs** produce thyrotrophic hormone (TSH). Thyrotrophs are more in the anterior and median part of the anterior lobe
    * **Gonadotrophs** produce two types of hormones having different action in male and female. In female these hormones stimulate growth of ovarian follicle called follicle stimulating hormone

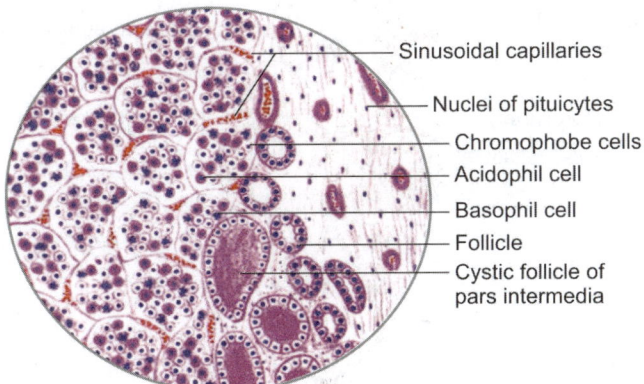

Fig. 48: Histology of pituitary gland.

(FSH), and also stimulates maturation of corpus luteum called luteinizing hormone (LH). In male, it stimulates interstitial cells of testis to produce androgen called interstitial cell stimulating hormone. They form about 10%. It is situated throughout the anterior lobe.

Pars intermedia
- Contains beta cells, chromophobe cells and other secretory cells
- The follicles of chromophobe cells are seen as cyst lined by epithelium and colloidal like material fill the cyst
- It secretes MSH and endorphin.

Pars tuberalis
- Contains a large number of blood vessels, undifferentiated cells arranged in the form of cords are present in-between
- **Intraglandular cleft** seen between pars anterior and pars intermedius.

Posterior Lobe
- Made of unmyelinated nerve fibers
- Nerve fibers are the axons from supraoptic and paraventricular nuclei located in hypothalamus
- Fenestrated plexus of blood capillaries are present
- No hormone is synthesized by posterior lobe
- It acts as storage and releasing center
- Supporting cells: Pituicytes (neuroglial cells), are non-excitatory cells situated between the axons
- **Herring bodies:** Secretory vesicles on terminals of nerve fibers.

Functions: hormones released are:
- Vasopressin (ADH): Reabsorption from distal convoluted tubules of kidney
- Oxytocin: Ejection of milk and contraction of smooth muscles of uterus.

24. Circle of Willis.

- The **circle of Willis** is an arterial circle
- Situated in the base of brain
- Related to interpeduncular fossa
- A communication is established between carotid and vertebrobasilar systems.
- **Formation:**
    - **Anteriorly:** Anterior communicating arteries from anterior cerebral
    - **Anterolaterally:** Anterior cerebral arteries from internal carotid
    - **Laterally:** Terminal part of internal carotid arteries
    - **Posterolaterally:** Posterior communicating arteries from internal carotid
    - **Posteriorly:** Posterior cerebral arteries from basilar.

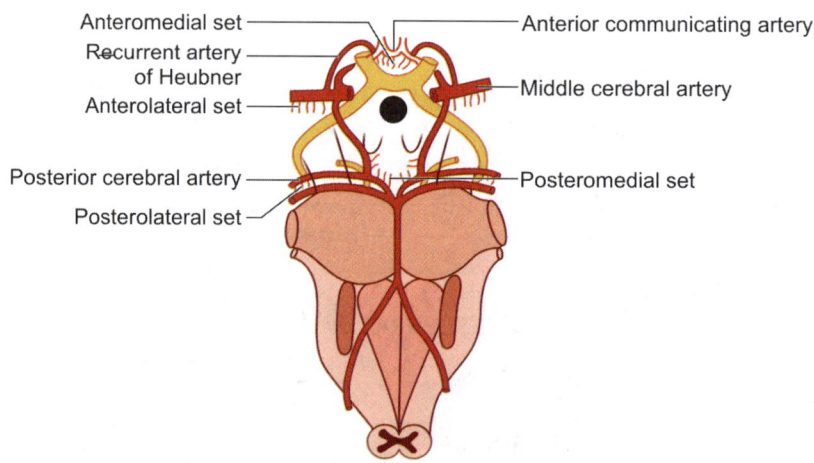

Fig. 49: Circle of Willis.

- **Central branches** from the primary arteries perforate the white matter and supply thalamus, the corpus striatum and internal capsule.
- **Central branches**—6 sets
  - **Anteromedial set**
    - Branches from anterior cerebral and anterior communicating arteries
    - It supplies corpus striatum and internal capsule, optic chiasma, lamina terminalis, the hypothalamus, septum pellucidum, and putamen and the head of the caudate nucleus.
  - **Anterolateral sets**
    - A pair of anterolateral set
    - Branches from middle cerebral and anterior cerebral
    - Pierces the anterior perforated substance
    - It has medial and lateral arteries
    - The branches from middle cerebral artery are known as **lateral striate or lenticulostriate arteries or Charcot's artery** of cerebral hemorrhage
    - They pierce through the anterior perforated substance and supply the corpus striatum, the anterior limb, genu and posterior limb of the internal capsule
    - The **medial striate artery**, from recurrent artery of Heubnar, a branch of anterior cerebral artery
    - Supplies the cranial part of the caudate nucleus and putamen and the anterior limb and genu of the internal capsule
  - **Posterolateral or thalamogeniculate sets**
    - A pair of posterolateral set
    - They are from posterior cerebral arteries
    - Supplies the cerebral peduncle, superior and inferior colliculi, pineal gland, the posterior thalamus and medial and lateral geniculate bodies.
  - **Posteromedial or thalamoperforator set**
    - It is given by the posterior cerebral and posterior communicating arteries
    - They pierce through posterior perforated substance
    - Supplies thalamus, hypothalamus, pituitary gland, and the mammillary bodies.

25. Microscopic structure of the lung.

The section shows from outer to inner are:
- **Pleura:** Made of mesothelial cells, with connective tissue
- **Alveoli**
  - The alveoli are thin-walled sac provide gaseous exchange
  - The alveoli are separated by septae
  - The **septae** contains connective tissue, elastic and collagen type III fibers
  - The three types of epithelial cell (pneumocytes) are present in the walls of alveoli
  - In addition it contains connective tissue with a network of capillaries
  - Adjacent alveoli are in close contact with each other frequently
  - The alveolar epithelium is a mosaic of types I and II pneumocytes.
  - **Type I pneumocytes**
    - Made of simple squamous epithelial cells
    - 90% of the alveolar area is formed by it.
    - The basal laminae of the pneumocytes and the endothelium of adjacent capillary fuse.
  - **Type II cells**
    - Are smaller and rounded cells
    - Protrude from the alveolar surface
    - Their cytoplasm contains numerous secretory lamellar bodies
    - The secretory bodies are the precursors of alveolar surfactant
    - **Inter alveolar pores of Kohn** are present to connect adjacent alveolar airspaces
    - These spaces also help for migration of macrophages.

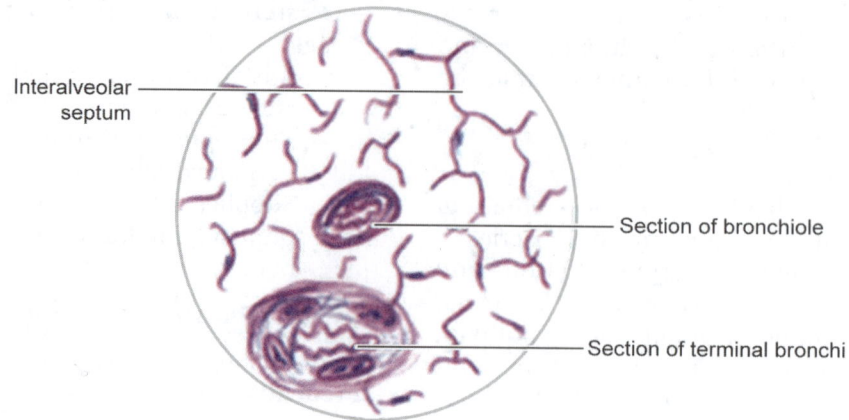

Fig. 50: Histology of lung.

- **Type III cells:** They are brush cells
- **Alveolar macrophages** are derived from circulating monocyte precursors.
  - The macrophages clean alveoli of invading organisms, and inhaled particles by phagocytosis
  - Hence they are also known as '**dust cells**'
  - The macrophages remove the extravasated red blood corpuscles in congestive heart failure, become brick red in colour and are termed **heart-failure cells**.
- **Bronchi**
  - Sections of lobar or secondary bronchi
  - Section of the **terminal bronchi** is seen provided with islands of cartilage
  - The lining epithelium of the bronchi are pseudostratified ciliated/simple ciliated/non-ciliated columnar epithelium
  - The cartilage is made of hyaline cartilage forming the wall of bronchi with few smooth muscle fibers.
- **Bronchioles**
  - Sections of lobular and terminal (respiratory) bronchioles are seen
  - They are lined by simple columnar/cuboidal epithelium
  - Bronchioles are identified by absence of cartilage and mucous glands and presence of more smooth muscle fibers.
- **Alveolar duct:** These are divisions of respiratory bronchi and enter a passage called atrium which is continued as alveolar sac.

26. Tympanic membrane.

- The tympanic cavity is separated from the external acoustic meatus by the tympanic membrane
- It forms the lateral wall of middle ear cavity
- It is thin, semi-transparent membrane
- **Shape:** Oval in shape, broader above than below
- **Position:** It is placed obliquely, making an angle of 55° with the floor of external acoustic meatus
- **Attachment:** The membrane is thickened at its circumference by fibrocartilage
  - It is attached to the groove in the medial end of tympanic plate
  - The tympanic sulcus is deficient superiorly
  - So from the ends of this notch, two folds—the anterior and posterior malleolar folds, get attached to the lateral process of the malleus.
- **Parts:** It has two parts
- **Pars flaccida:** The small triangular part of the membrane above the malleolar folds. It is lax and thin
- **Pars tensa:** The rest of the tympanic membrane is tense, and below the folds.

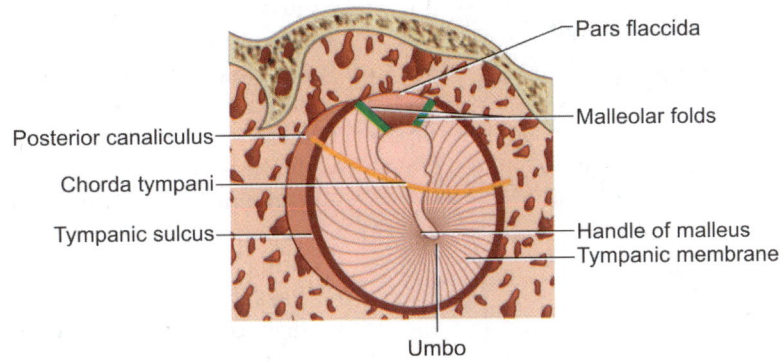

Fig. 51: Tympanic membrane.

- **Surfaces:**
  - The outer surface of the membrane is concave
  - The inner surface is convex and the point of maximum convexity is known as **umbo**. The handle of the malleus is attached to the umbo.
- **Histologically**, the tympanic membrane is made of 3 layers:
  1. An outer cuticular layer, lined by skin, the epithelium is stratified squamous
  2. An intermediate fibrous layer made up of inner circular and outer radiating fibers. The chorda tympani nerve passes in between the fibrous and mucous layer
  3. An inner mucous layer lined by flat cells.
- **Nerve supply**: The main nerve supplying the tympanic membrane is the auriculotemporal nerve, it is also supplied by the auricular branch of vagus, and glossopharyngeal through tympanic plexus
- **Blood supply**: Anterior tympanic and deep auricular branches of maxillary artery.
- **Development**
  - Outer layer ectodermal in origin from first cleft
  - Middle layer mesoderm of first arch
  - Inner layer endodermal in origin from first pouch (tubotympanic recess).
- **Applied anatomy**
  - Myringotomy—in case of collection of fluid/pus inside middle ear cavity the tympanic membrane is incised to let out the collected fluid
  - Myringoplasty is surgical procedure of replacement of tympanic membrane
  - When the living tympanic membrane is examined the reflected light extends anteroinferiorly from tip of the handle of malleus called the **cone of light**.

27. Second branchial arch.

- Each pharyngeal arch is made of mesenchyme which are invaded by neural crest cells
- Each arch is covered by an outer ectoderm and inner endoderm layers
- The neural crest cells of each arch contribute, the skeletal element and associated connective tissue
- Initially six arches appear, of which the fifth one disappears
- Second arch is also called as the **hyoid arch**
- It extends from midline of neck to the ear capsule
- The cartilage of the arch is **Reichert's cartilage**
- The cartilage gets ossified in some places to form bones and in some places the cartilage disappears and the fibrous sheath forms ligament
- The **nerve of the arch** is facial nerve
- The **artery of the arch** is stapedial artery which disappears later
- The mesodermal cells of the arch gives rise to musculature supplied by the nerve of the arch and it is retained even if they migrate

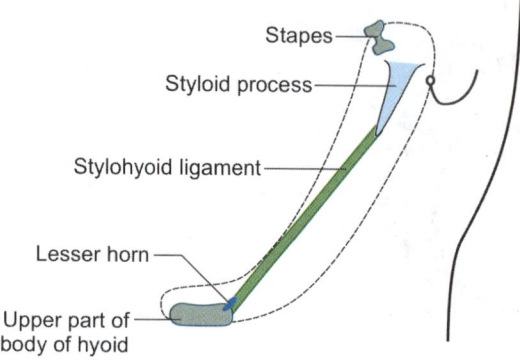

Fig. 52: Second arch derivatives.

Structures derived from it are ('S')

From cartilage		Muscles
Bones	Ligaments	
Stapes	**S**tylohyoid ligament	**S**tapedius
Styloid process of temporal bone		Muscles of facial expression
Lesser (**s**mall) horn of hyoid bone		Auricular muscles
Upper (**s**uperior) part of body of hyoid bone		Posterior belly of digastrics
		Stylohyoid
		Platysma
		Occipitofrontalis

28. Chorda tympani.

- It is a **branch** from facial nerve given within the facial canal
- It **contains** secreto motor fibers (parasympathetic) from superior salivatory nucleus and carry taste fibers from anterior two-third of tongue
- It **arises** about 6 mm above the stylomastoid foramen
- **Course**
  - It leaves the facial canal and reenters the tympanic cavity through posterior canaliculus
  - Runs medial to handle of malleus
  - Passes between fibrous and mucous layer of tympanic membrane
  - It leaves the tympanic cavity through anterior canaliculus
  - Enters the infratemporal fossa by passing through petrotympanic fissure
  - Reaches behind the capsule of temporomandibular joint
  - It grooves the medial side of spine of sphenoid posterolateral to tensor palati muscle
  - Runs forwards deep to lateral pterygoid muscle
  - It is crossed by the middle meningeal artery, auriculotemporal and inferior alveolar nerve.
- **Termination:** Deep to lateral pterygoid muscle it joins with the lingual nerve at an acute angle
- **Structures supplied**
  - Through lingual nerve it supplies secretomotor fibers to submandibular and sublingual glands

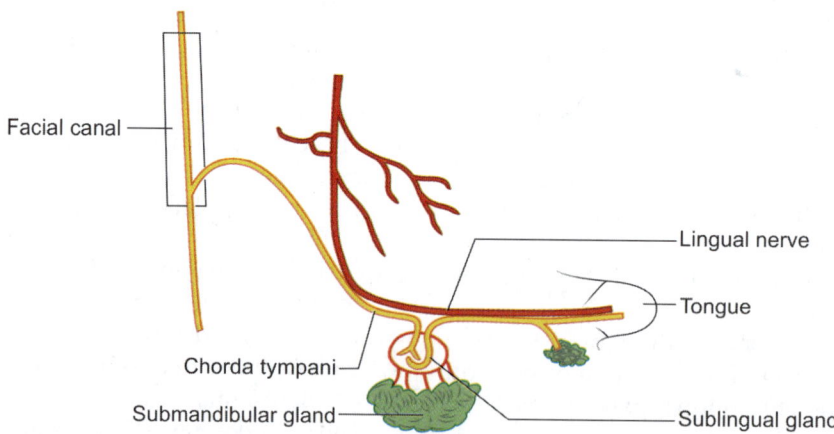

Fig. 53: Chorda tympani.

- Carries taste sensation from the mucous membrane of anterior two-third of tongue excluding the vallate papillae.
- **Applied anatomy:** The lingual nerve is very closely related to the 3rd molar tooth, just separated by mucous membrane. Care should be taken during extraction of the tooth. Injury to it results in loss of secretomotor fibers to the submandibular and sublingual glands, and taste sensation will be lost.

29. Amnion.

- Embryo blast or the inner cell mass are arranged as bilaminar disc
- The upper layer is called primitive ectoderm and inner layer endoderm
- The outer cell mass is arranged as inner cytotrophoblast and outer syncytiotrophoblast
- A space appear by 2nd week between the ectoderm and cytotrophoblast resulting in a cavity called amniotic cavity
- The roof of the cavity is formed by newly formed cell known as amnion cells/amnioblast
- The floor is formed by ectoderm lined by tall columnar cells
- The cavity contains fluid which has nutritive value
- With the extension of extraembryonic coelom, the amniotic cavity and yolk sac cavities are surrounded by extraembryonic mesoderm
- The mesoderm is continuous with chorion through the connecting stalk
- Due to the folding of the embryo, the amniotic cavity with fluid surrounds the embryo
- As the amniotic cavity increases, the extraembryonic coelom is completed obliterated.
- **Functions:**
  - Protection of fetus from external pressure and shock
  - It allows foetal movements
  - Maintains a constant temperature
  - The pressure exerted by the fluid helps for a proper growth and differentiation of the tissue of the embryo
  - The fluid prevents the adherence of skin with amnion.
- **Anomalies:**
  - Hydramnios—excess amount of fluid
  - Oligoamnios—diminution of amniotic fluid. Results in maldevelopment of fetus
  - Amniocentesis—the amniotic fluid is aspirated by a needle to find out sex of fetus and to analyze alpha-fetoprotein to diagnose neural tube defects.

30. Lateral pterygoid muscle.

It has 2 heads—upper and lower
- **Origin:**
  - Upper head—infratemporal crest and infratemporal surface of greater wing of sphenoid bone

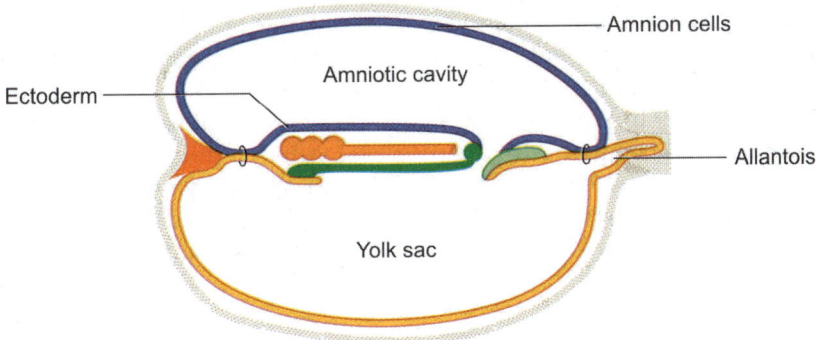

Fig. 54: Amnion.

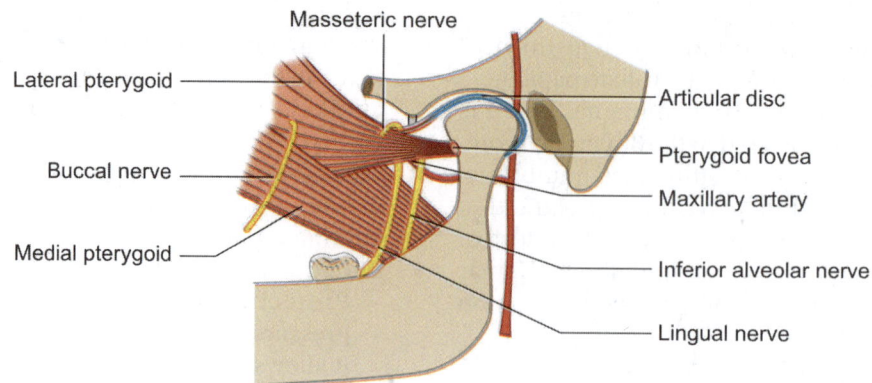

Fig. 55: Lateral pterygoid muscle.

- Lower head—lateral surface of lateral pterygoid plate.
- **Insertion:**
  - Pterygoid fovea along the anterior surface of neck of mandible
  - Articular capsule and disc of temporomandibular joint.
- **Nerve supply:** Pterygoid branch from anterior division of mandibular nerve.
- **Action:**
  - Depresses (opening of mouth) the mandible
  - Both pterygoids help in side to side - chewing movement
  - Lower head helps in protrusion of mandible.
- **Relations:**
  - Superficial—temporalis, 2nd part of maxillary artery, superficial part of medial pterygoid, ramus of mandible
  - Deep—middle meningeal artery Mandibular nerve and its branches, otic ganglion, chorda tympani, sphenomandibular ligament, deep head of medial pterygoid muscle
  - Upper border—masseteric nerve, deep temporal nerve
  - Lower border—lingual and inferior alveolar nerves
  - Between two heads—buccal branch of mandibular nerve emerges and maxillary artery dips in
- **Applied anatomy:** In wide yawning the head of mandible gets dislocated anteriorly. The jaw gets locked and patient cannot close the mouth.

31. Muscles of tongue.

- **Extrinsic muscles:**
  - Origin from outside the tongue and insertion into the tongue
  - Does not alter the shape of tongue
  - Extrinsic muscles are genioglossus, hyoglossus, chondroglossus, styloglossus, palatoglossus.
- **Intrinsic muscles:**
  - Origin and insertion both within the tongue
  - Alters the **shape** of the tongue
  - Intrinsic muscles are longitudinal, vertical, transverse muscles
  - All the muscles of the tongue are supplied by hypoglossal nerve **except** palatoglossus by cranial accessory through pharyngeal plexus.

S. No	Name of muscle	Origin	Insertion	Action
1	Genioglossus	Upper genial tubercle of mandible	Whole length of the ventral surface of the tongue from root to apex, intermingling with the intrinsic muscle	1. Protrusion of the tongue. It prevents falling back of the tongue. Hence known as safety muscle of the tongue 2. Central depression
2	Hyoglossus	From whole length of the upper border of the greater cornu and part of the body of the hyoid bone	Side of the tongue lateral to geniohyoid muscle	Depresses the tongue

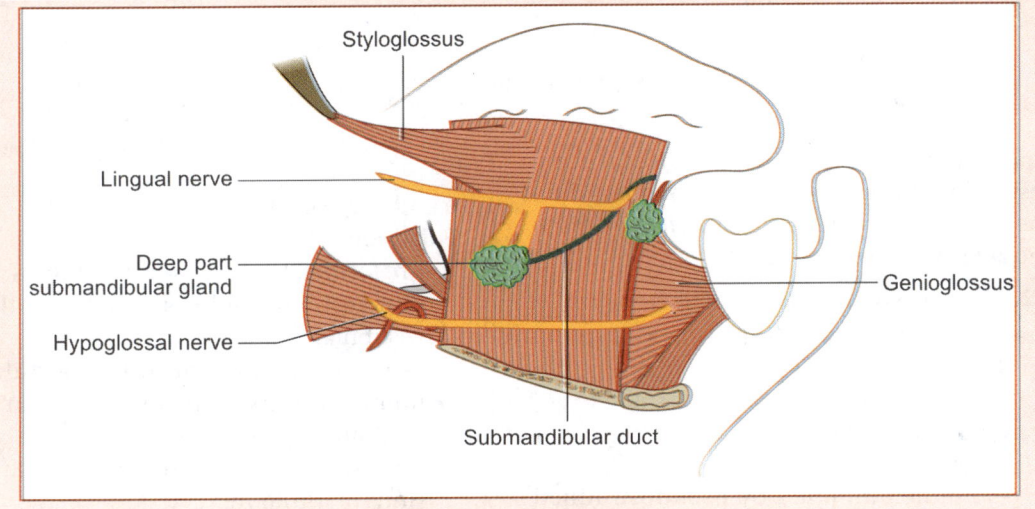

Fig. 56: Muscles of tongue.

S. No	Name of muscle	Origin	Insertion	Action
3	Chondroglossus	From base of lesser cornu of the hyoid bone	Merges with the intrinsic muscles	Depression of the tongue.
4	Styloglossus	Anterolateral surface of styloid process near the tip and upper part of stylohyoid ligament	1. The upper fibers longitudinal part merges with longitudinal muscle of tongue. 2. The lower oblique part decussates with hyoglossus.	Pulls the tongue upwards and backwards—retraction.
5	Palatoglossus	Oral surface of palatine aponeurosis	1. Some fibers to the dorsum of the tongue 2. Others interdigitate with the transverse muscle fibers.	1. Elevates the tongue. 2. Closes the oral cavity from oropharynx.
6	Longitudinal Superior	1. From the submucosa near the epiglottis 2. From the median septum of tongue	Inserted into the mucous membrane	Shortens the tongue by folding
	Inferior	From the root of the tongue	To the apex	
7	Transverse	From the median septum	The mucous membrane along the margin	Narrows and elongates the tongue
8	Vertical	From the dorsal surface	Ventral aspects of the tongue	Flattens and broadens the tongue

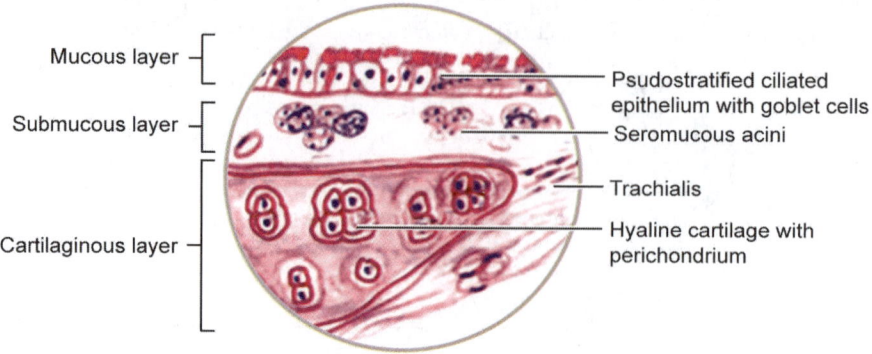

Fig. 57: Histology of trachea.

Applied anatomy: Injury to hypoglossal nerve results in paralysis of muscles of tongue. When the patient protrudes the tongue, it deviates to the side of lesion.

32. Microscopic structure of trachea.

Trachea is lined internally by:
- Mucous layer
- Submucous layer
- Cartilaginous layer
- **Mucous layer:**
  - Epithelium lined by pseudostratified ciliated columnar epithelium with goblet cells
  - Six types of epithelial cell are present in the trachea—ciliated columnar, goblet cell, Clara cell, basal cell, brush cell and neuroendocrine cell
  - From the underlying connective tissue of submucous layer the lymphocytes and mast cells enter.
- **Submucous layer:** Seromucous glands of tubuloacinar type, are present in this layer
- **Cartilage:** The trachea contains a framework of incomplete C shaped rings of hyaline cartilage connected by fibrous tissue. The gap is filled by the smooth muscle called trachialis.

33. Vocal cords.

- The cavity of the larynx is divided into three parts by two pairs of vocal folds—vestibular and vocal folds (cords).

Types

True and false vocal cords
- **False vocal cord**
  - Are formed by the **vestibular fold**
  - The vestibular fold is formed by the vestibular ligament
  - The lower end of quadrangular membrane is thickened to form vestibular ligament
  - **Situated** between the vestibule and sinus of the larynx
  - It **extends** from angle of thyroid cartilage to anterolateral surface of arytenoid cartilage
  - It is pink in **color**
  - They are named as false as they do not take part in phonation
  - The **lining epithelium** is ciliated columnar epithelium
  - The space between the two vestibular folds is known as **rima vestibule**.
- **True vocal cord (Fig. 58)**
  - Are formed by the vocal folds
  - **Situated** between the sinus and infraglottic part of the larynx
  - It **extends** between the angle of thyroid cartilage to tip of vocal process of arytenoid cartilage
  - Each fold **contains** mucous membrane, lamina propria, vocalis muscle, and the vocal ligament

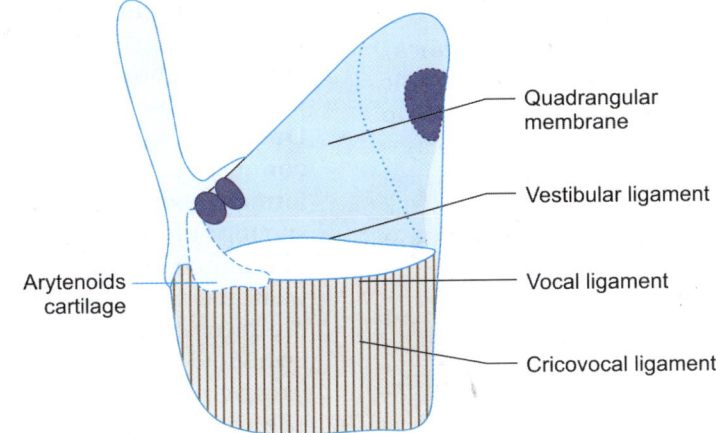

Fig. 58: Interior of larynx.

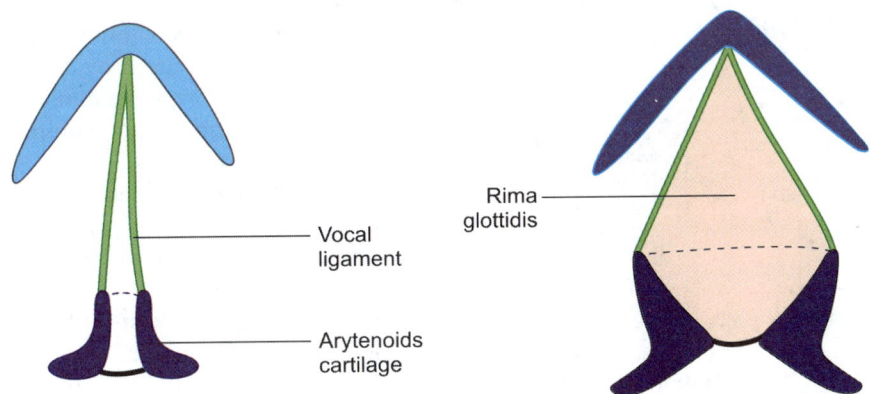

Fig. 59: Rima glottidis.

- It is pearly white in **colour** as the ligament is attached to the underlying lamina and absence of blood vessels
- The **lining epithelium** of vocal cord is stratified squamous epithelium
- The space between the two vocal cords is known as **rima glottidis or the glottis**
- The **rima glottidis** is bounded behind by the interarytenoid fold of mucous membrane
- The glottis is divided into two parts, an anterior **intermembranous part**, between the two vocal ligament which forms 3/5 of rima, and a posterior **intercartilagenous part** formed by the vocal processes of the arytenoid cartilages. There is change in the width and shape according to the movements of the vocal cords and arytenoid cartilages during respiration and phonation
- **Muscles acting on vocal cord:**
    - Tensor of vocal cord—cricothyroid:
    - Relaxor of vocal cord—vocalis, thyroarytenoid
    - Abductor of vocal cord—posterior cricoarytenoid:
    - Adductor—lateral cricoarytenoid, transverse arytenoids, oblique arytenoids.

Applied Anatomy

Vocal fold nodules called **singer's/clergyman's nodules** are due to chronic lesions of the vocal folds. The reason is due to repeated over use of the voice which increases the tension and forceful adduction of vocal fold. The nodule appears at the junction of the anterior third and the posterior two-thirds of the vocal ligament.

34. Microscopic structure and development of palatine tonsil.

- It is covered by **mucous membrane** of the oropharynx **(Fig. 60)**
- Lined by **non-keratinized stratified squamous epithelium**
- The mucous membrane invaginates into the underlining connective tissue called the **crypts**
- Around 10 – 12 crypts are seen and are filled with plugs of desquamated epithelial cells, lymphocytes and oral bacteria, which sometimes calcify
- Deep to mucous membrane, the connective tissue is made of network formed by collagen type III fibers which supports the tonsil
- The septae extends from the connective tissue merge with fibrous hemi capsule on the deep aspect of the tonsil
- Lymphoid follicles, are arranged along the lengths of tonsillar crypts
- The size of the follicle varies according to the activity of the tonsil
- The follicles contain lightly stained germinal center
- The mantle zones of follicle nearest to the mucosal surface are provided with, small lymphocytes, forming a dense cap
- The serous and mucous acini are in the deeper aspect of tonsil
- The epithelial cells covering the tonsil has intimate relation with lymphocytes and helps for direct transfer of antigen from external environment to tonsillar lymphoid tissue, resembling similar to M-fold (M cells) of gut.
- **Development of tonsil (Fig. 61)**
  - The palatine tonsil is **developed** from the ventral part of second pharyngeal pouch (endodermal)

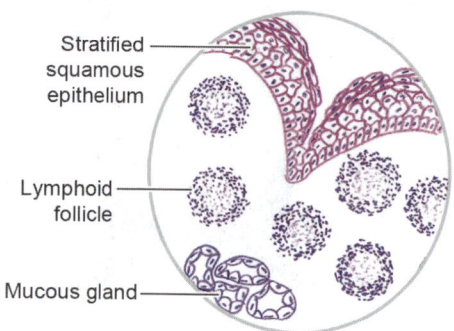

Fig. 60: Histology of tonsil.

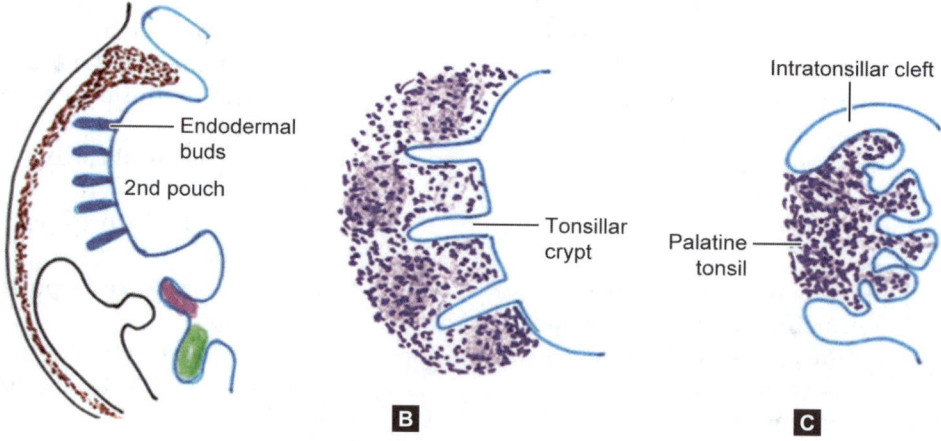

Figs. 61A to C: Development of tonsil.

- The endodermal cells proliferate and protrude into the surrounding mesenchyme as solid buds
- The central cells of the bud are destroyed to form tonsillar crypts
- **Tonsil stroma** is derived from the mesoderm of second pharyngeal arch
- **Lymphoid tissue** of tonsil develops from mesenchyme.
- The accumulation of lymphoid follicles produces inward bulging on the tonsil into the oropharynx
- The major part of the pouch gets obliterated except a part persists as **intratonsillar cleft**.

35. Hilum of lungs.
Refer essay Q. No. 3 – 2004.

36. Dentate nucleus.
- Dentate is one of the deep nuclei of cerebellum
- **Situated** on either cerebellar hemispheres within the whitematter
- It is the largest and laterally situated nucleus
- Shape: Like a crumpled bag and the hilum faces medially
- The interior of the nucleus is filled with white matter made up of efferent fibers
- The efferent fibers from nuclei form major part of the superior cerebellar peduncle.
- **Connection**:
  - **Efferent**
    - Dentatothalamic fibers—to the lateral and anterior part of ventral nuclei of thalamus, and from thalamus to motor cortex
    - Dentatorubral fibers—end in red nucleus
    - The descending fibers end in inferior olivary complex.
  - **Afferent**:
    - It receives fibers from premotor and supplementary motor cortex via pontocerebellar fibers
    - Fibers from cerebellar cortex.
- **Development/Morphology**: It belongs to neocerebellum.
- **Functions:** It regulates the motor functions through corticospinal and corticobulbar tracts.

37. Boundaries of tympanic cavity.
- Tympanic cavity is the middle ear cavity situated between external and internal ear
- It is situated within the petrous part of the temporal bone
- It is cuboidal in shape
- It **communicates** posteriorly with the mastoid antrum and the mastoid air cells, and anteriorly through the auditory tube with the nasopharynx
- Division: The space within the middle ear can be subdivided into three parts:
  1. **Mesotympanum or tympanic cavity proper**, which is opposite the tympanic membrane
  2. **Epitympanum or attic**, is portion superior to the membrane. The head of the malleus and the body and short process of the incus are present in this part
  3. **Hypotympanum**, related to the floor of the cavity, and is between the superior bulb of IJV and the lower margin of the tympanic membrane.

The boundaries (Fig. 62): It has roof, floor, medial, lateral, anterior and posterior walls.
- **Roof (tegmental wall):** It is formed by the bony plate the tegmen tympani of temporal bone. It separates the middle ear cavity from cranial cavity

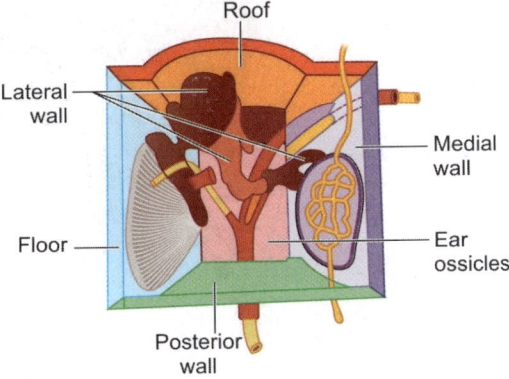

Fig. 62: Boundaries.

- **Floor (jugular wall):** The jugular fossa forms the floor. The superior bulb of the internal jugular vein is separated from the cavity by the fossa. Sometimes the wall may be incomplete, in which case, the mucous membrane and fibrous tissue separates the tympanic cavity and the vein
- **Lateral wall (membranous wall):** The lateral wall consists mainly of the tympanic membrane which is attached to the ring of bone. The anterior and posterior canaliculi are small openings for the passage of chorda tympani are present.
- **Medial wall (labyrinthine wall):** The features are (Fig. 63)
    - **Promontory:** Rounded elevation produced by the basal turn of cochlea. Below this a depression seen called sinus tympani
    - **Fenestra vestibule:** It is also called as oval window. It is posterosuperior to the promontory, with convexity facing upwards. It is covered by foot plate of stapes
    - **Fenestra cochlea:** Round window situated posteroinferiorly to promontory. It is closed by secondary tympanic membrane
    - **Prominence produced by facial canal**
       – seen superior to the oval window, and then curves down into the posterior wall of the cavity.
- **Anterior wall (carotid wall):** It is divided into a lower larger part forming carotid canal occupied by internal carotid artery and an upper smaller part. The small part is divided into two by a bony plate. The upper one is canal for tensor tympani and lower bony part of auditory tube.
- **Posterior wall (mastoid wall) (Fig. 64)**
  The features are:
    - Aditus to mastoid antrum
    - Fossa incudis to lodge the short process of incus
    - Pyramidal eminence for the stapedius muscle is situated in front of vertical part of facial canal.

Contents
- 3 ear ossicles—malleus, incus and stapes
- 2 muscles—tensor tympani, stapedius
- Nerve plexus, blood vessels
- Air.

Blood supply: Supplied by the middle meningeal artery, artery of pterygoid canal, anterior tympanic artery.

Applied anatomy:
- Infection of the mastoid antrum and mastoid air cells may spread into the middle cranial fossa through the petrosquamous fissure in children

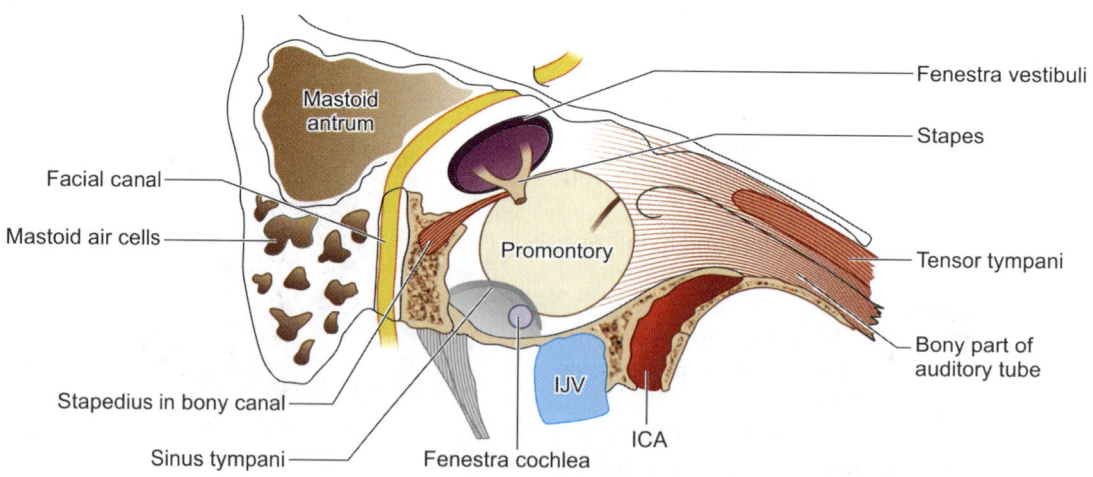

Fig. 63: Medial wall.

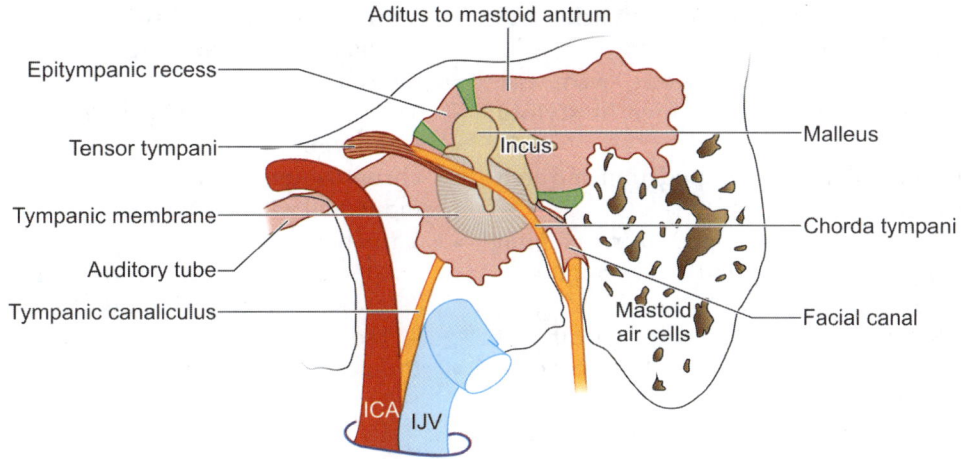

Fig. 64: Posterior wall.

- Perforation of the tympanic membrane may be due to otitis media, foreign bodies, trauma, or excessive pressure.

38. Styloid process.

- Styloid process is present in temporal bone
- Situated medial to mastoid process
- Passes between internal and external carotid arteries
- It extends just lateral to tonsillar fossa
- The tip extends medial to posterior border of ramus of mandible
- It has **two parts**—tympanohyal and stylohyal
- Tympanohyal (base) is covered by the tympanic plate
- Stylohyal projects outside
- It is crossed laterally by the facial nerve close to the base and apex by the external carotid artery

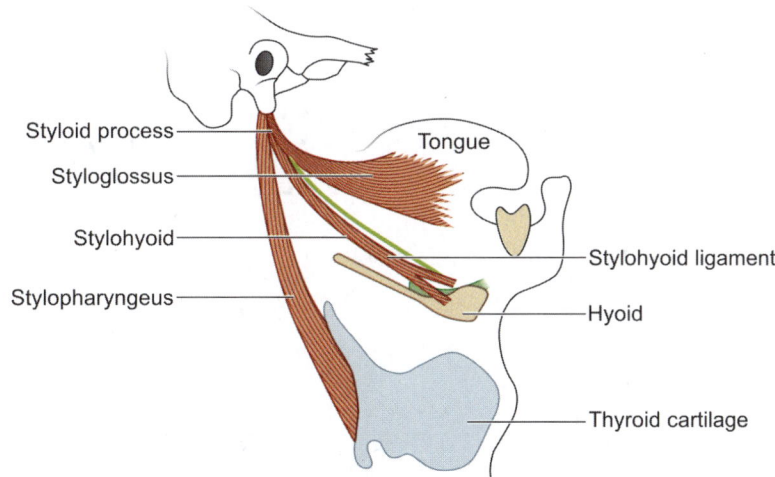

Fig. 65: Styloid apparatus.

- It gives attachment to three muscles and two ligaments
- The styloid process along with the structures attached is known as **styloid apparatus**
- Styloid process is **developed** from 2nd arch
- **Muscles attached** are –
  - Styloglossus developed from occipital myotomes supplied by hypoglossal nerve
  - Stylopharyngeus developed from 3rd arch supplied by glossopharyngeal nerve
  - Stylohyoid developed from 2nd arch supplied by facial nerve.
- **Ligaments** are –
  - Stylohyoid ligament developed from 2nd arch
  - Stylomandibular ligament thickening of deep cervical fascia.
- **Applied anatomy**: Eagle' syndrome – long styloid process with calcified stylohyoid ligament results in pain in oropharynx and neck. It radiates to the ear and increased during swallowing.

39. Klinefelter's syndrome.

- Klinefelter syndrome is a rare genetic condition which **affects male**
- Man has an **extra X chromosome**
- A total of 47 chromosomes will be present per cell
- This is referred to as **(47, XXY) syndrome**
- **Genotype**: Due to non-disjunction of XY chromosome present in the sperm. The individual will be 47, XXY.
- Karyotype:
  - Men with Klinefelter syndrome have the extra X chromosome - 47, XXY"
  - Mosaicism
- **Phenotype:**
  - Small testis and penis
  - Reduced intelligence
  - Reduced facial and body hair
  - Tall stature
  - Gynecomastia (development of breast).
- **Associated conditions**
  - Hypothyroidism
  - Infertility
  - Testicular cancer
  - Increased risk for male breast cancer
  - Osteoporosis.

40. Pleural recesses.

Refer essay Q. No. 3 – 2003.

MBBS Examination 2006

ANSWER ALL QUESTIONS

I. Essay questions (15/10 Marks)

1. Describe the pancreas under the following headings: (a) Morphology, (b) Relations, (c) Microscopic anatomy, (d) Development, and (e) Clinical anatomy.
2. Describe the shoulder joint under the following headings: Definition, articular surfaces, ligaments, movements and muscles causing the movements and applied anatomy.
3. Describe the uterus under the following headings: Position, parts, supports, structure, arterial supply, and applied anatomy.
4. Describe the extension, the bed, blood supply and lymphatic drainage of mammary gland. Add a note on its clinical importance.
5. Describe the formation, termination, course, tributaries and relations of portal vein.
6. Describe the internal capsule of brain under the following heading: Position, divisions, constituent fibers, blood supply and applied anatomy.
7. Describe the heart under the following headings: Position, coverings, internal features, conducting and skeletal systems and applied anatomy.
8. Describe the pharynx under the following headings: Extent, divisions, internal features, musculature, structures related and applied anatomy.
9. Define a typical intercostal nerve. Describe the course and distribution. Add a note on its clinical importance.
10. Describe the parotid gland under the following headings: (i) Extension, (ii) Features, (iii) Relations, (iv) Innervations, and (v) Applied aspects.

II. Short notes (5/3/2 Marks)

1. Microscopic structure of hyaline cartilage.
2. Prostatic part of urethra.
3. Adductor canal.
4. Paramesonephric duct.
5. Clavipectoral fascia.
6. Deep peroneal nerve.
7. Microscopic anatomy of fundus of stomach.
8. Anastomosis around elbow.
9. Femoral sheath.
10. Congenital anomalies of kidney.
11. Histology of compact bone.
12. Triceps brachii.
13. Second part of duodenum.
14. Trigone of urinary bladder.
15. Great saphenous vein.
16. Yolk sac.
17. Bronchopulmonary segments.
18. Fate of aortic arches.
19. Hyoglossus muscle.
20. Cerebellar peduncles.
21. Lateral wall of nose.
22. Microscopic structure of ganglions (spinal and sympathetic).
23. Blood supply and nerve supply of scalp.
24. Histology of palatine tonsil.
25. Development of interatrial septum.
26. Circle of Willis.
27. Lacrimal apparatus.

28. Turner's syndrome.
29. External jugular vein.
30. Histology of cerebellum.
31. Sternocleidomastoid.
32. Development of tongue.

I. ESSAY QUESTIONS

1. **Describe the pancreas under the following headings: (a) Morphology, (b) Relations, (c) Microscopic anatomy, (d) Development and (e) Clinical anatomy.**

Morphology

Type of Gland

- It is a compound acinar type of gland—majority exocrine and small part of endocrine.
- Ducts
  - Main duct (duct of Wirsung)
  - Accessory duct (duct of Santorini).
- Main duct **(Fig. 1)**
  - Lies near the posterior surface. It begins at the tail, runs left to right
  - Receives tributaries at right angles like a pattern of Herring bone appearance
  - It joins with the bile duct to form the hepato—pancreatic duct/ampulla of Vater which opens on the summit of the major duodenal papilla, along the posteromedial wall of 2nd part of duodenum. It is 8 – 10 cm distal to the pylorus of stomach.
- **Accessory duct**
  - Receives secretion from upper part of head of pancreas
  - Crosses in front of the main duct and communicates with it
  - Opens into the duodenum at minor duodenal papilla. It is 2 cm proximal to major duodenal papilla
  - The opening of the accessory duct lies medial and ventral to that of main duct.

Gross Features

It is lobulated, elongated, J-shaped gland.

- **Parts:** It has head, neck, body, tail and uncinate process **(Fig. 2).**
  - **Head:**
    - Enlarged, lies within the concavity of the duodenum
    - It is flattened
    - 4 borders—superior, inferior, right and left
    - 2 surfaces—anterior and posterior
    - 1 process—uncinate process.
  - **Neck:**
    - Constricted part, directed forwards, upwards and to the left
    - Two surfaces—anterior and posterior.
  - **Body:**
    - Elongated, directed upwards, backwards and to the left
    - Triangular in cross-section
    - 3 borders—superior, inferior and anterior.

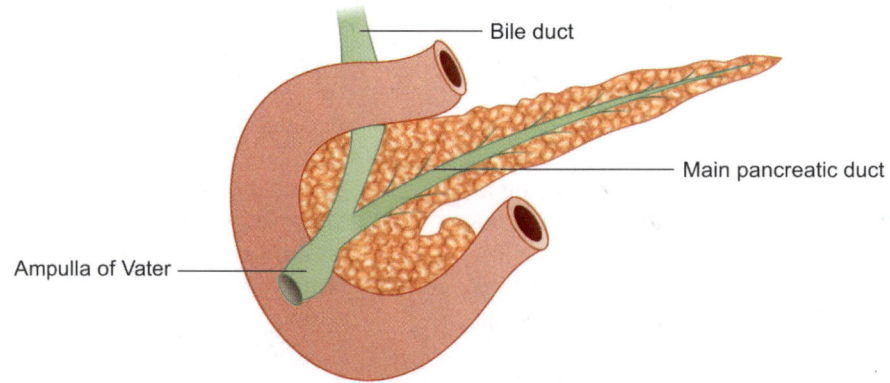

Fig. 1: Ducts of pancreas.

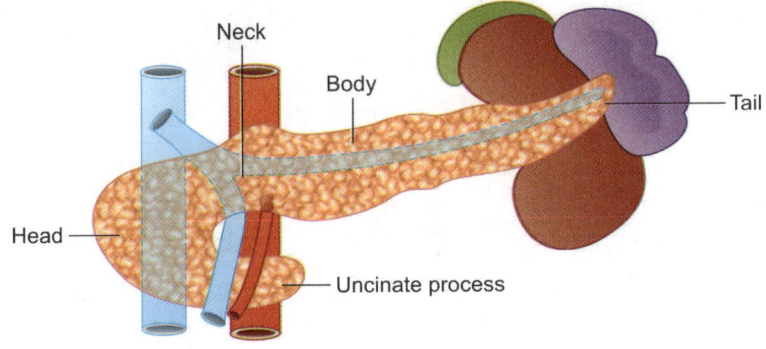

Fig. 2: Parts.

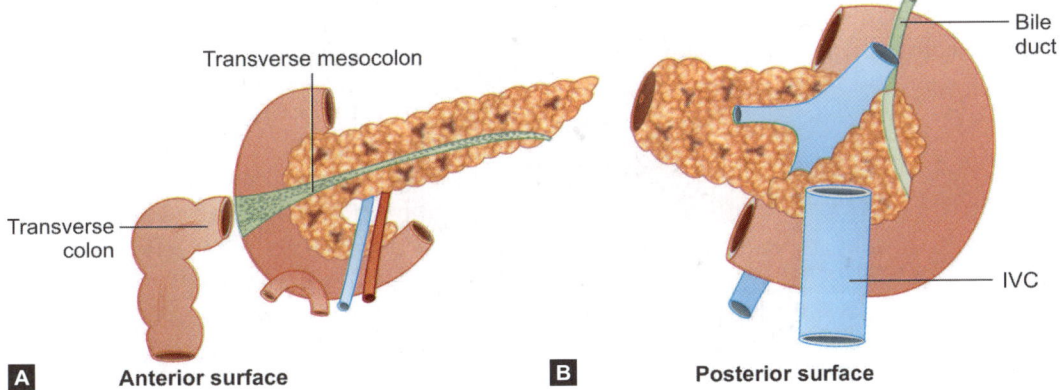

Figs. 3A and B: Relations of head.

- 3 surfaces—anterior, inferior and posterior.
- **Tail:** Left end, lies in the splenorenal ligament along with splenic vessels.

Relations

- **Head (Fig. 3)**
  - Anterior surface
    - First part of duodenum
    - Transverse colon
    - Transverse mesocolon
    - Jejunum.
  - Posterior surface
    - Inferior vena cava (IVC)
    - Terminal parts of renal veins
    - Right crus of diaphragm
    - Bile duct—embedded nearer to the posterior surface.
- **Uncinate process (Fig. 4)**
  - Anterior—superior mesenteric vessels
  - Posterior—aorta.

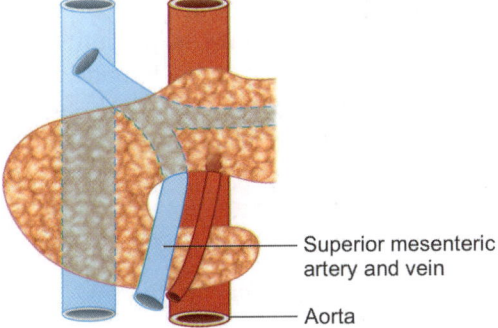

Fig. 4: Uncinate process.

- **Neck**
  - Anterior—lesser sac and pylorus
  - Posterior—superior mesenteric vein and portal vein.
- **Body (Figs. 5 and 6)**
  - Anterior border—gives attachment to transverse mesocolon

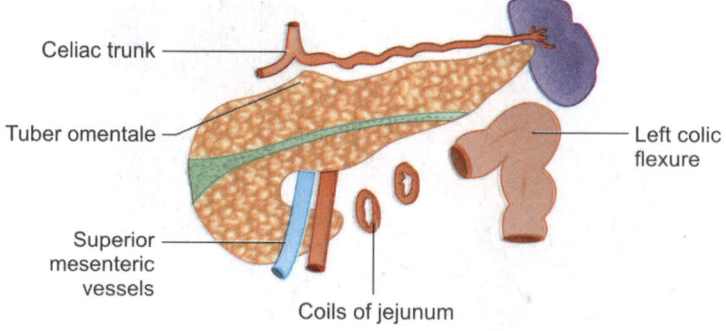

Fig. 5: Relations of body of pancreas.

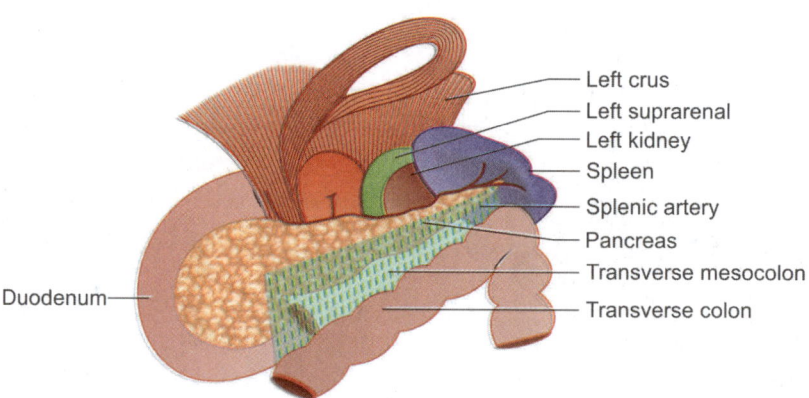

Fig. 6: Posterior relations.

- Superior border—a projection known as **tuber omentale** is present. It is related to coeliac trunk, hepatic artery and splenic artery
- Inferior border—superior mesenteric vessels.
- **Anterior surface**
  - Lesser sac
  - Stomach.
- **Posterior surface (Fig. 6)**
  - Aorta
  - Origin of superior mesenteric artery
  - Left crus of diaphragm
  - Left kidney across hilum
  - Left suprarenal gland
  - Left renal vessels
  - Splenic vein.
- **Inferior surface**
  - Duodenal flexure
  - Coils of jejunum
  - Left colic flexure.

- **Tail**
  - Lienorenal ligament
  - Splenic vessels
  - Spleen.

Microscopic Anatomy

Refer short notes 10 – 2003.

Development

Refer short notes 6 – 2005.

Applied Anatomy

- Carcinoma of head of pancreas is common. It results in jaundice, ascites
- Annular pancreas—obstructs the 2nd part of duodenum
- Pancreatitis—inflammation of pancreas presents with symptoms of fever and pain at the back
- Endoscopic retrograde cholangio pancreatography (ERCP), Magnetic

retrograde cholangiopancreatography (MRCP) are radiological procedures to out pattern of duct system.

2. **Describe the shoulder joint under the following headings: Definition, articular surfaces, ligaments, movements and muscles causing the movements and applied anatomy.**

Type (Definition)

Synovial, multi axial, and ball and socket variety.

Articulating Parts (Fig. 7)

- Glenoid cavity of scapula and the head of humerus
- **Glenoid cavity of scapula**: Pear shaped, concave, directed upwards, forwards and laterally. Anterior border is notched and the cavity is lined by articular cartilage which is thin at the centre and thick at the periphery. The cavity is deepened by the glenoidal labrum
- **Head of humerus:** Hemispherical, directed upwards, backwards and medially, lined by articular cartilage which is thick at the centre and thin at the periphery. It forms one-third of sphere.

Ligaments

- **Fibrous Capsule (Fig. 8):**
  - Medially attached to the margin of glenoid cavity beyond glenoidal labrum and encloses the origin of long head of biceps
  - Laterally to the anatomical neck of humerus

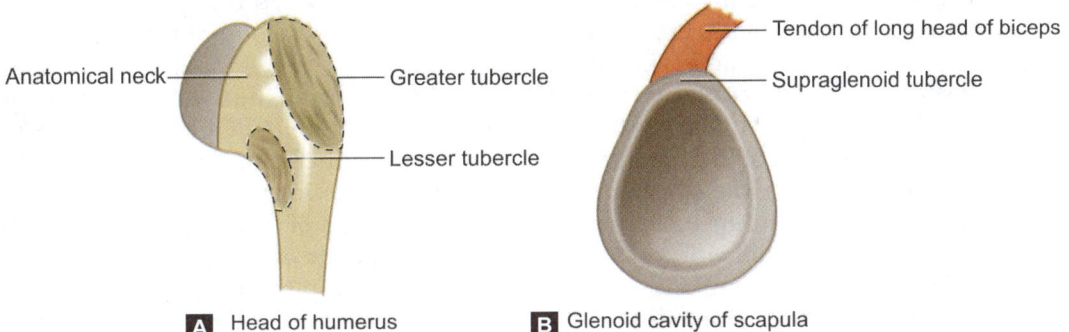

Figs. 7A and B: Articulating parts.

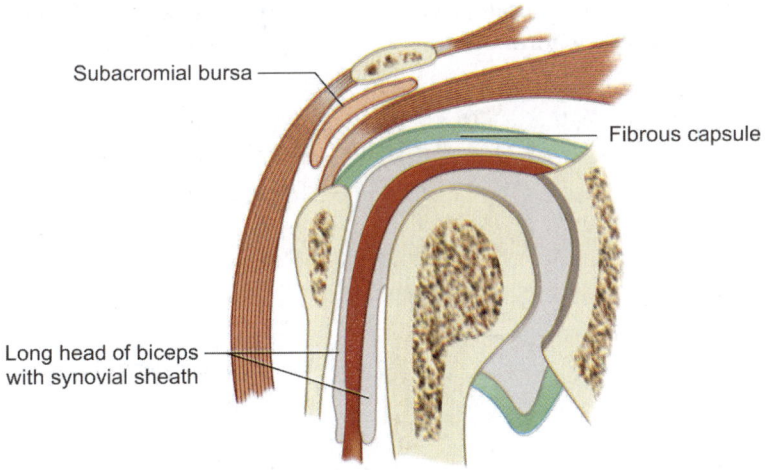

Fig. 8: Fibrous capsule.

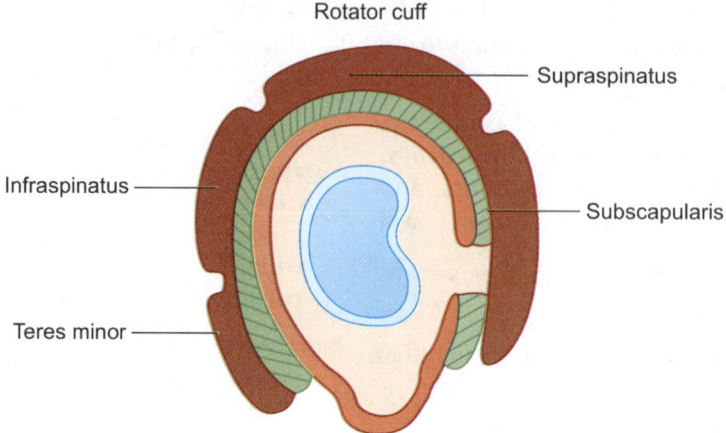

Fig. 9: Rotator cuff.

- Inferiorly extends for 1 cm below the anatomical neck
- The capsule is least supported inferiorly
- It is strengthened by the **rotator cuff** The muscles fuse with the capsule of the shoulder joint and is called as **musculotendinous cuff/rotator cuff of Codmann (Fig. 9)**
- The cuff usually collide against the coracoacromial arch when the humerus is abducted, flexed and internally rotated.
- Components of rotator cuff
   - Anteriorly—subscapularis
   - Superiorly—supraspinatus
   - Posteriorly—infraspinatus and teres minor
   - These tendons merge with lateral part of articular capsule to form the cuff
- It is supported inferiorly by the long head of triceps. The axillary nerve and posterior circumflex vessels intervene between triceps and the capsule
- The synovial membrane lines the capsule
- Three **openings** are present in the capsule. 1. Opening anteriorly communicating with subscapular bursa. 2. Opening for the passage of long head of biceps. 3. Posteriorly an inconstant opening communicating with infraspinatus bursa.

- **Transverse humeral ligament (Fig. 10)**
Between lesser tubercle and greater tubercle of humerus. It acts as a retinaculum and holds the tendon of long head of biceps brachii in position.

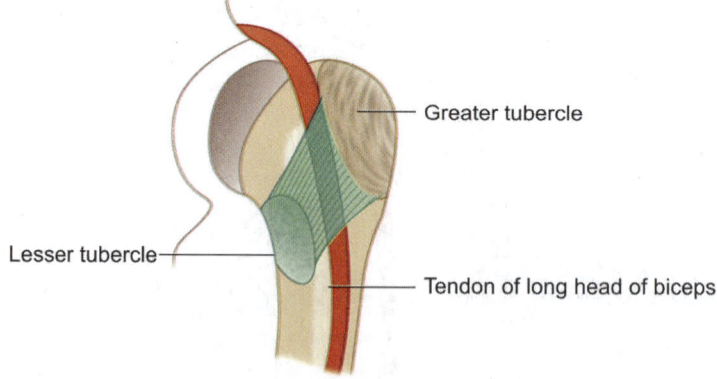

Fig. 10: Transverse humeral ligament.

- **Glenohumeral ligament (Fig. 11)**
  - It is seen inside the capsule
  - It is seen as 3 bands—superior, middle and inferior bands
  - These are thickening of the anterior aspect of the capsule
  - Extends between the anterior border of glenoid cavity to the anatomical neck of humerus and lesser tubercle
  - It is taut during abduction and rotation of humerus.
- **Coracohumeral ligament**: Extends from the base of coracoid process to the capsule between greater and lesser tubercles. Checks the lateral rotation of humerus.
- **Glenoidal labrum**
  - It is made of fibro cartilage, triangular in section
  - Attached to the margin of glenoid cavity
  - Helps to deepen the cavity.
- **Synovial sheath and bursae around the joint:**
  - The synovial membrane lines the fibrous capsule
  - A sheath envelops the tendon of the long head of biceps brachii and extends up to the surgical neck of humerus
  - Subacromial bursa—between supraspinatus below and coracoacromial arch and deltoid above. It is the largest bursa. It is also called as the sub deltoid bursa when it extends deep to deltoid
  - Subscapular bursa – between subscapularis and fibrous capsule. It communicates with the joint cavity
  - Infraspinatus bursa – occasionally present
  - Supraacromial bursa lies above the acromion process.

Movements and Muscles Producing

- **Flexion:**
  - Carrying the arm anteromedially
  - It is along horizontal plane
  - Muscles producing are: Clavicular head of pectoralis major, anterior fibers of deltoid, coracobrachialis, short head of biceps brachii.
- **Extension**: Muscles producing are—posterior fibers of deltoid, teres major, latissimus dorsi, sterno-costal fibers of pectoralis major.
- **Abduction**:
  - The arm is carried away from the trunk laterally till it comes in horizontal position
  - The abduction is further continued to raise the arm above the head and the arm moves a total of 180 degrees (overhead abduction)
    - 0 – 15 degrees: By supraspinatus
    - 15 – 90 degrees: By middle fibers of deltoid
    - Above 90 degrees: By trapezius and serratus anterior.
  - Up to 90 degrees, the movement is confined to the shoulder joint
  - For next 30 degrees, there is lateral rotation of humerus
  - Above 120 degrees the abduction is done by scapular movement along with the shoulder joint movement
  - For every 15 degrees of movement 10 degree is contributed by shoulder and 5 degrees by the scapular movement in the ratio of 2:1.
- **Adduction**: Muscles producing are Latissimus dorsi, subscapularis, infraspinatus, teres major and minor, pectoralis major, short head of biceps brachii, long head of triceps brachii
- **Medial rotation**: Pectoralis major, anterior fibers of deltoid, latissimus dorsi, teres major, subscapularis.

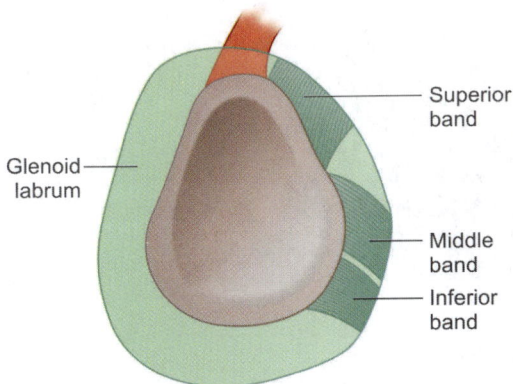

Fig. 11: Glenohumeral ligament.

- **Lateral rotation**:
  - Posterior fibers of deltoid, infraspinatus, teres minor
  - **Circumduction**: Successive movements as above.

Applied Anatomy

- **Subacromial bursitis**: Inflammatory reaction may be due to calcium deposition in the tendon of supraspinatus leading to irritation of the subacromial bursa
- **Calcified scapulohumeral bursitis**: Inflammation and calcification of the subacromial bursa results in pain, tenderness, and reduction in movements of shoulder joint
  - Rotator cuff disease
  - (Refer Short 4 – 2003)
  - **Dislocation:** It is the commonest joint to dislocate. Usually the dislocation is anteroinferior which lacks support. Posterior dislocation is usually due to violent movement as in epileptic seizures or electric shock
  - **Tear of glenoid labrum** commonly occur in the baseball players. The tear is due to sudden contraction of biceps
  - **Rupture of tendon of supraspinatus** leads to difficulty in initiation of abduction of shoulder.

3. **Describe the uterus under the following headings: Position, parts, supports, structure, arterial supply, and applied anatomy.**

Position, Parts, Supports, Applied anatomy-Refer Essay Q. No. 2 – Aug 2004.
- **Microstructure of uterus (Fig. 12):** It is made up of 3 layers—endometrium, myometrium, perimetrium
- **Endometrium** is mucous layer
  - Lined by columnar epithelium, and before puberty by ciliated columnar
  - Deep to epithelium the stroma contains numerous simple tubular glands lined by columnar epithelium
  - The endometrium undergoes cyclic changes according to the menstrual cycle
  - Glands are straight in postmenstrual phase, in proliferative phase elongates, and secretary phase become twisted.
- **Myometrium is** muscular layer
  - Bundles of smooth muscles in various direction
  - Arranged as three layers—outer longitudinal, middle circular, inner oblique
  - Middle circular layer contains blood vessels and hence called **stratum vasculare**
  - The inner oblique layer contraction helps to arrest the uterine bleeding

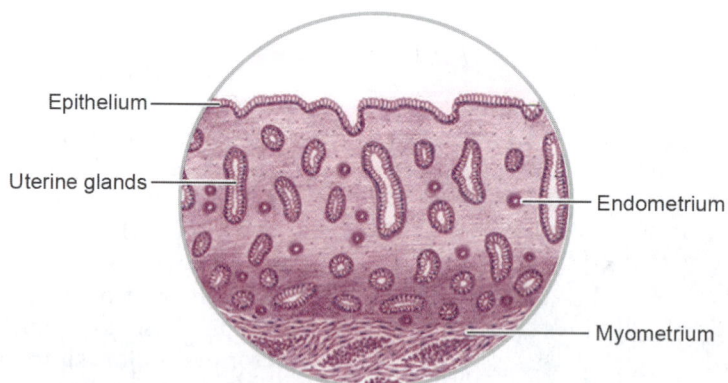

Fig. 12: Histology of uterus.

during placental separation. Hence the layer is named as **living ligature of the uterus**
- **Perimetrium** is serous layer formed by peritoneum.
- **Arterial supply: Uterine artery**
  - Branch from the anterior division of internal iliac artery
  - It is tortuous
  - It crosses the ureter and divides into an ascending and descending branch
  - The ascending branch runs along the lateral border of uterus within the broad ligament
  - It runs up to the hilum of ovary and anastomose with the ovarian artery
  - The smaller descending branch supplies cervix and anastomose with vaginal artery and take part in formation of **azygos artery of vagina**
  - The branches enter myometrium and supply circumferentially as anterior and posterior arcuate arteries
  - The terminal branches are tortuous called **helical arterioles**
  - The branches from helical arteriole enter the endometrium.

4. **Describe the extension, the bed, blood supply and lymphatic drainage of mammary gland. Add a note on its clinical importance.**

- The breast is secondary sexual feature of female and is present bilaterally
- Situated in the superficial fascia of pectoral region in both sexes
- In the male and pre-pubertal female, it is rudimentary
- Develops in female after puberty
- Enlarges during pregnancy and lactation
- Shape varies in adult female
- Mammary gland is a modified sweat gland. The mode of secretion is **apocrine** (milk fat) and **merocrine** (milk protein).

Extent (Fig. 13A)

- Horizontal—from lateral border of sternum to mid axillary line along 4th rib
- Vertical—from 2nd to 6th rib in mid-clavicular line
- A tail like projection extends from the upper and outer quadrant of the gland into axilla through an opening in the axillary fascia (Foramen of Langer) called the **axillary tail of Spence (Fig. 13B).**

Relations

Deep Relations (Mammary Bed) (Fig. 13A)

- Formed by
  - Medial two-third—pectoralis major
  - Lateral one-third—serratus anterior
  - Inferomedially—external oblique aponeurosis.
- Loose connective tissue intervening between the base of the gland and the deep fascia covering the mammary bed is known as **retromammary space**

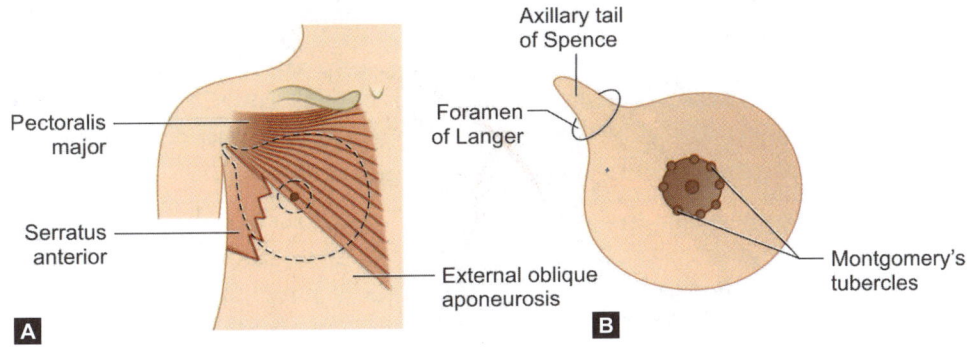

Figs. 13A and B: Extent and mammary bed.

- This space protects the gland from external injury
- The space is avascular
- Space allows free flow of lymphatics and is called as **lake of Marcelli.**

Superficial Features (in Skin)
- **Nipple**
    - It is a conical projection below the center of the breast
    - Level: 4th intercostal space in nulliparous women
    - It is pierced by 15 – 20 lactiferous ducts
    - Circular and longitudinal smooth muscle fibers are seen in the nipple. It has rich nerve supply.
- **Areola**
    - It is a pigmented circular area of skin around the base of the nipple
    - Melanocytes are more in the skin of the nipple and areola
    - Numerous sweat and sebaceous glands present open directly onto the skin
    - The secretion of the sebaceous glands are oily, act as a lubricant and protect the areola
    - The sebaceous glands are arranged around the margin of the areola circularly as small elevations, called Montgomery's tubercles
    - Hair follicles are absent in the sebaceous glands of the areola
    - Beneath the areola each lactiferous duct dilates to form lactiferous sinus.

Blood Supply (Fig. 14)
- **Laterally:** Lateral thoracic artery from 2nd part of axillary artery
- **Superiorly:** Superior thoracic artery branch from 1st part of axillary artery
- **Anteromedially:** Perforating branches of internal thoracic artery
- **Anterolaterally:** Perforating branches of 2nd, 3rd and 4th anterior intercostal arteries. The branch from second is large and supply the nipple, areola and upper part of breast.

Venous Drainage
- Venous plexus of Sappey is formed around the areola
- The veins from plexus and glandular tissue drain into the axillary, internal thoracic and intercostal veins
- The veins communicate with the internal vertebral venous plexus of Batson and with the veins of clavicle, humerus and cervical vertebrae.

Lymphatic Drainage
Refer Short notes 19 – 2005.

Applied Anatomy
Refer Short notes 19 – 2005.

---

5. Describe the formation, termination, course, tributaries and relations of portal vein.

Formation, termination, tributaries - Refer Short Notes 6 – Aug 2004.

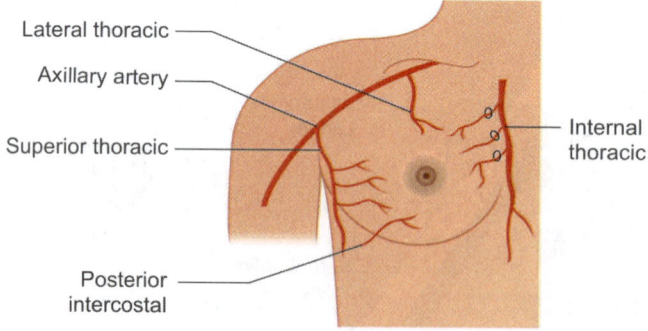

Fig. 14: Blood supply.

- **Course:**
  - It runs upwards and behind the neck of the pancreas
  - Next behind the first part of the duodenum
  - Above duodenum in the right free margin of the lesser omentum
  - The vein ends at the right end of the porta hepatis by dividing into right and left branches which enter the liver
  - The course of vein is divided into infra-, retro-, and supraduodenal parts.
- **Relations (Fig. 15):**
  - **Infraduodenal part:**
    - Anteriorly—neck of pancreas
    - Posteriorly—inferior vena cava.
  - **Retroduodenal part:**
    - Anteriorly—1st part of duodenum, bile duct, gastroduodenal artery
    - Posteriorly—inferior vena cava.
  - **Supraduodenal part:**
    - Anteriorly—hepatic artery, bile duct
    - Posteriorly—inferior vena cava, separated by epiploic foramen.
  - **At porta hepatis :**
    - The right branch is shorter and wider than the left branch
    - The left branch is longer and narrower than the right branch
    - Vein is posterior to right and left branches of hepatic artery and hepatic ducts.

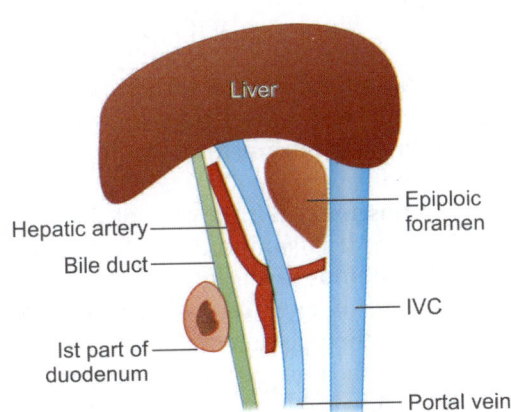

Fig. 15: Relations of portal vein.

6. **Describe the internal capsule of brain under the following heading: Position, divisions, constituent fibers, blood supply and applied anatomy.**

Refer Essay Q. No. 7 – 2005.

7. **Describe the heart under the following headings: Position, coverings, internal features, conducting and skeletal systems and applied anatomy.**

Position

- Situated in the middle mediastinum
- The heart is situated obliquely behind the body of sternum and costal cartilages
- One-third of the heart lies to the right and two-third lies to the left of the median plane.

Coverings

- The pericardium is a fibroserous sac which encloses the heart and the root of the great vessels.

  It consists of fibrous pericardium and serous pericardium.
  - **Fibrous pericardium**
    - It is a conical sac
    - Made up of fibrous tissue enclosing the heart.
  - **Serous pericardium**
    - It is a thin double layered serous membrane lined by mesothelium
    - The outer layer of serous pericardium is fused with the fibrous pericardium
    - Its inner layer is adherent to the heart
    - Between these two layers there is a thin capillary space called pericardial cavity filled with pericardial fluid
    - Pericardial sinuses are the spaces formed by the arrangement of the serosal layer.

Internal Features

Internal Features Right Atrium (Fig. 17)

- The internal aspect of right atrium is divided into:
  - Smooth posterior part or sinus venarum

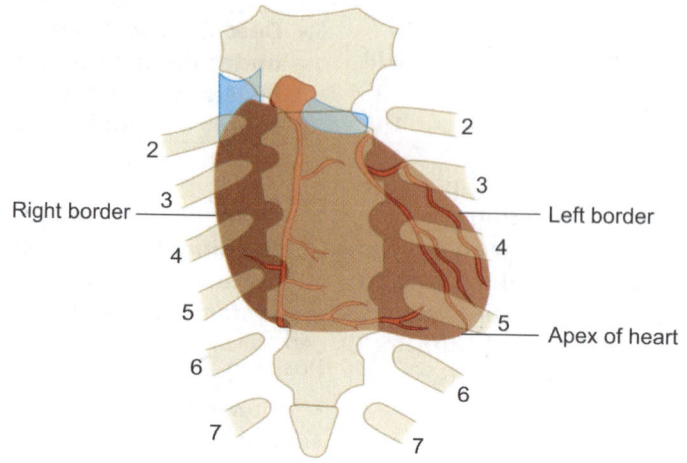

Fig. 16: Position of heart.

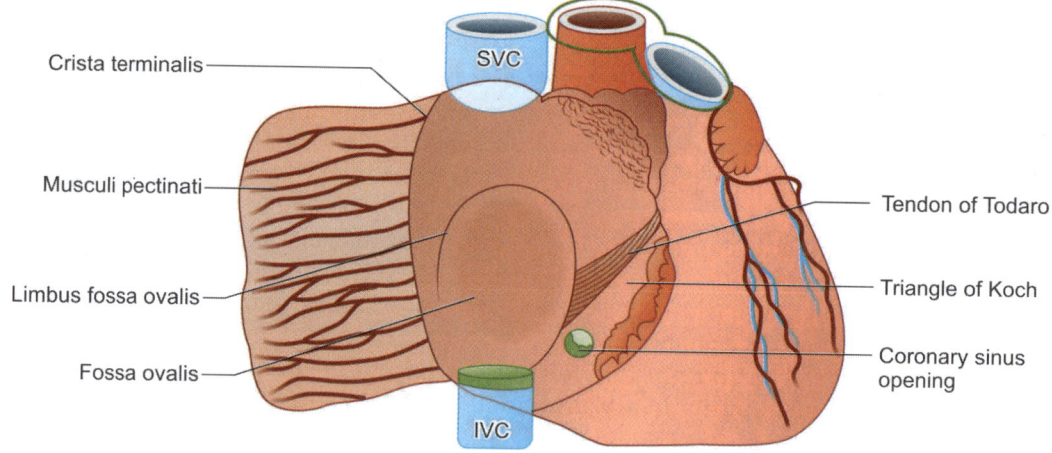

Fig. 17: Interior of right atrium.

- Rough anterior part or pectinate part
- Interatrial septum.

Smooth posterior part (sinus venosus):
- Posterosuperior part is the **opening of superior vena cava** not guarded by valve
- Posteroinferior part is the **opening of inferior vena cava** guarded by the eustachian valve.
  - The lateral part of the eustachian valve becomes continuous with the lower end of the crista terminalis
  - The valve is made of endocardium with few muscular fibers
  - It is large during fetal life, to direct oxygenated blood from the placenta into the left atrium through the foramen ovale
  - In postnatal life the size of the valve varies; it is sometimes cribriform or filamentous or absent.
- **Opening of coronary sinus:** Situated between the opening of the inferior vena cava and the right atrioventricular orifice. It is provided with a valve called Thebesian valve which prevents the regurgitation of blood into the coronary sinus.

- **Venae cordis minimae**
- **Anterior cardiac vein:** Opens into the anterior wall of the right atrium
- **Intervenous tubercle** is a very small projection, on the posterior wall of right atrium just below the opening of the superior vena cava.

Rough Anterior Part (Atrium Proper)

- **Crista terminalis** is a muscular ridge extending between the superior vena caval orifice and inferior vena caval orifice. It is represented externally as sulcus terminalis. In the upper part of this ridge close to orifice of SVC the SA node is situated
- From crista terminalis series of transverse muscular ridges called **musculi pectinati** pass forwards and downwards towards the atrioventricular orifice giving the appearance of the teeth of a comb
- In the auricle, the muscles are interconnected to form a reticular network.

Interatrial Septum

- It is obliquely placed between right atrium anteriorly and left atrium posteriorly
- The **fossa ovalis** is an oval shaped shallow depression above and to the left of the opening of inferior vena cava. It represents the remnant of septum primum
- The annulus ovalis or **limbus fossa ovalis** is the prominent margin of the fossa ovalis which surrounds the upper, anterior and posterior margins of the fossa, which is a remnant of the lower free margin of the septum secundum
- At the junction of the right atrium and right ventricle, AV orifice guarded by the tricuspid valve
- Tendon of Todaro is a subendocardial ridge extending dorsally from the central fibrous body to the left horn of the valve of the inferior vena cava
- **Triangle of Koch** is situated anteroinferiorly and is bounded by septal leaflet of tricuspid valve, tendon of Todaro and coronary sinus opening. AV node is situated in it
- Anterosuperiorly the non-coronary sinus (right posterior sinus) of the ascending aorta produces a bulge in the septal wall above the membranous septum called the **aortic mound/torus aorticus**
- **Internal features of right ventricle (Fig. 18):**
  - Is divided into an inflow and outflow tracts
  - Each part is with an opening.
- **Inflowing part:**
  - It is rough due to the presence of muscular ridges called trabeculae carneae
  - The trabeculae carneae are of three types—ridges, bridges, papillary muscles
  - One of the bridge in the right ventricle is prominent, called the **septomarginal trabecula or septal band**. It extends from ventricular septum to the anterior papillary muscle. Right bundle branch forms the content of septal band
  - Three papillary muscles are seen anterior from anterolateral ventricular wall, posterior from the inferior surface and septal small arises from septal wall
  - The apex of the papillary muscles give attachment for chordae tendinae
  - The chordae are collagenous threads covered by endothelium to support the cusps of the AV valves
  - The opening of the inflow tract is right AV orifice and the tricuspid valve guards the orifice.
- **Outflowing part:**
  - It is smooth and forms the upper conical part of the right ventricle called as **infundibulum/conus arteriosus**
  - The inflow and outflow tracts/parts are separated from each other by a muscular ridge called supraventricular crest
  - The outlet is guarded by pulmonary orifice with semilunar valves.

Internal Features of Left Atrium

- Musculi pectinati are present only in the auricle
- Four pulmonary veins and a few venae cordis minimi open into the left atrium.

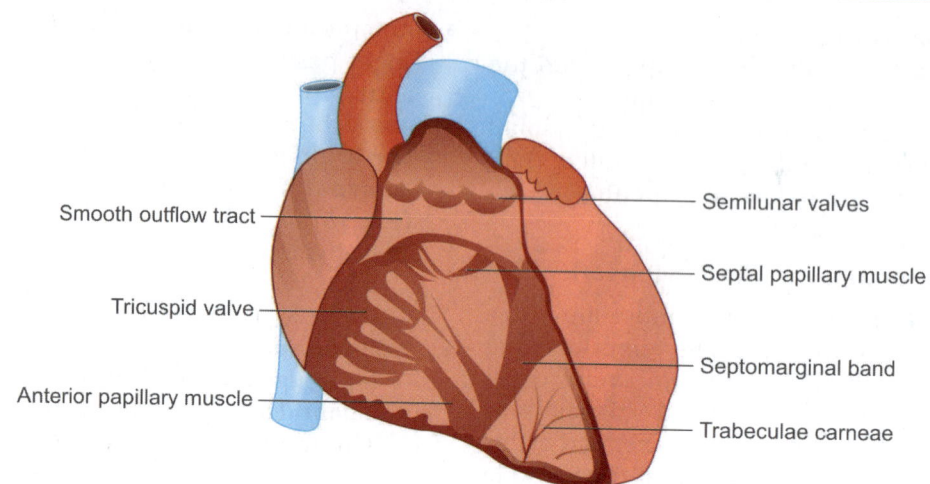

Fig. 18: Interior of right ventricle.

Internal Features of Left Ventricle
- The left ventricular wall is thick as it is concerned with systemic circulation
- The interior is divided into inflow and outflow tracts
- The inflow tract is more rougher than the right ventricle
- Two papillary muscles, anterior and posterior are present which are very thick
- Two orifices namely left atrioventricular orifice (mitral orifice) and aortic orifice are present
- The margin of the cusp is attached to the papillary muscles by chordae tendinae
- The semilunar valve having three cusps guards the aortic orifice.

Interventricular Septum
- It separates the right ventricle and left ventricle
- It is obliquely placed
- It bulges towards the right ventricle and so the right ventricle is crescentic and left ventricle is circular in shape
- Its upper part is thinner called **membranous part** and the lower part is thicker called **muscular part**.

Conducting System (Fig. 19)
- It is made up of specialized myocardial cells for propagation and conduction of cardiac impulses.

It has following parts:
- Sinoatrial node (pacemaker of the heart)
- Atrioventricular node
- Atrioventricular bundle
- The right and left bundle branches
- Purkinje fibers.
- **Sinoatrial node**
  - Is situated at the upper part of crista terminalis
  - The fibers are spindle shaped and loosely arranged
  - Are highly vascular
  - The fibers branch and are continuous with atrial fibers.
- **Atrioventricular node:** It is situated in the interatrial septum (triangle of Koch)
- **Atrioventricular bundle**
  - Starts from the AV node and reaches muscular part of interventricular septum
  - It divides into right and left bundle.
- **The right and left bundles**
  - The right branch passes through the moderator band and reaches the anterior papillary muscle and ramifies beneath the endocardium
  - The left branch ramifies similar way in the left ventricle.

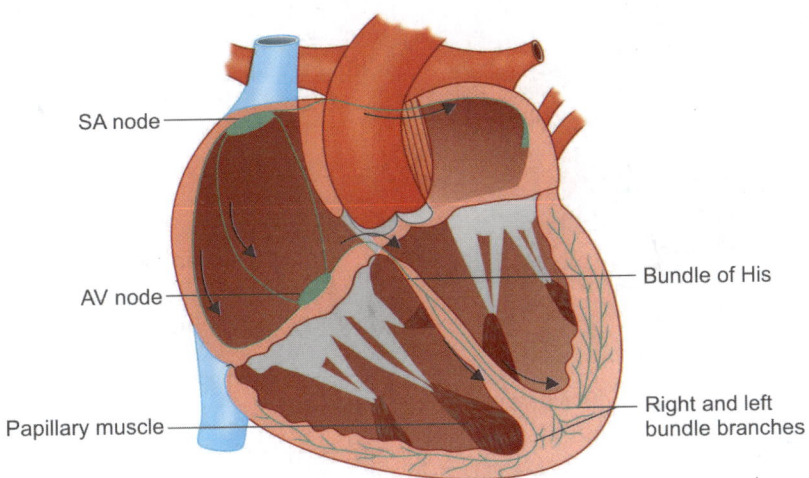

Fig. 19: Conducting system.

Fibrous Skeleton of Heart

- Fibrous rings surrounding the atrioventricular and arterial orifices constitute the fibrous skeleton of the heart
- The large mass of fibrous tissue is present between the atrioventricular rings behind and the aortic rings in front known as trigonum fibrosum dextrum (right fibrous trigone)
- A small mass of fibrous tissue is present between the aortic and mitral rings called as trigonum fibrosum sinistrum (left fibrous trigone).

Applied Anatomy

- Inflammation of pericardium is called pericarditis
- Valvular lesions - mitral stenosis – narrowing of mitral valve
- Mitral incompetence (regurgitation)— widening of mitral orifice
- Tricuspid stenosis
- Tricuspid incompetence
- Aortic stenosis
- Aortic incompetence
- Pulmonary stenosis
- Pulmonary incompetence
- Septal defects—ASD/VSD
- Tetralogy of Fallot—pulmonary stenosis, hypertrophy of right ventricle, interventricular septal defect and overriding of aorta.

8. **Describe the pharynx under the following headings: Extent, divisions, internal features, musculature, structures related and applied anatomy.**

Extent

- From base of skull to lower border of cricoid cartilage
- Vertebral level—lower border of C6
- Becomes continuous with esophagus.

Divisions

The anterior wall of pharynx is incomplete and it communicates with nasal, oral and laryngeal cavity. Hence by this the pharynx is subdivided into three parts:

- Nasopharynx—extends from base of skull to soft palate
- Oropharynx—from soft palate to epiglottis
- Laryngopharynx—from epiglottis to lower border of cricoid cartilage.

Internal Features

- **Nasopharynx (Fig. 20)**
  - **Auditory tube opening**—situated 1.2 cm behind and below the posterior end of inferior concha. Through this the

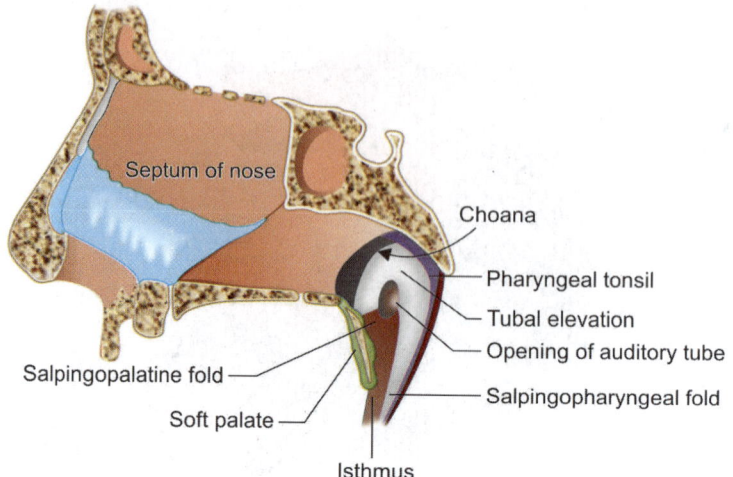

Fig. 20: Nasopharynx.

tympanic cavity communicates with nasopharynx
- **Tubal elevation**—produced by the pharyngeal end of auditory tube. Seen along the upper and posterior margins of the auditory opening. Used as a guide for the introduction of catheter into the eustachian tube
- **Tubal tonsil** sometimes collection of lymphoid tissue overlies the tubal elevation
- **Salpingopharyngeal fold** is a vertical mucosal fold, produced by salpingopharyngeus muscle that descends downwards from the tubal elevation
- **Salpingopalatine fold** is smaller in front of the auditory opening and extends from the anterosuperior angle of the tubal elevation to the soft palate
- The **levator veli palatini** produces an elevation around the tubal opening as it enters the soft palate
- **Pharyngeal recess** (fossa of Rosenmüller) is a depression behind the tubal elevation
- The **pharyngeal bursa** (bursa of Luschka), is a median blind recess which extends backwards and upwards. It is developed as diverticulum due to adhesion of the cranial end of notochord to the dorsal wall of pharyngeal part of foregut
- **Nasopharyngeal tonsil**—is a mucoid associated lymphoid tissue (MALT). Aggregation of lymphoid tissue in the roof and posterior wall, more prominent in children and atrophies in adults. When enlarged due to infection, it is known as **adenoids**
- **Pharyngeal hypophysis**—derived from Rathke's pouch. Histologically resemble adenohypophysis.
- **Oropharynx (Fig. 21)**
  - Is from soft palate to upper border of epiglottis
  - It communicates anteriorly with oral cavity through oropharyngeal isthmus
  - Laterally two folds are present—palatoglossal fold and palatopharyngeal fold produced by corresponding muscles underlying the folds
  - Between the folds a triangular depression called tonsillar fossa containing the palatine tonsil.
- **Laryngopharynx**
  - Is from the superior border of the epiglottis, to the inferior border of the cricoid cartilage

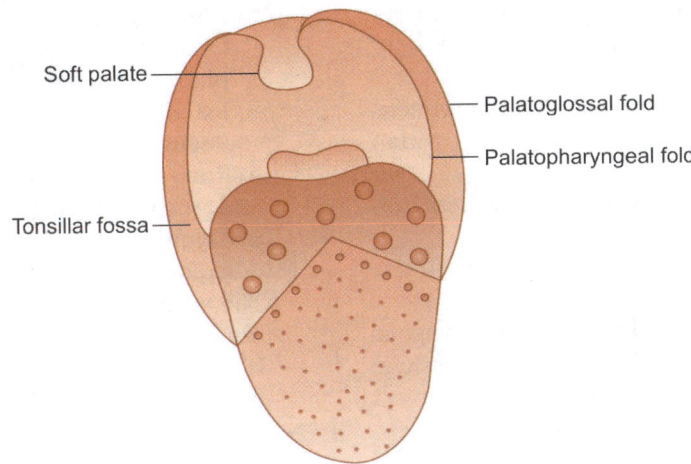

Fig. 21: Oropharynx.

- The anterior wall of laryngopharynx is formed by the larynx—inlet of larynx above, and posterior surface of arytenoids and cricoid cartilages below
- The inlet of the larynx is contributed anterosuperiorly by the epiglottis, posteriorly by the arytenoid cartilages of the larynx, and laterally by the aryepiglottic folds
- The piriform fossa is situated on each side of the laryngeal inlet. The boundaries of the fossa are—medially by the aryepiglottic fold and laterally by the thyroid cartilage and thyrohyoid membrane. Branches of the internal laryngeal nerve lie deep to the mucous membrane.

Musculature

The muscles are arranged as circular (constrictors) and vertical muscles
- Constrictors are three in number:
  i. Inferior constrictor
  ii. Middle constrictor
  iii. Superior constrictor
- **Inferior constrictor (Fig. 22):**
  - The pharynx is made up of inner circular and outer longitudinal muscular coat
  - The circular muscular layer forms the constrictors of pharynx

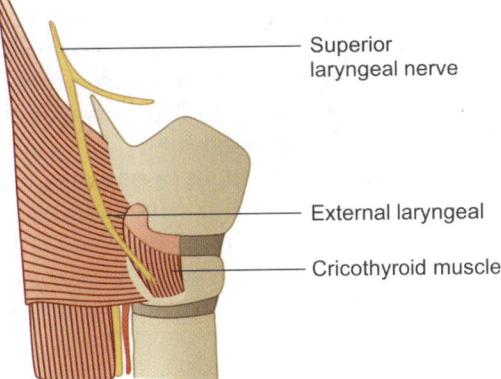

Fig. 22: Inferior constrictor.

- It has three constrictors—superior, middle and inferior arranged one overlapping the other
- The inferior constrictor is the thickest of the three constrictor muscles
- It has two parts, thyropharyngeus and cricopharyngeus.
- **Origin:**
  - Thyropharyngeus arises from the oblique line and inferior cornu of the lamina of the thyroid cartilage.
  - Cricopharyngeus arises from the lateral surface of arch of cricoid cartilage and the attachment is between the origin of cricothyroid

and the articular facet for the inferior horn of thyroid cartilage.
- **Insertion**:
  - The upper fibers of thyropharyngeus are oblique and ascend to overlap the middle constrictor
  - Thyropharyngeus is inserted into the pharyngeal raphe
  - Cricopharyngeus merges with the circular fibers of esophagus
  - According to some, cricopharyngeus consist of oblique upper superficial portion, called the **pars oblique**, and a transverse lower deeper portion, known as the **pars fundiformis**. The superficial part is inserted to the median raphe, while the deeper part, loops around, forming circular bundle
  - Killian's dehiscence (or Killian's triangle) is the weaker area between the oblique and transverse parts of cricopharyngeus. The diverticula occur in this weak area
  - The other thought by some is, that the area between cricopharyngeus and thyropharyngeus is weak as it is not supported by pharyngeal muscles and is called the dehiscence of Killian.
- **Nerve supply**:
  - Cranial accessory nerve through pharyngeal plexus
  - External laryngeal nerve
  - Recurrent laryngeal nerve.
- **Action**: Thyropharyngeus is propulsive and pushes the food, whereas cricopharyngeus has sphincteric action.

• **Middle constrictor (Fig. 23)**:
- The middle constrictor is a fan-shaped muscle
- It has **two parts**—cricopharyngeus and ceratopharyngeus
- **Origin**:
  - Chondropharyngeal part—arises from the lesser cornu of the hyoid and the lower part of the stylohyoid ligament
  - Ceratopharyngeal part—attached to the whole length of the upper border of the greater cornu of the hyoid bone.
- **Direction of the fibers**
  - The lower fibers are oblique, and the inferior constrictor overlaps the middle constrictor. It extends up to the lower end of the pharynx
  - The middle fibers are arranged transversely

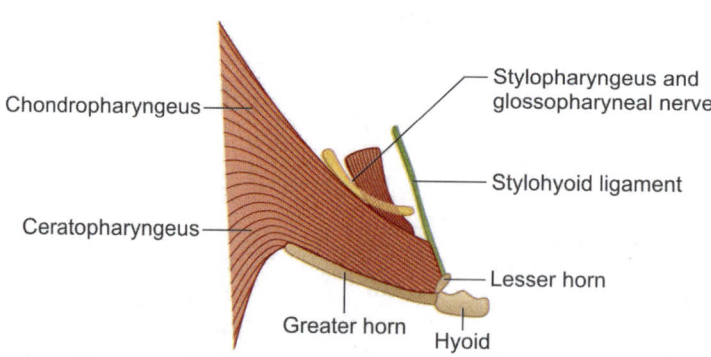

Fig. 23: Middle constrictor.

- The superior fibers are oblique and overlap the lower border of superior constrictor.
- **Insertion**: All fibers are inserted into the median pharyngeal raphe
- **Nerve supply**: Cranial accessory through pharyngeal plexus
- **Action**: Constricts the pharynx during swallowing.

- **Superior constrictor (Fig. 24):**
  - It is a quadrilateral muscle
  - It has **four parts**—pterygopharyngeus, buccopharyngeus, mylopharyngeus, glossopharyngeus.
  - **Origin**:
    - Pterygopharyngeus—attached to the pterygoid hamulus and lower part of posterior margin of the medial pterygoid plate
    - Buccopharyngeus—the posterior border of the pterygomandibular raphe
    - Mylopharyngeus—posterior end of the mylohyoid line of the mandible
    - Glossopharyngeus—to the side of the tongue
    - Palatopharyngeal sphincter in the upper border of the superior constrictor, encircles the pharynx. It produces an elevation called **passavants ridge**.
  - **Insertion**:
    - The fibers are inserted to median pharyngeal raphe
    - The upper fibers are attached to the pharyngeal tubercle on the basilar part of the occipital bone
    - A gap is seen above the upper border of the superior constrictor, separating muscle from the base of cranial cavity called **sinus of Morgagni** through which levator veli palatini, the pharyngotympanic tube pass.
  - **Nerve supply**: Cranial accessory nerve through pharyngeal plexus
  - **Action**: The superior constrictor constricts the upper part of the pharynx.

Vertical Muscles (Fig. 25)

Vertical muscles are three in number. They are:
i. Stylopharyngeus
ii. Palatopharyngeus
iii. Salpingopharyngeus

- **Stylopharyngeus**
  - Rounded above and flat below.
  - **Origin**: It arises from the base of the styloid process along its medial side.

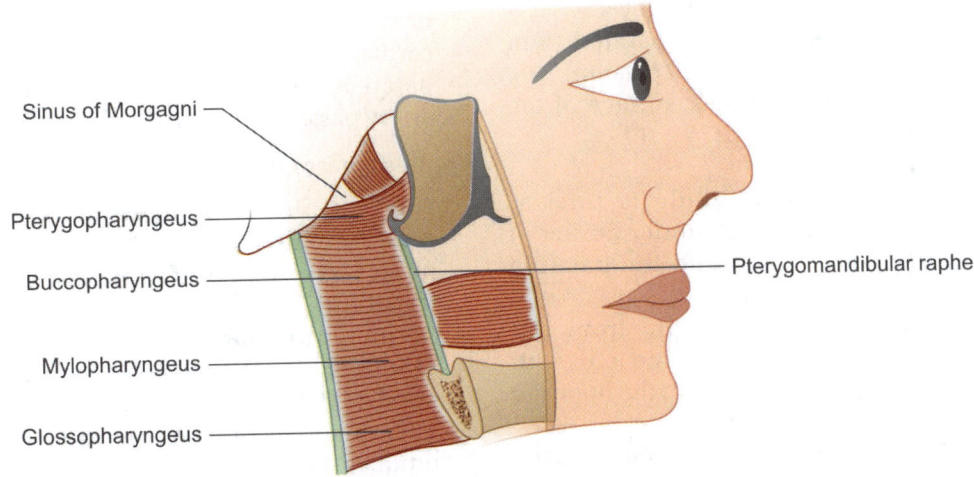

Fig. 24: Superior constrictor.

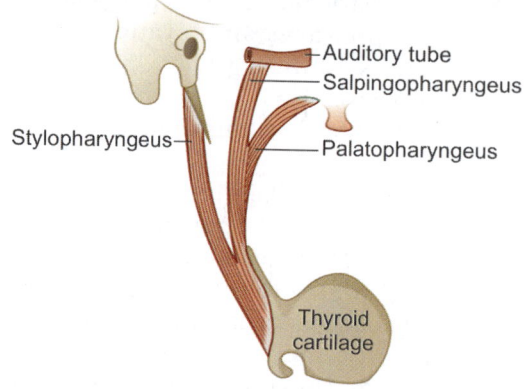

Fig. 25: Vertical muscles.

- **Course**
  - Descends along the side of the pharynx
  - Passes between the superior and middle constrictors.
- **Insertion:** Join with palatopharyngeus and are inserted to the posterior border of the thyroid cartilage.
- **Nerve supply**
  - Glossopharyngeal nerve
  - Action
  - Elevates the pharynx.
- **Palatopharyngeus**
  - Palatopharyngeus is composed of anterior and posterior bundles
  - The two bundles are separated from each other by levator veli palatini
  - Attached to the upper surface of the palatine aponeurosis
  - **Origin:**
    - The anterior bundle is thicker, arises from the posterior border of the hard palate and the palatine aponeurosis
    - The posterior bundle from the mucosa of the palate, and joins with the posterior bundle of the opposite muscle in the midline.
  - **Course:** The two bundles unite, and the fibers of salpingopharyngeus join with it. Passes laterally behind the tonsil, and joins with stylopharyngeus muscle
  - **Insertion:** Inserted to the posterior border of the thyroid cartilage
  - **Nerve supply:** Cranial accessory through pharyngeal plexus
  - **Action:** The palatopharyngeus pull the pharynx upwards, forwards and medially there by shortens the pharynx during deglutition.
- **Salpingopharyngeus**
  - **Origin:** Arises from the inferior surface of the cartilaginous part of the auditory tube close to its pharyngeal opening
  - **Insertion:** Passes downwards produces the salpingopharyngeal fold and join with palatopharyngeus
  - **Nerve supply:** Cranial accessory through pharyngeal plexus
  - **Action:** Elevates the pharynx.

Structures Related

- **Lower border of inferior constrictor**—recurrent laryngeal nerve and inferior laryngeal vessels
- **Between inferior and middle constrictor**—superior laryngeal vessels and internal laryngeal nerve
- **Between middle and superior constrictor**—stylopharyngeus muscle and glossopharyngeal nerve
- **Above upper border of superior constrictor** is the space called **sinus of Morgagni**. Through the space the cartilaginous part of auditory tube, levator palati muscle and ascending palatine artery pass.

Applied Anatomy

- Hypertrophy of pharyngeal tonsil is called adenoids. The child with adenoids have adenoid facies with mouth breathing
- In chronic tonsillitis, the pus accumulates in the peritonsillar space leading to peritonsillar abscess or quinsy
- The carcinoma of piriform fossa may not produce symptoms for a longer period and may produce pain in the ear
- Zenker's diverticulum/pharyngeal pouch—protrusion of mucous membrane

of pharynx through the Killian's dehiscence. It is due to neuromuscular incoordination in this region.

9. **Define a typical intercostal nerve. Describe the course and distribution. Add a note on its clinical importance.**

- **Definition**
    - The nerves lying between the ribs are named as **intercostal nerves**
    - They are 11 in number
    - They are formed by the **ventral rami of the thoracic nerves**.
- **Classification**
    - They are classified as (i) typical and (ii) atypical intercostal nerves.
        i. Typical nerves: The nerves which are confined to the thoracic wall are called as **typical intercostal nerves.** 3rd to 6th are **typical** as they are confined to thoracic wall.
        ii. Atypical nerves: The first and second nerves supply thoracic wall and in addition supply upper limb. The lower five (7 – 11) supply both thoracic and abdominal walls. Hence called as **atypical**.
- **Course:**
    - From intervertebral foramen enter the posterior part of intercostal space by passing in front of the neck of the corresponding rib
    - Lies in the endothoracic fascia between the costal pleura and posterior intercostal membrane
    - At the angle of the rib, the trunk passes forwards in the costal groove
    - The arrangement of structures in the groove, from above downwards **vein, artery and nerve**
    - Lies between intercostalis internus and intimus
    - Pierces internal intercostal muscle, anterior intercostal membrane, and pectoralis major
    - It is continued as anterior cutaneous nerve.
- **Distribution (Branches):**
    - **Communication**:
        - **Ganglionic branches:** Gray and white rami communicans connect each intercostal nerve with the corresponding sympathetic ganglion. **White ramus** carry pre-ganglionic sympathetic fibers to the ganglion. **Gray ramus** conveys post-ganglionic sympathetic fibers from the ganglion
        - **Intercostal nerves communicate** with the adjacent nerves in the

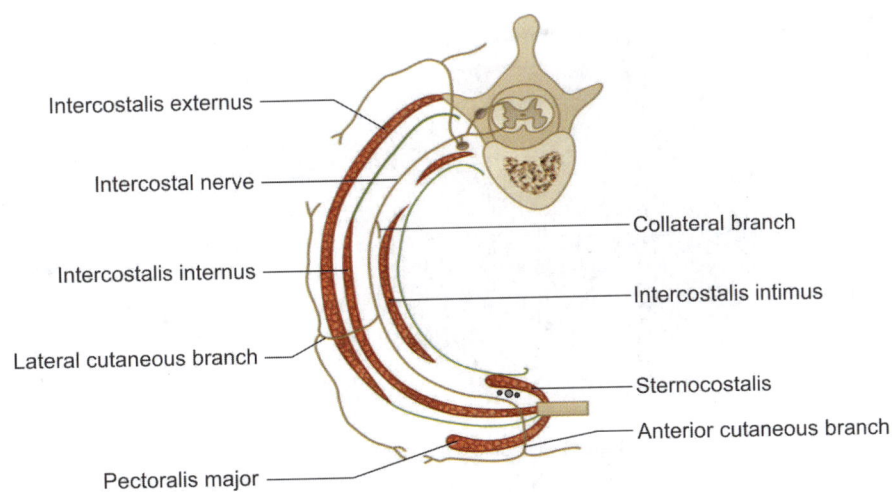

Fig. 26: Typical intercostal nerve.

anterior part of the space behind the costal cartilages.
- **Distribution:**
  - Muscular branches to the intercostal muscles.
  - Collateral branch:
    * Arises from the nerve near the angle of the rib
    * Collateral branch and the main trunk runs forward in the same intercostal space
    * In the anterior part of the space, the nerve may or may not unite with the main trunk
    * It is continued as additional anterior cutaneous nerve in the same space, if it fails to unite with main trunk.
  - Lateral cutaneous branch:
    * Arises near the angle of the rib
    * Pierces the internus and externus muscles in the mid axillary line
    * Divides into anterior and posterior branches
    * Anterior branch joins with the lateral branch of anterior cutaneous nerve
    * Posterior branch unites with the cutaneous branch of the dorsal ramus of the same thoracic spinal nerve.
  - Anterior cutaneous branch:
    * Continuation of the main trunk of the nerve
    * In the anterior part of the space, pierces internal intercostal muscle, anterior intercostal membrane, and pectoralis major
    * Terminates as anterior cutaneous nerve
    * Divides into medial and lateral cutaneous branches.
- **Applied Anatomy:**
  - **Paracentesis thoracis:** Needle is passed along the lower part of the space in the midaxillary line to avoid injury to the neurovascular bundle in draining pleural effusion
  - **Intercostal neuralgia:** Sharp burning pain in the area of skin supplied by the thoracic spinal nerves. Produced by rib fracture or a viral disease of the spinal ganglia called herpes zoster.

10. Describe the parotid gland under the following headings: (i) Extension, (ii) Features, (iii) Relations, (iv) Innervations and (v) Applied aspects.

Refer Essay Q. No. 4 – 2004.

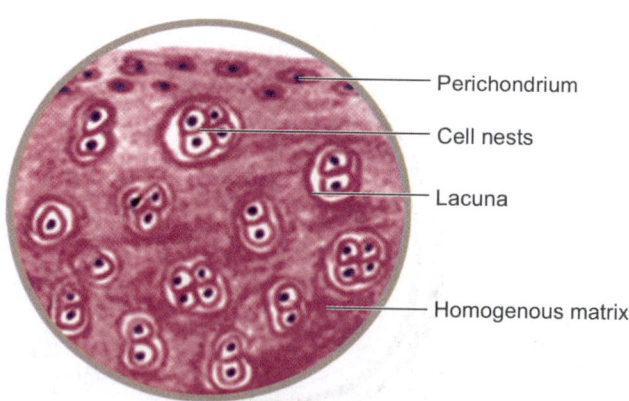

Fig. 27: Histology of hyaline cartilage.

II. SHORT NOTES

1. Microscopic structure of hyaline cartilage.

- Hyaline cartilage is so called because it has ground glass appearance
- It is covered by fibrous membrane called the **perichondrium**
- It is made of cells and matrix
- The **cells**—chondrocytes are round in the deeper part and flat towards perichondrium
- **Chondrocytes** are present in groups.
- Groups of cartilage cells are called cell-nests (isogenous cell groups).
- They are formed by division of a single parent cell, and separation is prevented by dense matrix
- The cells are surrounded by lacunae.
- The **matrix** contains fibers and ground substance
- The matrix is homogenous because the refractive index of fibers and ground substance are same.
- **Fibers:** Many collagen fibers type I are present in the matrix.
- Around cell nests, the matrix stains deeply called **territorial matrix** or lacunar capsule.
- The matrix lying in between the cell nests is called **interterritorial matrix**.
- An isogenous cell group, together with the pericellular matrix, is referred to as a **chondron**.
- **Property**: As age advances the hyaline cartilage can get ossified
- **Distribution:**
  - Costal cartilages
  - Articular cartilage
  - Skeletal framework of the larynx: Thyroid cartilage, cricoid cartilage and part of arytenoid cartilage
  - Trachea and large bronchi
  - Parts of the nasal septum and lateral wall of the nose
  - In growing bone epiphyseal plate
- **Function**: Resists tensional forces.

2. Prostatic part of urethra.

- It is a part of male urethra lying within the prostate gland
- **Commencement:** The preprostatic part is continued as prostatic part. It pierces the base of prostate at the junction of anterior one third and posterior two-third
- **Course:** Runs closer to the anterior surface of the gland, within the substance of the prostate
- **Termination:** Emerges from the prostate in front of apex, and continued as membranous part of urethra

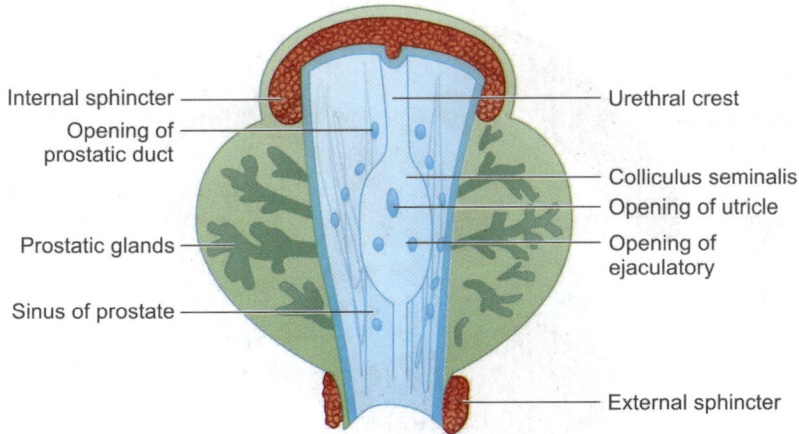

Fig. 28: Prostatic urethra.

- **Features in the posterior wall:**
  - A midline ridge is seen known as **urethral crest**
  - Hence the lumen of the prostatic urethra is crescent shaped in cross section
  - There is an elevation at the middle of the crest called **verumontanum (colliculus seminalis)**
  - In the middle of verumontanum a slit like opening is the orifice of **Prostatic utricle**
  - On each side of this orifice are the **openings of the ejaculatory ducts** which is formed by the union of vas deferens and duct of seminal vesicle
  - A shallow depression is present on each side of the crest—called **prostatic/urethral sinus**
  - Into the sinus about 15 – 20 ducts of prostate gland open.
- **Prostatic utricle:**
  - It is a blind sac 6 mm long; directed upwards and backwards
  - Its wall is made of fibrous tissue, muscle fibers and mucous membrane with glands
  - It is developmentally **remnant** of paramesophrenic duct (Mullerian duct)
  - It is **homologous** with the vagina of female; hence the name **vagina masculina**
  - According to some it is similar to uterus hence called as utricle.
- **Lining epithelium:** Up to colliculus seminalis it is lined by transitional epithelium, below it is lined by pseudostratified or stratified columnar epithelium
- **Applied anatomy:** Hypertrophy of median lobe can compress the prostatic part of the urethra resulting in symptoms of urinary retention.

3. Adductor canal.

It is an intermuscular tunnel in the thigh region
- **Other names:** Subsartorial canal or Hunter's canal named after John Hunter for treating popliteal aneurysm
- **Situation:** In distal two-third of medial side of thigh
- **Extent:** From apex of femoral triangle to tendinous opening in adductor magnus
- **Shape:** Triangular in section
- **Boundaries:**
  - **Posterior wall:** Adductor longus above and adductor magnus below
  - **Anterolateral wall:** Vastus medialis
  - **Roof:** Subsartorial fascia extending from anterior to posterior wall covering the femoral vessels, sartorius and the subsartorial plexus of nerves lie on the fascia.

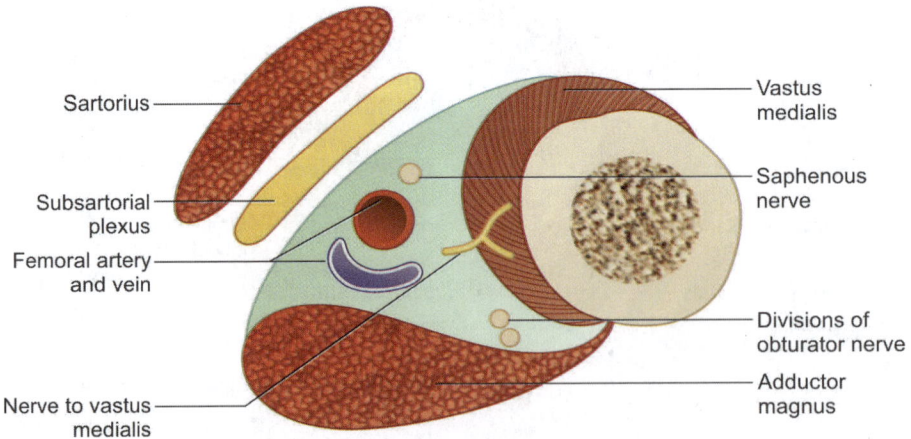

Fig. 29: Adductor canal.

- **Contents:** Femoral artery
  - Femoral vein is posterior to artery in the upper part and then it becomes lateral
  - Saphenous nerve crosses the artery from lateral to medial side
  - Nerve to vastus medialis
  - Descending genicular artery
  - Posterior division of obturator nerve.

Applied Anatomy

- Ligation of femoral artery to prevent bleeding from a distal cut end
- Ligation of femoral artery in popliteal artery aneurysm is done in subsartorial canal.

4. Paramesonephric duct.

- The paramesonephric ducts are developed in both sexes
- But it is the main genital duct in female
- It is also known as the **Mullerian duct**
- It is from intermediate mesoderm
- In the 6th week coelomic epithelium invaginates and appear like a longitudinal groove
- **Situation:**
  - Lateral to the mesonephric ridge
  - The margins of the groove gradually fuse to convert the groove into a duct
  - The cranial end of the duct opens into the coelomic cavity
  - Its caudal end is seen as a solid tube and later lumen is acquired as it descends to reach the definitive urogenital sinus.
- **Parts:** Each paramesonephric duct consists of three parts:
  i. Cephalic vertical part
  ii. Intermediate horizontal part
  iii. Caudal vertical part.
- **Derivatives in female**
  - The **cephalic vertical part** and most of the **intermediate horizontal parts** of each paramesonephric duct form the respective **uterine tube**
  - The commencement of the duct persists as the abdominal opening of the uterine tube through which it communicates with the coelomic cavity
  - Due the descent of the ovaries, the uterine tubes are pulled to the pelvic cavity and undergo a horizontal course
  - The **caudal vertical parts** of both paramesonephric ducts fuse in caudo-cranial direction
  - The partition between them completely disappears by the 3rd month
  - The single duct thus formed is the **uterovaginal canal**
  - The cranial part of this canal forms the entire **uterus**
  - The most cephalic point of fusion of the two ducts represents the site of the future fundus.
  - The caudal part of the uterovaginal canal is for the development of **vagina.**
- **Derivatives in male**
  - The paramesonephric duct disappears

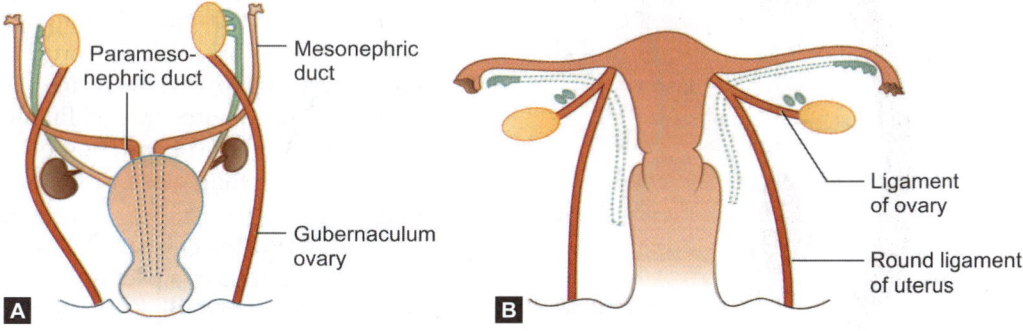

Figs. 30A and B: Paramesonephric duct.

- Cephalic end persists as **appendix of testis**
- Lower end represents the **prostatic utricle**.
- **Congenital anomalies:**
  - Duplication of uterus (uterus didelphys)—due to lack of fusion of the paramesonephric ducts
  - Uterus bicornis unicollis—uterus two horns and common vagina
  - Unicornuate—one of the paramesonephric duct development is rudimentary
  - Arcuate uterus—slightly indented in the middle
  - Septate uterus—failure of fusion of upper part of paramesonephric ducts.

5. Clavipectoral fascia.

- It is a fibrous sheet
- Extends from pectoralis minor to clavicle
- Situated deep to the clavicular part of pectoralis major muscle
- It extend over the axillary vessels and nerves
- **Extent**
  - **Above:** Splits into two as anterior and posterior layers, enclose subclavius and is attached to the corresponding lips of the groove for subclavius in the clavicle. The posterior layer is connected to deep cervical fascia thereby, attaches omohyoid to clavicle
  - **Below:** Splits to enclose pectoralis minor and is continued as suspensory ligament of axilla. (Gerdy's **ligament**) and blends with axillary fascia
  - **Medially:** Fuses with anterior intercostal membrane of upper two spaces
  - **Laterally:** Attached to coracoid process and merges with coracoclavicular ligament
  - The portion of the fascia between first rib and coracoid process is thickened to form **costocoracoid ligament**.
- **Structures piercing: (CALL)**
  - **C**ephalic vein
  - **A**cromiothoracic (thoracoacromial) artery
  - **L**ateral pectoral nerve
  - **L**ymphatics draining into the apical group of lymph node.

6. Deep peroneal nerve.

- **Formation:**
  - Deep peroneal nerve is one of the terminal branch of common peroneal nerve
  - The root value: dorsal division of ventral rami of L4, 5 S1, 2.
- **Course and termination (Fig. 32A):**
  - It origin is related to the lateral side of the neck of the fibula
  - It pierces the anterior inter muscular septum, the extensor digitorum longus and enters the anterior compartment
  - In the leg, it accompanies the anterior tibial artery
  - It is lateral to the artery in the upper part, anterior in the middle and again lateral in the lower part. Hence the nerve is called as **nervi hesitans**
  - The nerve terminates by dividing into **lateral and medial branches** on the dorsum of the foot, close to the ankle joint **(Fig. 32B)**
  - **Lateral terminal branch:** Turns laterally and ends in a pseudoganglion deep to the extensor digitorum brevis
  - **Medial terminal branch**: Ends by supplying the skin adjoining the first interdigital cleft.

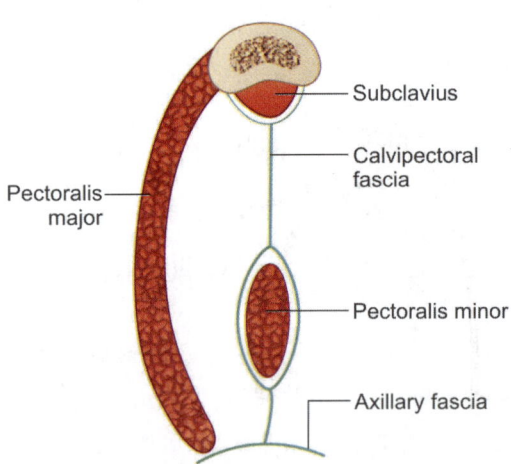

Fig. 31: Clavipectoral fascia.

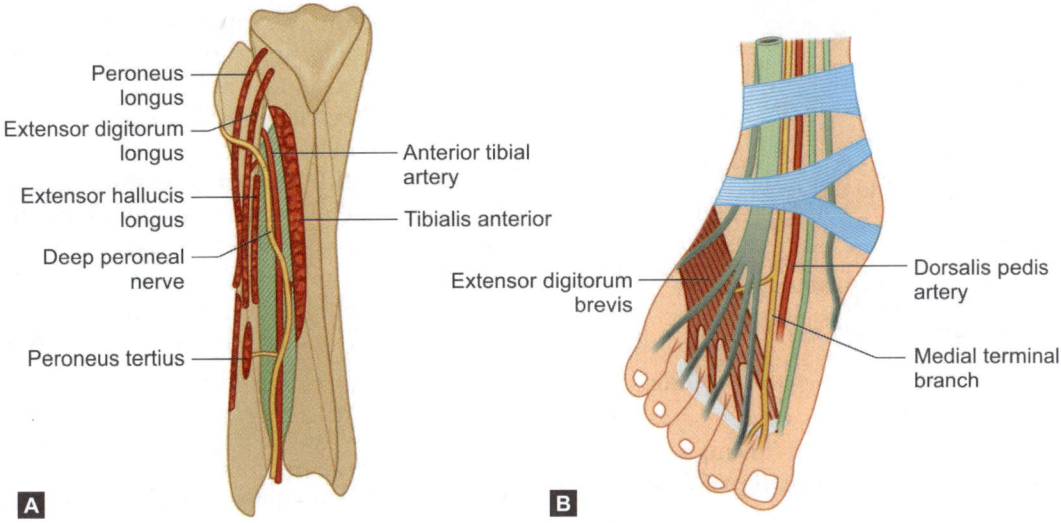

Figs. 32A and B: Deep peroneal nerve.

- **Relations**
  - Posterior
    - Interosseous membrane in the upper two-thirds
    - Lower end of tibia and ankle joint in the lower one-third.
  - Anterior
    - Covered by the adjoining muscles and
    - Deep fascia in upper two-thirds
    - The deep fascia and extensor retinacula in lower one-third.
  - Medial: Tibialis anterior.
  - Lateral
    - Extensor digitorum longus.
    - Peroneus tertius.
- **Branches**
  - **Muscular branches** supply:
    - Anterior compartment of the leg—tibialis anterior, extensor digitorum longus, extensor hallucis longus, peroneus tertius
    - Dorsum of the foot—extensor digitorum brevis, 1st dorsal interossei
  - **Cutaneous branch** supplies adjacent sides of the first and second toes (first interdigital cleft)
  - **Articular branches** supply the ankle joint, the tarsal joints, 1st metatarsophalangeal joints of the big toe and metatarsophalangeal joints of middle three toes.
- **Applied Anatomy:**
  - **Anterior leg syndrome:** Weakness of dorsiflexion of ankle and extension of all toes results due to excessive accumulation of tissue fluid in the anterior compartment of leg
  - **Foot drop:** Injury to deep peroneal nerve results in foot drop.

7. Microscopic anatomy of fundus of stomach.

Stomach is made up of 4 layers. Inner to outer are:

I. **Mucous layer**
   - Mucous folds or rugae are seen placed longitudinally, more towards greater curvature and pyloric part
   - The mucous layer is formed by epithelium, lamina propria, and muscularis mucosa
   - **Epithelium:** Lined by simple columnar epithelium. It presents depressions called gastric pits. The pits are deep extending to lamina up to muscularis mucosa and are lined by surface mucous cells

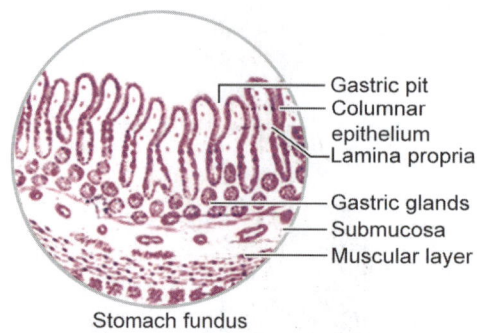

Fig. 33: Histology of stomach fundus.

- The **gastric pits, in fundus** are not deep and extend about one fourth of the thickness of mucous layer
- **Lamina propria:** Consists of vessels, nerves and gastric glands
- The glands are grouped as cardiac, principal, and pyloric glands
- The glands are packed in the lamina propria and long, tubular in the fundus and body
- **Muscularis mucosa:** Made up of inner circular and outer longitudinal smooth muscle fibers
- Each gastric **gland** is lined by :
  - **Zymogenic/chief/peptic cells:** Cuboidal cells, occupy the base of the gland and they synthesize digestive enzymes pepsin and lipase. They contain abundant zymogenic granules
  - **Oxyntic/parietal cells:** Situated along the lateral wall of the gland. They are large and oval in shape. Secrete HCl and the intrinsic factor for absorption of vitamin B12
  - **Neck mucous cells:** It is more in number in pyloric glands. Situated at the neck of glands, and lateral walls of base of gland. Secrete mucous
  - **Stem cells:** Are columnar, less in number, undergo mitotic division
  - **Neuroendocrine or enteroendocrine (Argentaffin cells):** Cells belong to Amine Precursor Uptake and Decarboxylation (APUD) system. They are found in fundus and body and situated in the deeper part of gland. They include:
    * **G cells:** Secrete gastrin
    * **D cells:** Secrete somatostatin
    * **ECL (enterochromaffin like cell):** Secrete histamine and serotonin.
II. **Submucous layer:** Consists of loose areolar tissue, containing collagen and elastic fibers, blood vessels, lymphatics and nerves. Meissner's plexus (submucosal plexus), of nerves are present.
III. **Muscular layer:** Consists of 3 layers of smooth muscle outer longitudinal, middle circular, inner oblique.
IV. **Serous layer:** Derived from visceral peritoneum formed by simple squamous mesothelium.

8. **Anastomosis around elbow.**

Anastomosis around the elbow joint connects the branches of brachial artery with the upper parts of the radial and ulnar arteries.
- **Functions:**
  - During flexion of elbow the blood flow through the brachial artery is reduced
  - This anastomosis helps to provide more blood flow to the distal part of limb
  - It supplies the ligaments and bones of the joint.
- **Divisions:** The anastomosis can be subdivided into vertical and horizontal anastomosis.
  - **Vertical:**
    - **In front of the lateral epicondyle of the humerus:** (Above) the anterior descending branch of the profunda brachii anastomose, below with the radial recurrent branch of the radial artery
    - **Behind the lateral epicondyle of the humerus:** The posterior descending branch of the profunda brachii artery (above) anastomoses with the interosseous recurrent branch of posterior interosseous artery from ulnar artery (below)
    - **In front of the medial epicondyle of the humerus:** The inferior ulnar

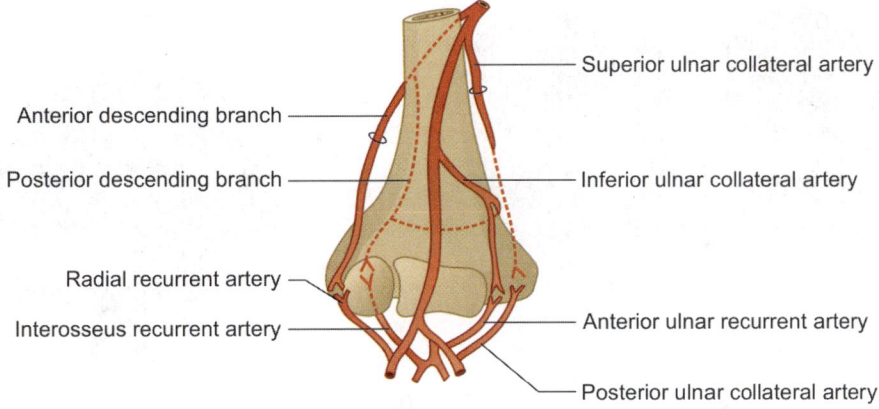

Fig. 34: Anastomosis around elbow.

collateral branch of the brachial artery (above) anastomoses with the anterior ulnar recurrent branch of the ulnar artery (below)
- **Behind the medial epicondyle of the humerus:** The superior ulnar collateral branch of the brachial artery (above) anastomoses with the posterior ulnar recurrent branch of the ulnar artery (below).
- **Horizontal**: Above the olecranon fossa.
  - Transverse branch of the posterior division of the inferior ulnar collateral branch of brachial artery anastomoses with posterior descending (middle collateral) branch of profunda brachii artery.

9. Femoral sheath.
Refer Short Notes 4 – 2005.

10. Congenital anomalies of kidney.
- **According to number:**
  - **Agenesis of one kidney:** The ureteric bud may fail to develop on one side, producing congenital absence of one kidney; the other kidney is normal
  - **Multiple kidneys:** More than one kidney may be present on one or both sides. This is due to early splitting of the ureteric bud.
- **According to position:**
  - **Pelvic kidney:** When the kidney fails to ascend, it occupies the pelvic cavity with normal functions

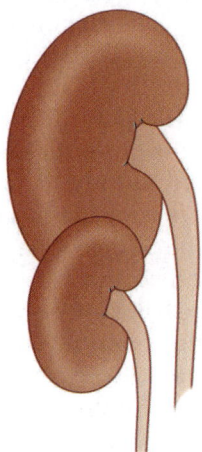

Fig. 35: Fused kidney.

- **Fused kidney:** Sometimes one kidney may be displaced from its own side and fuses with the kidney of the other side, although the ureter retains the normal position. In fused kidney, the higher one belongs to the normal side **(Fig. 35)**.
- **According to shape (Figs. 36A and B):**
  - **Horseshoe kidney:** In this anomaly, the lower poles of both kidneys are connected by an isthmus of kidney tissue which passes in front of the aorta and inferior vena cava. The ureters lie in front of the isthmus. The horse-shoe kidney is situated at a lower level than the normal one, because its ascent is arrested by the origin of the inferior mesenteric artery.

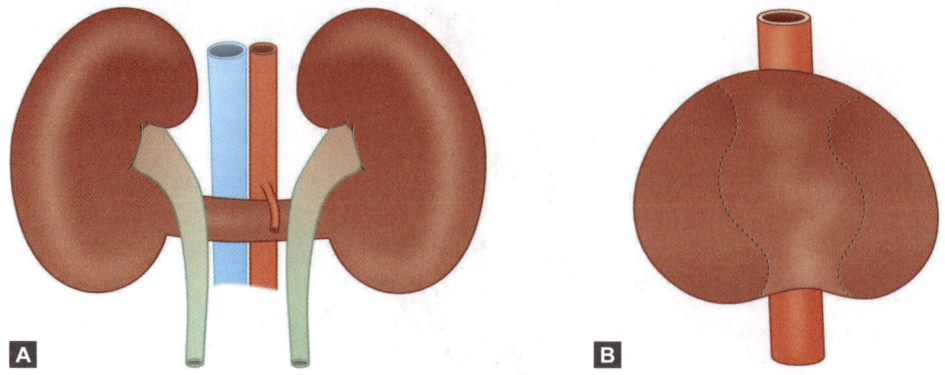

Figs. 36A and B: According to shape: (A) Horseshoe kidney; (B) Fused kidney.

- **Disc kidney:** This condition is due to complete fusion of both kidneys across the mid line, although the ureters descend to the respective side. The hilum of disc kidney lies in the median plane on the posterior surface
- **Lobulated kidney:** Fetal lobulations may exist in adult life. In such condition, the outline of the kidney is somewhat larger than normal.
- **According to failure of fusion of excretory and collecting tubules (Fig. 37):**
  - **Polycystic kidney:** Numerous cysts appear in the substance of kidney which are filled with urine. This condition is usually bilateral, and is the commonest of all anomalies. The polycystic kidney results from the failure of fusion of the secretory and collecting tubules. This anomaly is of two types: Adult and childhood
  - **Adult type:** Autosomal dominant; accounts for 90% of the polycystic kidney disease; disease is manifested above the age of 20 years
  - **Childhood type:** Autosomal recessive; rare; disease is manifested below the age of 20 years.
- **According to arterial supply:**
  - **Accessory renal artery:** The accessory artery is the precocious origin of a segmental artery.

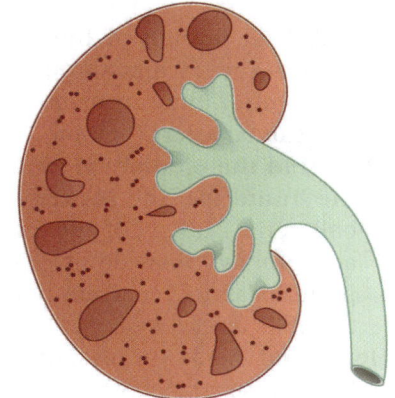

Fig. 37: Polycystic kidney.

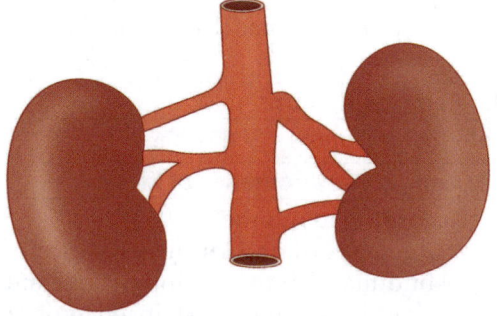

Fig. 38: Floating kidney.

- **According to mobility:**
  - **Floating kidney (Fig. 38):** A kidney may be suspended by a fold of peritoneum from the posterior abdominal wall.

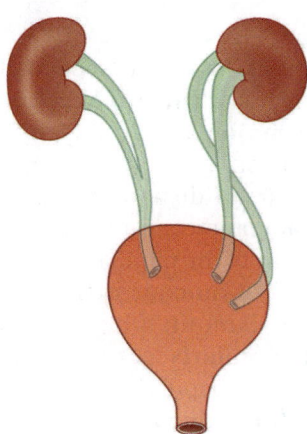

Fig. 39: Double ureter.

- Single kidney with double ureters (Fig. 39).

11. Histology of compact bone.
Refer Short Notes 1 – 2003.

12. Triceps brachii.
- It is situated in the extensor compartment of arm
- It arises as three heads
- **Origin:**
  - The **long head** arises from the infra glenoid tubercle of the scapula. The long head forms medial boundary for quadrangular space, lateral boundary for upper triangular space and medial boundary for lower triangular space
  - The **lateral head** arises from an oblique ridge on the posterior surface of the humerus present in the upper part of humerus. It forms lateral boundary for lower triangular space
  - The **medial head** arises from a large triangular area on the posterior surface of the humerus below the radial groove, and from medial and lateral intermuscular septae.
- **Insertion:**
  - The long and lateral heads converge and fuse to form a superficial flattened tendon
  - The tendon formed covers the medial head
  - Inserted into the posterior part of the superior surface of the olecranon process
  - Few deep fibers are inserted to the articular capsule of elbow joint known as **articularis cubiti** or subanconeus.
- **Nerve supply:** Each head receives a separate branch from the radial nerve (C7, C8).
- **Actions:**
  - Triceps is a powerful active extensor of the elbow

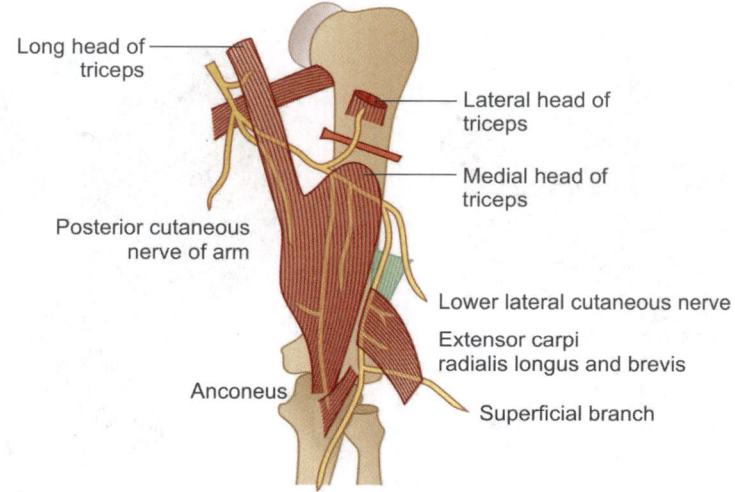

Fig. 40: Triceps brachii.

- The long head supports the head of humerus during abduction
- The articularis cubiti pulls the capsule of elbow joint during extension of forearm.

13. Second part of duodenum.

Second part of duodenum is vertical in position
- **Length:** 8 – 10 cm long,
- **Extent:** From superior duodenal flexure to inferior duodenal flexure, vertebral level of L_1, to the lower border of the L_3 vertebra
- **Peritoneal covering:** It is retroperitoneal and fixed. Its anterior surface is covered with peritoneum.
- **Relations (Figs. 41A and B):**
  - **Anteriorly:** Right lobe of the liver, transverse colon, root of the transverse mesocolon, small intestine
  - **Posteriorly:** Anterior surface of the right kidney, right renal vessels, right edge of the inferior vena cava, right psoas major
  - **Medially:** Head of the pancreas, ventral and dorsal anastomoses of superior and inferior pancreaticoduodenal arteries, bile duct joins with main pancreatic duct to form ampulla of Vater
  - **Laterally:** Right colic flexure.

- **Interior (Fig. 42):**
  - Circular folds are seen called plica circularis or **valve of Kerckring**
  - The **major duodenal papilla** is an elevation present posteromedially, 8 to 10 cm distal to the pylorus. The hepatopancreatic ampulla opens at the summit of the papilla
  - A fold of mucous membrane resembling a monk's hood called **plica semicircularis** seen covering the major duodenal papilla
  - The **minor duodenal papilla** is present anteromedial and 2 cm proximal

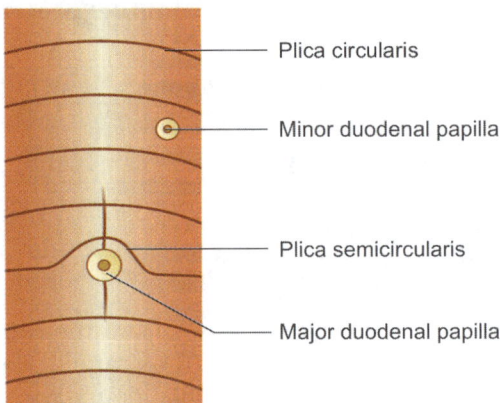

Fig. 42: Interior of second part.

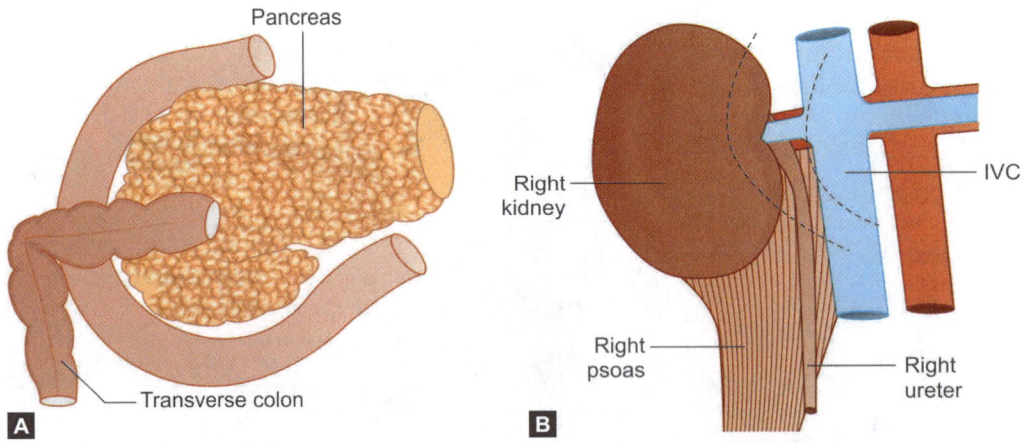

Figs. 41A and B: Second part of duodenum: (A) Anterior relations; (B) Posterior relations.

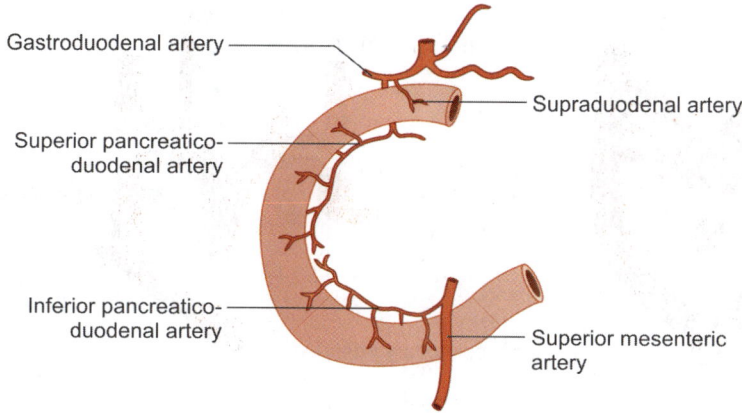

Fig. 43: Blood supply of second part of duodenum.

to major duodenal papilla and the accessory pancreatic duct opens.
- Plica longitudinalis a vertical fold extending from major duodenal papilla.
- **Blood supply (Fig. 43):**
  - Arterial supply: 2nd part is supplied by superior pancreaticoduodenal branch of gastroduodenal artery and inferior pancreaticoduodenal branch of superior mesenteric artery arteries
  - Venous drainage corresponding veins into portal vein.
- **Development:** Up to major duodenal papilla from foregut, and below it from midgut
- **Applied anatomy:**
  - Malignant growth of head of pancreas, annular pancreas encircling the second part of duodenum produces obstruction
  - Duodenal atresia may be caused due to annular pancreas. It is diagnosed by the **double bubble sign** in the ultrasound due to distension of stomach and first part of duodenum.

14. Trigone of urinary bladder.
Refer Essay Q. No. 2 – 2003.

15. Great saphenous vein.
Refer Short Notes 14 – 2005.

16. Yolk sac.
Refer Short Notes 2 – 2004.

17. Bronchopulmonary segment.
Refer Essay Q. No. 3 – 2004.

18. Fate of aortic arches.
- During fourth and fifth week, the pharyngeal arches appear
- Each pharyngeal arch receives artery from aortic arches which are derived from aortic sac
- The arteries of aortic arches end in the dorsal aorta
- During the sixth week a transverse septa appears within the aortic sac, termed the **aorticopulmonary septum**
- The aortic sac is divided by the spiral aorticopulmonary septum into pulmonary trunk and ascending aorta
- Initially six aortic arches appear
- Later the fifth one disappears
- The ascending aorta is connected to four arches and the pulmonary trunk to the sixth aortic arch
- **Fate of the aortic arches:**
  - **First arch:** Disappears leaving a small portion which persists as **maxillary artery**
  - **Second arch:** Disappears leaving hyoid **and stapedial arteries**, which disappear later
  - **Third arch: Common carotid** and first part of **internal carotid artery (ICA).**

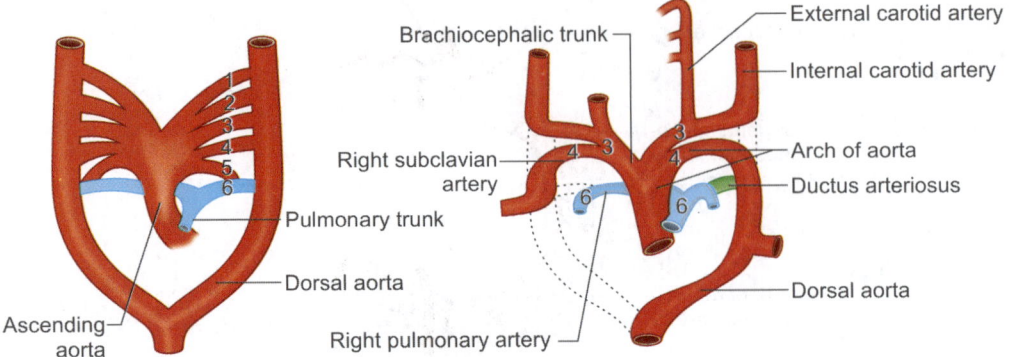

Fig. 44: Aortic arches.

- **Fourth arch**
  - Left side part of **arch of aorta**
  - Right side proximal part of **right subclavian artery**.
- **Sixth arch (pulmonary arch)**
  - Right side the distal part loses its connection with dorsal aorta and later disappears. The proximal part forms **right pulmonary artery**
  - Left side the distal part forms the **ductus arteriosus** in fetal life and proximal part the **left pulmonary artery**.

19. Hyoglossus muscle.

Refer Short Notes 15 – 2004.

20. Cerebellar peduncles.

The cerebellum is connected to other parts of nervous system by peduncles.

There are three peduncles—superior, middle, inferior cerebellar peduncles.

The middle cerebellar peduncle is larger and lateral, the inferior cerebellar peduncle is medial to it.

- **Inferior cerebellar peduncle** connects the medulla oblongata with cerebellum. Fibers entering the cerebellum (afferent fibers)
  - Posterior spinocerebellar tract from spinal cord

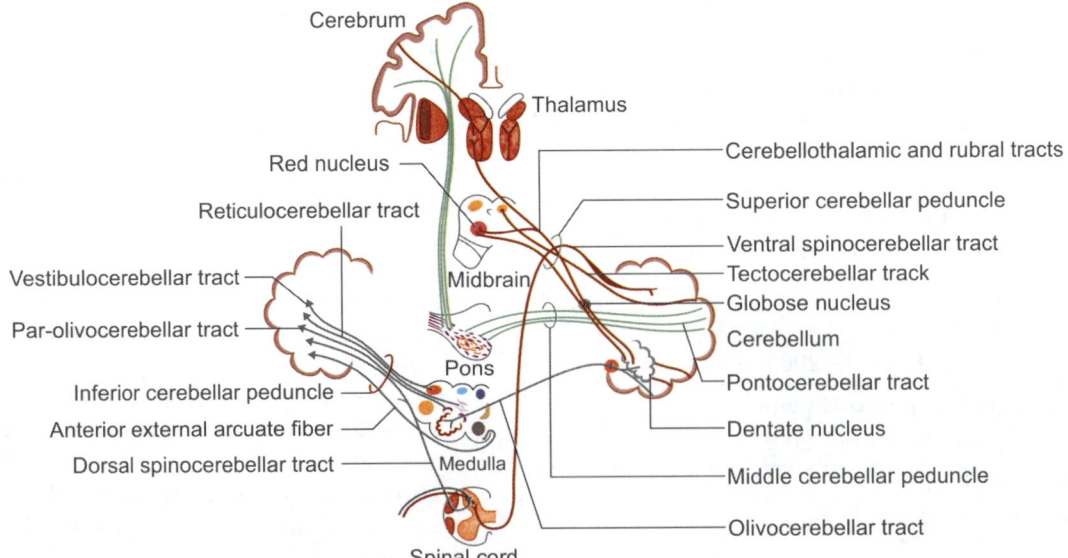

Fig. 45: Connections—cerebellar peduncles.

- Cuneocerebellar tract (posterior external arcuate fibers) from accessory cuneate nucleus
- Olivocerebellar fibers from inferior olivary nucleus
- Para olivocerebellar fibers from medial and dorsal accessory olivary nuclei
- Reticulocerebellar fibers from medulla
- Vestibulocerebellar fibers
- Anterior external arcuate fibers from Arcuate nucleus
- Stria medullaris from arcuate nucleus
- Trigeminocerebellar fibers from chief sensory and spinal nuclei of trigeminal.
• Fibers leaving the cerebellum (efferent)
  - Cerebelloolivary fibers
  - Cerebellovestibular fibers from fastigii nucleus
  - Cerebelloreticular fibers.
• **Middle cerebellar peduncle** connects pons with cerebellum (afferent fibers only)
  - Cortico-ponto-cerebellar fibers from all the lobes of cerebrum to pontine nuclei and from pons to cerebellum.
• **Superior cerebellar peduncle** connects midbrain with cerebellum
  Fibers entering the cerebellum (afferent)
  - Ventral spinocerebellar tract from spinal cord
  - Tectocerebellar fibers
  - Rubrocerebellar fibers from red nucleus.
  - Trigeminocerebellar fibers—from mesencephalic nucleus of trigeminal nerve.
• Fibers leaving the cerebellum (efferent)
  - Dentatorubral fibers from dentate nucleus to red nucleus
  - Cerebellothalamic fibers
  - Cerebelloreticular fibers (from dentate and fastigii nucleus).

21. Lateral wall of nose.

Refer Short Notes 16 – 2004.

22. Microscopic structure of ganglions (spinal and sympathetic).

• **Spinal (sensory) ganglion (Fig. 46A):**
  - The sensory ganglia includes the ganglion of dorsal roots of spinal nerves and the ganglia of the trigeminal, facial, glossopharyngeal and vagal cranial nerves
  - The ganglion are covered by connective tissue
  - Neurons of sensory ganglion are unipolar
  - They have spherical or oval soma/body of different size
  - The cytoplasm contains central nucleus
  - Neurons are arranged in group in-between bundles of myelinated and unmyelinated nerve fibers

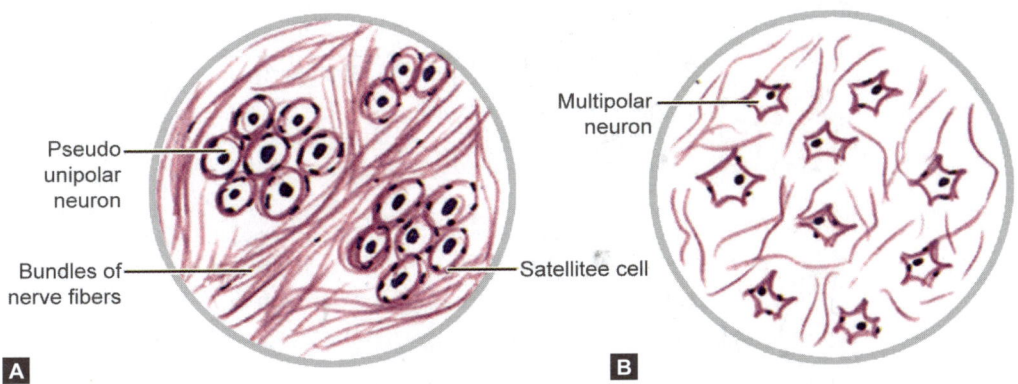

Fig. 46: Histology of ganglions: (A) Spinal/Sensory ganglion; (B) Sympathetic ganglion.

- The soma of each neuron is surrounded by a capsule formed by glial cells called **satellite cells**
- All of the cells in the ganglion are surrounded by vascular connective tissue.

- **Sympathetic (autonomic) ganglion (Fig. 46B)**
  - The neurons are multipolar
  - The nucleus is eccentrically situated
  - They are scattered
  - Surrounded by unmyelinated and myelinated nerve fibers which are scattered
  - The satellite cells are less in number.

23. Blood supply and nerve supply of scalp.

- **Motor nerve**:
  - **Anteriorly:** Frontal belly of occipitofrontalis is supplied by temporal branch of facial nerve
  - **Posteriorly:** Occipital belly of occipitofrontalis by posterior auricular branch of facial nerve.
- **Sensory nerve:** Four pairs of nerves supply the anterior half and posterior half of scalp **(Fig. 47)**.

  Anteriorly:
  - **Supratrochlear nerve**, branch of frontal nerve of ophthalmic division supplies paramedian part of forehead
  - **Supraorbital nerve**, branch of frontal nerve of ophthalmic division supplies the skin of forehead and anterior part of scalp as far as vertex
  - **Zygomaticotemporal nerve** from zygomatic nerve of maxillary division supplies skin of the anterior part of the temple
  - **Auriculotemporal nerve**, branch of mandibular division supplies hairy part of temple.

  Posteriorly:
  - **Third occipital nerve** (dorsal ramus of C_3) supply skin around external occipital protuberance
  - **Greater occipital nerve** (dorsal ramus of C_2) thickest cutaneous nerve of the body supplies skin of the back of scalp up to vertex
  - **Lesser occipital nerve** (ventral ramus of C_2) supply the scalp above and behind the ear
  - **Great auricular nerve** (ventral ramus of $C_{2,3}$) supplies lower part of auricle.

- **Blood supply (Fig. 48):**

  Arterial supply –
  - Scalp is supplied by branches of external and internal carotid arteries.
  - Five arteries supply the scalp
    i. Supratrochlear ⎫ from ophthalmic
    ii. Supraorbital   ⎭ artery ICA
    iii. Superficial temporal ⎫
    iv. Posterior auricular   ⎬ from external carotid artery (ECA)
    v. Occipital   ⎭

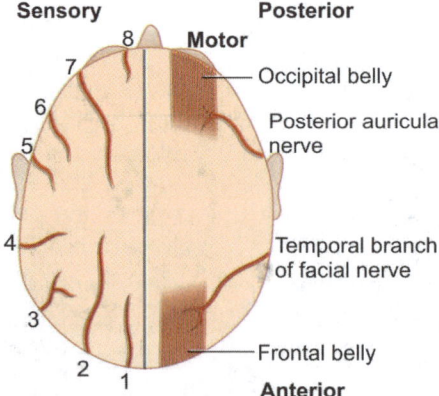

1. Supratrochlear
2. Supraorbital
3. Zygomatic temporal
4. Auriculotemporal
5. Great auricular
6. Lesser occipital
7. Greater occipital
8. Third occipital

Fig. 47: Nerve supply of scalp.

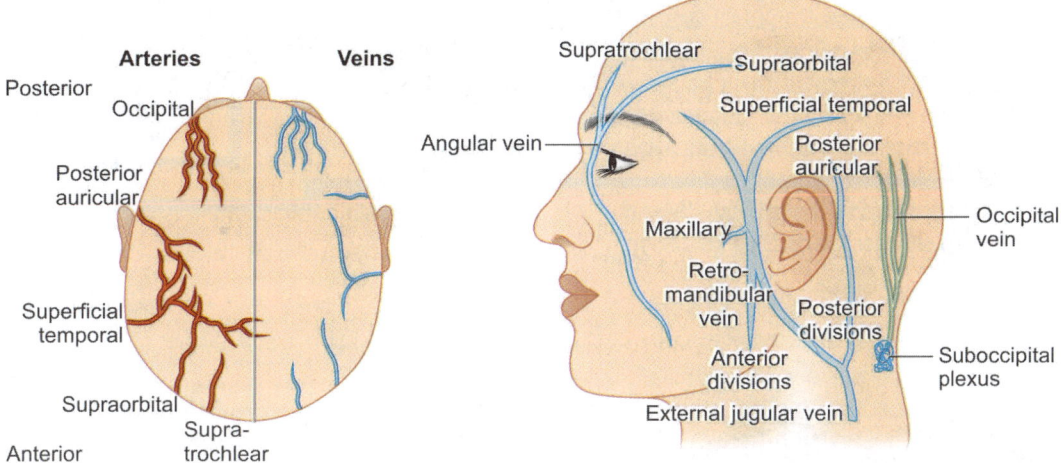

Fig. 48: Blood supply of scalp.

Venous Drainage
- Veins accompany the arteries
- Supratrochlear vein joins with supraorbital vein at the medial angle of eye to form angular vein
- Superficial temporal vein joins with maxillary vein to form retromandibular vein which in turn divides into anterior and posterior divisions
- Posterior auricular vein joins with posterior division of retromandibular vein to form external jugular vein
- Occipital veins drain into suboccipital plexus of veins
- Two **emissary veins** are present in scalp:
  i. Parietal emissary vein connects scalp with superior sagittal sinus
  ii. Mastoid emissary vein connects scalp with sigmoid sinus

Applied anatomy
- Scalp is richly supplied with blood vessels and there is anastomosis between the internal and external carotid arteries. Even a small wound will bleed profusely
- Superficial temporal veins is used for intravenous infusion in children
- The scalp is connected to the dural venous sinuses by emissary veins. So infection from scalp can spread resulting in thrombosis.

24. Histology of palatine tonsil.
Refer Short Notes 34 – 2005.

25. Development of interatrial septum.
- The interatrial septum is developed from septum primum and septum secundum
- From the roof of the primitive atrium the cells proliferate and grows downwards called **septum primum**
- It is a flap valve
- The atrioventricular canal is divided by the **septum intermedium** into a right and left atrioventricular openings
- A gap is seen between the septum primum and septum intermedium called **foramen primum**
- As the septum grows downwards it comes in contact with the septum intermedium thereby closing the foramen primum
- At the same time the cells in the upper part gets absorbed up by process of apoptosis and a newer opening is produced above the septum known as **foramen secundum**
- Another septum seen to the right of septum primum called **septum secundum.** It is rigid and free margin is crescent shaped. It covers the foramen secundum and overlaps the septum primum.

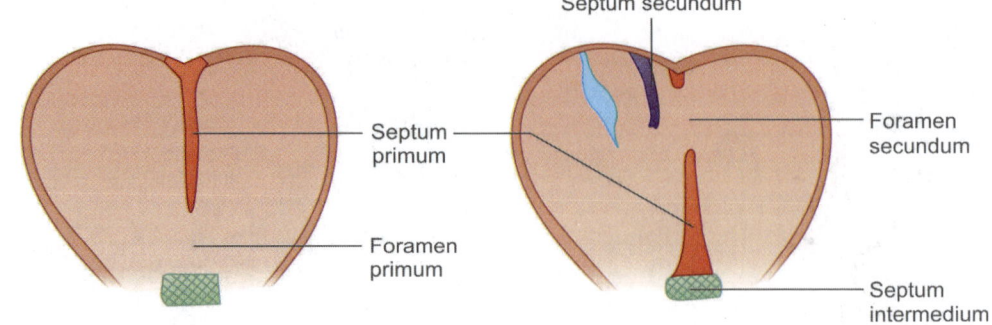

Fig. 49: Development of interatrial septum.

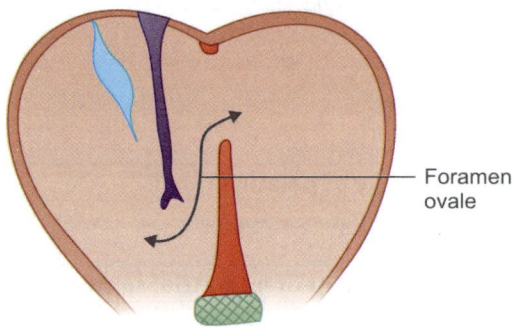

Fig. 50: Formation of foramen ovale.

- Now by the appearance of septum secundum the foramen is converted into intervalvular space called **foramen ovale**
- After birth, the intra-atrial pressures on both side become equal, the septum primum moves towards secundum and closes the foramen ovale
- The free crescentic margin of the septum secundum forms the border limbus fossa ovalis and the septum primum forms the fossa ovalis.

Congenital anomalies; atrial septal defect (ASD) may be due to
- Ostium primum—failure of fusion of endocardial cushions of the AV canal
- Ostium secundum defect—excessive absorption of septum primum or inadequate septum secundum
- Patent foramen ovale
- Probe patency of the foramen ovale

- Cor triloculare biventriculare—complete absence of atrial septum
- Premature closure of foramen ovale.

26. Circle of Willis.
Refer Short Notes 24 – 2005.

27. Lacrimal apparatus.
- The structures concerned with secretion and drainage of the lacrimal fluid constitute the lacrimal apparatus
- Components of lacrimal apparatus.
  - Lacrimal gland and its ducts
  - Conjunctival sac
  - Lacrimal puncta
  - Lacrimal canaliculi
  - Lacrimal sac
  - Nasolacrimal duct.
- **Lacrimal gland**
  - It is a serous type of gland
  - **Situated** in lacrimal fossa on the anterolateral part of the roof of the bony orbit
  - **Parts:** It has two parts separated by the aponeurosis of levator palpabrae superioris muscle **(Fig. 51)**
    i. Orbital part
    ii. Palpebral part
  - **Orbital part**
    - The size and shape is of an almond
    - Situation—related to anterolateral part of roof of the orbit and situated in the lacrimal fossa, on the medial surface of the zygomatic process of the frontal bone.

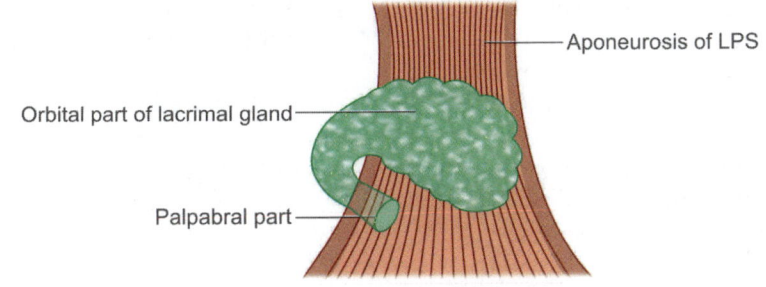

Fig. 51: Parts of lacrimal gland.

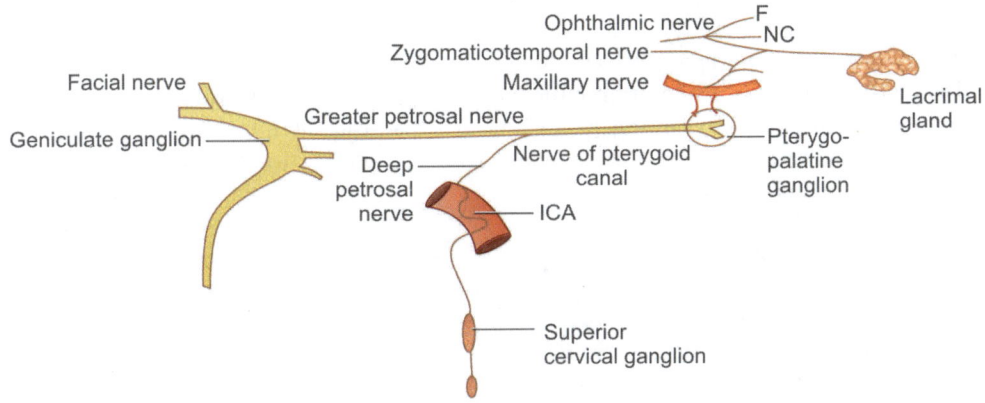

Fig. 52: Nerve supply of lacrimal gland.

- **Extent:** It lies above levator palpabrae superioris (LPA), anteriorly up to the orbital septum and posteriorly to the orbital fat
    - The palpebral part
    - Is one-third the size of the orbital part
    - Extends below the aponeurosis of levator palpabrae superioris and anteriorly to the lateral part of superior conjunctival fornix.
- **Duct:** The ducts of the orbital part pass through the palpebral part and open into the conjunctival sac
  Main ducts of the lacrimal gland is formed by, ducts from palpebral part about six in number and 4 to 5 ducts from the orbital part, open into the lateral part of superior fornix of the conjunctival sac.

Nerve supply
Secretomotor supply (Parasympathetic) (Fig. 52)
Lacrimatory nucleus in pons ----------- facial nerve -------- geniculate ganglion ------- greater petrosal nerve + deep petrosal nerve communicates nerve of pterygoid canal ----------- pterygopalatine ganglion relays maxillary nerve --- zygomaticotemporal ----------- lacrimal nerve ----- gland

Sympathetic supply
Postganglionic fibers from superior cervical ganglion ---- deep petrosal nerve (plexus around ICA)

- **Blood supply:** Lacrimal branch of ophthalmic artery.
- **Conjunctival sac**
    - The conjunctiva lining the deep surfaces of the eyelid called palpebral conjunctiva

- Lining the front of the eyeball is bulbar conjunctiva
- The potential space between the palpebral and bulbar conjunctiva is conjunctival sac.
- **Lacrimal puncta:** The puncta of the upper and lower lids, are directed towards the surface of the eye to collect tears.
- **Lacrimal canaliculi**
  - Each canaliculus, is about 10 mm long
  - Each canaliculus first passes vertically for about 2 mm from its punctum
  - Then the superior canaliculi bend downwards and medially
  - The inferior bends and pass horizontally
  - At the bend there is a dilatation called ampulla.
- **Lacrimal sac (Fig. 53)**
  - The lacrimal sac is dilated and closed upper end of the nasolacrimal duct
  - It is approximately 12 mm long and 5 mm wide
  - Lies in a fossa in between the anterior and posterior lacrimal crest formed by frontal process of maxilla and lacrimal bones
  - Its closed upper end is called fundus, and below continuous with nasolacrimal duct
  - The lacrimal canaliculi open into the upper part of the sac laterally

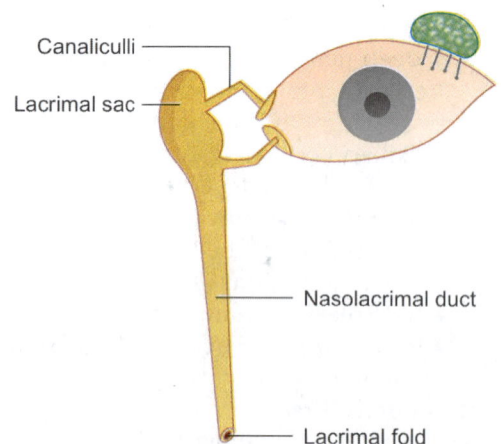

Fig. 53: Nasolacrimal duct.

- A dilatation is present at the level of opening of canaliculi called sinus of Meier
- It is covered by lacrimal fascia and is related to medial palpabral raphe in front and lacrimal part of orbicularis oculi behind
- Sac is surrounded by plexus of veins.
- **Nasolacrimal duct**
  - The nasolacrimal duct is approximately 18 mm long
  - Extends from the lacrimal sac to the inferior meatus of the nose
  - It opens into the inferior meatus at the junction of anterior one-third and posterior two-third
  - A fold of nasal mucous membrane (plica lacrimalis) is present just above its opening which acts as flap valve called **Hasner's valve**
  - The duct runs down in an osseous nasolacrimal canal formed by the maxilla, lacrimal bone and inferior nasal concha
  - It is narrowest in the middle
  - Duct is surrounded by plexus of veins
  - Direction—directed downwards, backwards and laterally.
- **Applied anatomy**
  - Removal of palpebral part of lacrimal gland is equal to removal of the entire gland, as the ducts pass through the palpebral part
  - Dacryocystitis: Inflammation of the lacrimal sac.

28. Turner's syndrome.

- **Turner syndrome** or **Ullrich – Turner syndrome**
- It is also known as "Gonadal dysgenesis"
- This condition occurs in about 1 in 2,500 female births
- One of the X chromosome is missing. 45, X, is most common.
  Genotype:
  - It is acrosomal anomaly in which complete or part of one of the sex chromosomes is absent (45, X0)
  - Turner mosaicism.

Phenotype:
- A low or indistinct hairline
- Shorter stature
- A broad chest and widely spaced nipples
- Wide neck (webbed neck)
- Because of absence of function ovary, women with this syndrome are usually infertile.
- **Complications:**
  - A heart murmur, sometimes associated with stenosis of aorta
  - Hypertension
  - Eye problems—cataract
  - Scoliosis occurs in 10 percent
  - Hashimoto thyroiditis
  - Obesity
  - Osteoporosis due to lack of estrogen
  - Renal defects.

29. External jugular vein.

- It is a superficial vein which drains the face and scalp
- **Formation:** Posterior division of retromandibular vein and posterior

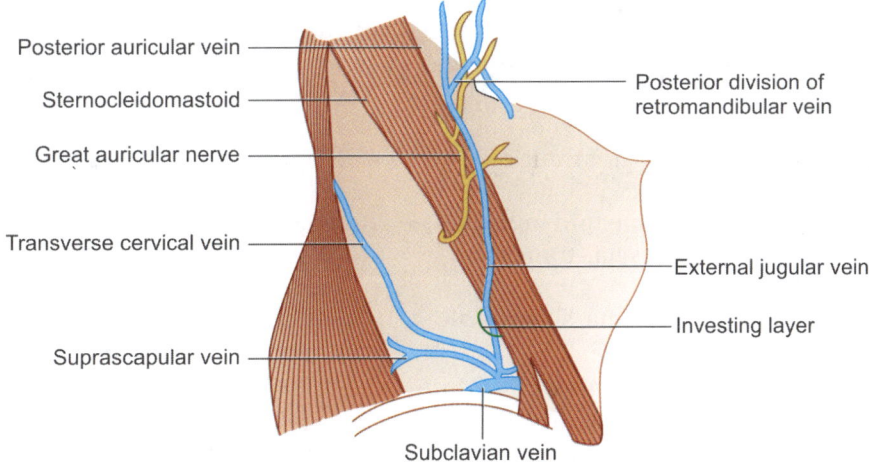

Fig. 54: External jugular vein.

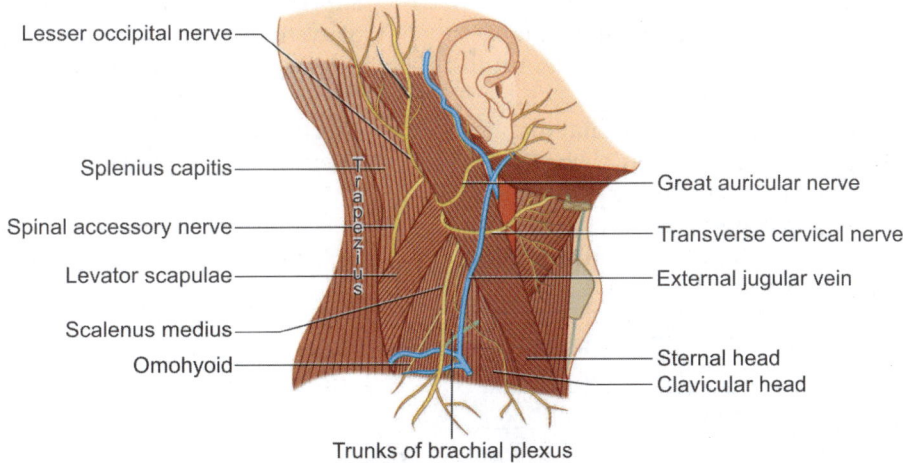

Fig. 55: Relations of sternocleidomastoid muscle.

auricular vein unite to form external jugular vein
- **Level of formation:** Formed at the level of the angle of mandible.
- **Course**
  - It descends downwards from angle of mandible to root of neck
  - It is superficial to sternocleidomastoid muscle
  - About 5 cm above the clavicle the investing layer of deep fascia is pierced by the vein
  - The fascia becomes adherent to the adventitial layer of the vein.
- **Termination**
  - Drains to subclavian vein
  - Near termination a dilatation is present called sinus.
- **Relations**
  - Descends parallel to great auricular nerve
  - Deep—sternocleidomastoid muscle separated by deep fascia, transverse cervical nerve
  - Superficial—skin, platysma, superficial fascia.
- **Tributaries**
  - Transverse cervical vein
  - Suprascapular vein
  - Anterior jugular vein.
- **Applied anatomy**
  - In a case of cut injury to the vein above it pierces the deep fascia, results in air embolism, as the vein cannot collapse due to the adherence of adventitial layer to the deep fascia
  - Venous pressure: The external jugular vein is distended when there is an increase in the venous pressure. The pressure can be raised by Valsalva's maneuver (forced expiration with closed mouth and nostrils).

30. Histology of cerebellum.
Refer Short Notes 18 – 2004.

31. Sternocleidomastoid.
- It is the key muscle of neck
- It divides the neck into anterior and posterior triangles
- It is a cruciate type of muscle
- It has two heads—sternal and clavicular head
- **Origin:**
  - Sternal head is tendinous in origin from upper part of anterior surface of manubrium sterni
  - Clavicular head from superior surface of medial one-third of clavicle
  - The two heads are separated by a gap called **lesser supraclavicular triangle**.
- **Insertion:** The sternal head spirals and passes behind the clavicular head and forms a rounded belly in the middle and the muscle inserted to the lateral surface of mastoid process and lateral half of superior nuchal line.
- **Nerve supply:**
  - Motor—spinal accessory
  - Proprioceptive impulses—ventral rami of C_2, C_3.
- **Relations:**
  - *Anterior border:* Forms boundary for the anterior triangles.
  - *Posterior border:*
    - Forms the anterior boundary for the posterior triangle
    - The four cutaneous branches emerge at the midpoint or just above the midpoint of the posterior border of the muscle and is called as **nerve point**.
  - *Superficial:* Skin, superficial fascia with platysma investing layer of deep fascia, external jugular vein, great auricular nerve, transverse cervical nerve, parotid gland
  - *Deep:*
    - 5 muscles—splenius capitis, levator scapulae, scalene muscles, posterior belly of digastric, infrahyoid muscles
    - 5 arteries—subclavian vessels, carotids (common, external and internal carotid arteries), supra scapular, transverse cervical arteries, occipital artery
    - 5 veins—internal jugular vein, anterior jugular vein, occipital, lingual and facial veins

- 5 nerves—cervical and brachial plexus, phrenic nerve, ansa cervicalis, spinal accessory nerve, and vagus.
- **Blood supply**: Superior thyroid, occipital, posterior auricular, and suprascapular arteries.
- **Actions:**
  - If one muscle contracts it tilts the head to same side and face to opposite side
  - If both side muscles act it helps to **draw the head forward** as in eating
  - When body is supine in position, contraction of both side muscles helps to lift the head.
- **Applied anatomy**:
  - Due to repeated painful contraction or shortening of sternocleidomastoid muscle results in a condition called **torticollis or Wry neck**
  - The branchial cyst is located along the anterior border of the muscle between the upper and middle third junction.

32. Development of tongue.

Refer Short Notes 20 – 2003.

MBBS Examination 2007

ANSWER ALL QUESTIONS

I. Essay questions   **(15/10 Marks)**

1. Describe the arches of foot under the following headings: (a) Bones forming, (b) Factors maintaining and (c) Applied anatomy.
2. Describe the stomach under the following headings: (a) Location and position, (b) Parts and relations, (c) Blood supply and (d) Microscopic and applied anatomy.
3. Describe the duodenum under the following headings: (a) Location and Extent, (b) Relations, (c) Blood supply, (d) Microscopic anatomy, (e) Development and (f) Applied anatomy.
4. Describe the axillary artery under the following headings: (a) Origin and Termination, (b) Course, (c) Relations (d) Branches.
5. Describe the sciatic nerve under the following headings: (a) Origin and Termination, (b) Course, (c) Relations and (d) Branches and applied anatomy.
6. Describe the tongue under the following headings. (a) Parts, (b) Muscles, (c) Nerve supply and (d) Lymphatic drainage.
7. Describe the sulci and gyri on the superolateral surface of cerebral hemisphere with functional areas.
8. Describe the thyroid gland under the following headings: (a) Gross anatomy, (b) Microscopic anatomy, (c) Applied anatomy and (d) Development.
9. Describe the facial nerve under the following headings: (a) Origin and termination, (b) Course and relations, (c) Branches and (d) Applied anatomy.
10. Describe the bronchopulmonary segments under the following headings: Definition, numbers, blood supply, nerve supply, and applied anatomy.

II. Short notes   **(5/4/3 Marks)**

1. Development of pancreas.
2. Cruciate ligaments of knee joint.
3. Microscopic structure of kidney.
4. Sesamoid bone.
5. Median nerve in hand.
6. Lymphatic drainage of stomach.
7. Adductor canal.
8. Descent of testis.
9. Anastomosis around elbow joint.
10. Development of urinary bladder.
11. Microscopic structure of ovary.
12. Spermatogenesis.
13. Boundaries and contents of quadrangular space.
14. Types of epiphysis with examples.
15. Femoral sheath formation, contents and applied anatomy.
16. Carpometacarpal joint of thumb.
17. Nerve supply of heart.
18. Buccinator.
19. Coronary sinus.
20. Medial surface of right lung.
21. Draw a well labeled diagram of c/s of pons at the level of facial colliculus.
22. Development of face and its anomalies.
23. Microscopic structure of pituitary gland
24. Derivatives of I pharyngeal arch.
25. Maxillary sinus.

26. Facial artery.
27. Structures derived from mesoderm of second branchial arch.
28. Microscopic structure of submandibular salivary gland.
29. Falx cerebri.
30. Styloid apparatus.
31. Circle of Willis.
32. Pericardium.

I. ESSAY QUESTIONS

1. Describe the arches of foot under the following headings. (a) Bones forming, (b) Factors maintaining and (c) Applied anatomy.

Refer Essay Q. No. 1 – Nov 2003.

2. Describe the stomach under the following headings: (a) Location and position, (b) Parts and relations, (c) Blood supply and (d) Microscopic and applied anatomy.

Location and Position

- It is expanded part of alimentary tract between esophagus and duodenum
- It is situated in the upper abdomen
- Extends from left upper quadrant to the right
- It is directed downwards, forwards and to the right

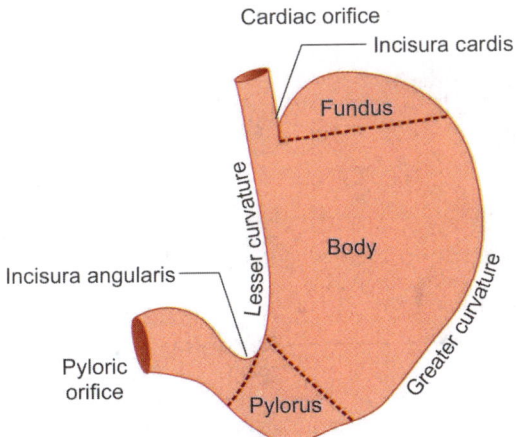

Fig. 1: Part and subdivisions of stomach.

- It is located in the left hypochondrium, epigastric and umbilical.

Presenting Parts and Relations (Fig. 1)

- It has two ends, two borders and two surfaces
- The **two ends** are the cardiac and pyloric ends with openings at each ends (cardiac and pyloric orifices)
- The **two borders** are lesser and greater curvatures
- The **two surfaces** are anterosuperior surface and posteroinferior surface.
- **Cardiac orifice:**
- It is situated at the left 7th costal cartilage, 2.5 cm to the left of the median plane, opposite T11
- It is 40 cm away from the incisor teeth. There is no demonstrable anatomical sphincter.
- **Relations**
- **Anteriorly:** covered by peritoneum and left lobe of liver
- **Posteriorly:** connected to left crus of diaphragm
- **Pyloric orifice:**
  - 1.25 cm to the right of mid line along transpyloric plane related to lower border of L1 vertebra
  - It is thicker and surrounded by circular muscle fibres called the pyloric sphincter
  - The pre-pyloric vein of Mayo runs superficial to this orifice.
  - Relations:
    - Anteriorly—peritoneum, quadrate lobe, falciform ligament
    - Posteriorly—neck of pancreas.
- **Lesser curvature:**
  - It is J shaped and it is more fixed and lies posteriorly
  - Incisura angularis is the most dependent part of lesser curvature
  - This border gives attachment to the two layers of lesser omentum and it is related to right and left gastric vessels.
- **Greater curvature:**
  - It forms the left border of the stomach.
  - It is more superficial and movable. It is four or five times greater than the lesser curvature

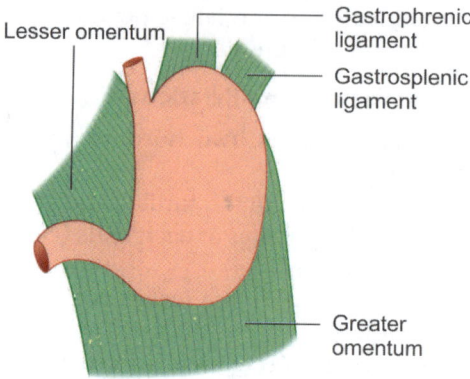

Fig. 2: Ligaments of the stomach.

- It starts at the cardiac notch on the left side of cardiac orifice, and reach the fifth intercostal space by passing upwards, backwards and to the left. Then it descends downwards to end in pyloric orifice
- The summit of the arch is called the fundus
- Opposite incisura angularis, the greater curvature bulges to form pyloric antrum.
- **Attachments**
  - **At the cardiac end:** Gastrophrenic ligament.
  - **At fundus:** Gastrosplenic ligament
  - **Remaining part:** Greater omentum.

- **Anterosuperior surface (Fig. 3):** It is entirely covered with peritoneum. It is related to:
  - On the right, to left lobe and quadrate lobe of liver
  - On the upper and left, to the diaphragm, left pleura and lung, sixth to ninth left costal cartilages
  - The middle triangular portion is directly in contact with anterior abdominal wall. This portion is called as the **gastric triangle**.

  The gastric triangle is bounded by the lower border of liver on the right side, left costal margin on the left side and transverse colon below. It is used for feeding the patient in case of obstruction of oesophagus (feeding gastrostomy).

- **Posteroinferior surface (Fig. 4)**
  It is covered with peritoneum. It is related to the **stomach bed** structures. The bed is formed by:
  - Left crus of diaphragm
  - Left suprarenal gland
  - Left kidney
  - Splenic artery
  - Anterior surface of pancreas
  - Anterior layer of transverse mesocolon
  - Gastric area of spleen

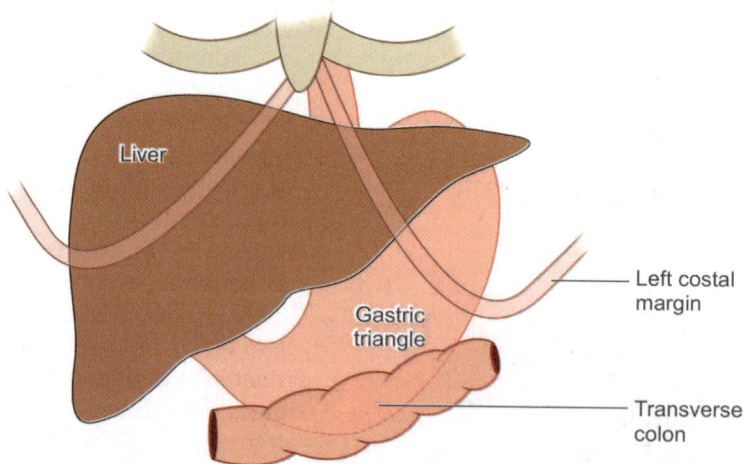

Fig. 3: Anterosuperior surface.

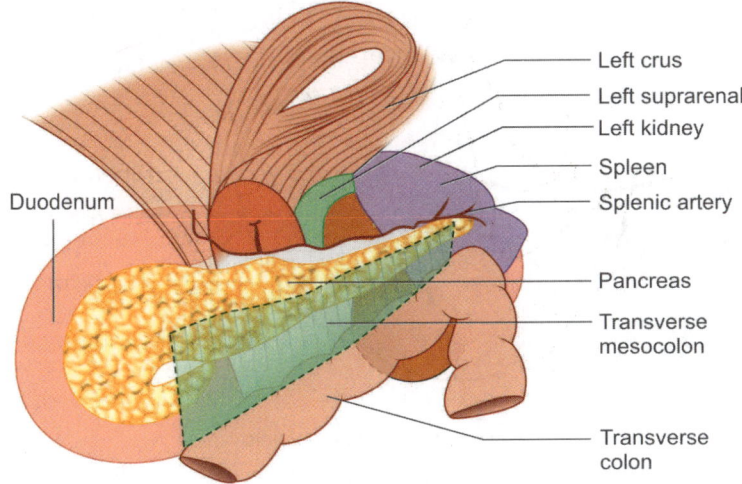

Fig. 4: Stomach bed.

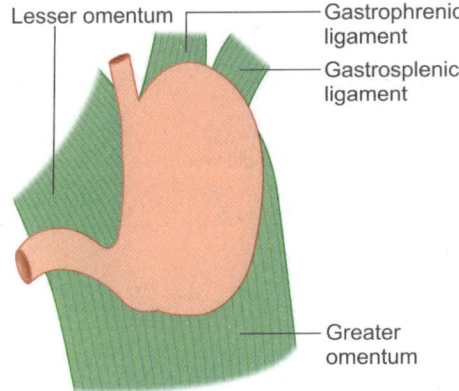

Fig. 5: Peritoneal relations.

- **Peritoneal relations (Fig. 5):**
  - **Lesser omentum:**
    - It is a fold of peritoneum made up of two layers
    - Attachment—between lesser curvature of stomach and proximal part of duodenum to porta hepatis of liver
    - Contents (a) along lesser curvature—right and left gastric vessels and gastric nerves. (b) along the right free margin—portal vein, hepatic artery, bile duct, nerve plexus, hepatic nodes.
  - **Greater omentum:**
    - It is a fold of peritoneum consisting of four layers
    - Attachment—between greater curvature and transverse colon
    - Contents—right and left gastro epiploic vessels, fat, areolar tissue and milky spots derived from macrophages.
  - **Gastrosplenic ligament/third omentum:**
    - It is a fold of peritoneum consisting of two layers
    - Attachments—connects fundus of stomach to hilum of spleen
    - Contents—short gastric vessels.
  - **Gastrophrenic ligament:**
    - It is a fold of peritoneum consisting of two layers
    - Attachment—between bare area of stomach to left crus of diaphragm
    - Contents—left gastric artery.

Blood Supply

- **Arterial supply (Fig. 6):** The stomach is supplied by six arteries which are derived from coeliac trunk either directly or through its branches.
  - **The left gastric artery**—(principal artery of the stomach) is a direct branch

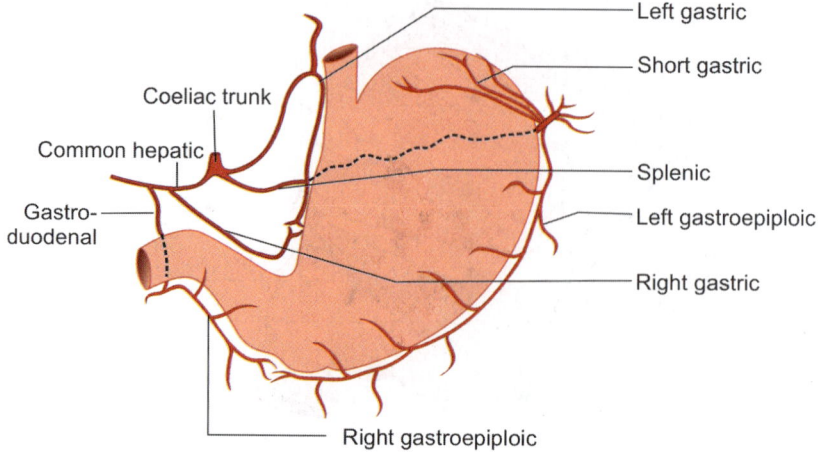

Fig. 6: Arterial supply.

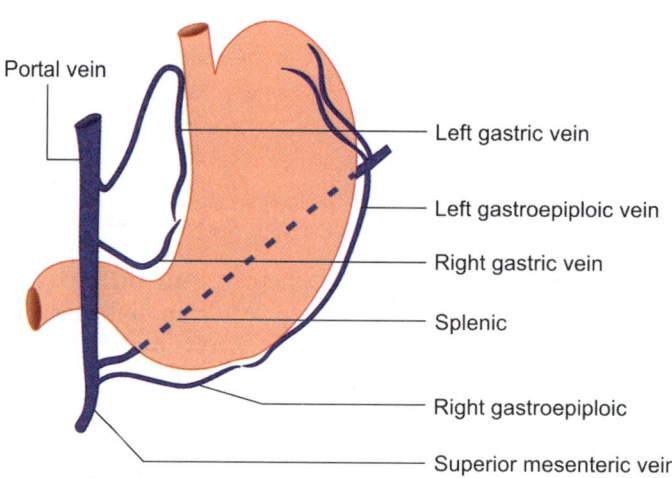

Fig. 7: Venous drainage.

of coeliac trunk. It enters the superior gastropancreatic fold, arches and then enters lesser omentum along lesser curvature and supplies two-third of the stomach
- **Right gastric artery**—arises from common hepatic artery, runs along lesser curvature within lesser omentum and anastomoses with left gastric artery
- **Short gastric arteries**—seen as 3 or 4 branches, arising from splenic artery and supplies fundus by passing through gastro splenic ligament
- **Right gastroepiploic artery**—arises from gastro duodenal artery, runs along the greater curvature within greater omentum and anastomoses with left gastro epiploic artery
- **Left gastroepiploic artery**—arises from splenic artery, runs along greater curvature within greater omentum
- **Posterior gastric artery**—from splenic artery and supplies the posterior wall of fundus.
- **Venous drainage (Fig. 7):** The veins of the stomach correspond to the arteries and drain directly or indirectly into the portal vein.

- Right and left gastric veins drain into the trunk of portal vein
- Short gastric and left gastroepiploic veins into splenic vein
- Right gastroepiploic vein into superior mesenteric vein.

Microscopic Anatomy (Figs. 8A and B)

It is made up of 4 layers. Inner to outer are
I. **Mucous layer**
   - Mucous folds or rugae are seen placed longitudinally, more towards greater curvature and pyloric part
   - The mucous layer is formed by epithelium, lamina propria, and muscularis mucosa
   - **Epithelium**: Lined by simple columnar epithelium. It presents depressions called gastric pits. The pits are deep extending to lamina up to muscularis mucosa and are lined by surface mucous cells.
   - The **gastric pits, in fundus** are not deep and extend about one fourth of the thickness of mucous layer. **In pylorus,** the gastric pit is deep and extend into the mucosa to about two third of its thickness
   - **Lamina propria**: Consists of vessels, nerves and gastric glands
   - The glands are grouped as cardiac, principal, and pyloric glands
   - The glands are packed in the lamina propria and long, tubular in the fundus and body
   - The pyloric glands are short and coiled.
   - Muscularis mucosa: Made up of inner circular and outer longitudinal smooth muscle fibers.
   - Each **gland** is lined by :
     - **Zymogenic/chief/peptic cells**: Cuboidal cells, occupy the base of the gland and they synthesize digestive enzymes pepsin and lipase. They contain abundant zymogenic granules
     - **Oxyntic/parietal cells:** Situated along the lateral wall of the gland. They are large and oval in shape. Secrete HCl and the intrinsic factor for absorption of vitamin B12
     - **Neck mucous cells**: It is more in number in pyloric glands, situated at the neck of glands, and lateral walls of base of gland. Secrete mucous
     - **Stem cells:** They are columnar, less in number, undergo mitotic division
     - **Neuroendocrine or enteroendocrine (Argentaffin cells)**: Cells belong to APUD system. They are found in fundus and body and situated in the deeper part of gland. They include:

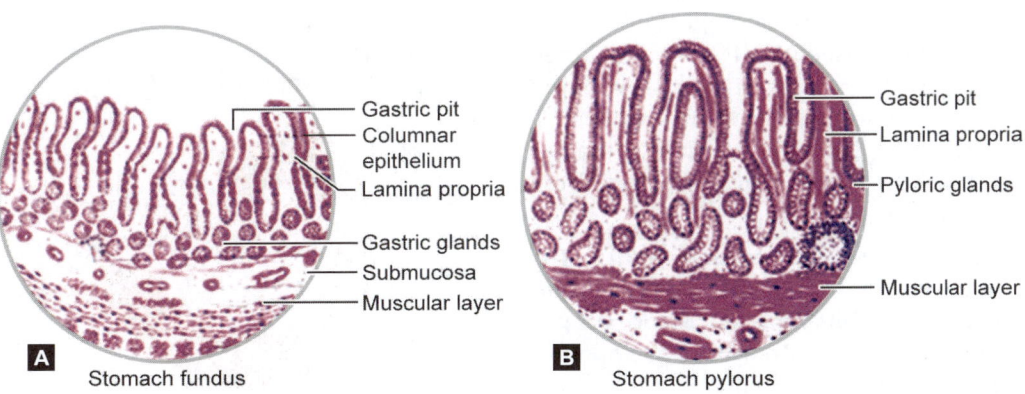

Figs. 8A and B: (A) Stomach fundus; (B) Stomach pylorus.

- G cells—secrete gastrin
- D cells—secrete somatostatin
- ECL (enterochromaffin like cell)—secrete histamine and serotonin
- Pylorus of stomach: The chief cells and oxyntic cells are few in number in the pylorus. More number of mucous secreting cells are present.

II. **Submucous layer:** Consists of loose areolar tissue, containing collagen and elastic fibers, blood vessels, lymphatics and nerves. Meissner's plexus (submucosal plexus), of nerves are present

III. **Muscular layer:** Consists of 3 layers of smooth muscle
Outer longitudinal, middle circular, inner oblique

IV. **Serous:** Derived from visceral peritoneum formed by simple squamous mesothelium.

Applied Anatomy

- Peptic ulcer: It is more common along the lesser curvature since the submucous plexus is absent and the vessels are long and slender. Occlusion of these vessels produce ischemia
- Pyloric stenosis is a congenital defect with neuromuscular incoordination of the pyloric sphincter
- Vagotomy is performed to reduce the secretion of HCl in case of peptic ulcer. **Vagotomy** may be:
  - **Truncal**—section of both vagal trunks. As the stomach becomes atonic the patient has to undergo either pyloroplasty or gastrojejunostomy
  - **Selective**—section of nerve of Latarjet. It results in delayed emptying as the motility of pyloric antrum is reduced
  - **Highly selective**—only smaller branches from gastric nerves to prevent delayed gastric emptying.

3. **Describe the duodenum under the following headings: (a) Location and Extent, (b) Relations, (c) Blood supply, (d) Microscopic anatomy, (e) Development and (f) Applied Anatomy.**

- Duodenum meaning 12 fingers breadth, 25 cm in length
- It is developed from foregut and midgut, hence supplied by both coeliac axis and superior mesenteric artery
- It forms the proximal and fixed part of small intestine
- It is C shaped enclosing the head of pancreas
- It is divided into 4 parts **(Fig. 9)**
- Proximal portion of 1st part alone is entirely covered by peritoneum. The rest of duodenum is retroperitoneal.

Location of Parts with Extent and Relations

- **First part:** Superior part
  - Extends from pyloric junction to superior duodenal flexure
  - **Features:**
    - Wider and more mobile
    - Mucosa more similar to gastric mucosa
    - Less number of circular folds
    - Supplied by end arteries; so, prone for peptic ulcers
    - A triangular projection called duodenal cap is seen after the barium meal
    - 5 cm in length.
  - **Relations (Fig. 10):**
    - **Anterior:** Quadrate lobe of liver, neck of gallbladder
    - **Posterior:** Gastroduodenal artery, bile duct, portal vein
    - **Superior:** Epiploic foramen
    - **Inferior:** Head and neck of the pancreas.
- **Second part**
Refer Short Notes 13 – 2006.

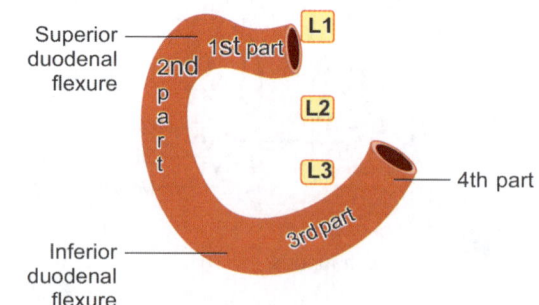

Fig. 9: Parts of duodenum.

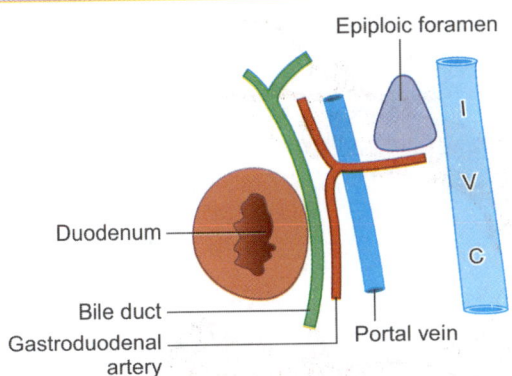

Fig. 10: Posterior relation of 1st part.

- It ends in duodenojejunal flexure
- 2.5 cm in length
- **Relations:**
  - **Anterior:** Transverse colon, transverse mesocolon, upper part of root of mesentery, stomach
  - **Posterior:** Aorta, left sympathetic chain, left renal vessels, left gonadal vessels, left psoas muscle
  - **Lateral:** Left kidney, left ureter
  - **Superior:** Body of pancreas.

Blood Supply

- **Arterial supply (Fig. 12)**
  - Up to the opening of the bile duct: Supplied by the superior pancreaticoduodenal artery branch of gastroduodenal artery
  - Below it: By the inferior pancreaticoduodenal artery branch of superior mesenteric artery
  - The superior and inferior arteries divide into anterior and posterior branches and situated in the groove between the head of pancreas and duodenum. The branches of superior and inferior anastomose with each other
  - Ist part also receives blood supply from:
    - Supraduodenal artery of Wilkie: Branch from gastroduodenal artery. It is an end artery.
    - Retroduodenal branch of gastroduodenal artery

- **Third part**: Horizontal part.
  - Extends from inferior duodenal flexure on the right side of L3 vertebra to left side of vertebra
  - 10 cm in length
  - It runs from right to left from right side of lower border of L3.
  - **Relations (Figs. 11A and B):**
    - **Anterior:** Superior mesenteric vessels, root of mesentery
    - **Posterior:** Right ureter, right psoas major, right gonadal vessels, inferior vena cava, abdominal aorta and origin of inferior mesenteric artery
    - **Superior:** Head of pancreas and uncinate process
    - **Inferior:** Coils of jejunum.
- **Fourth part**: Ascending part
  - Extends from L3 vertebra to upper border of L2 vertebra

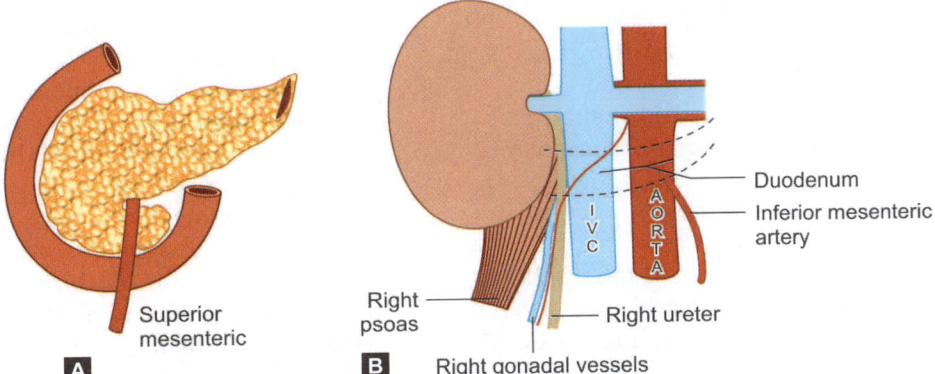

Figs. 11A and B: Relations of third part: (A) Anterior relations; (B) Posterior relations.

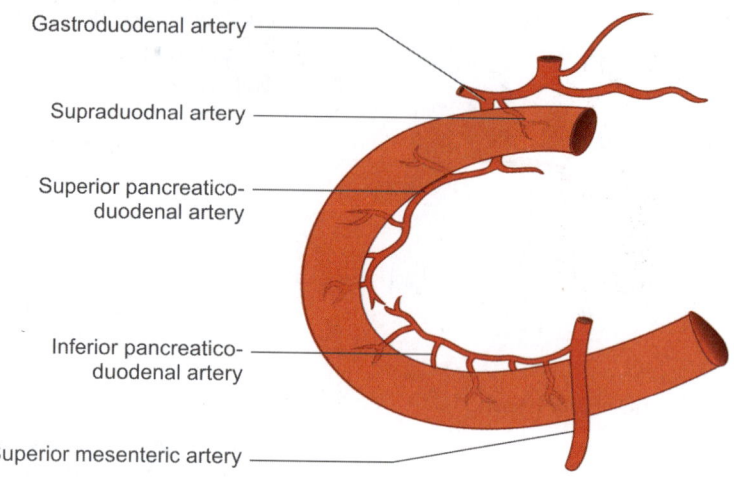

Fig. 12: Arterial supply.

- Infraduodenal artery – Branch of right gastroepiploic artery.
- **Venous drainage:** Splenic vein, superior mesenteric vein, portal vein.

Microscopic Structure

Refer Short Notes 9 – 2004.

Development of Duodenum

- The mucous membrane is from **endoderm** and muscular coat is from surrounding **splanchnic mesenchyme**
- The mucosa of duodenum is developed from **two sources**
- Second part up to opening of hepatopancreatic duct is from **distal part of foregut**
- Below that is from **proximal part of mid gut**
- The junction between the two parts is distal to the origin of hepatic bud
- Duodenum is supplied by celiac axis artery of foregut and superior mesenteric artery of midgut
- Developed by three stages
  - First stage: Rotation
    - The duodenum rotates to the right along with stomach
    - The rotation is due to rapid growth of the pancreas
  - Second stage: Fixation
    - The dorsal mesentry disappears
    - Gets fixed to posterior abdominal wall
    - The duodenum and pancreas become retroperitoneal except the proximal portion of duodenum
  - Third stage: Axial rotation
    - The second part of duodenum under goes rotation along with ventral pancreatic bud
    - It rotates to the right so the ventral and dorsal pancreatic buds fuse
    - The cells proliferate and the lumen is obliterated initially
    - Later the lumen is recanalized.
- Congenital anomaly
  - Duodenal atresia
    - Atresia in the **proximal part of duodenum** due to lack of recanalization of the duodenum
    - **Distal part atresia** may be due to malrotation, volvulus, or omphalocele
  - **Obstruction** of duodenum due to annular pancreas. Diagnosed by the observation of **double-bubble sign** on ultrasound, due to simultaneous distension of stomach and first part of duodenum.

Applied Anatomy

- Barium meal is a contrast X-ray taken after giving barium orally. Duodenal cap is seen as a triangular shadow, formed by the first part of duodenum
- The gastroduodenal artery is closely related to the first part of the duodenum along its posteromedial surface. The penetrating ulcers or tumor of the duodenum, may erode into the artery resulting in more bleeding from it and hence called as '**artery of hemorrhage**'.

4. Describe the axillary artery under the following headings: (a) Origin and Termination, (b) Course, (c) Relations and (d) Branches.

- It is the downward continuation of the subclavian artery
- Enters the axilla through cervicoaxillary canal
- **Origin:** It is continuation of subclavian artery from the outer border of the 1st rib
- **Termination:** it terminates at the lower border of the teres major by continuing down as the brachial artery
- **Course:** It runs downwards and laterally; direction varies with the position of the arm
- **Division:** The pectoralis minor crosses the artery and divides it into 3 parts (Fig. 13).
  - **1st part:** Lies proximal to pectoralis minor. From outer border of 1st rib to the medial border of pectoralis minor
  - **2nd part:** Deep to the muscle
  - **3rd part:** Distal to the muscle. From lateral border of pectoralis minor to the lower border of teres major.
- **Relations:**
  - 1st part (Fig. 14A):
    - The artery and cords of brachial plexus are enclosed in the axillary sheath
    - Posterior: Medial cord of brachial plexus
    - Lateral: Lateral and posterior cords of brachial plexus
    - Medial: Axillary vein
    - Anterior: Clavipectoral fascia and pectoralis major muscle.
  - 2nd part (Fig. 14B):
    - Lateral—lateral cord
    - Medial—medial cord and axillary vein
    - Posterior—posterior cord
    - Anterior—pectoralis minor and pectoralis major.
  - 3rd part (Fig. 15):
    - Medial: Axillary vein, medial cutaneous nerve of forearm, ulnar nerve, medial cutaneous nerve of arm
    - Lateral: Musculocutaneous nerve, coracobrachialis, median nerve
    - Posterior: Radial nerve, teres major, latissimus dorsi
    - Anterior: Pectoralis major, skin and fascia.
- **Branches:** 6 branches (Fig. 13)

  1st part
  1. **Superior thoracic artery:**
     - Small branch, runs downwards, forwards and medially
     - Supplies the pectoral muscles and wall of the thorax.

  2nd part
  2. **Thoracoacromial artery:**
     - Emerges at the upper border of pectoralis minor
     - Pierces the clavipectoral fascia
     - Gives 4 branches namely pectoral, deltoid, acromial and clavicular branches.
  3. **Lateral thoracic artery:**
     - It runs along the lower border of the pectoralis minor
     - In female, this is large and supplies the breast.

  3rd part
  4. **Subscapular artery:**
     - Largest branch, runs along the lower border of the subscapularis
     - Terminates near the inferior angle of the scapula
     - Supplies latissimus dorsi and serratus anterior

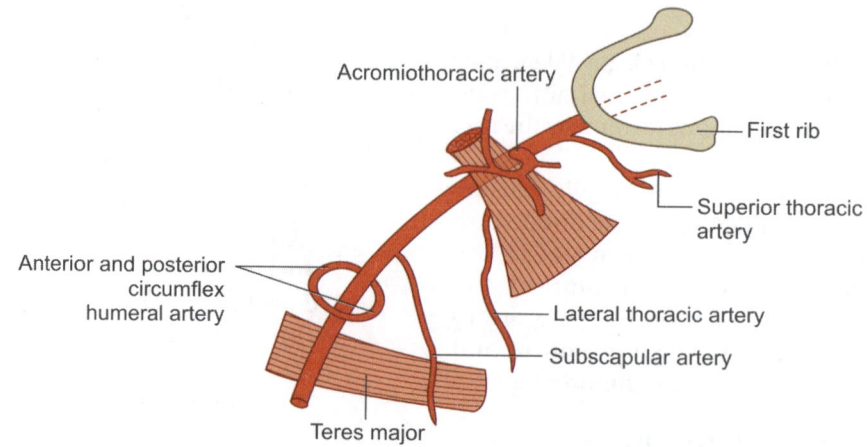

Fig. 13: Extent, division and branches of axillary artery.

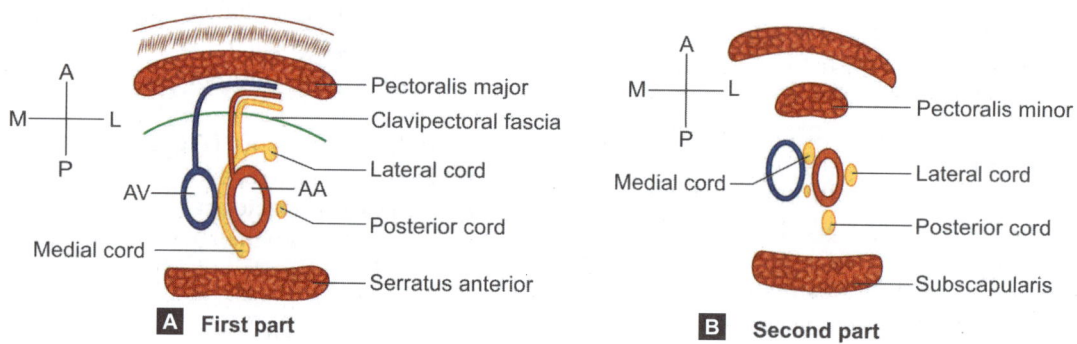

Figs. 14A and B: Relations of axillary artery.

- It gives a large branch called the circumflex scapular artery which passes through the upper triangular space, to take part in the anastomosis around the scapula.

5. **Anterior circumflex humeral artery:**
   - It passes laterally in front of the intertubercular sulcus of the humerus
   - Anastomoses with the posterior circumflex humeral artery around the surgical neck of humerus
   - Gives off an ascending branch, runs in the bicipital groove to supply the head of the humerus and shoulder joint.

6. **Posterior circumflex humeral artery:**
   - Larger branch; runs backwards accompanied by the axillary nerve
   - Passes through the quadrangular space
   - Anastomoses with the anterior circumflex humeral artery
   - It supplies the shoulder joint, deltoid and the muscles of the quadrangular space.

- **Applied anatomy**
  - **Compression of artery:** The third part of axillary artery can be compressed against humerus in case of profuse bleeding due to stab or bullet wound in axilla
  - **Aneurysm of axillary artery:** The first part of axillary artery may enlarge and compress the trunks of brachial plexus causing pain and anesthesia in the areas of the skin supplied by the affected nerve

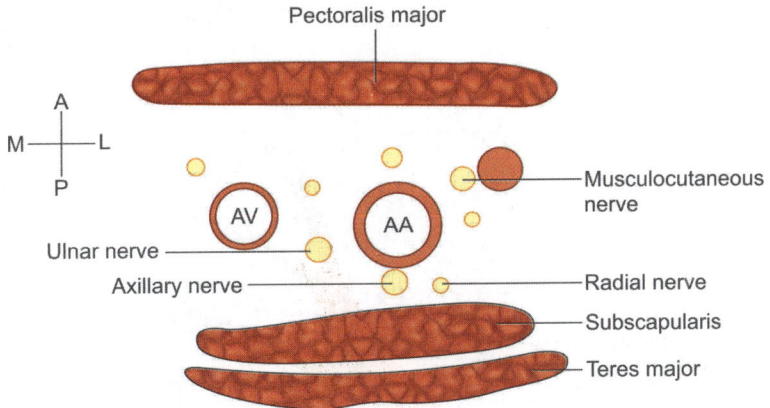

Fig. 15: Third part of axillary artery.

- **Collateral circulation**: Anastomoses around scapula is formed between subclavian and axillary arteries. Collateral circulation is established in case of ligation of axillary artery or vascular stenosis of axillary artery due to atherosclerosis. The direction of blood flow in the subscapular artery is reversed to reach the third part of axillary artery.

5. **Describe the sciatic nerve under the following headings: (a) Origin and Termination, (b) Course, (c) Relations and (d) Branches and applied anatomy.**

The sciatic nerve is the thickest nerve in the body; 2 cm wide.

- **Origin/Formation (root value):**
  - It is the largest branch of the sacral plexus formed in the pelvis
  - Root value: L_4, L_5, S_1, S_2, S_3
  - The nerve is made up of 2 components: Tibial and common peroneal components **(Fig. 16)**.
    - **Tibial component**: Formed by the ventral divisions of anterior primary rami of L_4, L_5, S_1, S_2, S_3
    - **Common peroneal component**: Formed by the dorsal divisions of anterior primary rami of L_4, L_5, S_1, S_2.
- **Termination:**
  - It terminates in the superior angle of popliteal fossa into tibial and common peroneal nerves
  - Sometimes the division may be above, in such a case, the tibial component passes below piriformis and the fibular component through the piriformis.
- **Course and relation (Fig. 17):**
  - **In the pelvis:**
    - It lies in front of the piriformis covered by its fascia
    - It emerges out of the pelvis via the greater sciatic foramen deep to piriformis and passes down between the greater trochanter and ischial tuberosity. Sometime it passes above or through piriformis.
  - **In the gluteal region:**
    - It runs downwards passing between the ischial tuberosity and the greater trochanter
    - Upper part of the nerve is under cover of gluteus maximus
    - Lies on dorsal surface of ischium separated by the nerve to quadratus femoris intervening in between
    - It then runs posterior to tendon of obturator internus, the gamelli and quadratus femoris
    - Obturator externus and the hip joint are separated by the quadratus femoris
    - The structures in the gluteal region mentioned above form the **sciatic bed**

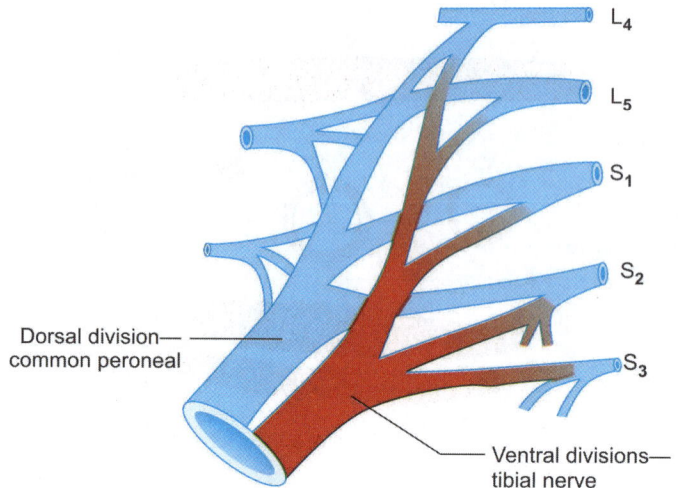

Fig. 16: Formation of sciatic nerve.

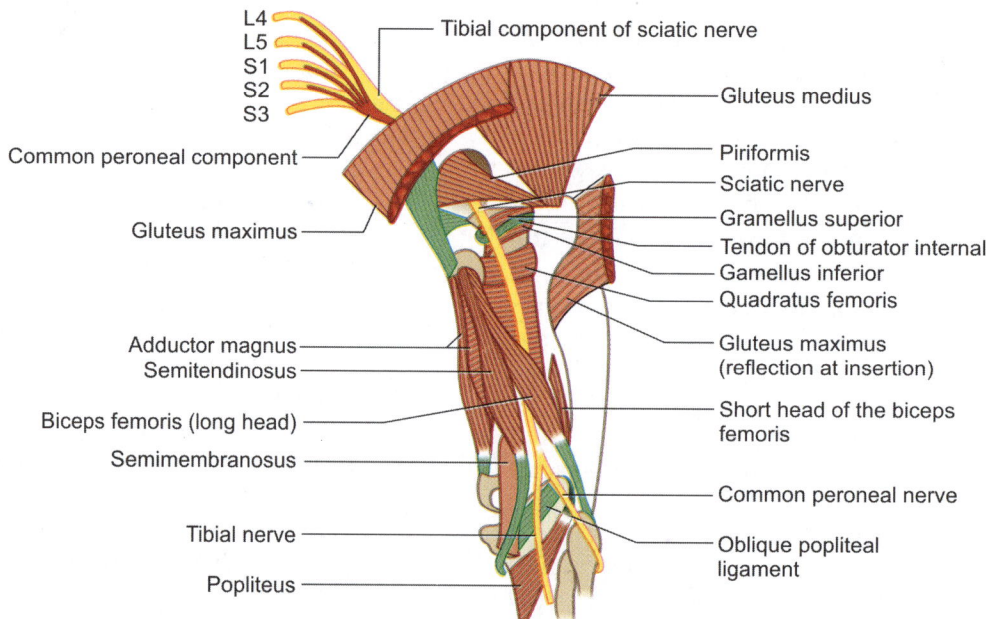

Fig. 17: Relations of sciatic nerve.

- The posterior cutaneous nerve of thigh and the inferior gluteal artery are medial to the nerve.
- **In the thigh:**
  - It enters the back of thigh at the lower border of the gluteus maximus
  - It lies on adductor magnus
- It runs vertically downwards up to the superior angle of the popliteal fossa at the junction of the upper two-third and the lower one-third of the thigh where it ends by dividing into two branches
- Long head of biceps femoris crosses the nerve close to termination.

- **Arterial supply**:
  - **Arteria nervi sciatica ischiadici** is the artery to the sciatic nerve
  - Situated either on the surface or within the nerve
  - It is a branch from internal iliac artery
  - It is persisting remnant of the axis artery of lower limb.
- **Branches:**
  - Articular branches to the hip joint
  - Muscular branches:
    - Tibial part supplies all the hamstring muscles namely the semitendinosus, semimembranosus, long head of biceps femoris and the ischial part of the adductor magnus
    - The common peroneal part supplies only the short head of the biceps femoris.
  - Terminal branches:
    - Tibial nerve
    - Common peroneal nerve.
- **Applied Anatomy**
  - The posterior dislocation of hip joint causes injury to the sciatic nerve. When the nerve is injured it results in excessive movement of foot and difficulty in walking
  - Compression of sciatic nerve can occur after sitting for a long time called "sleeping foot"
  - Sciatica: It is pain radiating along the cutaneous distribution of the sciatic nerve—pain is felt in the gluteal region or even higher, radiates along the back of thigh and lateral side of leg, to the dorsum of foot
  - Piriformis syndrome: Due to the hypertrophy of the muscle piriformis, the sciatic nerve is compressed, resulting in shooting pain along the course of the sciatic nerve in the gluteal region.
  - The nerve can be injured in total hip replacement (1% of cases)
  - Usual injury to sciatic nerve the most common part affected is common peroneal component resulting in foot drop and high stepping gait.

6. Describe the tongue under the following headings. (a) Parts, (b) Muscles, (c) Nerve supply and (d) Lymphatic drainage.

- The tongue is a muscular organ
- Situated in the oral and pharyngeal cavities
- It is covered by the mucous membrane
- Is held in position by the attachment of its muscles to the hyoid bone, mandible, styloid processes, soft palate and the pharyngeal wall.

Parts

- Root: Is attached to the hyoid bone and mandible
- Tip: Sharp anterior part, lies behind the central incisors
- Lateral borders in contact with gums and teeth
- 2 surfaces:
   i   Dorsal Surface
   ii Ventral Surface
- **Dorsal surface (superior surface) (Fig. 18A):**
  - Divide into two parts by a V shaped sulcus called the **sulcus terminalis**, 1. Anterior two-third oral/pre sulcal part and 2. Posterior one-third pharyngeal/post sulcal part
  - **Foramen cecum** is situated at the center of sulcus terminalis representing the upper end of thyroglossal duct
  - Anterior two-third part
    - In front of the palatoglossal arch, the foliate papillae are seen on either side as mucosal folds. The foliate papilla is vestigial in man.
    - The dorsal surface is covered by mucous membrane containing filiform, fungiform and circumvallate papillae.
  - Posterior one-third/postsulcal part
    - It forms the anterior wall of the oropharynx
    - Laterally its mucous membrane is continued onto the palatine tonsils and pharyngeal wall

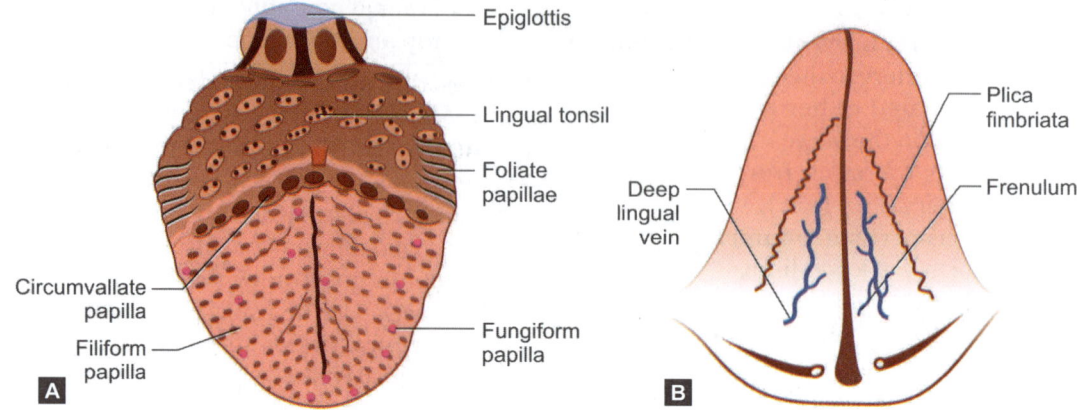

Figs. 18A and B: (A) Dorsum of tongue; (B) Ventral surface of tongue.

- Posteriorly the mucous membrane is reflected onto the epiglottis. Folds namely a median and two lateral glossoepiglottic folds are formed and the depressions formed between the folds are called **valleculae.**
- Papillae are absent in the pharyngeal part of the tongue.
  - Lymphoid nodules embedded in the submucosa produce elevations termed the **lingual tonsil.**
- **Ventral (inferior) surface (Fig. 18B):**
  - The mucosa on the inferior surface is smooth
  - It is connected to the floor of oral cavity and gums
  - Frenulum is a midline fold of mucous membrane connecting tongue to the floor of the oral cavity
  - The deep lingual vein, lies lateral to the frenulum on either side
  - The plica fimbriata, is a folded mucosal ridge lies lateral to the vein.

Muscles of Tongue

Refer Short Notes 31 – 2005.

Nerve Supply

Motor nerve supply

- **Somatomotor:** All the muscles of the tongue are supplied by hypoglossal nerve except palatoglossus which is supplied by the cranial accessory nerve
- **Secretomotor:** Preganglionic fibers from superior salivatory nucleus to facial nerve, chorda tympani and lingual nerve. From lingual it reaches submandibular ganglion and postganglionic fibers from ganglion reach tongue via lingual nerve to supply lingual glands
- **Vasomotor:** Postganglionic fibers from superior cervical ganglion reach tongue through plexus around lingual artery.

Sensory nerve supply

Areas supplied	General sensation (pain, temperature, touch)	Special sensation (Taste)
Anterior 2/3rd excluding vallate papillae	Lingual nerve branch of mandibular nerve	Chorda tympani branch of facial nerve
Posterior 1/3rd including vallate papillae	Glossopharyngeal	Glossopharyngeal
Posterior most end - vallecula	Internal laryngeal nerve branch of vagus	Internal laryngeal nerve branch of vagus

Lymphatic Drainage (Fig. 19)

- The lymph nodes draining tongue are submandibular group, submental nodes, jugulodigastric and jugulo-omohyoid group of nodes
- The lymphatic drainage of the tongue is divided into three main areas—marginal, central and dorsal
- Marginal and central vessels drain anterior two-third of the tongue

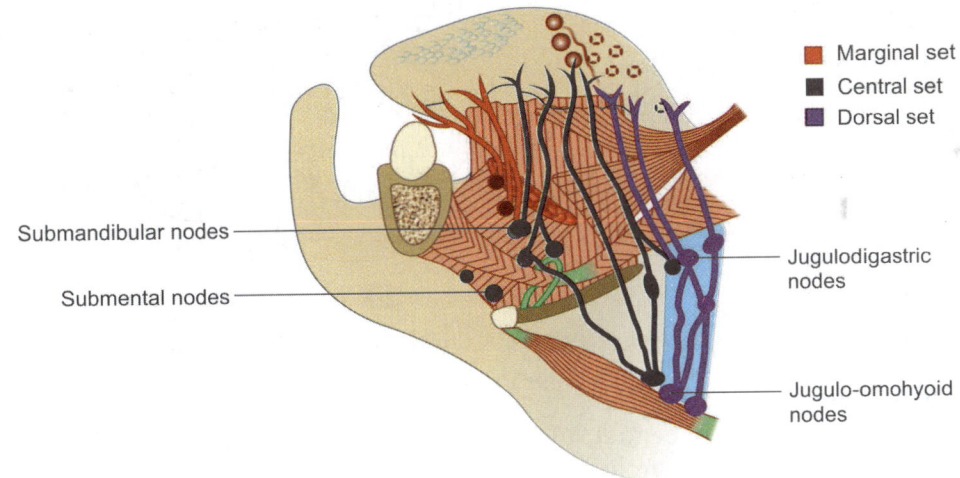

Fig. 19: Lymphatic drainage of tongue.

- The dorsal lymph vessels drain the posterior one-third of the tongue
- The central region is drained by both side vessels.
- **Marginal vessels**
  - **Areas drained**: The apex of the tongue and portion along the frenulum, and lateral margin
  - **Mode of drainage**
    - **From apex and frenulum** (i) vessels pierce mylohyoid end either the submental or submandibular nodes, or to the jugulo-omohyoid node and (ii) Some vessels cross midline and end in bilateral nodes
    - **From lateral margin** pierces mylohyoid muscle and end in submandibular nodes. Some vessels to jugulo-omohyoid or jugulo digastrics nodes.
- **Central lymphatic vessels**
  - **Areas drained**: Presulcal region
  - **Mode of drainage:** The lymph vessels pass along the lingual veins and drain to the deep cervical nodes, chiefly the jugulodigastric and jugulo-omohyoid nodes.
- **Dorsal lymph vessels**
  - **Areas drained**: Drain the postsulcal region and the circumvallate papillae
  - **Mode of drainage:** The vessels near the midline drain bilaterally. They reach the jugulodigastric and jugulo-omohyoid lymph nodes after piercing the pharyngeal wall.
- **Applied anatomy:** Central regions of tongue may drain bilaterally, and should be remembered in removal of malignant tumor of the tongue that are nearer the midline. Both cervical nodes may be involved.

7. Describe the sulci and gyri on the superolateral surface of cerebral hemisphere with functional areas.

- The superolateral surface of the brain are divided into four lobes by two imaginary lines and two sulci
- The two sulci are central sulcus and posterior ramus of lateral sulcus
- The two imaginary lines are:
  1. Connecting parieto-occipital sulcus in the superomedial border and pre-occipital notch inferolateral border, marked about 5 cm from the occipital pole
  2. Extension of posterior ramus of lateral sulcus to 1st imaginary line.

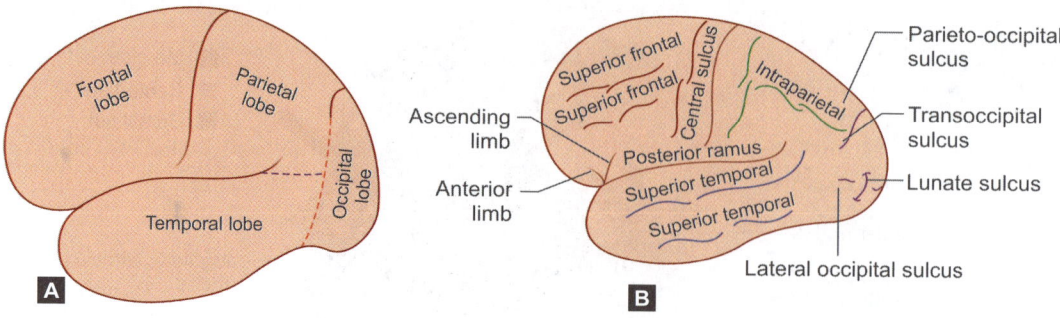

Figs. 20A and B: Superolateral surface of cerebrum: (A) Division-four lobes; (B) Sulci of superolateral surface.

- The **four lobes** are (Fig. 20A):
  1. The portion in front of central sulcus and above lateral sulcus—frontal lobe
  2. The portion behind the central sulcus and front of 1st imaginary line—parietal lobe
  3. The portion behind the 1st imaginary line—occipital lobe
  4. The portion below posterior ramus of lateral sulcus and 2nd imaginary line—temporal lobe.
- **Sulci and gyri**
  Central sulcus
  - It starts a little behind the midpoint between the frontal and occipital poles, in the superomedial border of the hemisphere
  - It extends into the medial surface and is surrounded by paracentral lobule
  - It is an example of limiting sulcus
  - It separates the motor area in the precentral gyrus from sensory area in the postcentral gyrus.

Lateral sulcus
- It is also called as **sylvian fissure**
- It has a short stem
- The stem reaching the lateral surface of the hemisphere, it divides into anterior horizontal, anterior ascending and posterior rami
- It is an example of secondary sulcus
- Insula is situated in the floor of the sulcus.

Frontal Lobe

- **Sulci (Fig. 20B)**
  - Precentral sulcus—runs parallel to central sulcus
  - The portion in front of precentral sulcus is divided into 3 by two sulci namely superior frontal and inferior frontal sulci.
- **Gyri (Fig. 21)**
  - Precentral—gyrus between central and precentral sulci
  - Superior frontal—gyrus above superior frontal sulcus

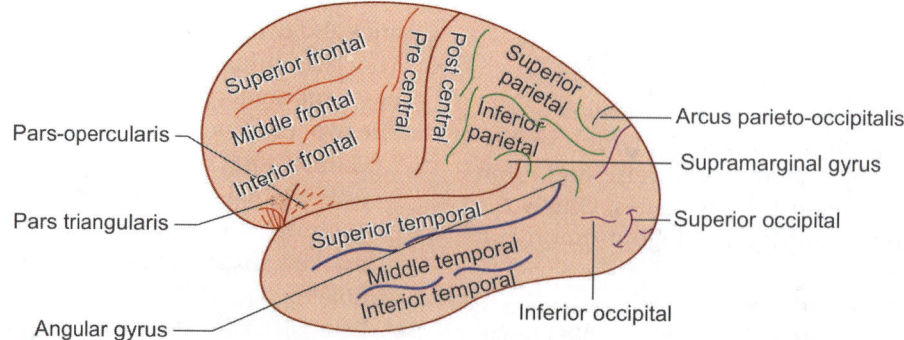

Fig. 21: Gyri of superolateral surface.

- Middle frontal gyrus—between superior and inferior frontal sulci
- Inferior frontal gyrus—below inferior frontal sulcus. Into this the anterior horizontal and anterior ascending rami of lateral sulcus enters. By these the inferior frontal gyri is divided into:
    - Pars orbitalis—anterior to anterior horizontal ramus
    - Pars triangularis—between anterior horizontal and ascending rami
    - Pars opercularis—between ascending and posterior rami of lateral sulcus.
- **Functional areas (Fig. 22A):**
  - Motor area (area 4)
      - It is situated in the precentral gyrus
      - In this area the opposite half of body is represented (homunculus) **(Fig. 22B)**
      - The representation is upside down, with representation of the head most laterally and the lower limb below knee on the medial surface of the hemisphere in the paracentral lobule
      - The axons of these cells form the corticospinal and corticobulbar tract
      - Lesion of primary motor area in one hemisphere produce paralysis of the extremities of the opposite half of the body.
  - **Premotor area (area 6 and 8)**
      - Situated in front of motor area, in the posterior part of superior, middle and inferior frontal gyri
      - It contributes for corticospinal fibers
      - Function of this area is preparation for movements and movements itself
      - Lesion of premotor area results in difficulty in performing skilled movements.
  - **Frontal eye field (areas 6, 8 and 9)**
      - The area 8 is predominantly frontal eye field
      - Situated anterior to premotor area, in the middle frontal gyrus
      - The function of this area is control of eye movements
      - Lesion of this area results in ipsilateral conjugate deviation of the eyes
  - **Prefrontal area (areas 9 to 12, 46)**
      - Situated in front part of frontal lobe
      - Function of this area is self-ordered working memory task, calculating, thinking and decision making, understanding time, normal expression of emotions
      - Lesion of this results in clownish behavior, euphoric, vulgar speech. "Frontal lobe syndrome", in which there is change in personality,

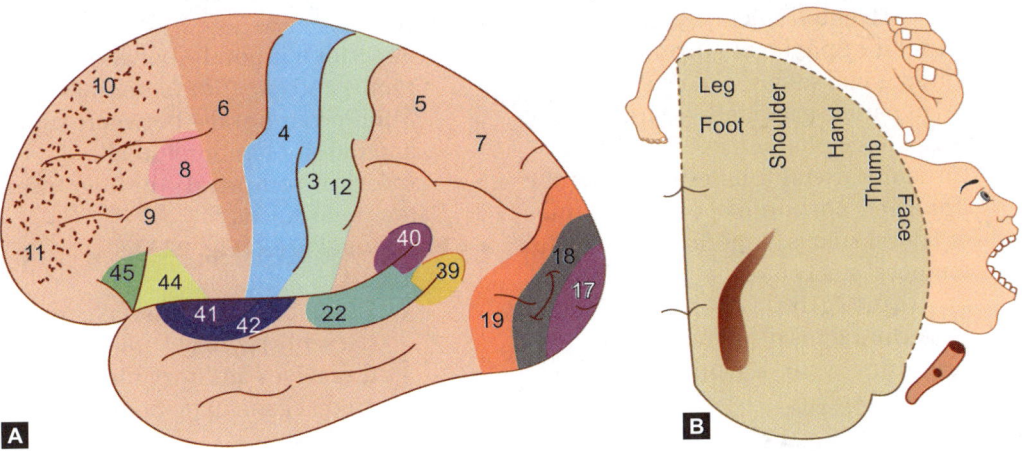

Figs. 22A and B: (A) Functional areas; (B) Homunculus.

with loss of reasoning, difficulty in understanding and judging, added with loss of individuality and social feelings (sympathy and empathy).
- **Motor speech area (area 45, 44)**
  - It is also called as **Broca's speech area**
  - Situated in pars triangularis and opercularis of inferior frontal gyrus
  - It is dominant on left hemisphere for right handed person
  - It is responsible for production of expressive speech/vocalization
  - It helps in formation of words with connections to adjacent primary motor area
  - Lesions- **Motor aphasia.** Though the patient can understand the language, cannot express in speech. Agrammatical and nonfluent speech. It is also called expressive aphasia.

Parietal Lobe

- **Sulci**
  - Postcentral sulcus—parallel and behind central sulcus
  - Intraparietal sulcus—runs horizontally from middle of post central sulcus and passes beyond parieto-occipital sulcus and joins with transoccipital sulcus.
- **Gyri**
  - Postcentral gyrus—between central and postcentral sulci
  - Superior parietal lobule—above intraparietal sulcus
  - Arcus parieto occipitalis—gyrus around parieto-occipital sulcus
  - Inferior parietal lobule—into this the upturned portion of posterior ramus of lateral sulcus, superior and inferior temporal sulci enter
  - Supramarginal gyrus—around posterior ramus of lateral sulcus
  - Angular gyrus—around superior temporal sulcus.

- **Functional areas:**
  Sensory area:
  Areas 3, 1, 2:
  - It is primary sensory area
  - Situated in the postcentral gyrus
  - Extends to medial surface in the paracentral lobule
  - It receives fibers from ventroposteromedial and ventroposterolateral nuclei of thalamus
  - Pyramidal cells in this areas give rise to corticospinal fibers.

  Area 39 (sensory speech area)
  - It is situated in angular gyrus of inferior parietal lobule
  - It stores visual images and recognizes objects by sight
  - Lesion—**word blindness**. Words are seen but not comprehended. **Alexia** (inability to read), **agraphia** (inability to write) and **acalculia** (inability to calculate), in the absence of aphasia.

  Area 40 (sensory speech area)
  - Situated in supramarginal gyrus of the inferior parietal lobule
  - Recognizes familiar objects with help of touch and proprioception
  - Lesion—produces **astereognosis.**

Temporal Lobe

- **Sulci**
  - Superior temporal sulcus
  - Inferior temporal sulcus.
- **Gyri**
  - Superior temporal—between posterior ramus and superior temporal sulcus
  - Middle temporal—between superior and inferior temporal sulci
  - Inferior temporal—below inferior temporal sulcus.
- **Functional area (Fig. 22A)**
  - Area 41
    - Situated in the transverse temporal (Heschl's) gyrus
    - It receives auditory radiation from medial geniculate body

- It helps to identify the direction, intensity, and distance of the sound.
- **Area 42**
  - It is associated auditory area
  - It is situated in the superior temporal gyrus
  - It is essential for interpretation of sound impulses.
- **Area 22 (Wernicke's area)—sensory speech area**
  - It is called as Wernicke's area
  - Situated in the superior temporal gyrus
  - Comprehends spoken language, recognizes familiar sounds and words
  - Lesion produces **word deafness**/sensory aphasia, unable to interpret spoken words.

Occipital Lobe

- **Sulci**
  - Transverse occipital
  - Calcarine sulcus occasionally seen at occipital pole
  - Lunate—in front of calcarine sulcus. It is limited above and below by polar sulci
  - Lateral occipital—in front of lunate sulcus.
- **Gyri**
  - Superior occipital gyrus—above lateral occipital sulcus
  - Inferior occipital gyrus—below lateral occipital sulcus
  - Gyrus descendens—between lunate and calcarine sulci.
- **Functional areas**

  Area 17
  - Situated in the posterior part of calcarine sulcus
  - It receives the optic radiation from lateral geniculate body
  - Lesion of this area results in homonymous hemianopia with macular sparing.

  Areas 18, 19
  - They are associated visual areas
  - They are called as occipital eye field
  - It helps to recognize the objects relating present and past visual experience.

8. **Describe the thyroid gland under the following headings: (a) Gross anatomy, (b) Microscopic anatomy, (c) Applied anatomy and (d) Development.**

Gross Anatomy

Refer Short Notes 17 – 2004.

Microscopic Anatomy

- The gland is covered by capsule – inner true capsule formed by condensation of connective tissue and outer false capsule contributed by pretracheal fascia
- Septa extends from capsule and divides the gland into irregular lobules
- The functional unit of thyroid gland is the follicle
- The follicles are surrounded by plexus of fenestrated capillaries, nerve and lymphatic
- Each follicle is lined by a single layered epithelium resting on basement membrane surrounding the colloid situated in the center of the follicle
- The colloid is a stored in the form of tri-iodothyronine and tetraiodothyronine
- The epithelium of each follicle is made up of two types of cells – follicular and C cells (parafollicular cells)
  - **Follicular cells**
    - Are more in number
    - Follicular cells vary depending on their level of activity

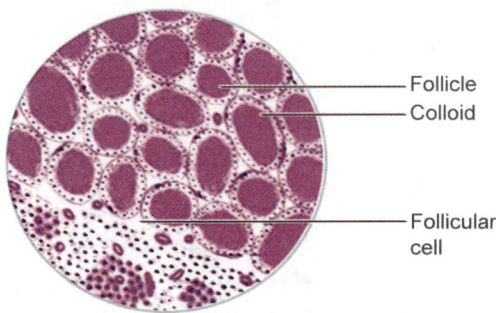

Fig. 23: Histology of thyroid.

- Inactive period the cells are squamous and when active low cuboidal/columnar
- They secrete T_3 and T_4.
– **Parafollicular cells/C (clear) cells**
  - Have pale-staining cytoplasm
  - C cells belong to amine precursor uptake and decarboxylation (APUD) system
  - They produce hormone calcitonin (thyrocalcitonin)
  - C cells are situated within the basement membrane of the thyroid follicles, but do not reach the lumen of the follicle
  - They occur singly or in clusters in between the follicular cells.

Applied Anatomy

- Goiter: enlargement of thyroid gland
- Hyperthyroidism: Exophthalmos, tachycardia, tremors and raised basal metabolic rate
- Hypothyroidism: Myxedema, bradycardia, edema, decreased basal metabolic rate
- During thyroidectomy: Gland should be removed with true capsule to avoid injury to the venous plexus lying between the true and false capsules
- Clinical significance during thyroidectomy
  – **Superior thyroid artery** is ligated **near** the apex of the gland as the external laryngeal nerve passes medial to lateral lobe
  – **Inferior thyroid artery** is ligated **away** from the gland to save the recurrent laryngeal nerve.

Development

Thyroid is developed from 3 sources.
  i. Before the fusion of tongue rudiments, the endodermal cells behind the tuberculum impar gives rise to an elevation called **median thyroid element**
  - The cells of thyroid element grow downwards into the substance of tongue, in front of hyoid, larynx and trachea
  - The downward growth is called the **thyroglossal duct (Fig. 24)**
  - It terminates by dividing into two in front of upper part of trachea
  - The two divisions give rise to isthmus and lateral lobes of thyroid gland
  - The thyroglossal duct disappears leaving the upper end as **foramen caecum**
  - Lower part sometimes persists as **pyramidal lobe**.
  ii. **Lateral thyroid element is** from caudal pharyngeal complex of the fourth pouch. It prevents the caudal migration of the thyroid gland
  iii. **Ultimobranchial body** from caudal pharyngeal complex **gives** rise to parafollicular cells.
- **Developmental anomalies**
  – **Thyroglossal cyst:** Persistence of the duct undergoes cystic changes. Seen in midline of neck and moves with deglutition
  – **Thyroglossal fistula:** Incision or rupture of thyroglossal cyst results in fistula
  – **Lingual thyroid:** Failure of formation of thyroglossal duct, the gland develops within the tongue
  – **Accessory thyroid gland:** Nodules of thyroid tissue found near the gland

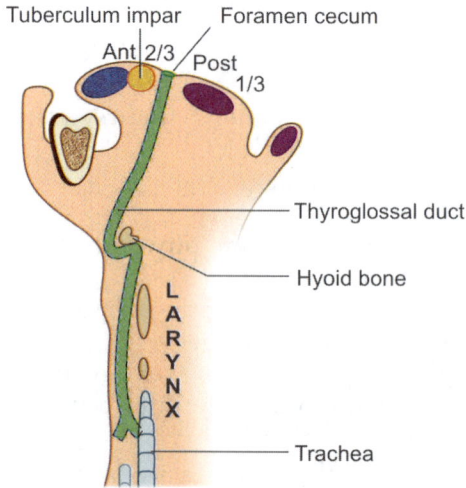

Fig. 24: Thyroglossal duct.

- **Ectopic thyroid:** Occasionally thyroid grows in posterior triangle of neck.

9. **Describe the facial nerve under the following headings: (a) Origin and termination, (b) Course and relations, (c) Branches and (d) Applied anatomy.**

- Facial nerve is the nerve of the second branchial arch
- It is the seventh cranial nerve
- It is a mixed type of nerve
- Structures supplied, origin & termination, Course & relations - Refer Short Note Q. No. 15 – 2003.
- Branches refer Short Note Q. No. 15 – 2003.
- **Temporal branch**
  - Emerges from superior border of parotid gland
  - Crosses the zygomatic arch
  - Supply the frontal belly of occipitofrontalis, orbicularis oculi and corrugator, and the anterior and superior auricular muscles.
- **Zygomatic branches**
  - Emerges from the anterior border of parotid gland
  - Are usually seen as many branches
  - They cross the zygomatic bone to reach the lateral angle of the eye
  - Supply orbicularis oculi.
- **Buccal branch**
  - Emerges from the anterior border of parotid gland
  - Upper deep branches supply levators of upper lip namely zygomaticus major and levator labii superioris, levator anguli oris, zygomaticus minor, levator labii superioris alaeque nasi and the small nasal muscles
  - Lower deep branches supply buccinator and orbicularis oris.
- **Marginal Mandibular**
  - They pass forwards and downwards towards the angle of the mandible
  - Descends into the neck below the angle
  - Then ascend upwards across the body of the mandible to reach the face
  - The branches supply risorius and the muscles of the lower lip and chin.

- **Cervical branch:** Emerges from the lower part of the parotid gland and supplies platysma.

Applied Anatomy
Facial Paralysis
Facial paralysis due to:
- **Upper motor neurone lesion:** Paralysis of the lower half of face on the contralateral side when frontalis is partially spared due to the bilateral innervation of the muscle of the upper part of the face
- **Lower motor neurone lesion:** Paralysis of muscles of one half of face on the ipsilateral side called **Bell's palsy.**

Bell's Palsy (Fig. 25)
- Bell's palsy is **due to** paralysis of one side muscles of facial expression
- **Level of lesion**
  - Ipsilateral lower motor neuron facial paralysis due to compression of facial nerve at stylomastoid foramen.
  - The **features** are:
    - Asymmetry of face
    - Loss of horizontal ridges on forehead
    - Inability to close the eyelid
    - Epiphora—tears fall over cheek
    - Widening of palpebral fissure
    - Deviation of angle of mouth to the opposite side
    - Drooling of saliva on the side of lesion
    - Collection of food in the vestibule
    - Disappearance of nasolabial fold.
  - **Muscles paralyzed** are muscles of facial expression**.**
  - Reasoning
    - Paralysis of **frontal belly of occipitofrontalis**—loss of horizontal folds on forehead
    - Paralysis of **orbicularis oculi** leads to inability to close the eyelid leading on to complications of dryness and ulceration of cornea. When a patient makes an attempt to close the eyelid the eyeballs roll upwards and is called **Bell's phenomenon**

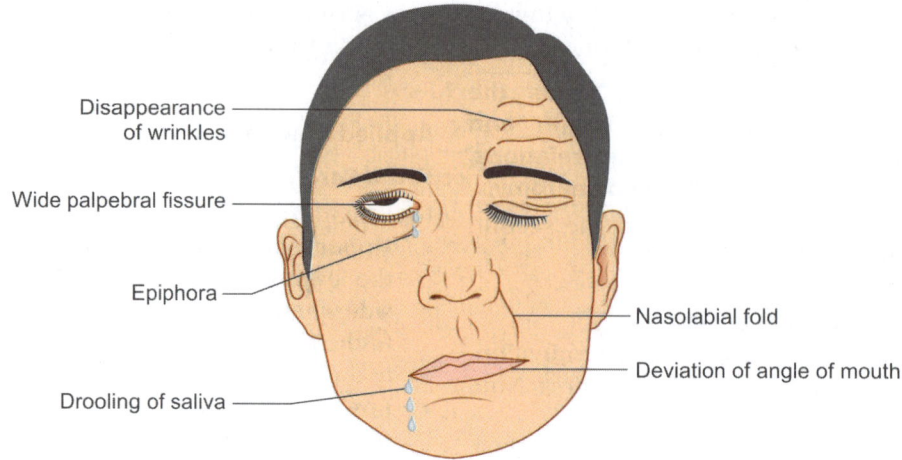

Fig. 25: Bell's palsy.

- Paralysis of **orbicularis oris**— deviation of angle of mouth to the opposite side and drooling of saliva
- Paralysis of **buccinator** results in, collection of food in the vestibule. Inability to play wind instrument. When patient makes an attempt to blow air there will be ballooning of cheek
- Paralysis of **levator labii superioris** —loss of nasolabial fold.

Crocodile Tears Syndrome

Lacrimation during eating occurs due to aberrant regeneration after trauma.

10. Describe the bronchopulmonary segments under the following headings: Definition, numbers, blood supply, nerve supply, and applied anatomy.

Refer Essay Q. No. 3 – 2004.

II. SHORT NOTES

1. Development of pancreas.

Refer Short Notes 6 – 2005.

2. Cruciate ligaments of knee joint.

- The cruciate ligaments are intracapsular but extrasynovial
- They cross each other like letter X
- They are named anterior and posterior according to their attachment to tibia.
- These are very thick and strong fibrous bands
- The ligaments are supplied by middle genicular vessels and nerves
- Both the ligaments remain tight throughout the movements of flexion and extension of knee joint
- Their attachment to femur is close to the axis of movements, they do not prevent flexion/extension of knee.
- **Anterior cruciate ligament (ACL):**
  - Begins from anterior part of intercondylar area of tibia
  - Runs upwards, backwards and laterally

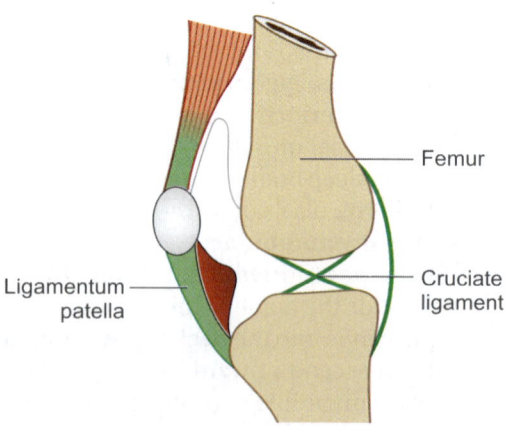

Fig. 26: Ligaments of knee joint.

- Above it is attached to the posterior part of medial surface of lateral condyle of femur
- It is taut during extension of knee and prevents hyperextension
- Acts as a pivot for rotatory movements of knee.

- **Posterior cruciate ligament (PCL):**
  - It is stronger than the anterior cruciate ligament
  - Begins from the posterior part of intercondylar area of tibia
  - Runs upwards, forwards and medially
  - Above is attached to the anterior part of the lateral surface of medial condyle of femur
  - It is taut during flexion of the knee.
- **Functions:**
  - The ligaments hold the two bones together
  - The anterior cruciate prevents femur sliding backwards on the upper surface of tibia
  - The posterior cruciate prevents femur sliding forwards on the superior surface of tibia.
- **Applied anatomy:**
  - Violent hyperextension of knee can result in sprain of anterior cruciate ligament
  - Posterior cruciate ligament may be injured in posterior dislocation of tibia
  - When the cruciate ligaments are ruptured, the tibia can be pulled excessively forwards or backwards at the lower end of femur
  - Injury to cruciate ligaments (in football and soccer) are always associated with injury to other structures. The result is an "**unhappy triad**" – (**3C**) collateral ligament, cruciate ligament, (semilunar) cartilage.

3. Microscopic structure of kidney.

- Kidney has an outer cortex and inner medulla **(Fig. 27)**
- **Cortex** contains proximal convoluted tubule (PCT), distal convoluted tubule (DCT), renal corpuscle, medullary ray
- **Medulla** formed by renal pyramids containing collecting ducts, thin segment of loop of Henle
- **Functional unit—nephron**
- Each nephron has **two parts**—renal corpuscle and renal tubules.
- **Parts of nephron:**
  - **Renal corpuscle/Malpighian corpuscle**—consists of
    - Glomerular plexus of capillaries formed by afferent and efferent arteriole
    - Bowman's capsule—is the dilated part of renal tubule. It has a parietal and visceral layer with space called urinary (Bowman's) space. It is lined by simple squamous epithelium and in addition the podocytes are seen in the visceral layer.

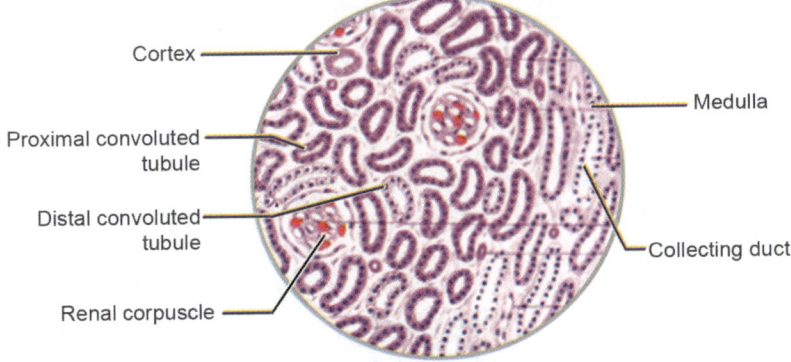

Fig. 27: Histology of kidney.

- Renal tubule consists of:
  - Proximal convoluted tubule
  - Loop of Henle
  - Descending and ascending limbs of loop of Henle
  - Distal convoluted tubule
  - Collecting tubule
  - Duct of Bellini
- PCT—pink stained tubules, lined by columnar cells with numerous microvilli giving a brush border appearance, and the lumen appear smaller
- Loop of Henle—thin segment by squamous cells and thick segment (descending and ascending limbs) cuboidal cells
- DCT light stained tubules, lined by cuboidal cells with less number of microvilli
- Collecting ducts by cuboidal/columnar cells.

4. Sesamoid bone.

Galen was the first person to use the term 'sesamoid'.
- **Features:**
  - These bones develop in tendons in close proximity to joints
  - They are devoid of periosteum
  - Ossify after birth
  - Lack Haversian system.
- **Functions:**
  - Direction of muscle pull may be altered by the sesamoid bone
  - Friction is reduced and alter pressure
  - Acts as pulley for muscle contraction.
- **Examples:**
  - Patella in quadriceps tendon
  - Fabella in lateral head of gastrocnemius
  - Pisiform in flexor carpi ulnaris
  - Two sesamoid in flexor hallucis brevis
  - Os peroneum in the tendon of peroneus longus
  - In the tendon of tibialis posterior
  - In the tendon of adductor pollicis
  - In the tendon of flexor pollicis brevis.

5. Median nerve in hand.

- **Course:**
  - Median nerve lies deep to flexor retinaculum in the carpal tunnel
  - Enters the palm through the tunnel
  - Superficial to flexor digitorum tendons
  - Distal to the retinaculum it enlarges and flattens
  - Immediately below the retinaculum, the nerve divides into lateral and medial divisions.
- **Branches of median nerve in the hand:**
  - **Muscular branches (Fig. 28)**
    - Recurrent branch for muscles forming thenar eminence—abductor

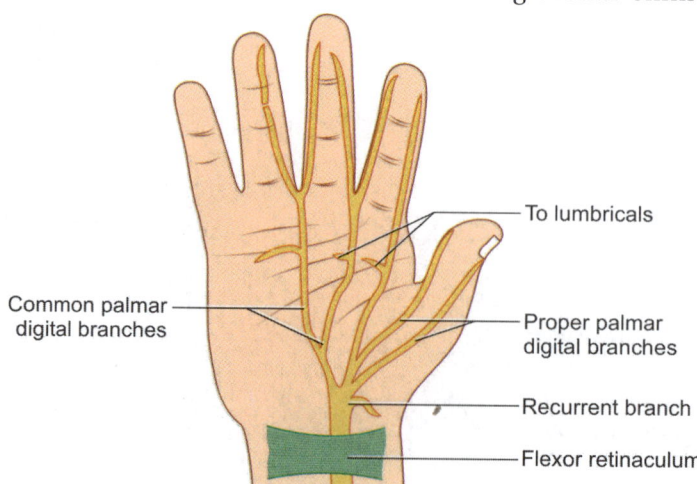

Fig. 28: Median nerve in hand.

pollicis brevis, flexor pollicis brevis and opponens pollicis
- Branches to 1st and 2nd lumbricals from the digital nerves.
- **Cutaneous branches**
  - Supply lateral three and a half digits
  - Two proper palmar digital branches to lateral and medial sides of thumb
  - One proper palmar digital branch to lateral side of index finger
  - Two common palmar digital branches one to adjacent sides of index and middle fingers and one to adjacent sides of middle and ring fingers
  - It also supplies the nail beds of corresponding digits.
- **Articular branches**—to carpometacarpal, intercarpal, intermetacarpal joints
- **Vascular branches**—to branches of radial and ulnar arteries.
- **Applied anatomy**
  - **Carpal tunnel syndrome**: Compression of median nerve in the carpal tunnel deep to flexor retinaculum results in carpal tunnel syndrome.
    - **Reason for compression**
      * By the swellings of synovial sheath
      * Narrowing of tunnel by arthritic changes in wrist joint
      * Dislocation of the underlying carpal bones
      * Edema due to pregnancy
      * Thickening of soft tissue as in myxedema.
    - **Effects of compression**
      * Results in pain, paraesthesia and numbness in the distribution of the nerve.
      * Paralysis of muscles of thenar eminence called **Ape thumb deformity**
      * Motor changes: loss of opposition
      * Sensory changes: there is loss of sensations on lateral 3½ digits including their nail beds if compression is prolonged
      * Vasomotor changes: The skin is warmer, due to arteriolar dilatation in the areas where there is loss of sensation
      * Trophic changes: long standing cases lead to dry and scaly skin.
- **Treatment**: Surgical division of flexor retinaculum to remove the compression.

6. **Lymphatic drainage of stomach.**

The stomach is **divided** into 4 areas for lymphatic drainage **(Fig. 29)**.

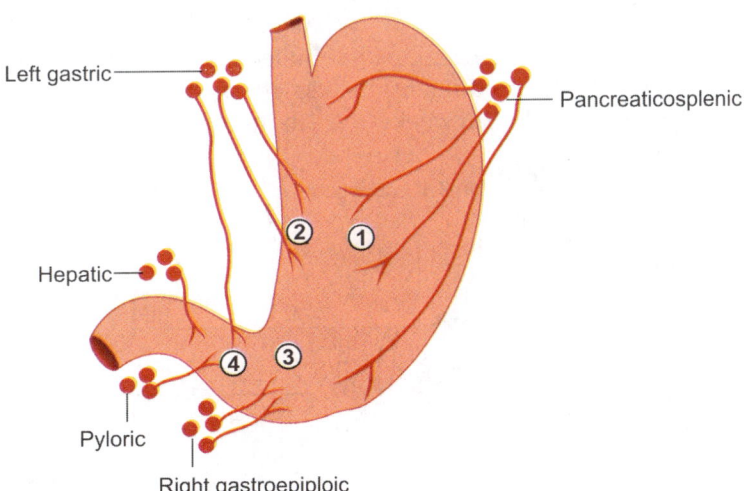

Fig. 29: Lymphatic drainage of stomach.

- A vertical line is drawn from cardiac orifice to greater curvature
- The portion to the right of the vertical line is divided into upper two-third and lower one-third
- The pyloric part is separated by a line extending from incisura angularis to lesser curvature
- **The four areas are:**
  i. Portion to the left of the vertical line
  ii. Upper two-third of the right part
  iii. Lower one-third of the right part
  iv. Pyloric part.
- **Drainage:**
  - Area 1 is drained by pancreaticosplenic nodes
  - Area 2 left gastric nodes
  - Area 3 right gastroepiploic nodes
  - Area 4 hepatic, pyloric and left gastric lymph nodes.
- **Applied anatomy:**
  - Carcinoma stomach spreading to the left supraclavicular nodes (Virchow's nodes) is known as Troisier's sign
  - Cancer stomach may spread into Esophagus and not into duodenum as the deep fibers of longitudinal muscle coat and circular fibers of stomach are not continuous with duodenum.

7. Adductor canal.
Refer Short Notes 3 – 2006.

8. Descent of testis.
- Testes is developed from the medulla of undifferentiated genital ridge by 7th week
- Developed retroperitoneally in the posterior abdominal wall
- By end of second month the testis and the mesonephros are attached to the posterior abdominal wall by the mesentry called urogenital mesentry
- The peritoneum of the abdominal cavity forms an evagination called the **processus vaginalis**
- There is a fibromuscular band called **gubernaculum testis**
- The upper end of the gubernaculum divides and is attached to lower pole of testis, processus vaginalis, mesonephric duct
- Lower end initially it extends up to inguinal region
- The lower end of the gubernaculum splits into many fibrous bands called **tail of Lockwood**
- When the testis begins to descend the gubernaculum grows towards the scrotal swelling
- The processus vaginalis follows the gubernaculum into the scrotal swellings
- **The tail of Lockwood is attached to (Fig. 30)**
  - Scrotum
  - Perineum
  - Symphysis pubis above penis
  - Saphenous opening of thigh
  - Anterior superior iliac spine
- As gubernaculum shortens, the testis is pulled along with processus vaginalis
- At 4th month the testis is in iliac fossa, 7th month deep inguinal ring, 8th month

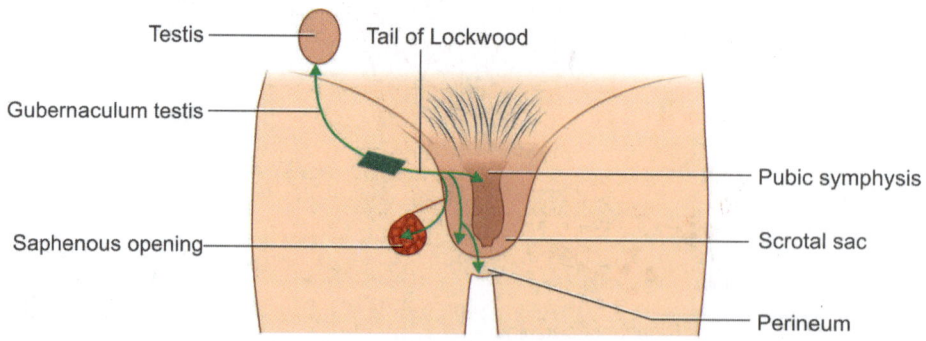

Fig. 30: Tail of lockwood.

traverses the inguinal canal, at or soon after birth reaches the scrotum
- The parietal layer of distal part of processus vaginalis persists as visceral layer of tunica vaginalis
- The proximal part of processus disappears.
- **Factors for descent**:
  - Gubernaculum testis
  - Intra-abdominal pressure
  - Intra-abdominal temperature
  - Uncurling of fetal curves
  - Hormone secreted by the fetal testis.
- Congenital anomaly:
  - **Cryptorchism** is a clinical condition in which one/both the testes are retained in the posterior abdominal wall
  - It is a congenital deformity
  - The testes fail to descend
  - Usually (in 95%) of the male child the testes reach the scrotal sac by birth
  - If not descended by 3 months of postnatal life, it does not reach the scrotum later
  - The undescended testes fail to produce mature sperms.

9. Anastomosis around elbow joint.

Refer Short Notes 8 – 2006.

10. Development of urinary bladder.

Development of urinary bladder is under two headings:

1. **Development of mucous membrane:**
   - Mucous membrane is developed from mesoderm and endoderm
   - Mucous membrane of urinary bladder is developed from three sources:
     i. Apex of bladder from allantoic diverticulum
     ii. Trigone of bladder is **mesodermal in origin**, from absorbed part of mesonephric duct
     iii. Rest of the part from **endoderm**, the vesicourethral canal.
   - From the hindgut a diverticulum extends into the connecting stalk called **allantoic diverticulum**
   - By the diverticulum the hind gut is divided into pre and post allantoic part
   - The post allantoic part is known as endodermal cloaca
   - The endodermal cloaca is divided into primitive urogenital sinus and primitive rectum by the urorectal septum
   - The primitive urogenital sinus in turn is divided into cephalic **vesicourethral part** and caudal **definitive urogenital sinus** by the opening of the mesonephric duct
   - The caudal part of mesonephric ducts gets absorbed into the urogenital sinus to form the **trigone**
   - **Apex of bladder** develops from absorption of allantoic diverticulum
   - **Rest** of the portion is from the endoderm of vesicourethral canal.

2. **Development of musculature:** Musculature from splanchnic layer of lateral plate mesoderm.

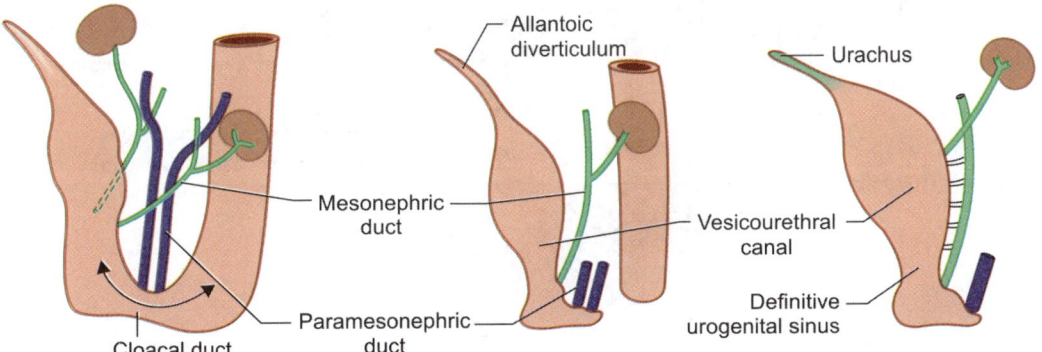

Fig. 31: Development of urinary bladder.

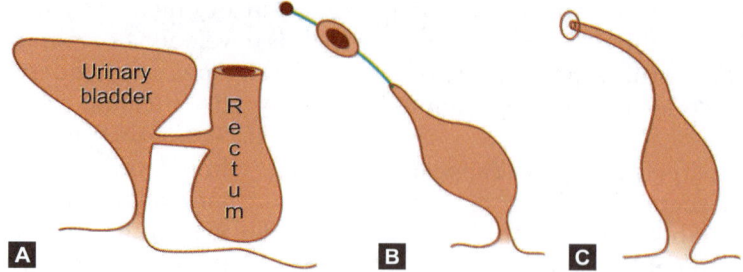

Figs. 32A to C: Congenital anomalies: (A) Rectovesical fistula; (B) Urachal cyst; (C) Urachal fistula.

- **Congenital anomalies**:
  - Vesicovaginal fistula
  - Rectovesical fistula **(Fig. 32A)**—incomplete development of urorectal septum
  - Urachal cyst **(Fig. 32B)**—intermediate portion of allantoic diverticulum remains patent
  - Urachal fistula **(Fig. 32C)**—entire allantoic diverticulum is patent and results in urinary fistula
  - Ectopic vesicae—defect in formation of anterior abdominal wall. The interior of bladder is exposed.

11. Microscopic structure of ovary.

The surface of the ovary is lined by a single layer of cuboidal epithelium called as germinal epithelium. Beneath the epithelium is **tunica albuginea** which is formed by condensation of connective tissue. The substance of the ovary has an **outer cortex** and an **inner medulla**.

- **Ovarian cortex:** The cortex has stroma and various stages of ovarian follicles namely, primordial follicles, primary follicles, secondary follicles, tertiary or graffian follicles and corpus luteum.
  - **Primordial follicle:** Consists of a primary oocyte surrounded by a single layer of flattened follicular cells
  - **Primary follicle**: The flattened follicular cells become columnar. Zona pellucida appears between the follicular cells and the oocyte
  - **Secondary follicle:** The follicular cells proliferate to form several layers of cells that constitute the membrana granulosa. The cells are now called as granulosa cells. Follicular cavity appears in the granulosa layer.

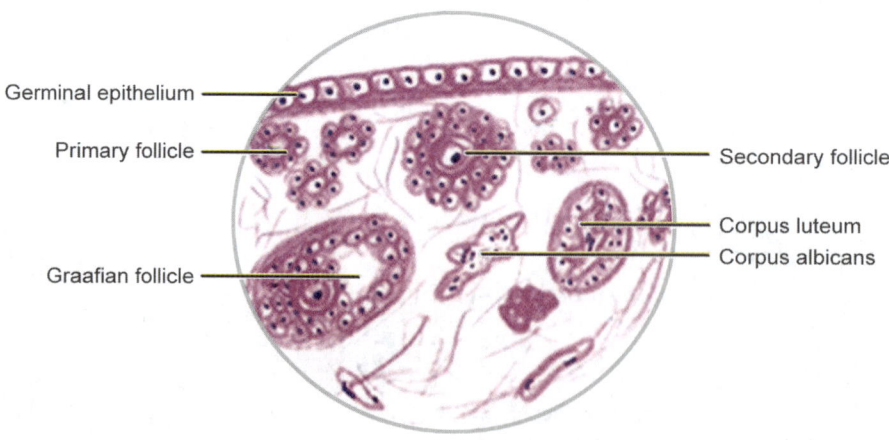

Fig. 33: Histology of ovary.

- **Tertiary/Graafian follicle:** The follicle and the cavity are enlarged. The oocyte (secondary oocyte) is pushed to the periphery. So, the granulosa cells attaching the oocyte to the wall of the follicle is called as membrana granulosa. The cells surrounding the oocyte is called as cumulus oophorus
- **Atretic follicle:** Though numerous follicles pass through various stages in a single cycle, only one matures to become a graafian follicle. All others that fail to mature degenerate and become atretic
- **Corpus luteum:** It is a yellow colored body formed from the ruptured follicle. Its cells are known as luteal cells. Corpus luteum persists for about 14 days and secretes progesterone. After this functional life, it degenerates and becomes a mass of white fibrous tissue called **corpus albicans**
- **Ovarian medulla:** It has connective tissue, blood vessels, nerves and lymphatics. Cells seen in the hilum of medulla are similar to the interstitial cells of the testis.

12. Spermatogenesis.

The process of maturation of male gametes is known as spermatogenesis **(Fig. 34)**. It occurs in 3 stages:

i. **Spermatocytosis**
   - The process of formation of primary spermatocyte from the primodial cell is called spermatocytosis
   - This process takes around **16 days**
   - Primodial germ cells divide by mitosis and form dark type A spermatogonia
   - It acts as stem cell
   - Each cell divides to form 2 cells, one dark type A and another light type A spermatogonia
   - Dark type A is kept as reserve
   - Light type A undergoes mitotic division and forms type B spermatogonia
   - Type B further divides to form 2 primary spermatocytes (46 + XY).

ii. **Meiosis**
   - In 1st meiotic/reduction division, the primary spermatocyte divides to form 2 secondary spermatocytes (22 + X/22 + Y)
   - Both cells contain equal amount of cytoplasm and the nuclear division is also equal

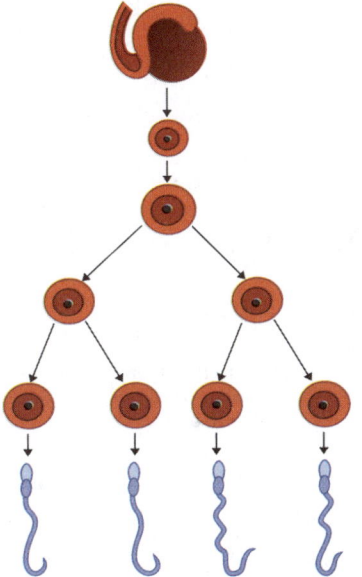 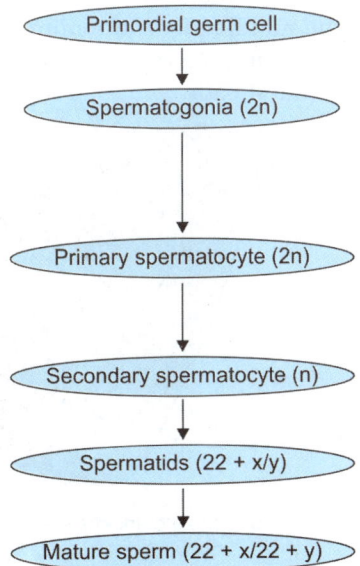

Fig. 34: Spermatogenesis.

- The secondary spermatocyte completes the second meiotic division immediately and forms 2 spermatids
- Each primary spermatocyte gives 4 spermatids, 2 with (22 + X) chromosomes and 2 with (22 + Y) chromosomes
- The meiosis **takes 24 days** (meiosis I 8 days + meiosis II 16 days) to complete.

iii. **Spermiogenesis**
- Morphological changes that happen in the conversion of spermatids to spermatozoa without cell division is called spermiogenesis
- It **takes 24 days** for spermatid to be converted spermatozoa
- Spermatid possesses a nucleus, Golgi apparatus, 2 centrioles, mitochondria and abundant cytoplasm.

Changes seen are
- Acrosomal granules of Golgi apparatus join and spread over the anterior pole of nucleus to form head cap. This covers two-third of nucleus
- The centrosome occupies the posterior pole of nucleus
- The centrosome divides into two centrioles. This gives rise to axial filament of the body and tail of the spermatozoa
- Around the middle piece, the mitochondria aggregate in spiral manner and forms mitochondrial sheath
- The spermatid elongates, and the nucleus evaginates from the cytoplasm
- The heads of immature spermatozoa plunge into cells of Sertoli
- When mature, they are set free into the lumen
- The whole process requires 64 days in man.

13. Boundaries and contents of quadrangular space.

It is an intermuscular space seen in the scapular region
It is undercover of deltoid.
- **Boundaries (Fig. 35)**
  - **Superior:** Subscapularis in front, capsule of the shoulder joint and teres minor behind
  - **Inferior:** Teres major
  - **Medial:** Long head of triceps
  - **Lateral:** Surgical neck of humerus.
- **Contents:** Axillary nerve, posterior circumflex humeral vessels
- **Applied Anatomy:** Dislocation of the shoulder or fracture of surgical neck of humerus results in injury to axillary nerve, leading to loss of rounded contour and flattening of shoulder and inability to abduct shoulder. There is loss of sensation over the upper part of lateral surface of arm called **regimental badge area.**

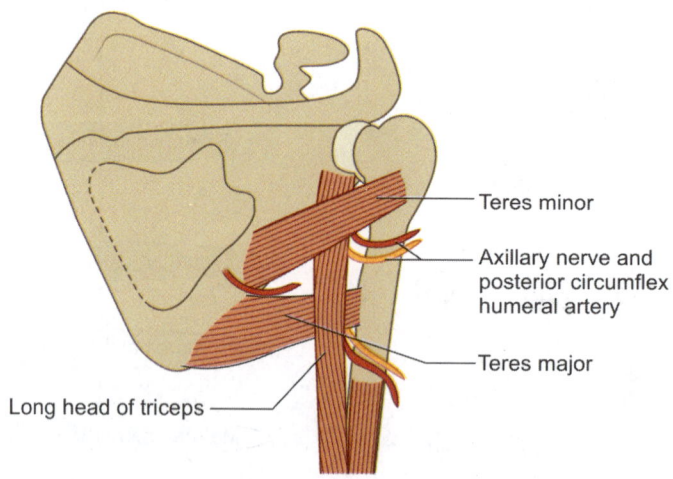

Fig. 35: Quadrangular space.

14. Types of epiphysis with examples.

- The upper and lower ends of long bones are called epiphysis
- The short long bones are provided with one epiphysis only
- They ossify from secondary centers
- The epiphysis is cartilaginous till the secondary center appear and ossify after birth
- It contains spongy bone and red marrow throughout life
- The center which appear first ossify and unites with the shaft later forming the growing end of long bone.

Types of Epiphysis

Pressure Epiphysis
- It is in the articular ends
- Takes part in transmission of weight
- For example, head of femur and humerus, lower end of radius.

Traction Epiphysis
- It is present in non-articular ends
- Does not help in the transmission of weight
- It provide attachment to one or more tendons
- Formed along the line of muscular pull
- It ossifies later than the pressure epiphysis
- For example, Trochanters of femur, tubercles and epicondyles of humerus.

Atavistic Epiphysis
- It is phylogenetically an independent bone
- In human becomes fused to an adjacent bone
- For example, coracoid process of scapula, os trigonum (posterior tubercle) of talus.

Aberrant Epiphysis
- Additional epiphysis may develop in long bones
- For example, Epiphysis at the head of the 1st metacarpal.

15. Femoral sheath formation, contents and applied anatomy.

Refer Short Notes 4 – 2005.

16. Carpometacarpal joint of thumb.

Refer Short Notes 16 – 2005.

17. Nerve supply of heart.

- Nerve supply to heart is from Cardiac plexus
- Formed by sympathetic and parasympathetic fibers.
- **Functions**
  - The parasympathetic supply atria and conducting systems
  - The sympathetic supply ventricular muscles in addition to the atria and conducting system
  - The nerves contain both afferent and efferent fibers except the cardiac branches from superior cervical sympathetic ganglia which contain only efferent fibers.
- **Nerves taking part** are
  - Recurrent laryngeal nerve
  - Vagus
  - Cervical sympathetic ganglia
  - Thoracic Sympathetic ganglia.

Parts
- Superficial
- Deep.

Superficial Cardiac Plexus

Situation: Below arch of aorta and anterior to right pulmonary artery.
- **Formation**
  - Superior cervical cardiac branch of left sympathetic chain
  - Inferior cervical cardiac branch of left vagus.
  - **Branches**
    - To deep cardiac plexus
    - Left anterior pulmonary plexus
    - Right Coronary plexus

Deep Cardiac Plexus
- **Situation**:
  - In front of bifurcation of trachea
  - Above the pulmonary trunk bifurcation
  - Posterior to arch of aorta.
- **Formation (Fig. 36)**: It is formed by branches from the cervical and upper

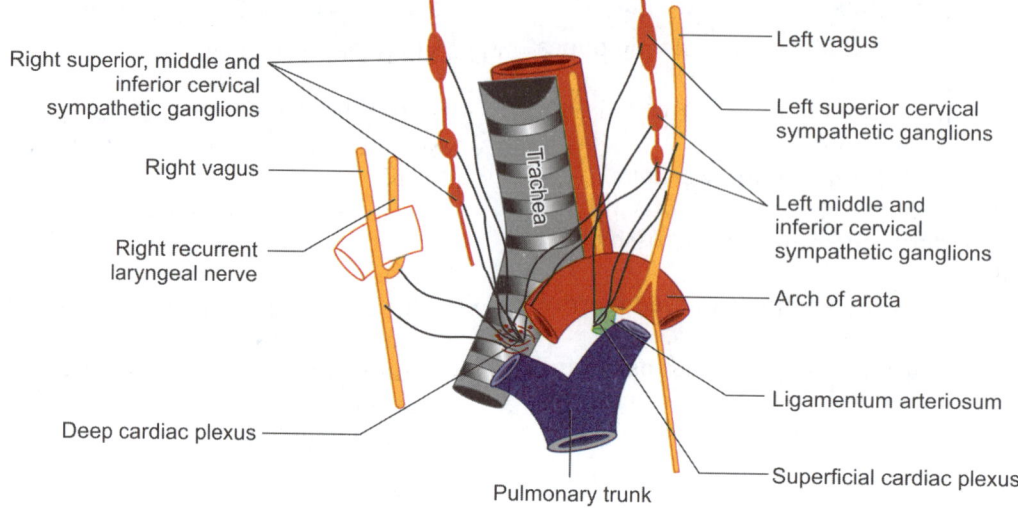

Fig. 36: Nerve supply of heart.

thoracic sympathetic ganglia, vagus and recurrent laryngeal nerve of both sides except that join the superficial plexus
- Cardiac branch from superior, middle, inferior cervical ganglia except superior cervical cardiac branch of left sympathetic trunk
- Upper 4 or 5 thoracic ganglia—both sides
- Cardiac branches of vagus except lower cardiac branch of left vagus
- Recurrent laryngeal branches of both sides
- **Branches**
  - **Right half**
    - Right anterior pulmonary plexus
    - Continued as right coronary plexus in front of pulmonary artery
    - Right atrium
    - Continued as left coronary plexus behind the artery.
  - **Left half**
    - To superficial plexus
    - Left anterior pulmonary plexus
    - Left atrium
    - Continued as left coronary plexus.
  - **Action of nerves:**
    - **Parasympathetic efferent fibers**
      * Decreases heart rate
      * Reduces force of cardiac contraction
      * Constricts coronary arteries.

- **Parasympathetic afferent fibers:** Depresses the cardiac activity.
- Sympathetic
  - **Sympathetic efferent fibers**
    - Increases the heart rate
    - Increases the force of cardiac contraction
    - Dilates the coronary arteries.
  - **Sympathetic afferent fibers:** Carry pain sensation from heart.
- **Applied anatomy:** Myocardial infarction: The pain is felt in the retrosternal region and radiates to the left arm.

18. Buccinator.

- Buccinator is the muscle of the cheek
- Shape: Quadrilateral
- Situated in the gap between the maxilla and the mandible
- It is also known as **trumpeter** or **whistling** muscle
- **Developed** from mesoderm of 2nd arch supplied by facial nerve
- **Attachment**
- **Origin**
  - Upper fibers are from the outer surfaces of the alveolar processes of the maxilla opposite the molar teeth
  - Lower fibers are attached to the outer surfaces of the alveolar processes

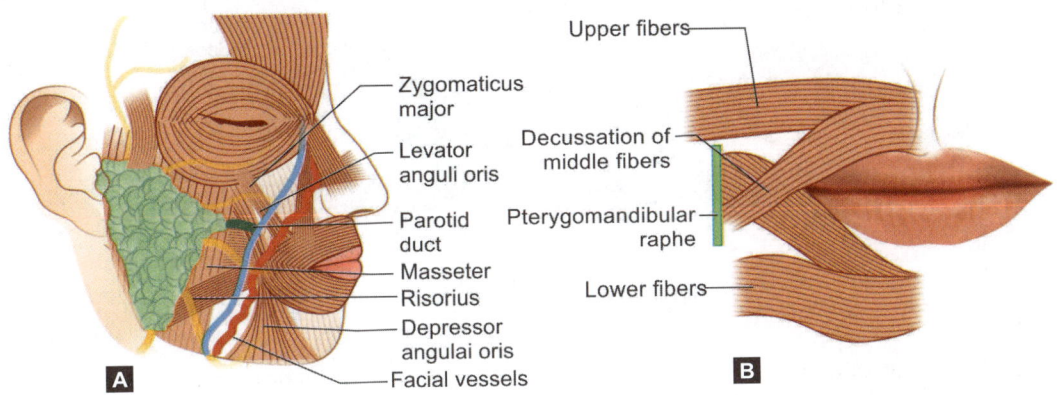

Figs. 37A and B: Buccinator.

of the mandible opposite the molar teeth
- Middle fibers are from the anterior margin of the pterygomandibular raphe.

- **Insertion**
  - The fibers of buccinator converge towards the modiolus near the angle of the mouth
  - The middle (pterygomandibular) fibers decussate, lower pterygomandibular fibers from below cross to the upper part of orbicularis oris, and upper pterygomandibular fibers from above cross to the lower part
  - The upper (maxillary) and lower (mandibular) fibres of buccinator, without decussation, continue forward to their corresponding lips.
- **Nerve supply:** Buccal branch of facial nerve.
- **Action**
  - The cheek is compressed against the teeth and gums during chewing by buccinator
  - When the cheeks are distended, the buccinator helps to blow the air out, which is important for playing wind instruments.
- **Relations**
  - **Deep**—pharyngeal constrictors
  - **Superficial**—covered by buccopharyngeal fascia, zygomaticus major, levator anguli oris, depressor anguli oris, risorius, facial artery and vein, branches of facial nerve, ramus of mandible and masseter. The muscle is pierced by parotid duct at the level of upper third molar.
- **Applied anatomy**
  - Paralysis of the muscle due to facial nerve injury results in collection of food in the vestibule
  - Cannot blow the air out
  - If a patient makes an attempt to blow air out there will be ballooning of cheek.

19. Coronary sinus.
Refer Essay Q. No. 5 – 2005.

20. Medial surface of right lung.
Refer Essay Q. No. 3 – 2004.

21. Draw a well labeled diagram of c/s of pons at the level of facial colliculus.
Refer Short Notes 13 – 2004.

22. Development of face and its anomalies.

Development of Face

- The face development begins at the end of 4th week
- It is developed from the facial eminences containing neural crest induced mesenchyme
- Face is developed from five mesenchymal elevations that bulge around the stomodeum
- These enlargements appear at 42nd day
- They are the frontonasal process (above), and a pair of mandibular arches and a pair of maxillary processes **(Fig. 38A)**

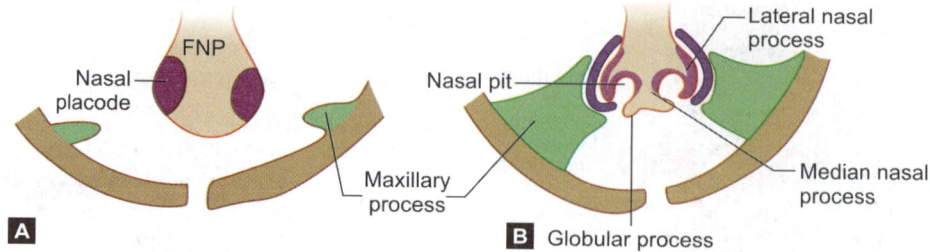

Figs. 38A and B: Development of face.

- **The frontonasal process** is the downward growth of proliferation of the mesenchyme in front of brain vesicles along with the ectoderm covering. It grows towards stomodeum.
  - In the frontonasal process an ectodermal thickening laterally on either side appear called **nasal placode**
  - By 5th week a depression appears below the surface of the nasal placode called the **nasal pit**
  - The nasal pits enlarge to form the **nasal cavity**
  - By the pit the frontonasal process is divided into two **lateral nasal processes** and a **median nasal process**
  - The lateral nasal processes form the **alae of nose**
  - The median nasal process grows down to form the **globular processes**. A triangular gap is seen in between the processes **(Fig. 38B)**
  - The globular processes join to form the **philtrum of the upper lip**.
- A pair of **maxillary processes** are from the dorsal portion of first pharyngeal arches
  - The maxillary processes grow medially and comes in contact with the lateral nasal process
  - The maxillary process fuse with the lateral nasal process. Before fusion a deep furrow is seen called nasolacrimal groove. The ectodermal cells submerge and later gets canalized to form **nasolacrimal duct**
  - The maxillary process continues to grow medially and joins with the medial nasal process (globular process) to form the **lateral part of upper lip**.
- A pair of **mandibular prominences**, the first pharyngeal arch is caudal to stomodeum
- The mandibular arches join to form the lower lip
- Initially the oral fissure extends from one ear to the other
- The **cheeks** are formed by union of the posterior parts of the maxillary and mandibular processes and the normal oral fissure is formed.

Congenital Anomalies

- **Cleft lip**: The cleft can be upper lip cleft or lower lip cleft **(Figs. 40A to C)**
  - **Upper lip cleft** is also known as **hare lip**. It is divided into central and lateral clefts
  - **Median upper lip cleft** is midline cleft. It is rare. It is due to failure of union of the two globular processes
  - **Lateral upper lip cleft** can be unilateral or bilateral. In **unilateral cleft** one of the maxillary process fails to join with the globular process. In **bilateral cleft** both the maxillary processes fail to join with globular processes
  - **Lower lip cleft** is rare. It is due to failure of fusion of mandibular arches.
- **Oblique facial cleft**: Due to failure of union of maxillary process with corresponding lateral nasal process. The nasolacrimal duct will be exposed to surface in this condition.

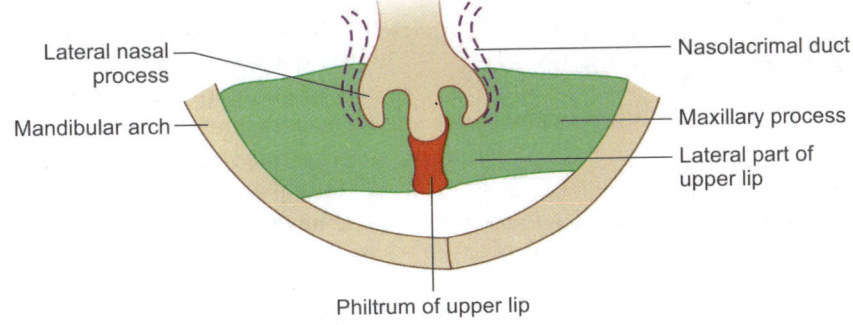

Fig. 39: Development of lips.

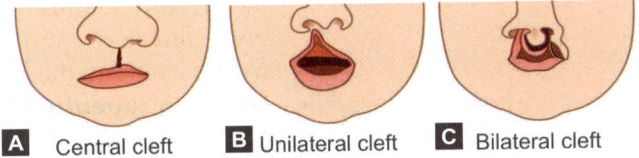

A Central cleft **B** Unilateral cleft **C** Bilateral cleft

Figs. 40A to C: Congenital anomalies.

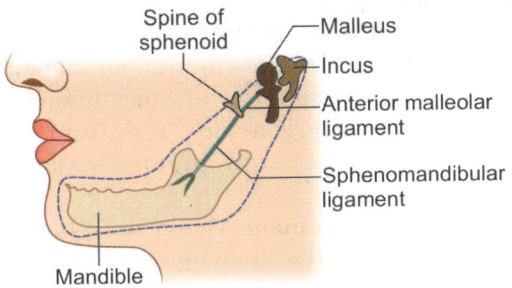

Fig. 41: First arch derivatives.

- **Macrostomia**: Large oral fissure. Due to incomplete union of maxillary process and mandibular arch
- **Microstomia**: Small mouth, due to over fusion of maxillary process and mandibular arch.

23. Microscopic structure of pituitary gland.

Refer Short Notes 23 – 2005.

24. Derivatives of I pharyngeal arch.

- Each pharyngeal arch is made of mesenchyme which are invaded by neural crest cells
- Each arch is covered by an outer ectoderm and inner endoderm
- The neural crest cells of each arch contribute, the skeletal element and associated connective tissue
- Initially six arches appear, of which the fifth one disappears
- First arch is also called as the **mandibular arch**
- The **dorsal portion** of the arch is the **maxillary process**
- It extends below the eye
- The **ventral part** is the **mandibular process**
- It extends from midline to ear capsule
- The cartilage of the mandibular process is **Meckel's cartilage**
- The cartilage gets ossified in some places to form bones and in some places the cartilage disappears and the fibrous sheath forms bones/ligaments
- The **nerve of the arch**—pre-trematic nerve is chorda tympani and post-trematic is mandibular nerve
- The mesodermal cells of the arch give rise to musculature supplied by the nerve of the arch and it is retained even if they migrate
- The **artery of the arch** is maxillary artery

- Structures derived are:

From maxillary process	From cartilage (Meckel's cartilage)		
	Bones	Ligaments	Muscles
Premaxilla Maxilla Zygomatic bone Part of temporal bone	Malleus Incus Body of the mandible (from mandibular foramen to mental foramen the cartilage disappears and the fibrous sheath form the body of mandible)	Anterior malleolar ligament Spheno-mandibular ligament	Muscles of mastication Anterior belly of digastrics Mylohyoid Tensor palati Tensor tympani

25. Maxillary sinus.

- The maxillary sinus/antrum, is the largest of the paranasal sinuses
- It is situated in the body of the maxilla
- **Shape**: Pyramidal in shape
- **Boundaries and relations**
  - The **floor** of the sinus is at a lower level, than the floor of the nasal cavity. The alveolar process and part of the palatine process of the maxilla form the floor. The roots of the teeth are related to it
  - The **roof** of the sinus forms the floor of the orbit. It contains the infraorbital canal
  - The **anterior wall** is facial surface of the maxilla
  - The **posterior wall** is formed by the infratemporal surface of the maxilla
  - The **apex** is directed laterally into the zygomatic process of the maxilla, and may invade into the zygomatic bone.
  - The **base/medial wall** related to the lateral wall of the nasal cavity.
- The **base** is deficient posterosuperiorly at the opening of maxillary sinus. The large opening is reduced by articulation of the perpendicular plate of the palatine bone posteriorly, the uncinate process of the ethmoid bone superiorly, the inferior nasal concha inferiorly, the lacrimal bone anteriorly, and the overlying nasal mucosa, to form the opening
- **Drainage/opening:** The sinus usually opens into the hiatus semilunaris of middle meatus. The opening is at a higher level than the floor.
- **Blood supply**
  - The **arterial supply** of the maxilla is mainly from the anterior, middle and posterior superior alveolar branches of maxillary artery and from the infraorbital and greater palatine arteries
  - **Venous drainage**: Veins corresponding to the arteries drain into the facial vein or pterygoid venous plexus.
- **Nerve supply**
  - **General sensation:** The infraorbital and anterior, middle and posterior superior alveolar branches of the maxillary nerve

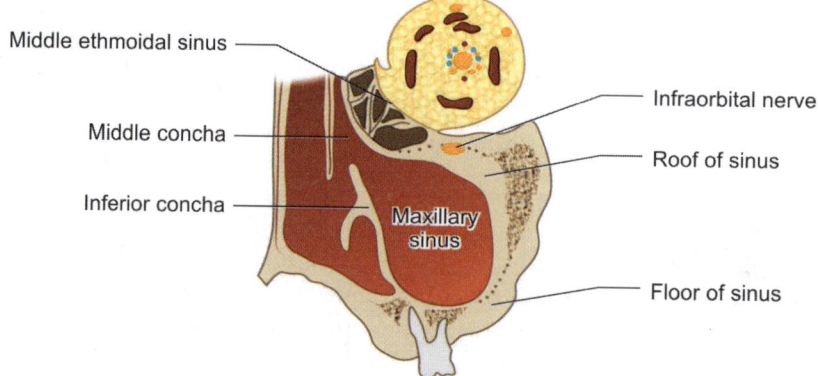

Fig. 42: Maxillary sinus.

- **Secretomotor fibers:** Nasal branches of the pterygopalatine ganglion.
- **Lymphatic drainage:** Submandibular nodes
- **Applied anatomy**
  - As the floor of the sinus is at a lower level drainage of the sinus is very difficult, often resulting in sinusitis. Drained by postural drainage
  - The walls of maxillary sinus is thin so the tumor from the maxillary sinus can spread. (i) Upward spread of the tumor may push up the orbital floor and displace the eyeball (ii) Medially spread into the nasal cavity, causing nasal obstruction and bleeding (iii) Project onto the cheek, causing swelling and numbness if the infraorbital nerve is damaged (iv) Project posteriorly into the infratemporal fossa, can compress pterygoid muscles causing difficulty in opening the mouth.

26. Facial artery.

- Chief artery supplying the face
- The artery runs forward in neck and reaches face. Hence the branches are classified as branches in neck and branches in face
- **Origin/formation:** One of the ventral branch of external carotid artery given above the greater horn of hyoid bone in the carotid triangle.

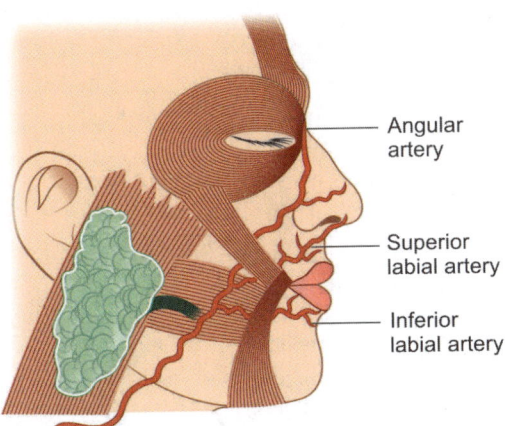

Fig. 43: Facial artery in face.

- **Course**
  - It ascends upwards deep to posterior belly of digastrics and reaches submandibular gland
  - It grooves submandibular the salivary gland posteriorly
  - It forms a loops between the gland and medial pterygoid muscle
  - Enters the face by winding around the base of mandible at anteroinferior angle of masseter
  - It runs forwards and medially reaches the angle of mouth
  - Then it ascends upwards to reach the medial angle of eye along the side of nose.
- **Termination:** Terminates by anastomosing with dorsal nasal branch of ophthalmic artery. After the lateral nasal branch, the continuation of the artery is named as **angular artery**
- **Nature of artery:** It is tortuous in course to accommodate to the movements of the face.
- **Branches in neck (TAGS)**
  - **T**onsillar branch—chief artery of tonsil
  - **A**scending palatine – supplies tonsil, palate, auditory tube
  - **G**landular—for submandibular gland
  - **S**ubmental artery—largest cervical branch. Supplies the skin in the submental region.
- **Branches in the face**
  - Premasseteric small and inconstant, runs along the anterior border of masseter
  - Inferior labial supplies mucous membrane, glands and muscles of lower lip
  - Superior labial supplies mucous membrane, glands and muscles of upper lip. In addition, it gives of alar and septal branches supplying anteroinferior part of septum of nose
  - Lateral nasal supplies dorsum and alae of the nose.
- **Relations**
  - **Superficial:** Skin, fat of cheek, zygomaticus major, risorius
  - **Deep:** Buccinator, levator anguli oris, levator labii superioris
  - **Posterior:** Facial vein.

- **Applied anatomy:**
  - Pulsation of the facial artery is felt at the anteroinferior angle of the masseter muscle. Often the anesthetists feel the pulsation of this artery to monitor the patient
  - The artery can be compressed against the base of mandible
  - The facial artery is used more in facial surgery, rhinoplasty and orofacial surgery. Artery used as a pedicle in flaps, e.g. nasolabial skin flaps, oral mucosal flaps, buccal mucosal flaps, musculomucosal flaps.

27. Structures derived from mesoderm of second branchial arch.

Refer Short Notes 27 – 2005.

28. Microscopic structure of submandibular salivary gland.

Refer Short Notes 1 – 2004.

29. Falx cerebri.

It is a fold formed by the meningeal layer of duramater

- **Shape:** It is a sickle shaped fold of duramater
- **Situation:** Situated in the median longitudinal fissure of brain
- **Parts:** 2 margins, 2 surfaces, 2 ends.
- **Attachment:**
  - Superior convex margin to the margins of superior sagittal sinus
  - The inferior concave margin is free
  - The anterior end is narrow attached to crista galli, frontal crest
  - Posterior broader attached to the superior layer of tentorium cerebelli
  - Surfaces are related to medial surface of cerebral hemispheres.
- **Sinuses related**
  - Superior sagittal sinus along the superior border
  - Inferior sagittal sinus along the concave free border
  - Straight sinus between the falx cerebri and tentorium cerebelli.
- **Nerve supply**
  - Anterior and posterior ethmoidal nerves
  - The supra tentorial part of falx cerebri is supplied by the nervus tentori (recurrent branch of the intracranial part of ophthalmic nerve)
- **Function:** Stabilizes the brain within the cranial cavity
- **Applied anatomy:**
  - In case of space occupying lesion or increase in the intracranial fossa may result in herniation of cerebrum below falx cerebri
  - The stimulation of the falx, during the intra cranial surgeries, may trigger trigeminocardiac reflex.

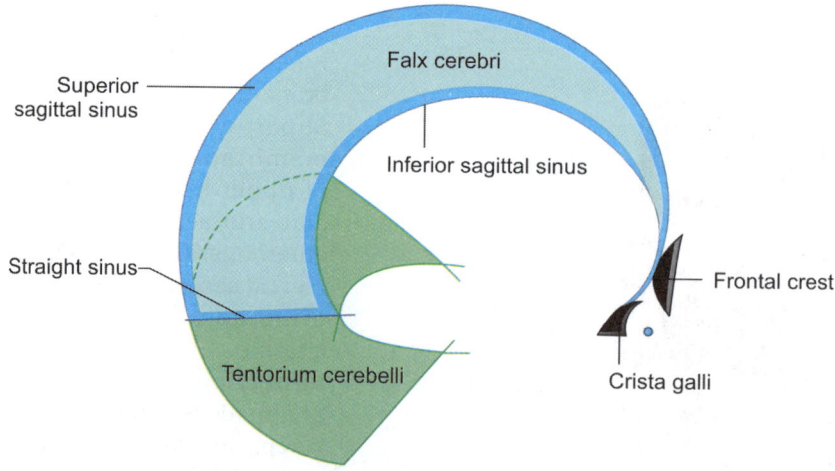

Fig. 44: Falx cerebri.

30. Styloid apparatus.

Refer Short Notes 38 – 2005.

31. Circle of Willis.

Refer Short Notes 24 – 2005.

32. Pericardium.

The pericardium is a fibroserous sac which encloses the heart and the root of the great vessels.
- It consists of
  - Fibrous pericardium
  - Serous pericardium

Fibrous Pericardium

- It is a conical sac
- Made up of fibrous tissue enclosing the heart.

Attachment

- Inferiorly it is firmly attached to the central tendon of diaphragm
- Anteriorly it is attached by superior and inferior sterno pericardial ligaments to the body of sternum
- Above it is continuous with pretracheal fascia
- Internally the parietal layer of serous pericardium lines the surface
- These attachments help to maintain the position of the heart, functioning as the **'cardiac seat belt'**

- The fibrous pericardium is **pierced** by ascending aorta, pulmonary veins, SVC, IVC and pulmonary trunk. The fibrous pericardium merges with adventitial layer of vessels. All these vessels receive extensions of the fibrous pericardium except IVC.

Serous Pericardium

- It is a thin double layered serous membrane lined by mesothelium
- The outer layer of serous pericardium is fused with the fibrous pericardium
- Its inner layer is adherent to the heart
- Between these two layers there is a thin capillary space called pericardial cavity filled with pericardial fluid
- Pericardial sinuses are the spaces formed by the arrangement of the serosal layer
- It is arranged as two 'tubes'. The aorta and pulmonary trunk are in one tube, and the superior and inferior venae cava and the four pulmonary veins form the second tube
- The **pericardial sinuses** are:
  - Transverse sinus
  - Oblique sinuses.
- **Transverse sinus:** The transverse sinus is a passage between the two pericardial 'tubes' mentioned above
- **Boundaries**: In front: The aorta and pulmonary trunk.

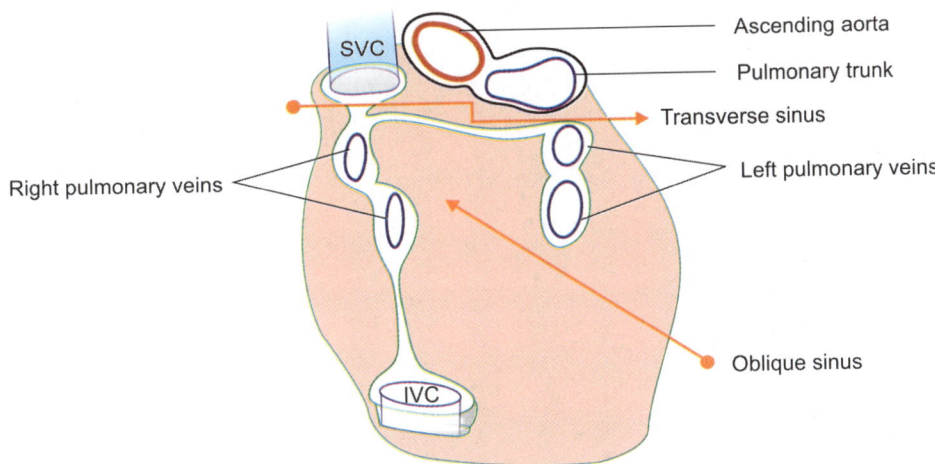

Fig. 45: Pericardial sinuses.

- Behind: The atria and great veins
- Above: Bifurcation of pulmonary trunk
- Below: Upper surface of left atrium
- **Function:** It helps to ligate the great vessels temporarily by passing ligature through this space.

- **Oblique sinus:**
  - It is a blind sac lying behind the left atrium
  - It is inverted "J" shaped.
  - **Boundaries**:
    - **Left side:** Left pulmonary veins.
    - **Right side:** Right pulmonary veins and Superior and inferior vena cava
    - **Anteriorly:** Left atrium
    - **Posteriorly:** Fibrous pericardium and posterior mediastinum
    - **Above:** Upper margin of left atrium
    - **Below:** Opens downwards and laterally
- It is also called as **cardiac bursa,** facilitates expansion of left atrium
- **Blood supply:**
  - Arterial supply:
    - **Fibrous** and parietal layer by the branches of internal thoracic artery and descending thoracic artery
    - Visceral layer by coronary arteries.
  - Venous drainage:
    - Fibrous and parietal layer drained by azygous and internal thoracic veins
    - Visceral layer drains into coronary sinus.
- **Nerve supply**
  - Fibrous and parietal layer by phrenic nerves, intercostal nerves (pain sensitive)
  - Visceral layer by vagus and sympathetic nerves via coronary plexus (not sensitive to pain).
- **Lymphatic drainage:** Mediastinal lymph nodes
- **Applied anatomy**:
  - Pericarditis—inflammation of pericardium
  - Inflammation of serous pericardium – **Pericarditis**—leads to accumulation of pericardial fluid—more fluid can compress the heart leading to **cardiac tamponade**
  - Aspiration of excessive amount of pericardial fluid from the pericardial cavity—**paracentesis.**

MBBS Examination 2008

ANSWER ALL QUESTIONS

I. Essay questions   **(15/10 Marks)**

1. Describe the formation, course, relations, branches of distribution and effects of injury of median nerve.
2. Describe the pancreas under the following headings: Parts, relations, blood supply, development and histology.
3. Describe the hip joint under the following headings: (a) Type of joint and bones taking part, (b) Ligaments, (c) Relations, (d) Muscles producing the action and (e) Applied anatomy.
4. Describe the prostate under the following headings: (a) Situation and lobes, (b) Blood supply, (c) Histology, (d) Age changes and (e) Applied anatomy.
5. Describe the cavernous sinus under the following headings: Situation, extent, boundaries, relations, contents, connections and applied anatomy.
6. Describe the right lung under the following headings: Surfaces, borders, impressions, fissures, lobes, hilum and bronchopulmonary segments.
7. Describe the muscles of mastication under the following headings: (a) Origin, (b) Insertion, (c) Relations, (d) Nerve supply and (e) Action.
8. Describe the blood supply and venous drainage of the heart.

II. Short notes   **(5/4 Marks)**

1. Lower end of humerus.
2. Trisomy 21.
3. Cutaneous innervations of hand.
4. Abductors of hip joint and their role in gait.
5. Saphenous vein.
6. Ligaments of liver.
7. Structure of kidney.
8. Inguinal ligament.
9. Rectus sheath.
10. Coeliac ganglion.
11. Lesser sac.
12. Ischiorectal fossa.
13. Mesentery.
14. Development of diaphragm.
15. Lumbrical muscles of the hand.
16. Cubital fossa.
17. Erb's paralysis.
18. Menstrual cycle.
19. Dorsalis pedis artery.
20. Inguinal canal.
21. Rhomboid fossa.
22. Maxillary air sinus.
23. Labelled diagram of superolateral surface of cerebrum, indicating major functional areas.
24. Histology of retina.
25. Coronary sinus.
26. Ansa cervicalis.
27. Blood supply of spinal cord.
28. Derivatives of I branchial arch.
29. Medial wall of middle ear.
30. Hyoglossus muscle—attachments and relations.
31. Histology of esophagus.
32. Tonsil.
33. Derivatives of II pharyngeal arch.
34. Lumbar puncture.
35. Vocal cords.
36. Lacrimal apparatus.
37. Paranasal air sinuses.
38. Blood supply of thyroid gland.
39. Middle meningeal artery.
40. Karyotyping chromosomes.

III. Short answer questions (2 Marks each)

1. Name of muscles of II layer of sole of the foot.
2. Name the bursae around the patella.
3. Name the abductors of the wrist joint.
4. Indicate the terminal branches of posterior cord of brachial plexus.
5. Indicate the tributaries of left renal vein.
6. Name the two most common positions of appendix.
7. Indicate the structure of the free border of lesser omentum.
8. Name the arteries of the spermatic cord.
9. Name the nerves closely related to humerus.
10. Name three structures at the transpyloric plane.
11. Name the bones meeting at pterion.
12. Indicate the sinuses of the pericardium.
13. Name the terminal branches of internal thoracic artery.
14. Indicate the paleocerebellar deep nuclei.
15. Name the muscles attached to the cricoid cartilage.
16. Name two sensory thalamic nuclei.
17. Name the structures passing through internal acoustic meatus.
18. Name the two parts of orbicularis oculi.
19. Name the lingual papillae.
20. Indicate the venous sinuses related to the falx cerebri.

I. ESSAY QUESTIONS

1. Describe the formation, course, relations, branches of distribution and effects of injury of median nerve.

- The median nerve is also known as **labourer nerve**
- It mainly supplies the flexors of forearm
- It arises from the brachial plexus as two roots one from medial cord and the other from lateral cord
- Root value is ventral rami of C5 to C8 and T1 segments of spinal cord.

Formation

Median nerve is formed by the union of two roots:
1. Lateral root from lateral cord (C5, C6, C7)
2. Medial root from medial cord (C8, T1).

Course and Relations

- **In axilla (Fig. 1):**
  - The medial root crosses the axillary artery to join the lateral root
  - The nerve runs on the lateral side of the axillary artery
  - No branch is given by the nerve in the axilla.
- **In arm (Fig. 2):**
  - The median nerve continues to run on the lateral side of the brachial artery
  - At the level of insertion of coracobrachialis (middle of arm) the nerve crosses in front the artery from lateral to medial.

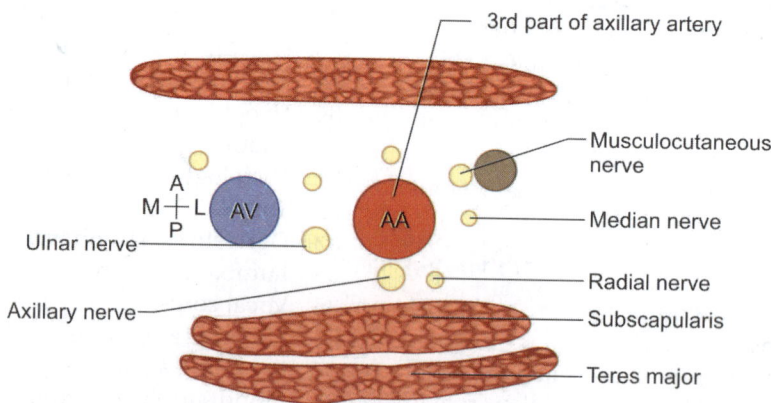

Fig. 1: Relations in axilla.

- **Elbow (cubital fossa) (Fig. 3):**
  - It is deep to the bicipital aponeurosis, and lies on brachialis and medial to the brachial artery
  - It leaves the fossa between the two heads of pronator teres.
- **In the forearm:**
  - It crosses the ulnar artery and lies lateral to the artery
  - The nerve is separated from the artery by deep head of pronator teres
  - It then passes deep to the fibrous arch of flexor digitorum superficialis and is adherent to the under surface of the muscle
  - Here it lies between the flexor digitorum superficialis and profundus muscles
  - About 5 cm above the above flexor retinaculum it becomes superficial
  - It lies in between the tendon of flexor digitorum superficialis and flexor carpi radialis
  - It is placed deep and lateral to palmaris longus
  - The nerve is accompanied by median branch of anterior interosseous artery
  - It then enters the palm deep to the flexor retinaculum (**Fig. 4**).
- **In Palm (Fig. 5):**
  - Distal to the retinaculum the nerve enlarges and flattens
  - The nerve terminates by dividing into four or five palmar cutaneous branches.

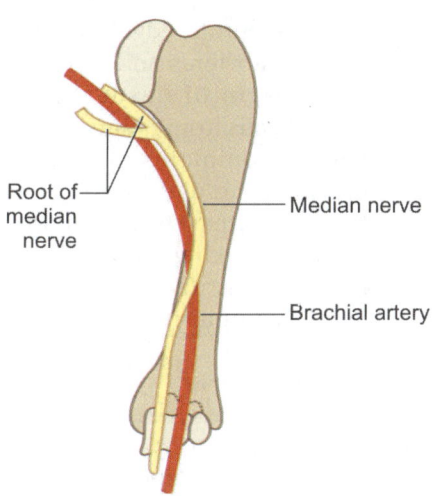

Fig. 2: Median nerve in arm.

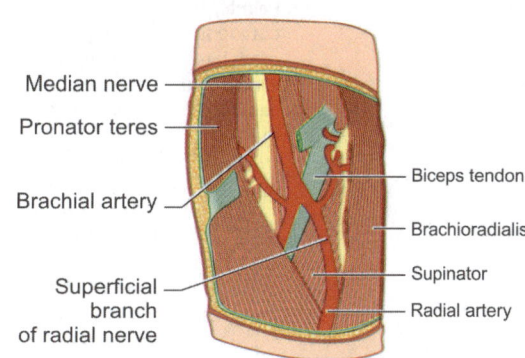

Fig. 3: In cubital fossa.

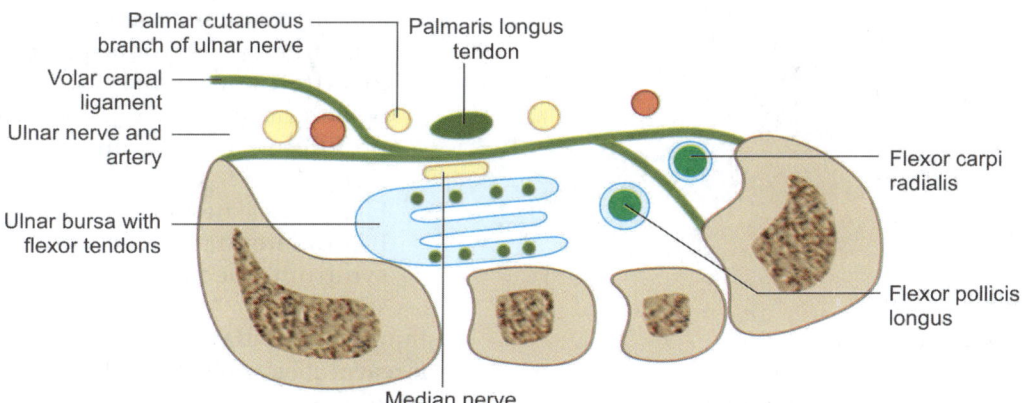

Fig. 4: Deep to flexor retinaculum.

Branches and Distribution

Type of fiber	Arm	Elbow (cubital fossa)	Forearm	Palm
Muscular	Nerve to pronator teres proximal to elbow joint	Nerves to pronator teres, flexor carpi radialis, flexor digitorum superficialis and palmaris longus	Anterior interosseous nerve supplies: Lateral half of flexor digitorum profundus, pronator quadratus, and flexor pollicis longus. Branch to flexor digitorum superficialis of index finger	Recurrent branch for abductor pollicis brevis, flexor pollicis brevis and opponens pollicis. 1st and 2nd lumbricals are supplied by the digital nerves
Cutaneous	—	—	Palmar cutaneous branch to thenar and central palmar skin	Lateral branch: Two digital branches to lateral and medial sides of thumb, a branch to lateral side of index finger. Medial branch: Two to adjacent sides of index, middle and ring fingers
Articular		Elbow joint, Superior radioulnar joint	Wrist, inferior radioulnar, and carpal joints	
Vascular	Brachial		Radial and ulnar arteries	Digital arteries
Secretomotor fibers				Sweat glands

Applied Anatomy

- **Injury at elbow:**
  - Pronator syndrome:
    - Compression of median nerve can occur in four areas.

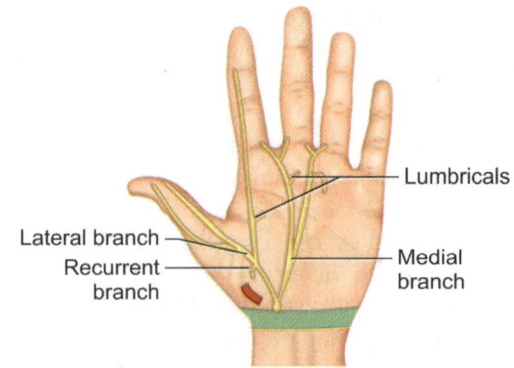

Fig. 5: In palm.

- (i) Struther's ligament, (ii) posterior to bicipital aponeurosis, (iii) aponeurotic edge of ulnar head of pronator teres and (iv) aponeurotic origin of flexor digitorum superficialis from radius
- Patient complains of pain in the proximal part of forearm
- Pain is increased in pronation of forearm, flexing elbow, flexion of middle finger all against resistance
- Sensory impairment on the palm of hand.
- **Injury in the forearm**
  - **Anterior interosseous nerve syndrome:**
    - The syndrome is due to compression of anterior interosseous nerve by (i) external pressure, (ii) aponeurotic edge of deep head of pronator teres and (iii) aponeurotic origin of radial head of flexor digitorum superficialis
    - Results in weakness of flexor pollicis longus and flexor digitorum profundus to index and middle finger
    - Effect is weakness of pinch grip
    - It is differentiated from pronator syndrome because there is no sensory loss.
  - Injury of **median nerve is at mid forearm** affects only the tendon of flexor digitorum superficialis to index finger and results in **pointing index finger.**

- **Injury at wrist**
  - **Laceration of median nerve:**
    - The median nerve is commonly affected from laceration at wrist
    - Results in weakness of thenar muscles and 1st and 2nd lumbricals
    - The effect of it is flattening of lateral part of hand as thenar muscles are affected

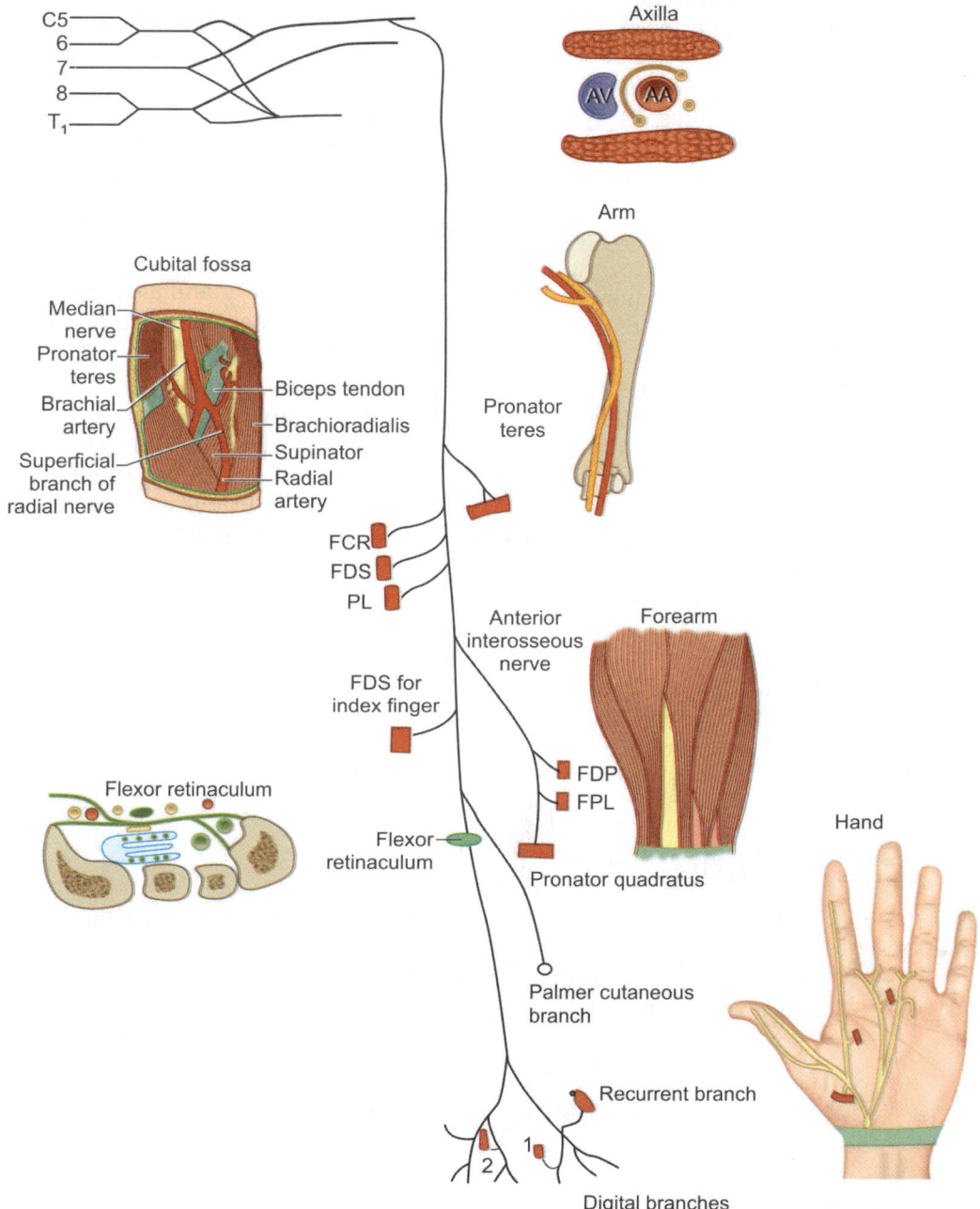

Fig. 6: Course and branches of median nerve.
Abbreviations: FCR, Flexor Carpi Radialis; FDS, Flexor Digitorum Superficialis; PL, Palmaris Longus; FDP, Flexor Digitorum Profundus; FPL, Flexor Pollicis Longus.

- The opposition of thumb is lost
- There is sensory loss over lateral three and a half fingers
- **Carpal tunnel syndrome**:
  - Compression of median nerve in the carpal tunnel deep to flexor retinaculum results in carpal tunnel syndrome.
  - **Reason for compression**
    * By the swellings of synovial sheath
    * Narrowing of tunnel by arthritic changes in wrist joint
    * Dislocation of the underlying carpal bones
    * Edema due to pregnancy
    * Thickening of soft tissue as in myxedema.
  - **Effects of compression**
    * Results in pain, paresthesia and numbness in the distribution of the nerve
    * Paralysis of muscles of thenar eminence called **Ape thumb deformity**
    * Motor changes: Loss of opposition
    * Sensory changes: There is loss of sensations on lateral 3½ digits including their nail beds if compression is prolonged
    * Vasomotor changes: The skin is warmer, due to arteriolar dilatation in the areas where there is loss of sensation
    * Trophic changes: Longstanding cases lead to dry and scaly skin.

Treatment: Surgical division of flexor retinaculum to remove the compression.

2. **Describe the pancreas under the following headings: Parts, relations, blood supply, development and histology.**

(Parts, Relations, Histology, Development – Refer Essay Q. No. 1 – 2006)

Blood supply: The gland is supplied by the branches of coeliac axis and superior mesenteric artery.

- **Arterial supply (Fig. 7)**
  - Head and uncinate process:
    - Superior pancreaticoduodenal artery is branch from gastroduodenal artery. It divides into anterior and posterior branches
    - Inferior pancreaticoduodenal artery branch of superior mesenteric artery. It divides into anterior and posterior branches which anastomose with the corresponding branches of superior pancreaticoduodenal artery

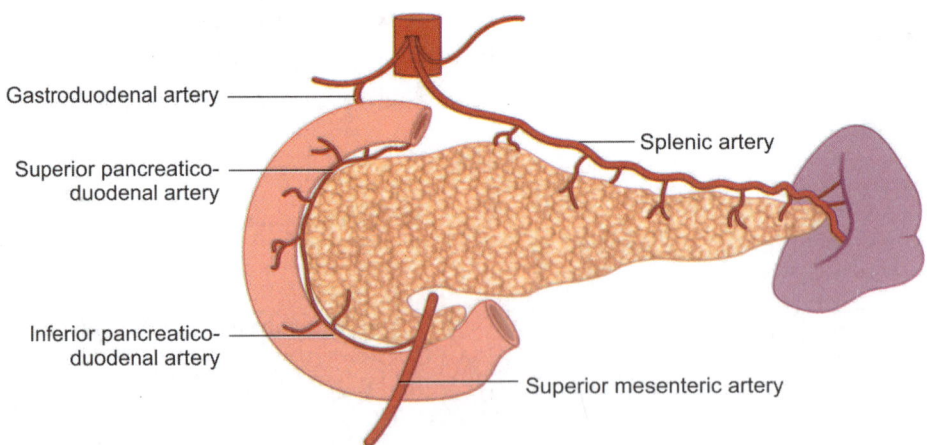

Fig. 7: Arterial supply of pancreas.

- The anastomosis is along the duodenopancreatic groove.
- The neck, body and tail are supplied by branches from splenic artery
- One of the branch from splenic artery is large and accompanies the main pancreatic duct
- A dorsal pancreatic branch from splenic artery, runs along posterior surface of body. It divides into right and left branch. The left branch runs along the inferior border of tail and is called **arteria pancreatica magna**
- The tail of pancreas is supplied by the arteria caudae pancreatis
- Capillary plexus supply the islets
- Blood from islets drain into acinar network forming **insularacinar portal system**.
- **Venous drainage**: Drains into splenic, superior mesenteric and portal veins.
- **Applied anatomy**:
  - Pancreatitis may cause aneurysm of superior mesenteric artery due to inflammation or thrombosis of the superior mesenteric vein as the superior mesenteric vessels are in between the body of pancreas and the uncinate process
  - Pancreas has rich blood supply and is prone for bleeding if injured or inflamed. Blood can appear in the flanks or in the groins.

3. **Describe the hip joint under the following headings: (a) Type of joint and bones taking part, (b) Ligaments, (c) Relations, (d) Muscles producing the action and (e) Applied anatomy.**

(a) Type of joint and bones taking part, (b) Ligaments, (d) Muscles producing the action and (e) Applied anatomy Refer Essay Q. No. 1 – 2004]

Relations (Fig. 8)

- **Anteriorly:** Pectineus, psoas tendon, iliacus, femoral nerve in between iliopsoas, femoral artery on psoas tendon, femoral vein on pectineus
- **Posteriorly:** Piriformis, obturator internus tendon with gamelli, quadratus femoris, gluteus maximus, sciatic nerve, superior gluteal nerve and vessels, inferior gluteal nerve and vessels, posterior cutaneous nerve of thigh, nerve to quadrates femoris.

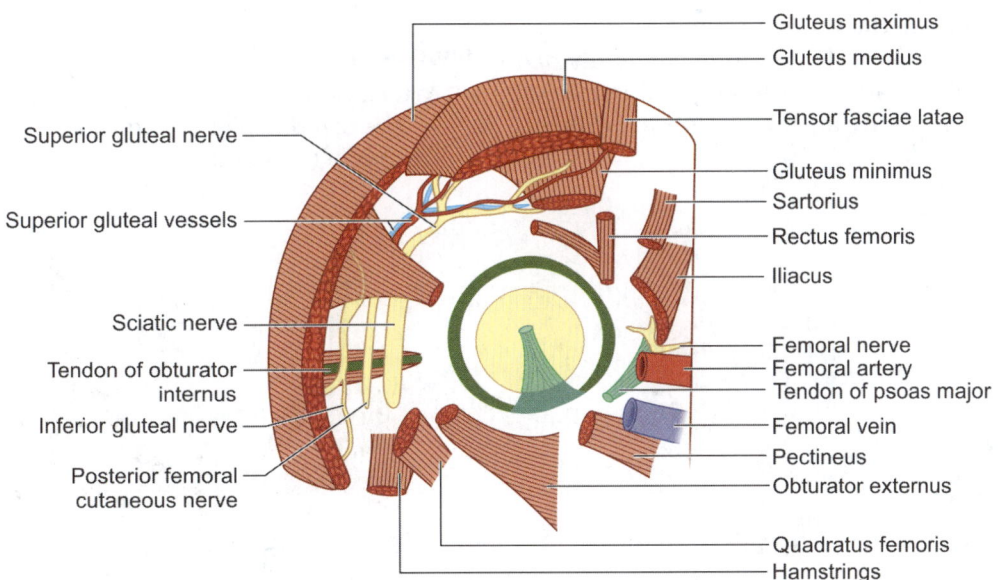

Fig. 8: Relations of hip joint.

- **Superiorly:** Reflected head of rectus femoris, gluteus medius and minimus
- **Inferiorly:** Pectineus, obturator externus.

4. Describe the prostate under the following headings: (a) Situation and lobes, (b) Blood supply, (c) Histology, (d) Age changes and (e) Applied anatomy.

- The prostate is a pyramidal fibromuscular gland
- It surrounds the proximal part of male urethra extending from base of bladder to the membranous urethra
- It corresponds to paraurethral glands of skene in female.

Situation and Lobes

- **Situation (Fig. 9A):**
  - It lies in the lesser pelvis
  - The base of the prostate is below the neck of the urinary bladder
  - Anterior surface is 2 cm behind the lower border of the pubic symphysis and pubic arch
  - Apex is directed down and is above urogenital diaphragm
  - Posterior surface is in front of the ampulla of the rectum.
- **Lobes of the Prostate**
  - Anatomically, the prostate is divided into 3 lobes, in fetal gland before 20 weeks five anatomical lobes are identified
  - **Anterior lobe:** The portion of the gland, lying in front of the urethra. It contains muscular tissue
  - **Median lobe:** The portion of the gland between the two ejaculatory ducts and the urethra. It forms the **uvula vesicae** at the apex of the trigone of bladder
  - **Lateral lobes:** The two lateral (right and left) lobes are separated by the urethra and form the main mass of the prostate
  - **Posterior lobe:** The rear part of the lateral lobes, which can be palpated through the rectum during a digital rectal examination.
- **Zonal anatomy in prostate:** The glandular tissue may be divided into:
  - 70%--- peripheral zone---carcinoma
  - 25%---central zone---rarely involved in any disease
  - 5%---transitional---Benign prostatic hypertrophy.
- **Structures passing through prostate (Fig. 10):**
  - **Prostatic urethra:** (Refer Short Notes 2 – 2006)
  - **Prostatic utricle:** (Refer Short Notes 2 – 2006)
  - **Ejaculatory ducts:** Passes posterolateral to median lobe.

Blood Supply

- **Arterial supply**
  - The arteries pierce and extend to the apex of the gland

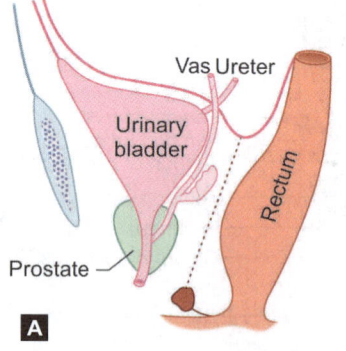
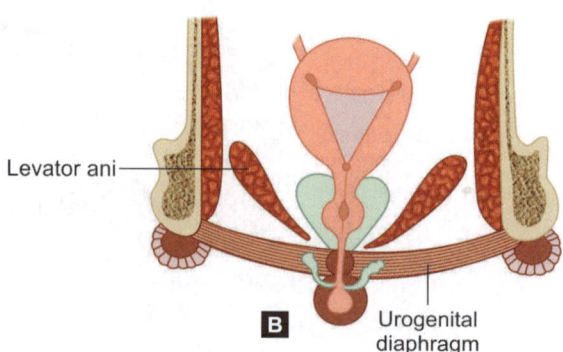

Figs. 9A and B: Prostate gland: (A) Situation; (B) Relations.

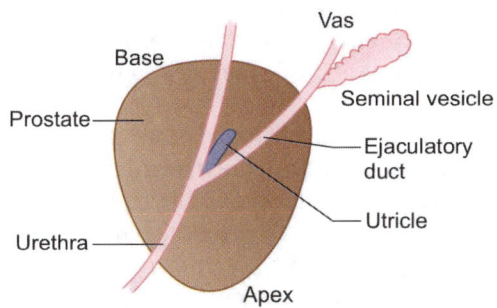

Fig. 10: Structures passing through prostate.

- The inferior vesical branch of internal iliac artery
- Internal pudendal artery from internal iliac artery
- Middle rectal artery.
- **Venous drainage**
  - The veins drain into a plexus around the anterolateral aspects of the prostate
  - Drains into vesical and internal iliac veins
  - A few veins communicate with internal vertebral venous plexus called **para vertebral venous plexus of Batson.**

Histology (Fig. 11)

- Prostate consists of ¼ fibrous, ¼ muscular and ½ glandular tissues

- **Fibrous muscular tissue**:
  - It contains collagen and smooth muscle fibers. It is thickened at periphery to form the capsule. It extends into the gland and divides the glandular tissue into follicles
  - The smooth muscle fibers arranged as two sheets. Inner sheet around the prostatic urethra and outer sheet deep to capsule. These two layers are connected by the radiating fibers.
- **Glandular tissue:**
  - Arranged in 3 concentric layers
    1. Inner **mucous glands**: Simple tubular, open in prostatic sinus above the colliculus
    2. Middle **submucous glands:** Less follicles and small ducts open in the sinus at the level of the colliculus
    3. Outer **main glands:** Numerous follicles and longer ducts open in the sinus below the colliculus.
  - The follicles are lined by simple columnar epithelium and infoldings are seen after puberty
  - In old age, the folding disappear and are filled with starch like material called **corpora amylacea**
  - The number of ducts are 12 – 20

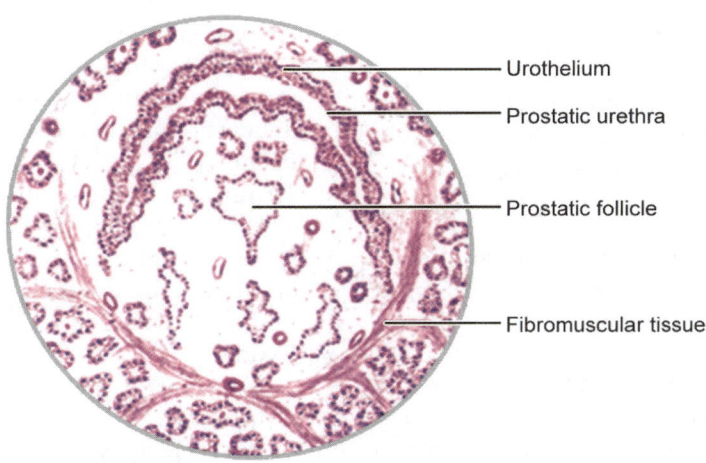

Fig. 11: Histology of prostate gland.

- A fibrous capsule intervenes between main glands and submucous glands. It separates the prostate into an outer and an inner zone
- **Carcinoma** usually affects the outer zone
- **Benign enlargement** of prostate affects the inner zone. The fibrous capsule acts as a surgical capsule and enucleation of hypertrophied mass is done.

Age Changes

- **At birth**
  - A large part of the prostate is formed by the ducts
  - Follicles are small seen as small buds on the ducts.
- **At puberty**
  - Between the ages of approximately 14 and 18 years, the prostate gland enlarges twice its size
  - The growth is in glandular tissue and branching of the ducts
  - The mucous cells are lost
  - The glandular secretory cells secrete acid phosphatase, prostate specific antigen.
- **After 40 years:**
  - The glandular epithelium grows more and form infoldings into the lumen of the follicles
  - Follicular lumen becomes irregular
  - After 45 years the infoldings disappear and **corpora amylacea** increase in number
  - The prostate is either enlarged called the benign hypertrophy or reduced in size called the senile atrophy.

Applied Anatomy

- **Senile enlargement of prostate:** After 50 years of age, the prostate is often enlarged due to benign hypertrophy or due to the formation of an adenoma. This causes retention of urine due to distortion of the urethra
- Digital examination of the rectum is very helpful in the diagnosis of an enlarged prostate
- Prostatectomy: Removal of prostate (transurethral resection of prostate)
- Inflammation of prostate is referred to as prostatitis
- Prostatic carcinoma: The malignant prostate feels hard and irregular
- Cancer cells metastasize by venous route (through internal vertebral venous plexus to vertebral vein), or through lymphatic route to distant nodes.

5. Describe the cavernous sinus under the following headings: Situation, extent, boundaries, relations, contents, connections and applied anatomy.

- The dural venous sinuses are veins draining the brain, meninges, and skull bones
- Situated between the endosteal and meningeal layers of dura mater
- CSF is drained into the venous system through arachnoid villi and granulations which open into the sinuses
- **Features:**
  - Lined by endothelium
  - No valves
  - No muscular tissue in their walls
  - Connected to extracranial veins by emissary veins
  - Not seen as a tube like veins and so no lumen
  - The cerebrospinal fluid drains into these sinuses.
- **Cavernous Sinus:** It is called as cavernous meaning spongy appearance because delicate strands of tissue seen traversing inside
- **Situation:** In the middle cranial fossa along the lateral side of the body of the sphenoid bone.
- **Shape and measurement:** It is cuboidal in shape measuring $2 \times 1 \times 1$ cm.
- **Extent**
  - **Anteriorly:** Medial end of superior orbital fissure
  - **Posteriorly:** Apex of petrous part of temporal bone.

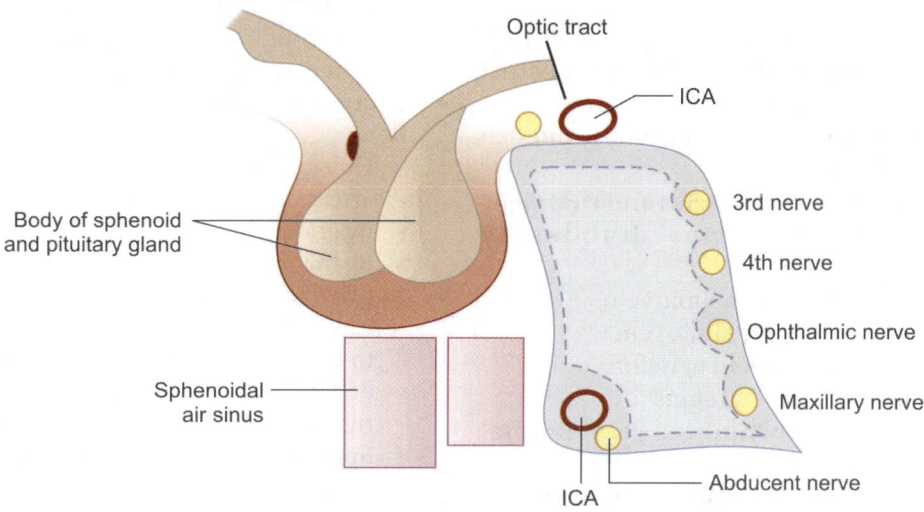

Fig. 12: Cavernous sinus.

- **Boundaries:** It has a roof, floor, medial and lateral walls, anterior and posterior ends.
- **Relations**
  - **Roof**
    - Formed by meningeal layer
    - It is related to the optic tract
    - It is pierced behind by oculomotor nerve and in front internal carotid artery
  - **Medial wall (Fig. 12)**
    - Body of the sphenoid
    - Pituitary fossa with pituitary gland
    - Sphenoidal air sinus
  - **Lateral wall (Fig. 13)**
    - Uncus of the temporal lobe
    - Four nerves are embedded in the lateral wall from above downwards are:
      i. Oculomotor nerve—pierces the roof and runs forward and divides into two divisions
      ii. Trochlear nerve—runs forwards and laterally
      iii. Ophthalmic nerve—runs forwards and divides into 3 branches

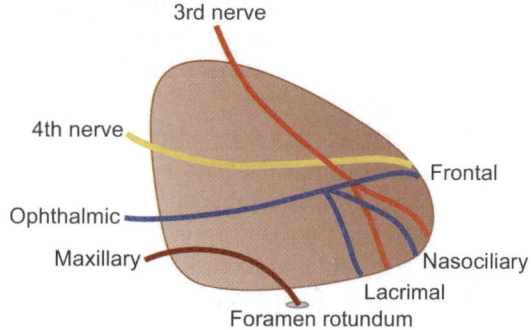

Fig. 13: Lateral wall.

namely frontal, lacrimal and nasociliary nerves.
      iv. Maxillary nerve—leaves the lateral wall to pass through foramen rotundum.
  - **Floor**
    - Formed by endosteal layer
    - Related to foramen lacerum
    - Junction of body and greater wing of sphenoid bone.
  - **Anterior end:** Superior orbital fissure and structures passing through it
  - **Posterior end:** Apex of petrous temporal bone, cavum trigeminale with trigeminal ganglion.

- **Content**
  - Internal carotid artery
  - Sympathetic plexus around it (internal carotid nerve)
  - Abducent nerve inferolateral to internal carotid artery.
- **Connections: Tributaries and Drainage**
  - **Tributaries (veins draining to cavernous sinus)**
    - Superior ophthalmic vein
    - Inferior ophthalmic vein
    - The central vein of retina
    - Sphenoparietal sinus
    - Middle meningeal vein (frontal tributary)
    - Superficial middle cerebral vein
    - Inferior cerebral vein.
  - **Drainage (veins carrying blood from cavernous sinus) (Fig. 14)**
    - With pterygoid venous plexus through emissary veins passing via foramen ovale, lacerum and vesalius
    - With transverse sinus through superior petrosal sinus
    - With internal jugular vein through inferior petrosal sinus
    - With facial vein indirectly through pterygoid plexus and directly through superior ophthalmic vein
    - With opposite cavernous sinus through anterior and posterior intercavernous sinuses.
- **Factors helping propulsion of blood flow:**
  - Due to pulsation of the internal carotid artery
  - By gravity
  - By the position of the head.
- **Applied anatomy**
  - Cavernous sinus thrombosis: Due to its connections to the danger area of face, any infection from here will reach cavernous sinus either through ophthalmic veins or through emissary veins resulting in thrombosis. Exophthalmos, papilledema, opthalmoplegia occur due to the involvement of cranial nerves related to the sinus
  - When there is injury to the internal carotid artery in the cavernous sinus arteriovenous anastomosis is established producing pulsating exophthalmos.

6. **Describe the right lung under the following headings: Surfaces, borders, impressions, fissures, lobes, hilum and bronchopulmonary segments.**

Surfaces, borders, impressions, fissures, lobes, hilum and bronchopulmonary segments.
Refer Essay Q. No. 3 – 2004.

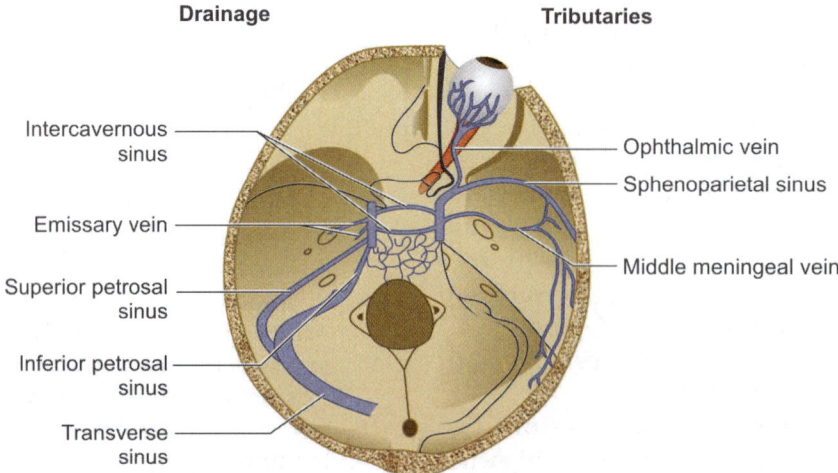

Fig. 14: Connections of cavernous sinus.

- Azygos lobe of the lung:
  - Azygos lobe is occasionally seen in the right lung
  - It is also called as **lobe of Wrisberg**
  - It is a supernumerary lobe of the right lung
  - It is present in 1% of people
  - Sometimes a fissure of variable depth containing the terminal part of the azygos vein separates the **medial part of the upper lobe of right lung**
  - From the mediastinal pleura a fold extends enclosing the vein along the free margin called **meso azygos**
  - The portion of lung medial to meso azygos is called the **'lobe of the azygos vein'**
  - The lobe varies in size, and sometimes includes the apex of the lung
  - The bronchus for the lobe is derived from apical bronchus of upper lobe
  - Radiographically, a pleural effusion may be restricted to the azygos fissure
  - **Development:** Due to descent of the heart before the azygos vein lie medial to the lung, thus bringing the vein close to the apex of right lung.

7. **Describe the muscles of mastication under the following headings: (a) Origin, (b) Insertion, (c) Relations, (d) Nerve supply and (e) Action.**

- The muscles of mastication produce movement of the mandible at temporomandibular joint
- They are developed from 1st pharyngeal arch
- Supplied by mandibular nerve
- The muscles included are—masseter, temporalis, lateral pterygoid, medial pterygoid muscles.

	Name of muscle	Origin	Insertion	Nerve supply	Action
1	Masseter	Superficial layer: Anterior ⅔ of lower border of zygomatic arch Middle layer: Posterior ⅓ of lower border of zygomatic arch and anterior ⅔ of inner surface of zygomatic arch Deep layer: Inner surface of zygomatic arch	Lateral surface of ramus of mandible	Masseteric branch of anterior division of mandibular nerve.	Elevates the mandible Deep fibres retract the mandible

Contd...

Contd...

	Name of muscle	Origin	Insertion	Nerve supply	Action	
2	Temporalis	Temporal fossa and temporal fascia covering the muscle.	Coronoid process	Deep temporal branches of anterior division of mandibular nerve	Elevates the mandible Posterior fibers retract the mandible	
3	Lateral pterygoid	**Upper head**—infratemporal crest and infratemporal surface of greater wing of sphenoid bone **Lower head**—lateral surface of lateral pterygoid plate	Pterygoid fovea in the anterior surface of neck of mandible. Articular capsule and disc of TM joint	Pterygoid branches of anterior division of mandibular nerve	Depression of mandible Both pterygoids help in side to side chewing movement. Lower head helps in protrusion of mandible	
4.	Medial pterygoid	Superficial head - Tuberosity of maxilla. Deep head—medial surface of lateral pterygoid plate	Medial surface of ramus and angle of mandible below mandibular foramen	Nerve to medial pterygoid branch from trunk of mandibular nerve	Elevates the mandible Both pterygoids help in side to side chewing movement Helps in protrusion of mandible	

- **Relations:**
  - **Masseter:**
    - Superficial—skin, zygomaticus major, parotid gland and duct, facial nerve branches, risorius, transverse facial artery
    - Deep—tendon of temporalis, ramus of mandible, masseteric nerve and vessels
    - Anteroinferior border—facial artery.
  - **Temporalis:**
    - Superficial—masseter, zygomatic arch, temporal fascia, superficial temporal vessels, temporal branch of facial nerve, auriculotemporal nerve
    - Deep—temporal fossa, deep temporal nerve.
  - **Lateral pterygoid muscle:**
    - Superficial—temporalis, 2nd part of maxillary artery, superficial part of medial pterygoid, ramus of mandible
    - Deep—middle meningeal artery Mandibular nerve and its branches, otic ganglion, chorda tympani, sphenomandibular ligament, deep head of medial pterygoid muscle
    - Upper border—masseteric nerve, deep temporal nerve
    - Lower border—lingual and inferior alveolar nerves

- Between two heads—buccal branch of Mandibular nerve emerges and maxillary artery dips in.
- **Medial pterygoid:**
  - Medial surface—tensor palati and superior constrictor
  - Lateral surface—ramus of mandible, sphenomandibular ligament, maxillary artery, inferior alveolar nerve and vessels.

8. **Describe the blood supply and venous drainage of the heart.**

Refer Essay Q. No. 5 – 2005.

II. SHORT NOTES

1. Lower end of humerus.

- The lower end of humerus is a modified condyle
- The distal end of the humerus has articular and non-articular parts.
- The **articular part** includes the following:
  - **Capitulum:** It is a lateral rounded convex projection. It is present in anterior and inferior surfaces and articulates with upper surface of the head of the radius
  - **Trochlea:** It is a medial pulley-shaped surface. It covers anterior, inferior and posterior surfaces. It articulates with the trochlear notch of the ulna
  - The medial edge of the trochlea is projecting about 6 mm more than the rest of the bone. This is responsible for formation of the **carrying angle**.
- The **nonarticular part** includes the following:
  - **Medial epicondyle:**
    - It is a prominent projection on the medial side of the lower end of humerus
    - It is very superficial and can easily be palpated on the medial side of the elbow
    - The ulnar nerve lies behind the medial epicondyle
    - The anterior surface gives attachment of common origin of superficial flexors of forearm.
  - **Lateral epicondyle:**
    - It is smaller and less prominent than the medial epicondyle
    - Rough muscular impression in the anterolateral surface is for attachment of superficial group of extensors of forearm
    - On the posterior surface anconeus takes origin.

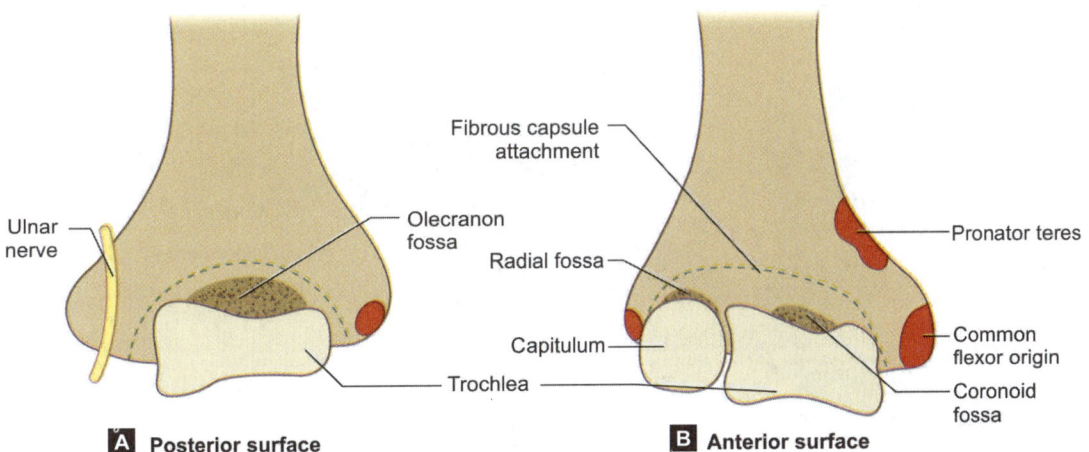

Figs. 15A and B: Lower end of humerus.

- **Coronoid fossa:**
  - It is a small hollow on the anterior aspect above the trochlea
  - The coronoid process of the ulna comes in contact when the elbow is flexed.
- **Radial fossa:**
  - It is a depression seen on the anterior aspect above the capitulum
  - It accommodates the head of the radius in full flexion of elbow.
- **Olecranon fossa:**
  - It is present on the posterior aspect above the trochlea
  - The olecranon process of the ulna is accommodated in the fossa during extension of elbow.
- **Applied anatomy**
  - Supracondylar fracture—is common in children, when they fall on the outstretched hands with elbow slightly flexed. The median nerve and brachial artery can be injured
  - The medial epicondyle has a separate ossification center, which is often mistaken for fracture
  - The ulnar nerve curves behind the medial epicondyle, which may be injured in the fracture lower end of humerus.

2. Trisomy 21.

Refer Short Notes 22 – 2005.

3. Cutaneous innervations of hand.

- **Palmar surface:**
  - **Median nerve:**
    - *The palmar cutaneous branch*
      * The branch is given off in the forearm about 3 cm proximal to the flexor retinaculum, passes superficial to the retinaculum
      * The branches supply the thenar skin, and the central palmar skin.
    - *Palmar digital branches*
      * The median nerve passes deep to the flexor retinaculum and terminates by dividing into four or five digital branches
      * Lateral branch: Two digital branches to lateral and medial sides of thumb, a branch to lateral side of index finger
      * Medial branch: Two to adjacent sides of index, middle and ring fingers.
  - **Ulnar nerve:**
    - *The palmar cutaneous branch:* Passes superficial to flexor retinaculum and supplies the skin of the medial aspect of the palm
    - *Palmar digital branches:*
      * Two **palmar digital nerves** are from superficial terminal branch of ulnar nerve

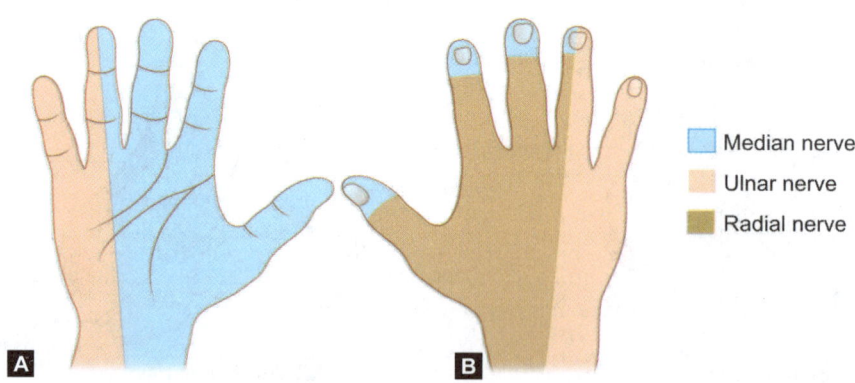

Figs. 16A and B: Cutaneous innervation of hand: (A) Palmar surface; (B) Dorsal surface.

* Medial branch supplies the medial side of the little finger
* Lateral branch is a common palmar digital nerve. It divides into two proper digital nerves to supply the interdigital cleft between the little and the ring fingers.

- **Dorsum of hand**
  - **Radial nerve**
    - The dorsum of the hand is supplied by the superficial terminal branch of the radial nerve
    - Dorsal digital nerves: There are usually four or five small dorsal digital nerves
    - The first supplies lateral side of thumb
    - Second supplies medial side of thumb
    - Third to the lateral side of index finger
    - The fourth and fifth branches divides into two and supply adjacent sides of index, middle and ring fingers
    - The digital branches reach in the thumb up to root of nail. In the index middle of middle phalanx, and the middle and ring fingers up to proximal interphalangeal joint.
  - **Median nerve**: Distal to base of proximal phalanges of the lateral three and a half digits, the skin and nail bed are supplied by the dorsal branches from palmar digital nerves of the median nerve.
  - **Ulnar nerve**
    - Arises 5 cm above the wrist
    - Passes dorsally deep to flexor carpi ulnaris
    - The dorsal branch of ulnar nerve divides into two dorsal digital branches
    - The medial side of little finger is supplied by a medial branch
    - The interdigital cleft between the little and ring fingers is supplied by the lateral branch
    - In the little finger the dorsal branch supplies up to base of distal phalanx and ring finger up to base of middle phalanx
  - The nail beds of the medial on and half fingers by the palmar digital branch of ulnar nerve.

4. **Abductors of hip joint and their role in gait.**

- The abductors of hip joint are:
  - **Chief muscles**: Gluteus medius, Gluteus minimus
  - **Accessory muscles**: Tensor fascia lata and sartorius
  - Abduction is **limited** by: (i) Pubofemoral ligament, (ii) Tension of adductors and (iii) Iliofemoral ligament
  - **Axis**: Movement of abduction takes place around anteroposterior axis which passes through the head of femur.
- **Stages in gait**
  - When the foot of opposite side is raised from the ground in walking or running, the gluteus medius and minimus, acts from below (femur), and helps to maintain upright position of the trunk
  - The body weight pulls the pelvis downwards on the opposite side
  - It is prevented by the muscles on the supporting side
  - The pelvis is raised on the unsupported side from dropping by the powerful action of the muscles
  - The downward tilt of pelvis on the unsupported side due to the gravity is minimized
  - The pelvis tilts alternately from side to side during walking
  - This **action depends** on the following conditions: (i) the nerve supply of both muscles must be normal (ii) the neck of the femur should be intact (iii) the hip joint should be normal (iv) neck shaft angle of femur should be normal
  - **Trendelenburg's sign**: In paralysis of glutei muscles, congenital dislocation of hip or coxa vera the supporting mechanism is affected and the pelvis sinks down on the unopposed side
  - Paralysis of gluteus medius or minimus results in lurching gait.

5. Saphenous vein

Refer Short Notes 14 – 2005.

6. Ligaments of liver.

- The ligaments of the liver attaches—liver to the diaphragm, anterior abdominal wall and other viscera which are produced by the peritoneal reflections
- **Falciform ligament**
  - Is a sickle-shaped fold of peritoneum which connects the liver to the anterior abdominal wall
  - The liver is anatomically divided into right and left lobes by the falciform ligament
  - The two layers extend from posterior surface of the anterior abdominal wall and diaphragm to the anterior and superior surface of the liver
  - Ligamentum teres, run along the lower free border of the falciform ligament. It is formed by the obliterated left umbilical vein
  - Above it is continuous with superior layer of coronary ligament on the right side, and left triangular ligament on the left side.
- **Coronary ligament**
  - The peritoneum extends from diaphragm to the posterior surface of the right lobe of liver
  - It is seen as two layers—superior and inferior layers
  - The two layers form boundary for the bare area of the liver
  - On the right side the two layers are continuous with right triangular ligament
  - On the left side two layers unite immediately to form left triangular ligament.
- **Triangular ligaments**
  - **Right triangular ligament** contributes for the apex of the bare area of liver
  - The coronary ligaments are continued as triangular ligament
  - **Left triangular ligament** is a short triangular fold, connects left lobe of liver to diaphragm
  - It is anterior to abdominal part of esophagus, upper end of lesser omentum, and fundus of stomach
  - It is continuous with the falciform ligament and lesser omentum
  - It is important factor for stability of the left lobe of liver.
- **Lesser omentum**
  - It connects lesser curvature of stomach and proximal part of duodenum to liver
  - It is attached to the fissure for ligamentum venosum and porta hepatis in the inferior surface of liver, along L shaped line
  - The vertical limb is attached to fissure for ligamentum venosum and contains the obliterated ductus venosus
  - The horizontal limb to the porta hepatis
- **Ligamentum venosum**: It is obliterated ductus venosus which persists in fetal life

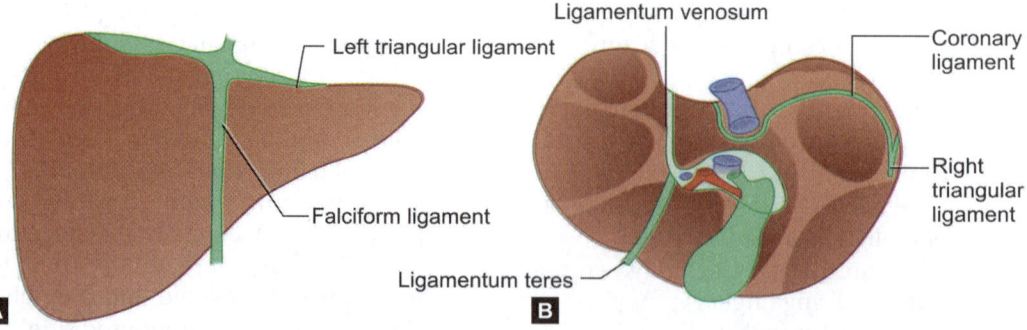

Figs. 17A and B: Ligaments of liver.

connecting left branch of portal vein with left hepatic vein.
- **Applied anatomy:**
  - Left lobe of liver becomes unstable by division of left triangular ligament
  - To expose inferior vena cava, the right lobe of liver is allowed to be pulled forwards after surgical division of coronary ligaments
  - To control extrahepatically the left hepatic vein, ligamentum venosum is used as a guide by the surgeons.

7. Structure of kidney.

Refer Short Notes 3 – 2007

8. Inguinal ligament.

- It is also known as **Poupart's ligament**.
- **Formation:** The lower border of aponeurosis of external oblique muscle is thick and curved inwards to form the ligament
- **Extent:** Extends from the anterior superior iliac spine to the pubic tubercle
- **Length:** 12 – 14 cm.
- **Direction:**
  - The lateral part is oblique, directed downwards and medially
  - The medial part is horizontal
  - It is inclined at 40 degrees to the horizontal plane.
- **Surfaces:**
  - **Superior surface** is grooved and forms the 'floor' of the inguinal canal and supports its contents
  - **Lower surface** is continuous with the fascia lata.
- **Extensions:**
  - **Lacunar ligament:** At the medial end, some fibres extend backwards and upwards to attach to the pectineal line. It is also known as **Gimbernat's ligament**. it is about 2 cm from apex to its base
  - **Reflected part of the inguinal ligament:** Few fibers pass superomedially from pubic tubercle deep to the superficial inguinal ring to join the linea alba. It is also called as **Colle's ligament**
  - **Pectineal ligament of Cooper:** From the base of lacunar ligament, a fibrous band extends laterally up to pubic eminence.
- **Structures attached to inguinal ligament:**
  - Origin of internal oblique from lateral two-third of grooved surface
  - Transversus abdominis from lateral one-third
  - Cremaster muscle from middle of ligament
  - Fascia lata lower surface.

9. Rectus sheath.

Refer Short Notes 6 – 2003.

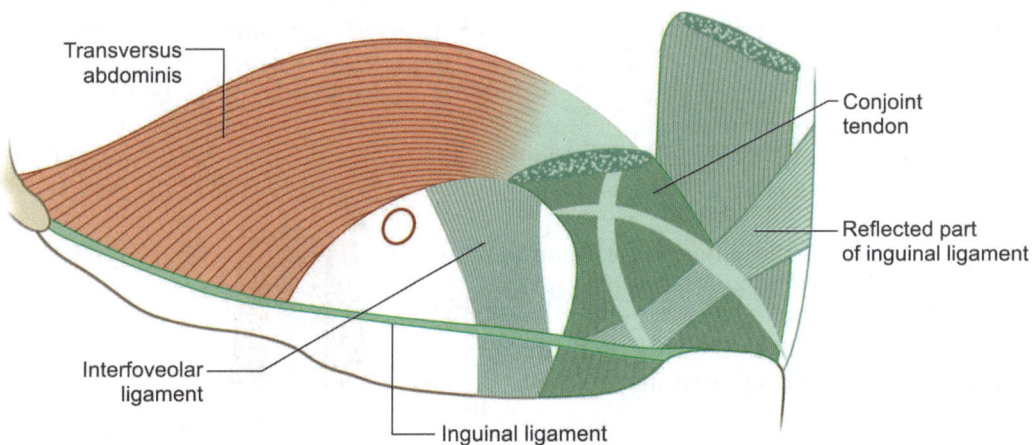

Fig. 18: Inguinal ligament.

10. Celiac ganglion.

- It is an autonomic ganglion situated in the abdominal cavity
- It is seen as an irregular mass
- **Situations:**
  - The coeliac ganglia are situated on either side overlapping the edges of abdominal aorta
  - The suprarenal glands are adjacent to it
  - Crura of the diaphragm are lateral to ganglion.
- **Relations:**
  - The right ganglion is behind the inferior vena cava
  - The left ganglion is behind the origin of the splenic artery.
- **Communication:**
  - The greater splanchnic nerve enter the upper part of ganglion
  - An offshoot from lower part of the ganglion is termed as aorticorenal ganglion
  - The ipsilateral lesser splanchnic nerve terminate with it
  - The renal plexus is formed from ganglion.

11. Lesser sac.

Refer Short Notes 10 – 2005.

12. Ischiorectal fossa.

Refer Short Notes 8 – 2003.

13. Mesentery.

- It is a fold of peritoneum suspending the jejunum and ileum
- It is made of two layers namely antero-superior and posteroinferior
- The mesentery extends from the posterior abdominal wall which is a broad, and fan-shaped
- The breadth of the mesentery is maximum in the central part (broadest at mid ileum) and is about 20 cm
- Gradually diminishes towards both the ends. It is shortest at jejunum and terminal part of ileum.
- **Border:**
  - The **attached border** or **root of the mesentery** is 15 cm long
  - Is directed obliquely downwards and to the right
  - The superior mesenteric artery runs along the root of mesentery
  - It **extends** from the duodenojejunal flexure on the left side of vertebra L_2 to the upper part of right sacroiliac joint.
  - Structures **crossed (Fig. 19)**
    - 3rd part of the duodenum
    - Abdominal aorta
    - Inferior vena cava
    - Right ureter
    - Right psoas major
    - Right gonadal vessels.
  - The **free or intestinal border** is 6 meters long; it is attached to the gut.
- **Contents:**
  - Jejunal and ileal branches of the superior mesenteric artery
  - Accompanying veins
  - Autonomic nerve plexuses
  - Lymphatics or lacteals
  - 100 – 200 lymph nodes
  - Loose areolar tissue
  - Fat—present close to root of jejunal mesentery, and in ileum throughout the mesentery
  - Occasional contents—suspensory muscle of duodenum (Trietz), accessory suprarenal tissue.
- **Development:** Remnant of dorsal mesentery
- **Function:** Mobility of intestine
- **Applied anatomy:** Mesenteric cyst a cystic swelling arising from the mesenteric lymph nodes. It presents clinically as a

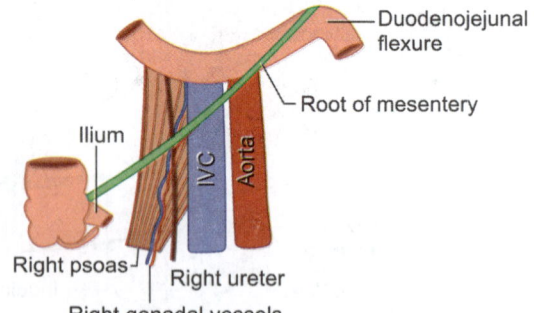

Fig. 19: Structures crossed by root of mesentery.

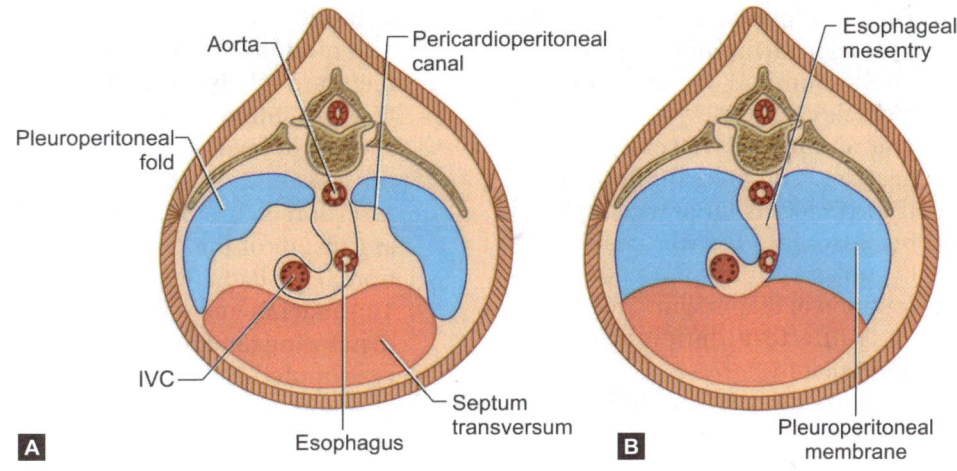

Figs. 20A and B: Development of diaphragm.

small painless, fluctuant, mobile swelling near the umbilicus.

14. Development of diaphragm.

- The diaphragm is developed from four sources:
  i. Septum transversum
  ii. A pair of pleuroperitoneal membranes
  iii. The mesentery of the esophagus
  iv. Body wall
- **Septum transversum (Fig. 20A):**
  - It is a thick mesodermal tissue situated between yolk sac and thoracic cavity
  - During fourth week it is situated opposite to cervical somites
  - It receives the nerve supply from C3 to C5 cervical segments
  - By sixth week it descends to the level of thoracic somites
  - The dorsal part of the embryo grows more than the ventral part and the septum descends down to the normal position
  - The septum transversum forms the central tendon of diaphragm.
- **Pleuroperitoneal membranes (Fig. 20B):**
  - Crescent shaped folds extend from caudal part of pericardioperitoneal canals of either side, called pleuroperitoneal membrane
  - By 7th week it unites with septum transversum and mesentery of esophagus
  - The connection between pleural and peritoneal cavities (pericardioperitoneal canal) are closed.
- **Mesentery of esophagus:**
  - By third month the dorsal bands appear at the level of L1
  - The crura of the diaphragm is developed from the mesentery.
- **Body wall (Fig. 21):**
  - Peripheral part is developed from mesenchyme of thoracic wall
  - Hence the lower intercostal nerves supply the periphery of diaphragm.
- **Congenital anomaly:**
  - Diaphragmatic hernia:
    - Most common malformation occurring in 1 per 2000 newborns

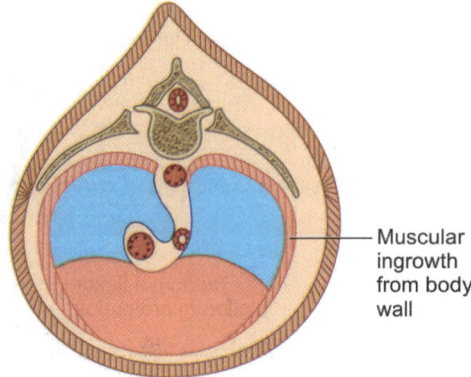

Fig. 21: Development of peripheral part.

- The pleuroperitoneal membrane fail to develop on one or both sides
- The abdominal viscera enter the thoracic cavity
- The abdominal viscera push the heart and compress the lung
- If the defect is large usually it will be associated with pulmonary hypoplasia.
– Eventration of diaphragm:
  - It is due to a deficiency of the musculature
  - Usually in the left half of the diaphragm
  - If the deficiency is present, the diaphragm shows paradoxical movement during respiration.

15. Lumbrical muscles of the hand.

- There are four lumbricals and are numbered from lateral to medial side
- 1st and 2nd are unipennate, 3rd and 4th are bipennate muscles.
- **Origin:**
  – Lumbricals 1 and 2: From the tendons of flexor digitorum profundus for index and middle fingers along its lateral side
  – Lumbricals 3 and 4: From adjacent sides of tendons of flexor digitorum profundus for middle, ring and little fingers.
- **Insertion:**
  – The tendons cross the radial side of metacarpophalangeal joints
  – Inserted into the lateral side of dorsal surface of bases of middle and distal phalanges
  – Insertion is through the dorsal digital expansion of the corresponding digit from second to fifth
  – The attachment to dorsal expansion as **distal wing tendon**.
- **Nerve supply:**
  – First and second lumbricals by median nerve
  – Third and fourth lumbricals by deep branch of ulnar nerve.
- **Actions:** Lumbricals flex the metacarpophalangeal joints and extend the interphalangeal joints.
- **Applied anatomy:**
  – **Claw hand:** Due to paralysis of lumbricals supplied by the ulnar and median nerve
  – In claw hand there is hyper extension at metacarpophalangeal joints and hyperflexion at interphalangeal joints of all fingers
  – In **ulnar nerve injury** at elbow: Results in ulnar claw hand with marked clawing at the medial two fingers due

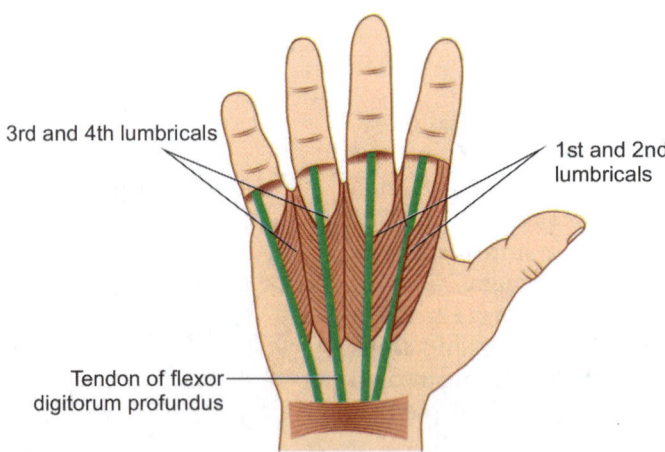

Fig. 22: Lumbrical muscles.

to paralysis of medial two lumbricals and interosseous muscles
- In **median nerve injury** lateral two lumbricals are paralyzed resulting in claw hand with inability to flex lateral two metacarpophalangeal joints.

16. Cubital fossa

- **Situation:** The cubital fossa is in the middle of the upper part of the anterior aspect of the forearm.
- **Boundaries:**
  - **Laterally:** Medial border of the brachioradialis
  - **Medially:** Lateral border of the pronator teres
  - **Base or superior border:** Is an imaginary line, joining the two epicondyles of the humerus
  - **Apex:** It is directed downwards, and is formed by the meeting point of the lateral and medial borders
  - **Roof:** The roof of the fossa is formed by the deep fascia of the forearm, the bicipital aponeurosis. The aponeurosis an expansion from the medial border of tendon of biceps muscle. The median cubital vein lies on the deep fascia, and the medial cutaneous nerve of the forearm crosses the vein
  - **Floor:** Brachialis and supinator.
- **Contents:** From medial to lateral, (**MBBS**)
  - Median nerve
    - Lies medial to brachial artery
    - It leaves the cubital fossa by passing in between the superficial and deep heads of pronator teres
    - The deep head of pronator separates the nerve from the ulnar artery
    - The anterior interosseous nerve is given as it leaves the fossa between the two heads of pronator.
  - **B**rachial artery terminal part
    - The artery ends at the level of neck of radius
    - It terminates by dividing into radial and ulnar arteries
    - The radial recurrent branch arises from radial artery in the fossa
    - The common interosseous artery arises from ulnar artery in the fossa.
  - **B**iceps brachii tendon
    - It is situated lateral to the artery
    - It is inserted to the posterior part of radial tuberosity.
  - **S**uperficial branch of radial nerve.
    - At the level of lateral epicondyle, the radial nerve terminates by dividing into superficial and deep branches
    - The deep branch passes between the two heads of supinator.
  - Beginning of radial and ulnar arteries
  - **Applied anatomy**:
    - The median cubital vein is used for venae puncture, or cardiac catheterization as it overlies the bicipital aponeurosis
    - The brachial artery pulsation can be felt medial to the tendon of biceps.

17. Erb's paralysis.

Refer applied anatomy of Essay Q. No. 3 – 2005.

18. Menstrual cycle.

- The structural changes occurring periodically in the endometrium of uterus is known as menstrual cycle
- The cycle has degenerative, proliferative and growth phases
- The cycle is repeated every 28 days
- It persists for 3 to 4 days

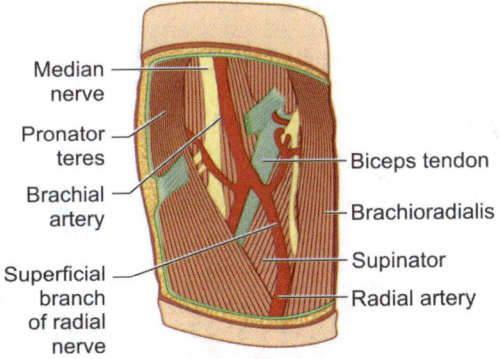

Fig. 23: Cubital fossa.

- The endometrial changes in each cycle is divided into three phases—proliferative, secretory and menstrual phases.
- **Proliferative (follicular) phase**
  - This phase takes about 4 days to repair
  - The epithelium proliferates
  - It grows about 1 to 3 mm in thickness
  - The epithelium of endometrium and glands become columnar
  - The glands enlarge, increase in length and become straight
  - The cells of endometrium are arranged as three layers—stratum compactum, stratum spongiosum, stratum basale
  - The changes are due to the estrogen derived from maturing ovarian follicles
  - Ovulation occurs at the end of this phase.
- **Secretory (Progestational) phase**
  - In the secretory phase there is growth of endometrium to about 5 to 7mm in thickness
  - The increase in thickness is due to:
    - Increase in tissue fluid
    - Glands enlarge and become dilated and tortuous
    - Increase in size of stromal cells.
  - The stratum is converted to decidua called decidual reaction
  - The spiral arteries in the spongy and compactum layers increase and become tortuous
  - The changes are due to the actions of progesterone and estrogen of corpus luteum
  - At the end of this phase there is regression of endometrium due to the reduction of progesterone level.
- **Menstrual phase**
  - This phase lasts for 3 to 5 days
  - The spiral arteries become more coiled and blood flow is reduced due to regression of the endometrium
  - Vasoconstriction of the arteries followed by vasodilatation results in damage to endometrium
  - The bleeding from capillaries with shedding of endometrium in bits occur
  - The blood loss is about 50 to 60 mL.

19. Dorsalis pedis artery

- It is the dorsal artery of the foot
- **Formation:** Distal to the ankle, the anterior tibial artery is continued as dorsalis pedis artery.
- **Course:**
  - It extends up to the proximal end of the first intermetatarsal space
  - It dips in between the heads of the first dorsal interosseous muscle.
- **Termination:** It completes the plantar arterial arch by anastomosing with the lateral plantar artery.
- **Relations:**
  - Posterior—capsule of the talocrural joint, talus, navicular and intermediate cuneiform bones
  - Anterior—the skin, fascia, inferior extensor retinaculum, extensor hallucis brevis
  - Medial—tendon of extensor hallucis longus
  - Lateral—tendon of extensor digitorum longus and medial terminal branch of the deep peroneal nerve.
- **Surface anatomy:** The pulsation of the dorsal artery is felt from the midpoint between the malleoli to the proximal end of the first inter metatarsal space.
- **Branches:**
  - Tarsal arteries:
    - The tarsal arteries are lateral and medial

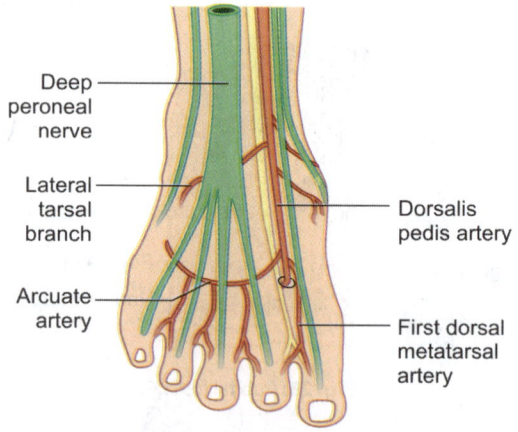

Fig. 24: Dorsalis pedis artery.

- The **lateral** tarsal artery passes laterally under extensor digitorum brevis
- It supplies the muscle and the joints of tarsal bones
- Anastomoses with the branches of the arcuate, lateral malleolar and lateral plantar arteries and the perforating branch of the peroneal artery
- Medial tarsal arteries are two or three in number, join the medial malleolar network.
  - **Arcuate artery:**
    - It runs laterally over the bases of metatarsal bones
    - It anastomoses with lateral tarsal artery
    - It gives rise to second, third and fourth dorsal metatarsal arteries
    - Each artery reach the interdigital cleft and divides into two dorsal digital branches to supply the contiguous sides of 2nd to 5th toes
    - The perforating arteries connect metatarsal branches with plantar arch.
  - **First dorsal metatarsal artery:**
    - It arises from dorsalis pedis artery just before it dips into sole
    - At the cleft between the first and second toes it divides
    - One branch supplies the medial side of the big toe. The other divides to supply the adjoining sides of the great and the second toe.
- **Applied anatomy**
  - Peripheral arterial pulse is usually palpated at dorsalis pedis artery because it is superficial
  - Any thrombosis or insufficiency causes diminished pulse
  - The pulsation is felt from the midpoint between malleoli to the proximal end of first intermetatarsal space.

20. Inguinal canal.

Inguinal canal is an musculoaponeurotic canal
- **Length:** 4 cm long
- It is an oblique canal
- **Situation:** Situated in the groin, present a little above the medial half of the inguinal ligament
- **Extent:** It extends from the deep inguinal ring to the superficial inguinal ring
- It is larger in males and is produced due to descent of testis
- **Boundaries (Fig. 25):** It has an inlet (deep inguinal ring), an outlet (superficial inguinal ring), roof, floor, anterior wall, and posterior wall.
  - Roof—by the arching fibres of internal oblique and transversus abdominis muscle
  - Floor—by the upper grooved surface of inguinal ligament and the lacunar ligament medially
  - Anterior wall—skin, superficial fascia, external oblique aponeurosis and in the lateral ⅓ in addition by fleshy fibers of internal oblique
  - Posterior wall is formed by—fascia transversalis, conjoint tendon, and reflected part of inguinal ligament medially **(Fig. 26)**.
- **Openings of the canal:**
  - *Superficial inguinal ring* **(Fig. 27)**
    - Opening in the external oblique aponeurosis
    - Situation: Superolateral to pubic crest
    - Shape: Is triangular
    - Size: It is smaller in female
    - From the margins of the crura of the ring, the aponeurosis is continued as external spermatic fascia.
    - Boundaries: Base is formed by pubic crest and apex by intercrural fibers, the medial and lateral crura are attached to the pubic symphysis and tubercle respectively

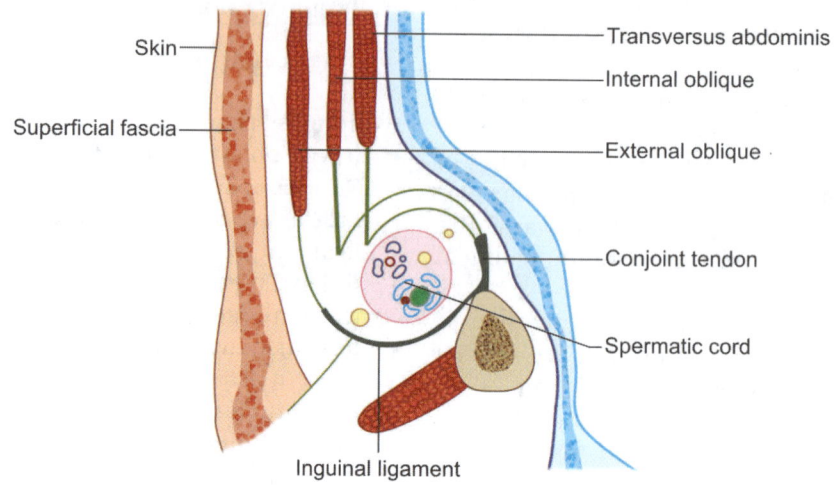

Fig. 25: Boundaries of inguinal canal (sagittal section).

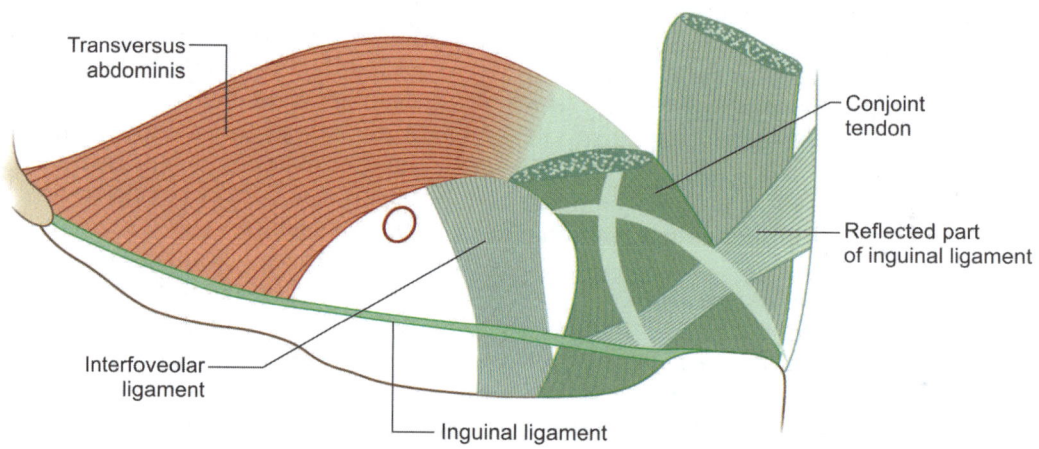

Fig. 26: Posterior wall of inguinal canal.

- Strengthened: By conjoint tendon and reflected part of inguinal ligament
- Structures passing: Spermatic cord in male, round ligament of uterus in female, and ilioinguinal nerve.
- *Deep inguinal ring*
  - It is an opening seen in transversalis fascia
  - Situation: 1.25 cm above mid inguinal point
- Shape: It is oval and vertically placed
- It is large in male
- Related medially to inferior epigastric artery and interfoveolar ligament
- Strengthened: By fleshy fibers of internal oblique muscle
- Structures passing: Spermatic cord in male, round ligament of uterus in female.

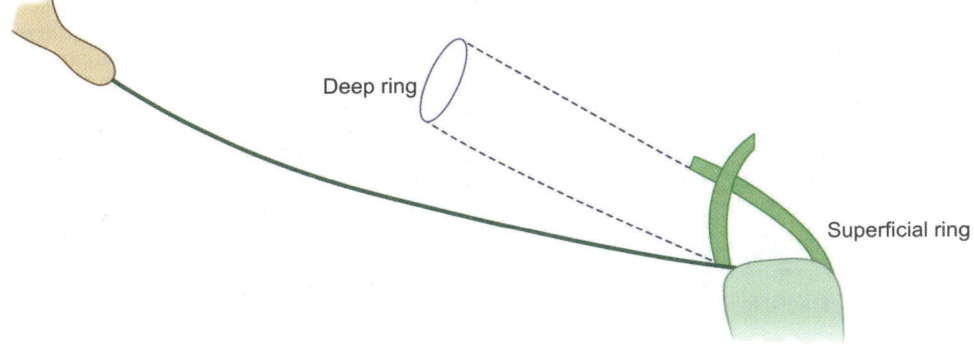

Fig. 27: Openings of inguinal canal.

- The **contents** of the inguinal canal are:
  - **In males:** Spermatic cord, ilioinguinal nerve
  - **In females:**
    - Round ligament of uterus, ilioinguinal nerve
    - The ilioinguinal nerve enters the canal by piercing the posterior wall.
- **Defensive mechanism of inguinal canal:**
  - **Flap valve:** The canal is obliquely placed with the two rings in different planes. So, in increased intra-abdominal pressure, the posterior wall of the canal comes in contact with the anterior wall, obliterating the canal
  - **Ball-valve mechanism:** In increased intra-abdominal pressure, the cremaster muscle contracts and pulls the testis towards the superficial ring, thus closing the outlet like a plug
  - **Demi-sphincters:** The arching fibers of internal oblique and transversus abdominis act as demi sphincters whenever there is increase in intra-abdominal pressure and obliterates the canal by bringing the roof in contact with the floor of the canal.
- **Applied Anatomy:** Inguinal hernia: Abnormal protrusion of abdominal contents with peritoneal sac through the inguinal canal is known as inguinal hernia. Types—(a) oblique hernia and (b) direct hernia
- **Oblique hernia**
  - Are indirect hernias
  - Are mostly congenital
  - Enters the canal through deep inguinal ring
  - It reaches the scrotum if processus vaginalis is patent. Then it is called as **complete oblique inguinal hernia**
  - The hernial sac lies lateral to inferior epigastric artery

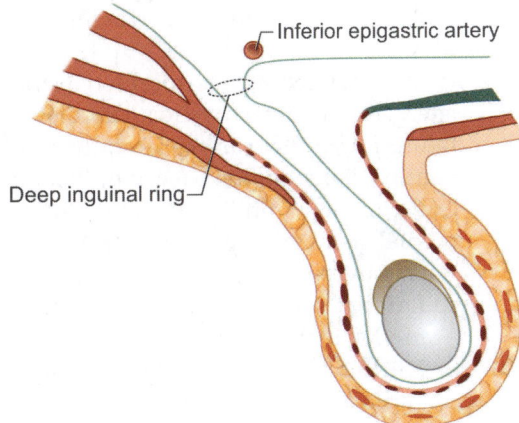

Fig. 28: Coverings of indirect inguinal hernia.

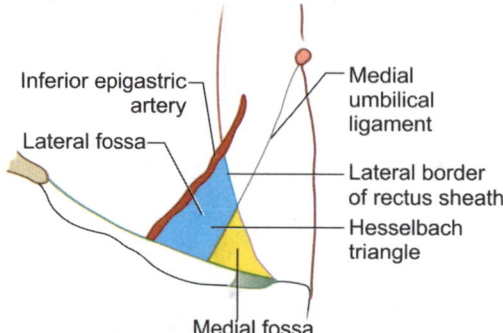

Fig. 29: Hesselbach triangle.

1	Medial type	(i) Peritoneum, (ii) Extraperitoneal tissue, (iii) Fascia transversalis, (iv) Conjoint tendon and reflected part of inguinal ligament, (v) External spermatic fascia, (vi) Dartos and (vii) Skin
2	Lateral type	(i) Peritoneum, (ii) Extraperitoneal tissue, (iii) Fascia transversalis, (iv) Cremaster and fascia, (v) External spermatic fascia, (vi) Dartos and (vii) Skin

- The **coverings of the hernia** are (i) peritoneum, (ii) extraperitoneal tissue, (iii) internal spermatic fascia, (iv) cremaster and fascia, (v) external spermatic fascia, (vi) dartos and (vii) skin.
- **Types of oblique inguinal hernia:**
  - **Vaginal:** Entire processus vaginalis is patent. Hernia reaches bottom of scrotum. Tunica vaginalis forms part of the hernia sac
  - **Funicular:** Proximal part of processus is patent, common type
  - **Infantile:** Peritoneal recess extends from vaginal sac to superficial ring.
- **Direct hernia**
  - Enters the canal through Hesselbach triangle
  - **Hesselbach triangle** is bounded by the lateral border of rectus sheath medially, inferior epigastric artery laterally, and inguinal ligament the base. It is divided by the medial umbilical ligament into a medial and lateral fossa **(Fig. 29)**.
  - It has two types:
    1. **Lateral type**—sac enters through medial inguinal fossa.
    2. **Medial type**—sac enters through supravesical fossa.
  - The hernial sac lies medial to inferior epigastric artery. The **coverings of the hernia** are:

21. Rhomboid Fossa.

- Floor of fourth ventricle is also called as rhomboid fossa as it is diamond/rhomboid in shape
- Formed by dorsal surface of the lower pons and dorsal surface of upper medulla **(Fig. 30)**
- The floor is lined by ependyma.
- Divided into:
  - Upper triangular: Pontine part
  - Lower triangular: Medullary part.
- **Features in the floor (Fig. 31)**
  - **Median sulcus**—divides the floor into two equal halves
  - **Medial eminence**—on either side of median sulcus is the median eminence
    - In the pontine part the facial colliculus produced by abducent nucleus and facial nerve fibers
    - In the medullary part the hypoglossal triangle formed by hypoglossal nucleus.

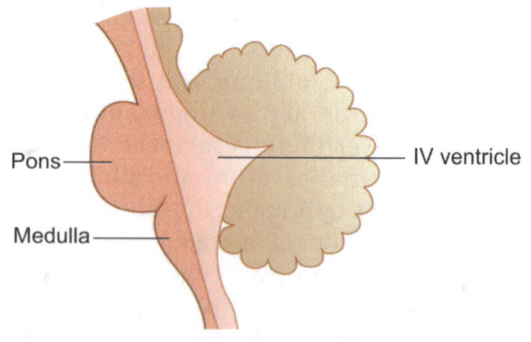

Fig. 30: IV ventricle.

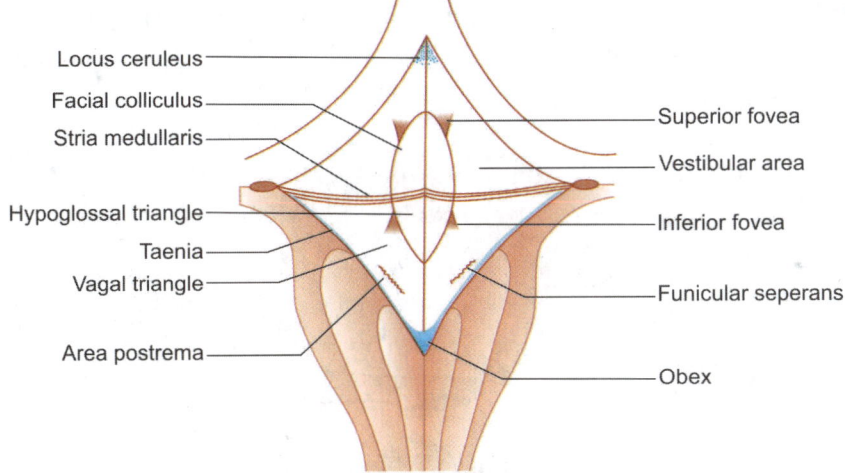

Fig. 31: Rhomboid fossa.

- **Sulcus limitans**—median eminence is limited laterally by sulcus limitans
- The sulcus limitans expands above and below to enclose **superior and inferior fovea**
- A bluish discoloration is seen at the upper part of sulcus limitans known as **locus coeruleus,** produced by **substantia ferruginia**
- Lateral to sulcus limitans is **vestibular area** deep to which the four vestibular nuclei lie
- Below and lateral to hypoglossal triangle is the **vagal triangle** deep to it the dorsal vagal nucleus is situated
- A translucent ridge is seen crossing the lower part of the floor called **funiculus separans**
- **Area postrema** is situated between funiculus separans and gracile tubercle. The blood brain barrier is absent in this area and stimulation of the area results in vomiting
- The ependyma is thickened along the inferolateral wall called **taenia**
- The taenia is united to form **obex** forming the posterior limit
- The **stria medullaris** emerge from the median sulcus and pass laterally to reach the cerebellum through inferior cerebellar peduncle. It divides the floor into a pontine upper part and medullary lower part
- The lower part of the floor resembles a pen nib and hence is called as **calamus scriptorius.**

- **Applied anatomy:**
  - Brain tumor can block the foramen Magendie and Luschka resulting in headache, vomiting, and papilloedema due to increase in intracranial pressure
  - Obstruction of flow of CSF, or overproduction, or problem with its absorption results in accumulation of CSF, in the ventricles resulting in a condition called hydrocephalus.

22. Maxillary air sinus.

Refer Short Notes 25 – 2007.

23. Labelled diagram of superolateral surface of cerebrum, indicating major functional areas.

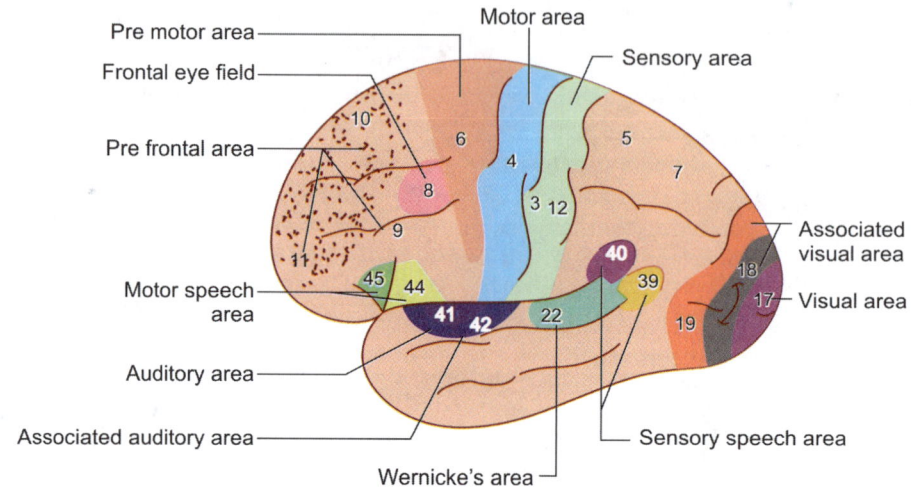

Fig. 32: Functional areas—superolateral surface.

24. Histology of retina.

Retina is made up of ten layers (Fig. 33):
1. **Retinal pigment epithelium**
   - The cells are flat and hexagonal
   - 4 – 6 million number of cells in the human retina
   - Numerous melanosomes are present in the cytoplasm
   - Long microvilli from apex of the cells protrude between, the outer segments of rods and cones.
   - **Functions**
   - They engulf the tips of rods and cones undergoing lysosomal destruction
   - Light reaching the outer retina is absorbed by this layer, and helps to maintain the quality of image

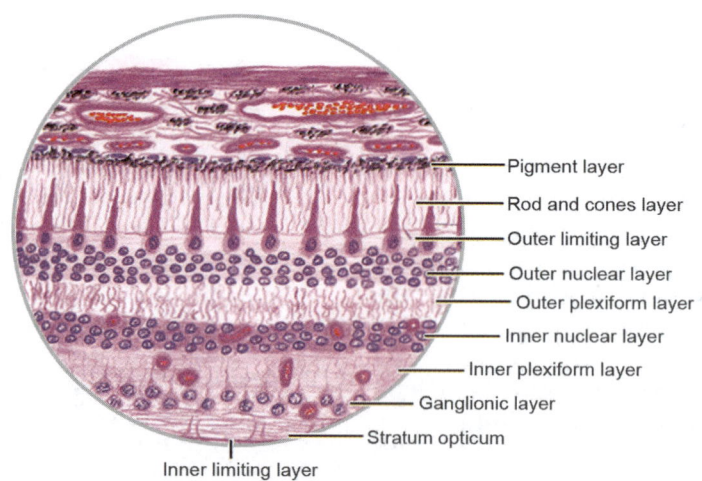

Fig. 33: Histology of retina.

- The pigment epithelium acts as blood-retinal barrier between the retina and the vascular system of the choroid by the tight junctions between the adjacent cells
- This layer helps to repair the bleached visual pigment.

2. **Rods and cones**
   - About 4.6 million cones and 92 million rods are present in the human retina
   - **Outer segments** of rods and cones are cylindrical, filled with membranous discs formed by deep infoldings of the plasma membrane
   - The **inner segment** of both rods and cones has an outer and inner parts. The outer **ellipsoid** contains mitochondria, and an inner **myoid** contains endoplasmic reticulum.
3. **Outer limiting layer:** This layer is formed by microvilli of Muller cells project into the space between the rod and cone inner segments.
4. **Outer nuclear layer:** The nuclei of the rods and cones form the outer nuclear layer
5. **Outer plexiform layer:** Cone pedicle or rod spherule, synapse with adjacent bipolar and horizontal cells and with other cone or rod cells
6. **Inner nuclear layer:** The soma of horizontal cells and bipolar cells are located
7. **Inner plexiform layer:** Axons of horizontal and bipolar cells synapse with dendrites of ganglion cells or amacrine cells
8. **Ganglion cell layer:** 0.7 – 1.5 million ganglion cells are present in the human retina. Soma of the ganglion cells, form the ganglion cell layer of the retina
9. **Stratum opticum:** Ganglion cell axons, are continued as the optic nerve
10. **Internal limiting membrane:** This layer is formed by the processes of Muller cell which spreads into a terminal foot plate and connects with neighboring glial cells.

25. Coronary sinus.
Refer Essay 5 – 2005.

26. Ansa cervicalis.
- It is a nerve loop and a content of the carotid triangle
- **Location**: It is embedded on the anterior surface of the carotid sheath
- **Formation**: By union of:
  - Descendens cervicalis (inferior root of ansa) - $C_2 C_3$ fibers
  - It is formed by ventral rami of $C_2 C_3$ fibers. It is first lateral to internal jugular vein and then winds around the vein a little below the middle of neck
  - Descendens hypoglossi (superior root of ansa) – C_1
  - Formed by C_1 fibers passing through hypoglossal nerve. It is given off when the hypoglossal nerve curves around the occipital artery. Both the roots join anterior to carotid sheath.
- **Branches to** strap muscles of the neck namely:
  - Sternohyoid
  - Sternothyroid
  - Inferior belly of omohyoid
  - Branch to join the cardiac and phrenic nerves
  - Before the inferior root joins the loop, supplies the superior belly of omohyoid muscle.

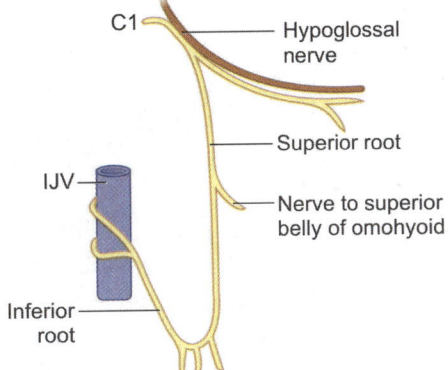

Fig. 34: Ansa cervicalis.

- **Applied anatomy**: The larynx may deviate towards the normal side in swallowing, due to unilateral paralysis of the infra hyoid muscles which depresses the larynx.

27. Blood supply of spinal cord.

Arterial Supply

- Spinal cord is supplied by:
  - Branches of vertebral arteries—anterior and posterior spinal arteries
  - Segmental arteries
  - Radicular arteries.
- **Spinal arteries**: Two spinal arteries branch from fourth part of vertebral artery.
  - **The anterior spinal artery** unites with the opposite artery to form a single anterior spinal artery, related to anteromedian fissure
  - **Two posterior spinal arteries**, each in turn divides into two branches and runs medial and lateral sides of dorsal nerve roots
  - The anterior spinal artery supplies anterior ⅔ of the spinal cord and posterior ⅓ by the posterior spinal arteries
  - The three arteries communicate around the spinal cord forming pial plexus called the **vasa corona**
  - The arteries descend and are reinforced at intervals by the anterior and posterior radicular arteries forming longitudinal chain throughout the length of the spinal cord.
- **Segmental arteries**:
  - Spinal arteries can supply up to cervical segment of spinal cord
  - Therefore, the segmental branches are received from vertebral, deep cervical, posterior intercostal, lumbar arteries
  - They join the anterior and posterior spinal arteries at various intervals
  - These branches enter through the corresponding intervertebral foramen.
- **Radicular arteries**:
  - The radicular arteries provide blood supply to the thoracic, lumbar, sacral, and coccygeal segments of the spinal cord
  - There are anterior and posterior radicular arteries
  - The anterior are long and less in number, whereas posterior are many and small
  - The **anterior radicular arteries** divide into a short ascending and a long descending branch and anastomose with each other and anterior spinal

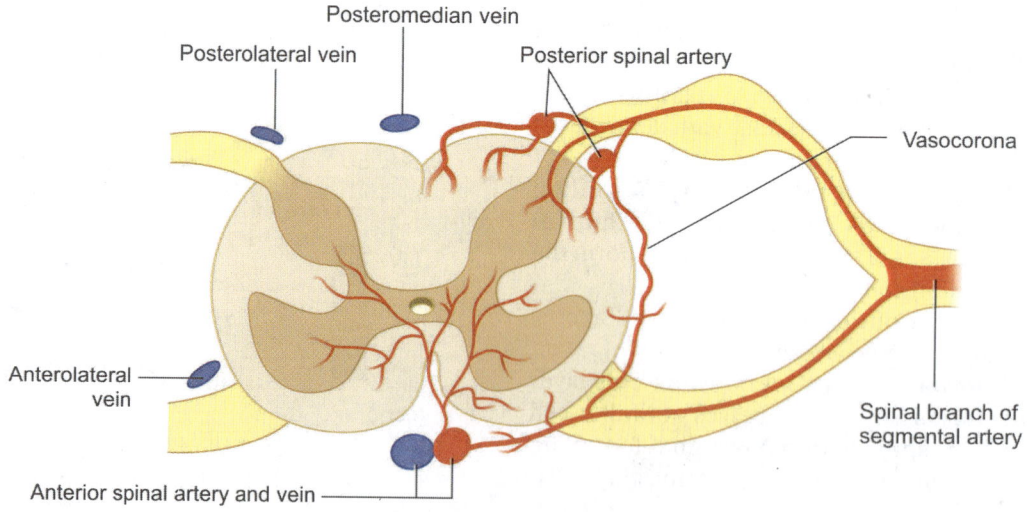

Fig. 35: Blood supply of spinal cord.

artery forming anterior longitudinal trunk
- There are about eight anterior radicular arteries and are present in cervical, thoracic and lumbar regions
- Largest radicular artery called **arteria radicularis magna/Adamkiewicz artery** arises from lower thoracic or upper lumbar level. It provides blood supply to the lower ⅔ of spinal cord.
- The **posterior radicular arteries** are around 10 – 20 in number
- Join the posterior spinal arteries and form a pair of posterior arterial trunk.
- **Venous drainage**
  - Six longitudinal venous chain drain the spinal cord
  - One along anteromedian fissure, one along posteromedian sulcus, two lateral venous channels behind the ventral roots, and two lateral venous channel in front of dorsal roots
  - These venous channels communicate with internal venous plexus and drain to basilar plexus, azygos, and vena cava.
- **Applied anatomy:** Anterior spinal artery syndrome—the anterior spinal artery may be occluded by thrombosis affecting the blood supply to the anterior two third of spinal cord. This may lead to loss of motor functions as the nuclei in the anterior horn and corticospinal tract will be affected.

There will be loss of pain and temperature on both sides due to involvement of spinothalamic tracts.

28. Derivatives of I branchial arch.
Refer Short Notes 24 – 2007.

29. Medial wall of middle ear.
Refer Short Notes 37 – 2005.

30. Hyoglossus muscle—attachments and relations.
Refer Short Notes 15 – 2004.

31. Histology of esophagus.
It is made up of 4 layers—from inner to outward are mucous, submucous, muscular, adventitial layer.
- **Mucous layer:**
  - Epithelium—lined by non-keratinized stratified squamous epithelium
  - Lamina propria—Lymphoid follicles are diffusely present
  - Muscularis mucosae is composed mainly of longitudinal smooth muscle
- **Submucous layer:** The submucosa loosely connects the mucosa and the muscularis externa. It contains larger blood vessels, nerves and mucous glands. Esophageal glands are small tubuloacinar glands. They are composed mostly of mucous cells
- **Muscular/muscularis externa layer:** Consists of the outer longitudinal and inner circular layers. The upper one-third of the esophagus, is formed by skeletal

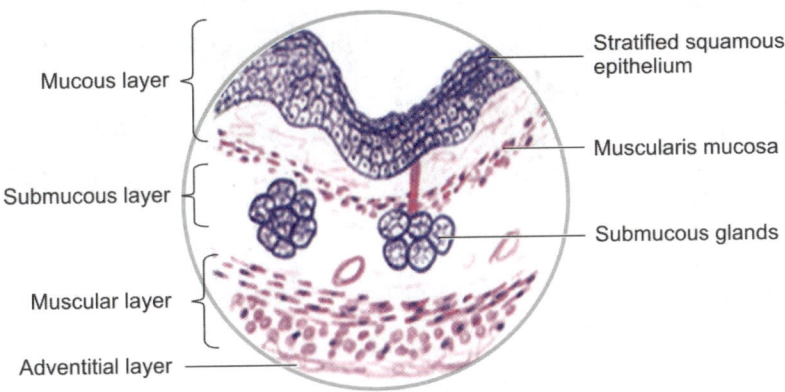

Fig. 36: Histology of esophagus.

muscle; middle one-third, smooth muscle fascicles intermingle with striated muscle, and the lower one-third contains only smooth muscle
- **Adventitial layer:** Separate the esophagus from surrounding structures.

32. Tonsil.

- It forms part of Waldeyer's ring
- **Situation:** In the lateral wall of the oropharynx, in the tonsillar fossa bounded by palatoglossal and palatopharyngeal folds
- **Shape:** The palatine tonsil is an oval lymphoid tissue
- **Size:** Varies according to the age and pathological conditions. In children there is rapid increase in size, and reach a maximum at puberty. Then starts to involute. A little lymphoid tissue remains in old age
- **Parts:** 2 borders, 2 surfaces, 2 poles
- **Relations**
  - **Anterior border** is related to palatoglossal fold
  - **Posterior border** to palatopharyngeal fold
  - **Upper pole** to the soft palate
  - **Lower pole** to the tongue

- **Medial surface:**
  - Covered by mucous membrane of oropharynx
  - Lined by stratified squamous epithelium
  - Surface presents a pitted appearance. The pits, are called the crypts
  - The crypts are 10 – 20 in number
  - A deep tonsillar cleft opens in the upper part of this surface called supratonsillar/intratonsillar cleft
  - The upper wall of the cleft extends into the soft palate containing lymphoid tissue.
- **Lateral surface (Fig. 37)**
  - Lateral aspect is covered by fibrous hemi capsule contributed by pharyngobasilar fascia
  - The capsule is related to **tonsillar bed**, contributed by the superior constrictor, the anterior fibers of palatopharyngeus, and styloglossus lateral to palatoglossus
  - The tonsillar branch of facial artery, accompanied by venae comitantes pierces the superior constrictor to enter the tonsil

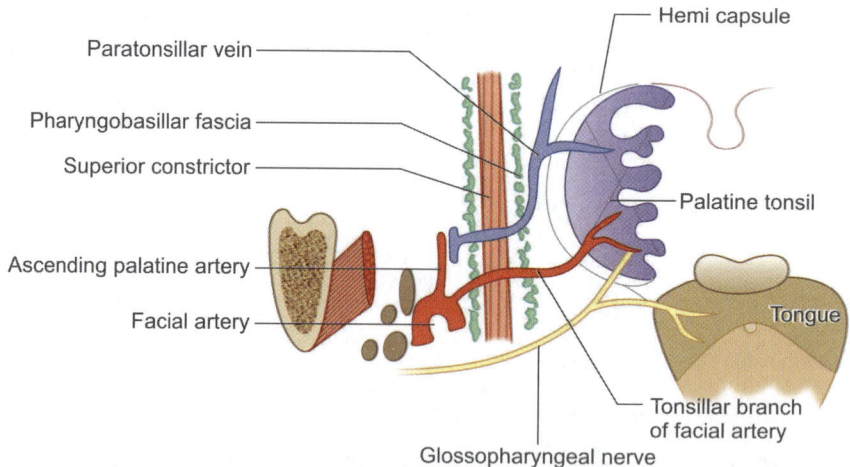

Fig. 37: Lateral relations of tonsil.

- The external palatine or para tonsillar vein, situated lateral to the tonsillar hemi capsule
- The tonsil is separated from the ascending palatine artery, the glossopharyngeal nerve by the muscular wall of the fossa
- The internal carotid artery lies approximately 25 mm posterolateral to the tonsil.

- **Blood supply**
  - **Arterial supply:** The tonsil is supplied by **five** arteries **(Fig. 38)**
    - Three arteries at its lower pole:
      1. The **largest is the tonsillar artery**, branch of the facial artery
      2. Anteroinferiorly dorsal lingual branches of the lingual artery
      3. Posteroinferiorly branch from the ascending palatine artery.
    - Two arteries in its upper pole:
      1. Posterosuperiorly branches from the ascending pharyngeal artery
      2. Superiorly the descending palatine artery from the greater and lesser palatine arteries.
  - **Venous drainage:** External palatine (Para tonsillar) veins, join the pharyngeal venous plexus, facial or internal jugular vein

- **Nerve supply:** Glossopharyngeal and lesser palatine nerves.
- **Applied anatomy**:
  - Bleeding during tonsillectomy may be from paratonsillar vein from the upper angle of the tonsillar fossa
  - Tonsillectomy is surgical removal of tonsil in a repeated acute tonsillitis
  - Referred pain to the ear in case of infection or inflammation of tonsil as both are supplied by the glossopharyngeal nerve.

33. Derivatives of II pharyngeal arch.
Refer Short Notes 27 – 2005.

34. Lumbar puncture.
- It is a procedure by which CSF is withdrawn from spinal subarachnoid space
- It is also used to introduce medicines into the subarachnoid space as in spinal anesthesia
- The CSF is taken by inserting a long lumbar needle into the space
- **Procedure**:
  - **Position of patient**: Lies on right/left lateral with vertebral column completely flexed. The flexed position pulls the spinal cord up
  - **Level of puncture**: The needle to be passed in between spine of third and

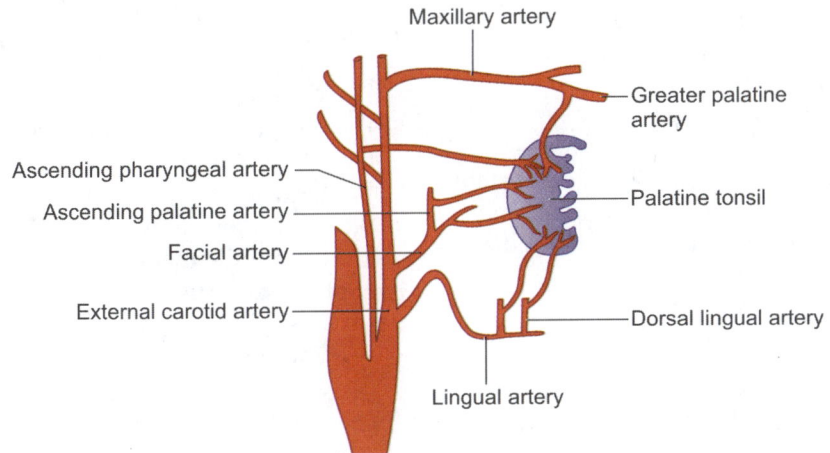

Fig. 38: Arterial supply of tonsil.

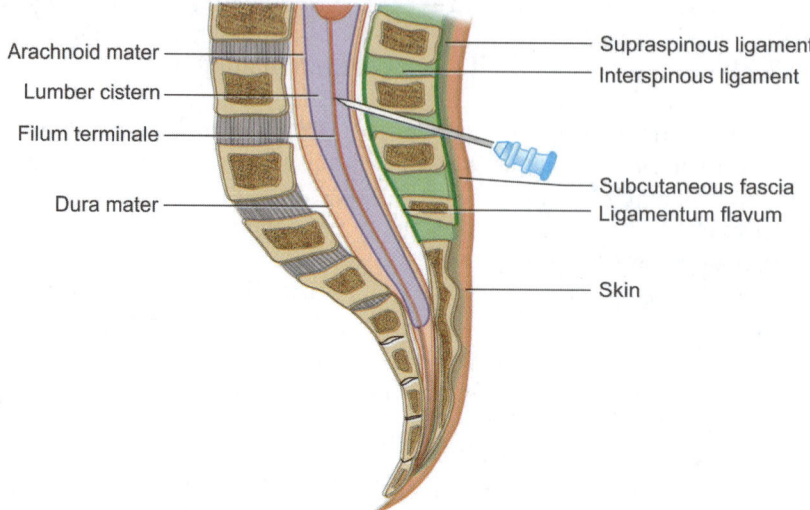

Fig. 39: Lumbar puncture.

fourth lumbar vertebra because the spinal cord ends at lower border of L_1.

- **Structures pierced by needle**:
  - Skin
  - Superficial fascia
  - Supraspinous ligament
  - Interspinous ligament
  - Ligamentum flavum
  - Spinal dura mater
  - Spinal arachnoid mater.
- **Uses of lumbar puncture**:
  - To introduce medicine (antibiotics), chemotherapy
  - Inject dye and CT/MRI pictures taken to find out the lesion
  - Spinal anesthesia
  - Diagnose diseases
  - Check intracranial pressure.
- **Applied anatomy**: Positive queckenstedt's sign indicates that there is some block in the subarachnoid space. The block may be due to some tumor of meninges.

35. Vocal cords.
Refer Short Notes 33 – 2005.

36. Lacrimal apparatus.
Refer Short Notes 27 – 2006.

37. Paranasal air sinuses.
- The paranasal sinuses are the frontal, ethmoidal, sphenoidal and maxillary sinuses
- They all open by small openings into the lateral wall of the nasal cavity
- The **functions** of the paranasal sinuses are add some resonance to the voice, and reduces the bony weight of skull
- The sinuses are incompletely developed or not formed at birth.
- At the time of eruption of the permanent teeth and after puberty they enlarge.
- **Frontal sinus**
  - It is a paired sinus
  - **Situated** between the inner and outer tables of frontal bone behind super ciliary arches
  - **Drainage:** Opens through ethmoidal infundibulum into the anterior part of the middle meatus.
- **Sphenoidal sinus**
  - It is a paired sinus
  - **Situated** in the body of sphenoid bone divided by bony septa into two
  - **Drainage:** Drains into sphenoethmoidal recess of lateral wall of nasal cavity.

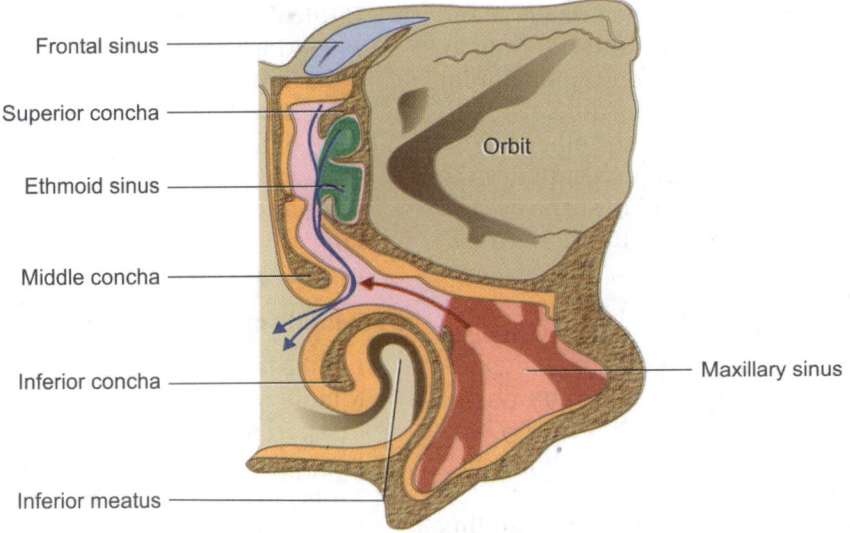

Fig. 40: Paranasal sinuses.

- **Ethmoid sinus**
  - **Situated** in the labyrinth of ethmoid bone. Variations are seen in the number and size of the cavities. There are about three large to 18 small sinuses on each side
  - It is **divided** into three groups—anterior, middle, and posterior ethmoidal sinuses.
- **Anterior ethmoidal sinus:** 11 anterior ethmoidal air cells drain into either the ethmoidal infundibulum or the frontonasal duct.
  - **Middle ethmoidal sinus:** There are usually three or less middle ethmoidal air cells. Opening is seen in the middle meatus or above the bulla ethmoidalis
  - **Posterior ethmoidal sinus:** Seven posterior ethmoidal air cells, opens into the superior meatus.
- **Maxillary sinus**
  - The maxillary sinus/antrum, is the largest of the paranasal sinuses
  - It is situated in the body of the maxilla
  - **Drainage/opening:** The sinus usually opens into the middle meatus, through the hiatus semilunaris. The floor is at a lowerer level than the openings of the sinus. The opening is large and is reduced by articulation of the perpendicular plate of the palatine bone posteriorly, the uncinate process of the ethmoid bone above, the inferior nasal concha below, the lacrimal bone anteriorly.
- **Applied anatomy:** The walls of maxillary sinus is thin so the tumor from the maxillary sinus spreads. (1) Upward spread of the tumor may push up the orbital floor and displace the eyeball; (2) Medially spread into the nasal cavity, causing nasal obstruction and bleeding; (3) Project onto the cheek, causing swelling and numbness if the infraorbital nerve is damaged and (4) Project posteriorly into the infratemporal fossa, causing difficulty in opening the mouth.

38. Blood supply of thyroid gland.

- **Arterial supply (Fig. 41A)**
  - **Superior thyroid artery**
    - From external carotid artery at the level of greater horn of hyoid bone
    - The external laryngeal nerve is closely related to superior thyroid artery
    - It artery after piercing the thyroid fascia divides into anterior and posterior branches

- The anterior surface of the gland is supplied by the anterior branch, and runs along the upper border of isthmus. It anastomoses with superior thyroid of the other side
- The posterior branch supplies the lateral and medial surfaces and anastomose with inferior thyroid artery.
- **Inferior thyroid artery**
  - From thyrocervical trunk of subclavian artery
  - The inferior thyroid artery passes anterior to vertebral artery and behind the carotid sheath to reach the base of the gland
  - It divides into superior ascending and inferior branches and supply corresponding surfaces of the gland
  - The superior ascending branch anastomose with superior thyroid and also supplies the parathyroid glands
  - The inferior branch is related to the recurrent laryngeal nerve. Supplies inferior and posterior surfaces of the gland
  - The artery is not accompanied by the vein.
- **Arteria thyroidea ima** from arch of aorta or brachiocephalic trunk.
- **Venous drainage (Fig. 41B)**
  - Venous plexus deep to true capsule
  - Superior thyroid veins emerge from upper part and drains into internal jugular vein
  - Middle thyroid veins from lower part of the gland and ends in internal jugular vein
  - Inferior thyroid vein of both side unite and a common trunk formed drains into left brachiocephalic vein or superior vena cava
  - Fourth Kocher's vein if present seen between middle and inferior and drain into internal jugular vein.
- **Clinical significance**
  - During thyroidectomy
    - Superior thyroid artery is ligated **near** the apex of the gland as the external laryngeal nerve passes medial to lateral lobe
    - Inferior thyroid artery is ligated **away** from the gland to save the recurrent laryngeal nerve.

39. Middle meningeal artery.

- It is the largest of the meningeal arteries
- Middle meningeal artery is branch from first part of maxillary artery
- It supplies the meninges of brain and main supply to the skull bones of the vault
- It is extradural in course.
- **Origin (Fig. 42):**
  - It is given in the infratemporal fossa
  - Below the lower border of lateral pterygoid muscle.
- **Course:**
  - **Extracranial:**
    - It ascends upwards deep to lateral pterygoid
    - It is encircled by two roots of auriculotemporal nerve
    - It enters the middle cranial fossa through foramen spinosum
    - It is accompanied by nervus spinosus of mandibular nerve.
  - **Intracranial:**
    - It runs anterolaterally in relation to the squamous part of temporal bone
    - It divides into a larger anterior (frontal) and a smaller posterior (parietal) branches.
- **Branches (Fig. 43):**
  - **Anterior division**
    - It runs forwards in the greater wing of sphenoid bone and terminates at the pterion into many branches
    - Few branches ascend upwards up to vertex
    - Other branches are directed backwards

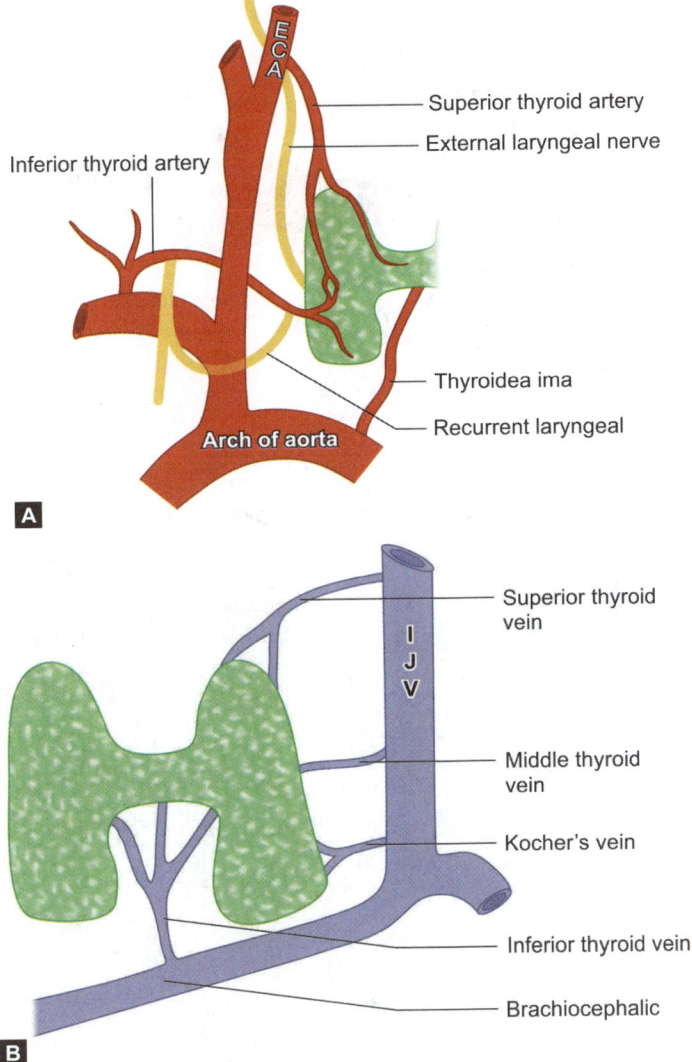

Figs. 41A and B: Blood supply of thyroid: (A) Arterial supply of thyroid; (B) Venous drainage of thyroid.

- One of the branch runs parallel and about 15 mm behind to the coronal suture
- It corresponds to the precentral sulcus.
- **Posterior branch**
  - Runs backwards in relation to squamous temporal bone and extend upto mastoid angle
  - It terminates by dividing into branches to supply posterior part of cranium and meninges.

- **Ganglionic branch:** Supplies trigeminal ganglion
- **Petrosal branch:** Enters through greater petrosal hiatus to supply facial nerve and geniculate ganglion
- **Superior tympanic:** To supply the tensor tympani muscle and mucous membrane of the canal
- **Temporal branch:** Anastomose with deep temporal branch of maxillary artery in the infratemporal fossa

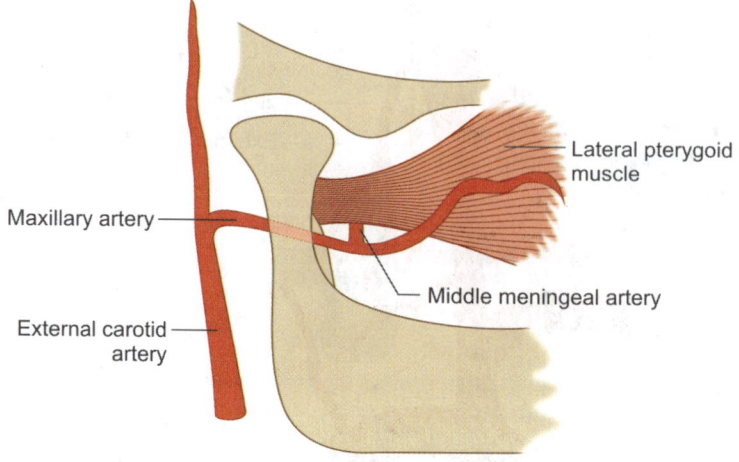

Fig. 42: Origin of middle meningeal artery.

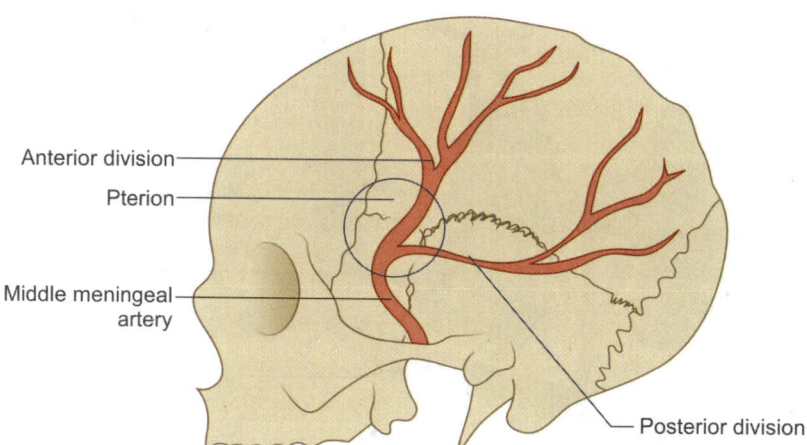

Fig. 43: Course and branches.

- **Anastomotic branch:** Pass through the lateral part of superior orbital fissure and anastomose with recurrent branch of lacrimal artery.
- **Applied anatomy:**
  - Fracture leads to laceration of middle meningeal artery. It results in extradural hematoma
  - The hematoma separates the dura from the underlying periosteum. The effect of lesion is similar to intracranial lesion. Trephining or Burr hole to be done to evacuate the blood collected extradurally

- **Surface marking:** A point 3.5 cm above the midpoint of zygomatic bone used for trephining which corresponds to the anterior branch of middle meningeal artery.

40. Karyotyping chromosomes.

- Karyotyping is a test to examine the chromosomes in a sample of cells
- It helps to identify the genetic problems due to disorder or disease
- **Uses of test**
  - Number of chromosomes are counted
  - Structural change in chromosome can be identified.

- The **tissues used** for the test:
  - Amniotic fluid
  - Peripheral blood (lymphocytes)
  - Bone marrow
  - Placenta—chorionic villi
  - Skin (fibroblasts).
- The test is **done for**
  - The couple with history of miscarriage
  - Children with delayed milestones
  - Chromosomal abnormalities in developing fetus
  - Ambiguous genitalia
  - Multiple congenital defects
  - Leukemia.
- **Method**:
  - The tissue taken from above mentioned, is allowed to grow in a culture medium and incubated in the laboratory
  - The cells are arrested in the metaphase and fixed
  - Metaphase spread is stained and photographed
  - Individual chromosome is cut and arranged according to length of chromosome
  - The karyotype is then analyzed.
- **Normal result**:
  - Female 44 autosomes and 2 sex chromosomes (xx)
  - Male 44 autosomes and 2 sex chromosomes (xy)
- **Abnormal results** due to genetic conditions. Example: Down syndrome, Klinefelter syndrome, trisomy 18, Turner syndrome.

III. SHORT ANSWER QUESTIONS

1. **Name of muscles of II layer of sole of the foot.**

Layers	Tendons	Muscles	Nerve supply
Second	Tendon of flexor hallucis longus Tendon of flexor digitorum longus	Flexor accessorius Lumbricals—four in number	Lateral plantar 1st—Medial plantar 2nd, 3rd, 4th—Lateral plantar

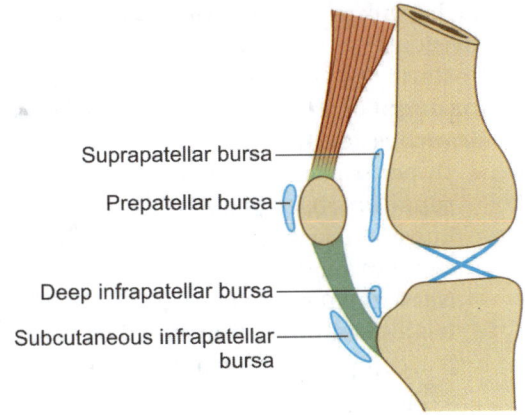

Fig. 44: Bursae related to patella.

2. **Name the bursae around the patella.**
- Subcutaneous prepatellar bursa
- Subcutaneous infrapatellar bursa
- Deep infrapatellar bursa
- Suprapatellar bursa
- **Applied anatomy:**
  - Housemaid's knee—inflammation of prepatellar bursa
  - Clergyman's knee—inflammation of subcutaneous infrapatellar bursa.

3. **Name the abductors of the wrist joint.**
- Abduction is also known as radial deviation
- Range of movement is 15°
- It occurs in midcarpal joint
- The capitate rotates around anteroposterior axis and scaphoid around transverse axis
- Muscles producing: Flexor carpi radialis, extensor carpi radialis longus and brevis
- Associated with abductor pollicis longus and extensor pollicis brevis.

4. **Indicate the terminal branches of posterior cord of brachial plexus.**
- The anterior primary rami of C5, C6, C7, C8 and T1 contribute for brachial plexus
- Roots C5 and C6 join to form the upper trunk. Root C7 forms the middle trunk. Roots C8 and T1 join to form the lower trunk

- Each trunk divides into ventral and dorsal divisions
- **Posterior cord** is formed by the union of the dorsal divisions of all the three trunks.
- **Branches** are (ULNAR):
  - **U**pper subscapular nerve (C5, C6): It supplies subscapularis
  - **L**ower subscapular nerve (C5, C6): It supplies subscapularis and teres major
  - **N**erve to latissimus dorsi (C6, C7, C8): It is also known as thoracodorsal nerve. It accompanies subscapular artery and supplies latissimus dorsi
  - **A**xillary nerve (C5, C6): Also called as circumflex nerve. Winds around the surgical neck of humerus along with posterior circumflex humeral artery. It supplies deltoid and teres minor muscles. It is continued as upper lateral cutaneous nerve of arm
  - **R**adial nerve (C5-C8, T1): It passes behind the arm and enters the spiral groove by passing through the lower triangular space. It is nerve of extensor compartments of arm and forearm.

5. Indicate the tributaries of left renal vein.

- The left renal vein is longer than the right vein
- It crosses the abdominal aorta from left to right
- Ends in the inferior vena cava
- The vein crosses in between aorta and superior mesenteric artery
- **Tributaries:**
  - Left suprarenal vein
  - Left gonadal vein.
- **Applied anatomy:**
  - Varicocele of left testicular vein is common than on the right side
  - The **reasons** are:
    - The left gonadal vein ends at right angles
    - The left renal vein is compressed in-between aorta and superior mesenteric artery
    - Compression by loaded sigmoid colon.

6. Name the two most common positions of appendix.

The position of the appendix depends on the direction of its tip
- Retrocecal/retrocolic (12°clock)—commonest position. Behind the cecum
- Pelvic (4°clock) second commonest position towards pelvis.

7. Indicate the structure of the free border of lesser omentum.

- The attachment of the lesser omentum extends from lesser curvature of stomach and proximal part of duodenum to the visceral surface of liver
- The right margin of lesser omentum forms the free border.
- The structures in the free border are
  - Portal vein posteriorly
  - Hepatic artery anterior and to left
  - Bile duct anterior and to right.

8. Name the arteries of the spermatic cord.

- Spermatic cord is a tubular sheath containing vas deferens, vessels, nerves of testis and epididymis
- The arteries of the cord are:
  - Testicular artery—branch of abdominal aorta
  - Artery to vas—branch from superior/inferior vesical artery
  - Artery to cremaster—from inferior epigastric artery.

9. Name the nerves closely related to humerus.

Three nerves are directly related to the humerus:
- Axillary nerve at the surgical neck
- Radial nerve at the radial groove
- Ulnar nerve behind the medial epicondyle.

10. Name three structures at the transpyloric plane.

- It is also known as **Addison's plane**
- Horizontal plane midway between the suprasternal notch and the upper end of symphysis pubis or midway between the Xiphisternal joint and the umbilicus

- The plane passes through:
  - Tips of both 9th costal cartilages
  - Lower border of L1 vertebra
  - Pylorus of stomach
  - Fundus of gallbladder
  - Lower end of spinal cord
  - Hila of both kidneys. On the left side through upper part and right side through lower part of hilum
  - Origin of superior mesenteric artery.

11. Name the bones meeting at pterion.

- Pterion is an **H-shaped sutural junction.**
- Four bones meet on one side
  Formation: superiorly by the frontal and parietal bones and inferiorly by the greater wing of the sphenoid and squamous temporal.

12. Indicate the sinuses of the pericardium.

- Pericardial sinuses are the spaces formed by the arrangement of the serosal layer
- It is arranged as two 'tubes'. The aorta and pulmonary trunk are in one tube, and the superior and inferior venae cava and the four pulmonary veins form the second tube
- The **pericardial sinuses** are:
  - Transverse sinus
  - Oblique sinuses
  - The transverse sinus is a passage between the two pericardial 'tubes' mentioned above
  - Oblique sinus is a blind sac lying behind the left atrium. It is inverted "J" shaped.

13. Name the terminal branches of internal thoracic artery.

- The internal thoracic artery is from first part of subclavian artery about 2 cm above the sternal end of clavicle
- Runs vertically downwards, about 1 cm from lateral border of sternum
- Terminates at sixth intercostal space
- The venae comitantes accompany the artery.
- Divides into two terminal branches:
  1. Musculophrenic artery and
  2. Superior epigastric artery.

14. Indicate the paleocerebellar deep nuclei.

Paleocerebellum
- Made up of the anterior lobe except lingula and the pyramid and uvula of inferior vermis
- Its connections are chiefly spino-cerebellar
- It controls tone, posture and crude movements of the limbs.
  - **E**mboliformis nucleus—paleocerebellum
  - **G**lobosus nucleus—paleocerebellum.

15. Name the muscles attached to the cricoid cartilage.

- Cricoid is an unpaired cartilage of larynx
- It has a narrow anterior arch and broader posterior lamina
- **Lamina** has a ridge in the center and it gives attachment to the tendon of esophagus
- On either side of ridge the posterior cricoarytenoid muscle is attached
- **Arch:** Superior border of the arch gives attachment for lateral cricoarytenoid muscle
- To the external surface the cricothyroid muscle and cricopharyngeal part of inferior constrictor are attached.

16. Name two sensory thalamic nuclei.

- Anterior group—anterior medial, anterior dorsal and anterior ventral
- Medial group—medial dorsal and medial ventral
- Lateral group—divided into ventral and lateral.
- Lateral—lateral dorsal, lateral posterior and pulvinar
- Ventral—ventral anterior, ventral lateral and ventral posteromedial and ventral posterolateral.

17. Name the structures passing through internal acoustic meatus.

- Internal acoustic meatus is present in the posterior surface of petrous part of temporal bone
- It is an opening in the posterior cranial fossa

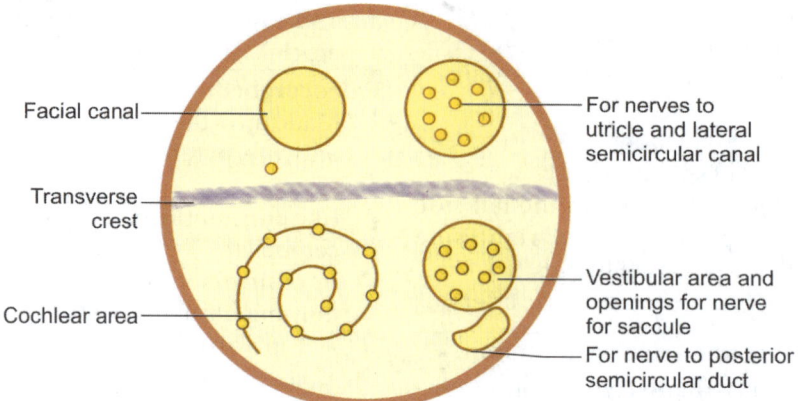

Fig. 45: Internal acoustic meatus.

- It lies anterosuperior to jugular foramen
- It is separated from the internal ear by a vertical plate
- **Features:**
  - It is divided by a transverse crest unequally
  - **Above the crest:** anteriorly is the opening of facial canal, posteriorly the opening for the nerves to utricle and anterior and lateral semicircular ducts
  - **Below the crest:** anteriorly cochlear area, made of small holes arranged spirally and posteriorly vestibular area containing openings for nerves for saccule and more posteroinferiorly a single opening for the nerve to posterior semicircular duct
  - The **length** of internal acoustic meatus is about 7 mm at birth and 11 mm in adult
  - **Structures passing** are
    - Motor and sensory (nervus intermedius) roots of facial nerve
    - Vestibulocochlear nerve
    - Labyrinthine artery branch from basilar artery.

18. Name the two parts of orbicularis oculi.

- It is one of the muscle of facial expression, **developed** from 2nd branchial arch, supplied by facial nerve
- It is a muscle which surrounds the circumference of the orbit and eyelids and extends to anterior temporal, infraorbital cheek and super ciliary regions.

- **Parts**
  - Orbital part
  - Palpebral part
  - Lacrimal part.

19. Name the lingual papillae.

- Papillae are projections of the mucosa covering the dorsal surface of the tongue
- They are present only in the presulcal part of the tongue
- Functions: It gives roughness, increase the surface area, and gustatory
- There are four types of papillae, namely—filiform, fungiform, foliate and circumvallate papillae
- All the papillae are provided with taste buds except the filiform papillae.

20. Indicate the venous sinuses related to the falx cerebri.

- It is a fold formed by the meningeal layer of duramater
- It is a sickle shaped fold of duramater
- It has superior convex margin inferior concave margin is free, posterior broader attached to the superior layer of tentorium cerebelli
- **Sinuses related**
  - Superior sagittal sinus along the superior border
  - Inferior sagittal sinus along the concave free border
  - Straight sinus between the falx cerebri and tentorium cerebelli.

MBBS Examination 2009

ANSWER ALL QUESTIONS

I. Essay questions (15/10 Marks)

1. Describe uterus under the following headings: (a) Position and parts, (b) Relations, (c) Blood supply, (d) Ligaments and supports, (e) Development, (f) Histology and (g) Applied anatomy.
2. Describe hip joint under the following headings: (a) Articular, surfaces, (b) Ligaments, (c) Relations, (d) Muscles and movements and (e) Applied anatomy.
3. Describe the mammary gland and give its blood supply lymphatic drainage and applied anatomy.
4. Describe the relations, blood supply and microscopic structure of duodenum.
5. Explain thyroid gland under the following headings: (a) Location and parts, (b) Coverings, (c) Relations, (d) Blood supply, (e) Histology, (f) Development and (g) Applied anatomy.
6. Explain the typical intercostal space.
7. Describe tongue under the following headings: Situation and parts, blood supply, lymphatic drainage, histology and development.
8. Describe the interior of right atrium and correlate it with its development.

II. Short notes (5/4 Marks)

1. Great saphenous vein.
2. Blood supply of long bone.
3. Karyotyping.
4. Lesser sac.
5. Thoracolumbar fascia.
6. Histology of duodenum.
7. Axillary lymph nodes.
8. Popliteal fossa.
9. Neural tube.
10. Celiac trunk.
11. Femoral sheath.
12. Subtalar joints.
13. Histology of spleen.
14. Development of urinary bladder.
15. Superficial perineal pouch.
16. Arteria profunda brachii.
17. Turner's syndrome.
18. Lesser sac.
19. Popliteus muscle.
20. Dorsalis pedis artery.
21. Development of face.
22. Otic ganglion.
23. Cerebellar peduncles.
24. Right atrium.
25. Extraocular muscles.
26. Palatine tonsil.
27. Nerve supply of tongue.
28. Tympanic membrane.
29. Bronchopulmonary segments.
30. Ansa cervicalis.
31. Ciliary ganglion.
32. Facial artery.
33. Interpeduncular fossa.
34. Midline structures of the neck.
35. Histology of cornea.
36. Pleural recesses.
37. Development of thyroid gland.
38. Lateral medullary syndrome.
39. Subclavian triangle.
40. TS at the level of superior colliculus of midbrain.

III. Short answer questions (3/2 Marks)

1. Enumerate the contents of spermatic cord.
2. Enumerate the bare areas of liver.
3. Name four tributaries of inferior vena cava.
4. Nerve supply of the lumbricals of the hand.
5. Name the muscles supplied by the obturator nerve.
6. Erb's point.
7. Name the contents of superficial perineal pouch.
8. Name the bones forming medial longitudinal arch of foot.
9. Enumerate four structures related to the anterior surface of left kidney.
10. Name four derivatives of ectoderm.
11. Name the structures piercing clavipectoral fascia.
12. Give the action of lumbrical muscle.
13. Name the structures deep to flexor retinaculum of hand.
14. Give the boundaries of epiploic foramen.
15. Give the significance of Douglas pouch.
16. What is annular pancreas?
17. Name the branches of external iliac artery.
18. Name the structures piercing oblique popliteal ligament.
19. Name the arteries forming trochanteric anastomosis.
20. Name the contents of subsartorial canal.
21. Draw and label the histology of trachea.
22. Name the structures present in the lateral wall of cavernous sinus.
23. Nerve supply of larynx.
24. Parts of corpus callosum.
25. Four derivatives of ectoderm.
26. Enumerate four branches of 1st part of maxillary artery.
27. Structures passing through the foramen ovale. (MALE)
28. Tributaries of coronary sinus.
29. Name the bones forming the nasal septum.
30. Name muscles of mastication.
31. What is ligamentum arteriosum?
32. Significance of pyriform fossa.
33. Name the muscles of mastication.
34. Give the sub divisions of mediastinum.
35. What are Hassall's corpuscles?
36. Name the splanchnic nerves in the thoracic region.
37. What is danger area of face?
38. Give the attachment of suprapleural membrane.
39. What is insula?
40. What is visual stria?

I. ESSAY QUESTIONS

1. Describe uterus under the following headings: (a) Position and parts, (b) Relations, (c) Blood supply, (d) Ligaments and supports, (e) Development, (f) Histology and (g) Applied anatomy.

a, b, d and g - Refer Essay Q. No. 2 – 2004
f - Refer Essay Q. No. 3 – 2006.

(c) Blood Supply

- **Arterial supply:**
Refer Essay Q. No. 3 – 2006.
- **Venous drainage:**
  - Uterine vein pass along the artery in the broad ligament and drain to internal iliac vein
  - The uterine venous plexus anastomoses with ovarian and vaginal venous plexus.

(e) Development (Fig. 1)

- It is mesodermal in origin
- Uterus is developed from paramesonephric duct
- The paramesonephric (Mullerian) ducts are developed in both sexes in the 6th week
- Each paramesonephric duct consists of three parts:
  1. Cephalic vertical part
  2. Intermediate horizontal part
  3. Caudal vertical part
     Caudal vertical parts of both paramesonephric ducts fuse in caudocranial direction.

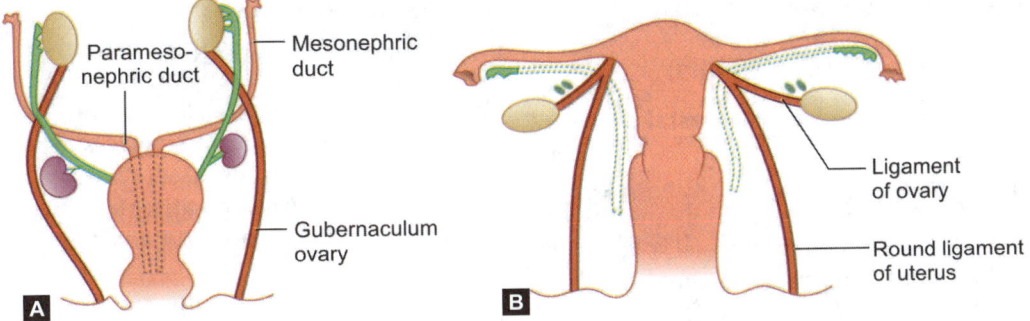

Figs. 1A and B: Development of uterus.

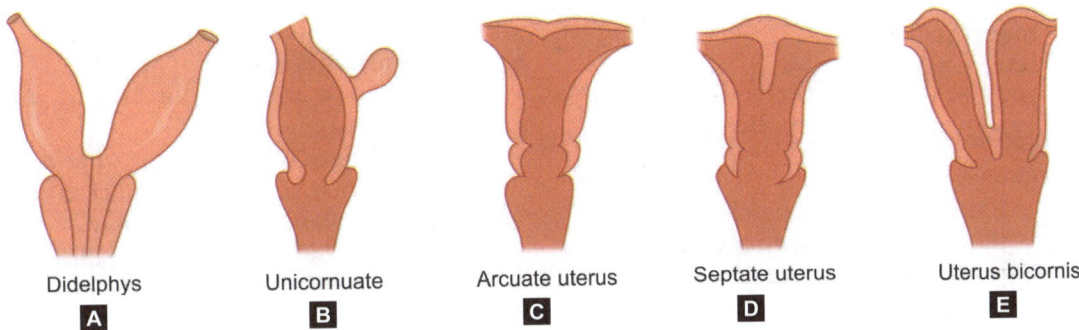

Figs. 2A to E: Congenital anomalies.

- By the 3rd month the partition between them disappears
- The single canal thus formed is the utero-vaginal canal
- The cranial part of this canal forms the entire uterus
- The most cephalic point of fusion of the two ducts form the fundus
- Portion of the vagina developed from the caudal part of the utero-vaginal canal
- The endometrium is developed from mesoderm, the myometrium is from surrounding mesenchyme and perimetrium from peritoneum.
- **Congenital anomalies (Fig. 2):**
  - Duplication of uterus (uterus didelphys)—due to lack of fusion of the paramesonephric ducts
  - Uterus bicornis unicollis—uterus two horns and common vagina
  - Unicornuate—one of the paramesonephric duct development is rudimentary
  - Arcuate uterus—slightly indented in the middle
  - Septate uterus—failure of fusion of upper part of paramesonephric ducts.

2. **Describe hip joint under the following headings: (a) Articular surfaces, (b) Ligaments, (c) Relations, (d) Muscles and movements and (e) Applied Anatomy.**

a, b, d, e - Refer Essay Q. No. 1 – 2004
c - Refer Essay Q. No. 3 – 2008.

3. **Describe the mammary gland and give its blood supply lymphatic drainage and applied anatomy.**

Refer Essay Q. No. 4 – 2006.

4. **Describe the relations, blood supply and microscopic structure of duodenum.**

Refer Essay Q. No. 3 – 2007.

5. **Explain thyroid gland under the following headings: (a) Location and parts, (b) Coverings, (c) Relations, (d) Blood supply, (e) Histology, (f) Development and (g) Applied anatomy.**

a, b, c - Refer Short Notes 17 – 2004
d - Refer Short Notes 38 – 2008
e, f, g - Refer Essay Q. No. 8 – 2007.

6. Explain the typical intercostal space.

Definition

- Space between two ribs and costal cartilages is called intercostal space
- There are 11 intercostal spaces
- 3rd to 6th spaces are called as **typical intercostal** spaces.

Contents

- Intercostal muscles
- Intercostal nerve
- Intercostal vessels.

Intercostal Muscles (Fig. 3)

- **External intercostal**
  - **Extent:** From the tubercles of the ribs, to the costal cartilages. Anteriorly modified to form the **external intercostal membrane** which is aponeurotic extending from costal cartilage to sternum
  - **Origin:** Each muscle arises from the lower border of one rib
  - **Insertion:** To the upper border of the lower rib
  - **Direction of fibers:** Fibers are directed at the back of the thorax, obliquely downwards and laterally, and at the front downwards, forwards and medially.

- **Internal intercostal**
  - **Extent:** Anteriorly from sternum to the posterior costal angles. Posteriorly an aponeurotic layer, called the **internal intercostal membrane** replaces from angle to superior costotransverse ligament
  - **Origin:** Each muscle arises from the floor of a costal groove and adjacent costal cartilage
  - **Insertion:** Into the upper border of the lower rib
  - **Direction of fibers:** Fibers are directed obliquely, at right angles to those of the external intercostal muscles.

- **Innermost intercostal**
  - **Extent:** In the middle half of the intercostal spaces
  - **Attachment:** The muscles pass between the internal surfaces of adjacent ribs (from rib above to the rib below)
  - **Direction of fibers:** Fibres are directed obliquely, similar to internal intercostal muscle.

Intercostal Nerve

Refer Essay Q. No. 9 – 2006.

Intercostal Vessels

Arteries

- **Anterior intercostal arteries (Fig. 4A)**
  - Usually two anterior intercostal arteries in each space
  - The anterior intercostal arteries are branches of internal thoracic artery
  - Sometimes a single artery divides into two branches
  - One artery passes along the upper, and other along the lower part of intercostal space
  - They pass laterally and anastomose with the corresponding posterior intercostal arteries and their collateral branches
  - The arteries passes at first between the pleura and the internal intercostal, then between the innermost and the internal intercostal

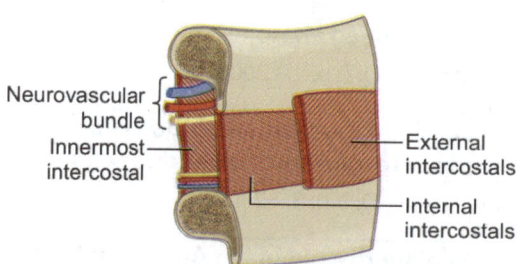

Fig. 3: Intercostal muscles.

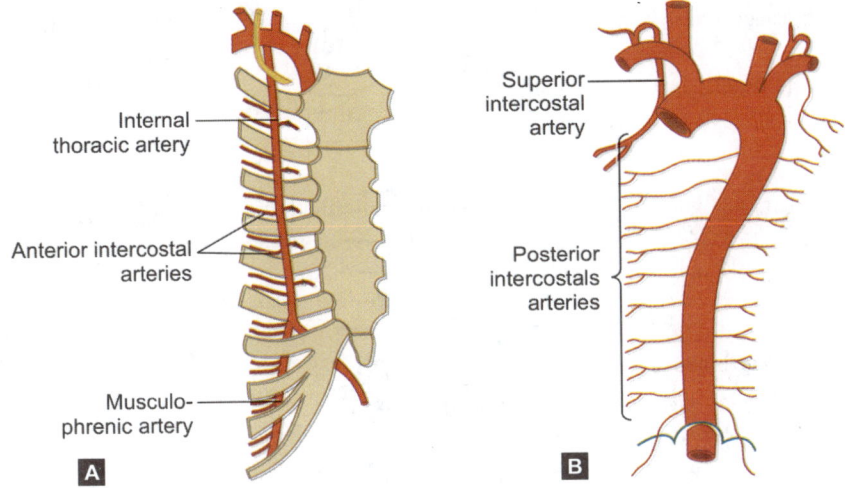

Figs. 4A and B: (A) Anterior intercostal arteries; (B) Posterior intercostal arteries.

- They supply the intercostal muscles, the pectoral muscles, breast and skin.
- **Posterior intercostal artery (Fig. 4B)**
  - One posterior intercostal artery in each space
  - The arteries of typical space arise from the descending thoracic aorta
  - As the aorta is to the left of midline, the right posterior intercostal arteries are longer, and traverse the vertebral bodies behind the esophagus, thoracic duct and azygos vein **(Fig. 5)**
  - Left posterior intercostal arteries run behind on the bodies of vertebra
  - Each artery passes obliquely towards the angle of the rib above and continues forward in its costal groove
  - Up to the costal angle lies between the pleura and internal intercostal membrane, then between the internal intercostal and innermost intercostal muscles
  - Anastomoses with an anterior intercostal artery
  - A collateral branch is given near the costal angle and runs downwards to the upper border of the rib to anastomose with lower anterior intercostal artery.

Veins (Fig. 6)
- **Anterior intercostal veins:** End in the internal thoracic vein
- **Posterior intercostal veins**

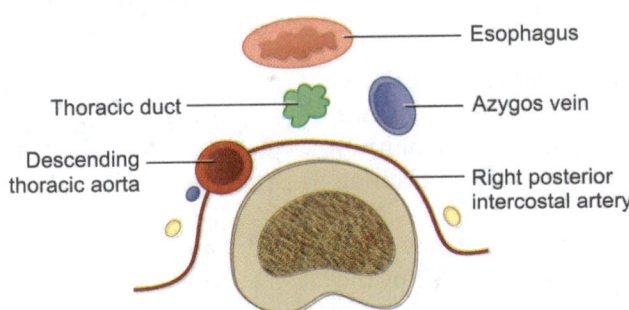

Fig. 5: Relations of posterior intercostal artery.

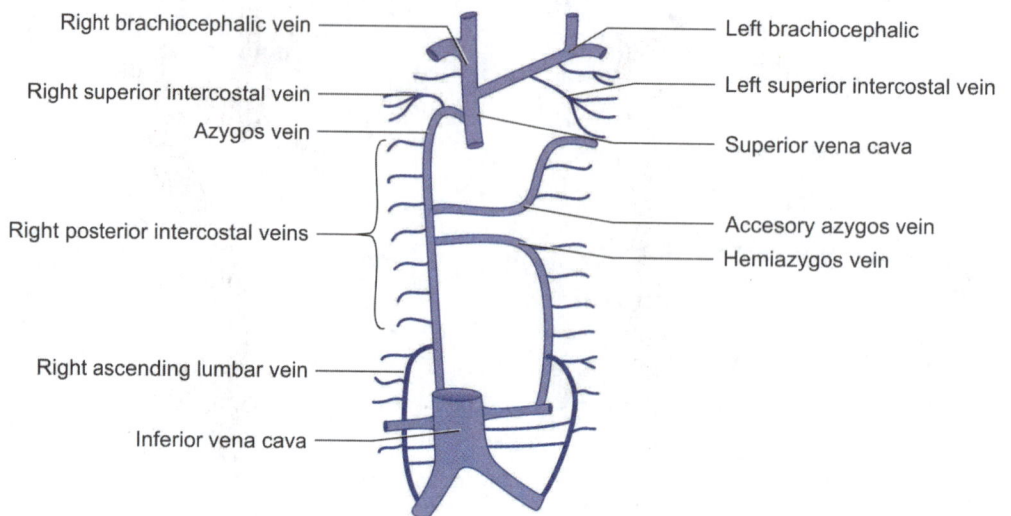

Fig. 6: Venous drainge—posterior intercostal veins.

Right side
- First right posterior intercostal vein to right brachiocephalic vein
- Right superior intercostal vein is formed by the union of second, third and fourth posterior intercostal veins ends in azygos vein
- Fifth and sixth right posterior intercostal veins to azygos vein.

Left side
- First left posterior intercostal vein to left brachiocephalic vein
- Left superior intercostal vein is formed by the union of second, third and fourth posterior intercostal veins and ends in left brachiocephalic vein
- Fifth and sixth ends in accessory azygos vein.

- **Applied anatomy**
  - **Paracentesis thoracis:** Needle is passed along the lower part of the space in the mid axillary line to avoid injury to the neurovascular bundle in draining pleural effusion
  - **Intercostal neuralgia:** Sharp burning pain in the area of skin supplied by the thoracic spinal nerves due to herpes zoster which is a viral disease of the spinal ganglia with pain and vesicular eruptions along the dermatomes of the affected nerves.

7. **Describe the tongue under the following headings: Situation and parts, Blood supply, Lymphatic drainage, Histology and development.**

Situation and parts, lymphatic drainage- Refer Essay Q. No. 6 – 2007.

Blood Supply of Tongue

Arterial Supply

The tongue is supplied by lingual and branches from it, facial artery and ascending pharyngeal artery. Main artery of tongue is lingual artery.

- **Lingual artery (Fig. 7)**
  - It is a branch from the external carotid artery
  - It dips in between hyoglossus and middle constrictor accompanied by the lingual veins reaches the floor of the mouth
  - Then it passes between the genioglossus and longitudinal muscle and extends up to the tip of the tongue
  - Near the tip it terminates by anastomosing with the opposite lingual artery
  - It forms plexus in the submucosa and supply the muscles of tongue.

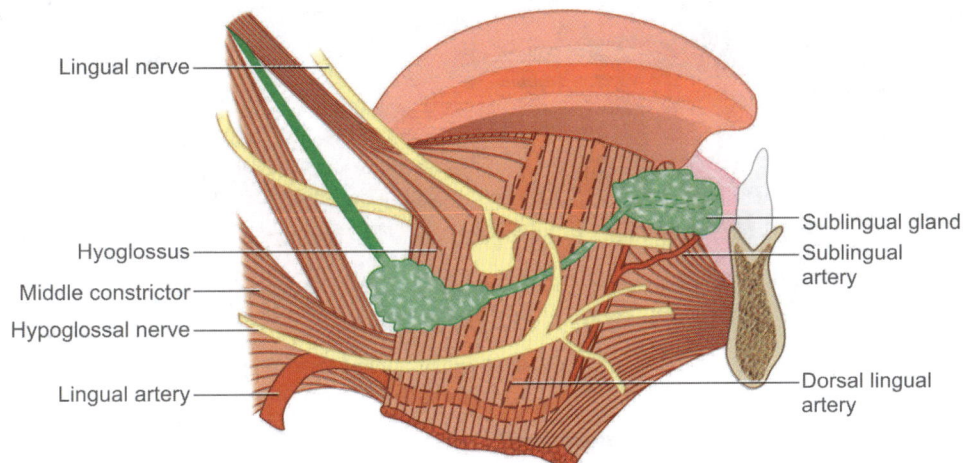

Fig. 7: Lingual artery.

- **Dorsal lingual artery:**
  - Branch from lingual artery
  - Usually seen as two or three branches
  - Supply the posterior part of dorsum of tongue
  - It anastomose with opposite artery.
- **Deep lingual artery**
  - Continuation of the lingual artery
  - Supply the inferior surface of tongue.
- **Arteries to supply root of tongue**
  - Ascending palatine artery
  - Tonsillar branch of facial artery
  - Ascending pharyngeal artery.
- **Venous drainage**
  - The **dorsal lingual vein** drain dorsum and side of the tongue. It accompanies the lingual artery
  - The **deep lingual vein** starts from the tip of the tongue drain the inferior surface of tongue. It accompanies the hypoglossal nerve as vena comitans nervi hypoglossai
  - The dorsal lingual vein and deep lingual vein join to form the **lingual vein**
  - The lingual vein drains to the internal jugular vein.

Histology of Tongue (Fig. 8)

- It is made of mucous and muscular layers
- The submucosa is absent
- The mucous membrane is adherent to the muscular coat.
- **Mucous layer**
  - **Epithelium:** Mucous membrane is lined by stratified squamous epithelium
  - It is non-keratinized in the posterior part of tongue and keratinized over filiform papillae
  - The **lamina propria** contains dense fibrous connective tissue, elastic fibers, nerve and lymph plexus, blood vessels and lingual glands
  - The mucous membrane projects in the dorsal surface to form papillae
  - There are four types of **papillae**—filiform, fungiform, vallate, foliate papillae
  - **Taste buds** are present in all the papillae except filiform papilla
  - The taste buds are present in the epithelium of mucous membrane
  - They are made of sustentacular cell surrounding the neuroepithelial cells. They converge on gustatory pore. The gustatory nerve fibers spirals around the neuroepithelial cells
  - **Muscular coat** made of skeletal muscle arranged as irregular bundles.

Development

Refer Short Notes 20 – 2003.

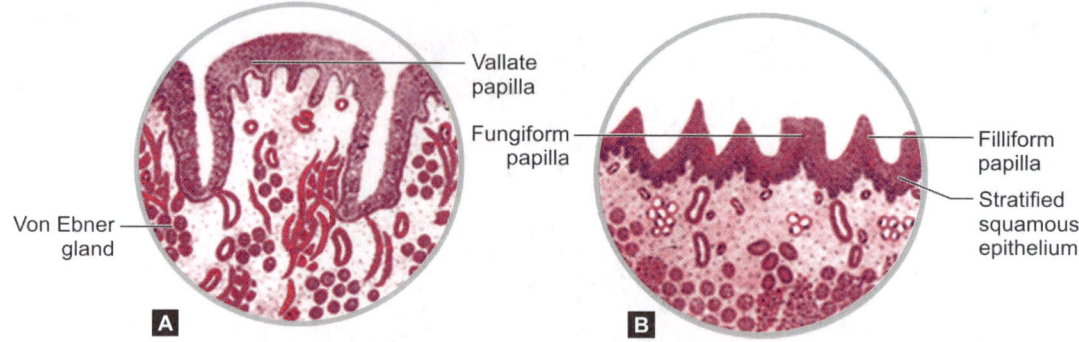

Figs. 8A and B: Histology of tongue.

8. Describe the interior of right atrium and correlate it with its development.

Interior of right atrium
Refer Essay Q. No. 7 – 2006
- **Development** is under two headings: 1. Development of atrium, 2. Development of interatrial septum.
1. **Development of right atrium:**
   - It is developed from three sources
   - **Smooth part behind crista terminalis** is from absorption of enlarged right horn of sinus venosus
   - Septum spurium and upper part of right venous valve persist as **crista terminalis**
   - Lower part of right venous valve forms the **valve of IVC and coronary sinus**
   - The **rough anterior part** is from right half of primitive atrium
   - A small ventral part from right half of atrioventricular canal.
2. **Development of interatrial septum:**
Refer short notes on Q. No. 25 – 2006.

II. SHORT NOTES

1. Great saphenous vein.
Refer Short Notes 14 – 2005.

2. Blood supply of long bone.
The long bone is supplied by the following four sets of arteries:
1. **Nutrient artery**
   - It enters the middle of the shaft (diaphysis) through a nutrient foramen, runs obliquely through the cortex, and then divides into ascending and descending branches in the medullary cavity
   - Each branch then subdivides into a number of smaller parallel vessels close to endosteal surface and enter metaphysis and form hair-pin loops
   - Near epiphysis they anastomose with terminal branches of metaphyseal and epiphyseal arteries
   - The nutrient artery supplies the medullary cavity containing bone marrow and inner two-thirds of the outer shell of compact bone of diaphysis and metaphysis
   - The oblique direction of nutrient foramen in the shaft is opposite to the growing end of the long bone
   (Towards the elbow I flow, away from the knee).
2. **Periosteal artery:**
   - They are numerous and branch out beneath the periosteum
   - Periosteal arteries enter the bone through Volkmann's canals, and outer one-third of the cortex is supplied by it.
3. **Metaphyseal (Juxta-epiphyseal) artery:** They are derived from neighboring arteries and enter the metaphysis directly along the attachment of joint capsule
4. **Epiphyseal artery:** They are derived from arterial anastomosis around the joint. They enter the epiphysis either directly or after piercing the epiphyseal cartilage.

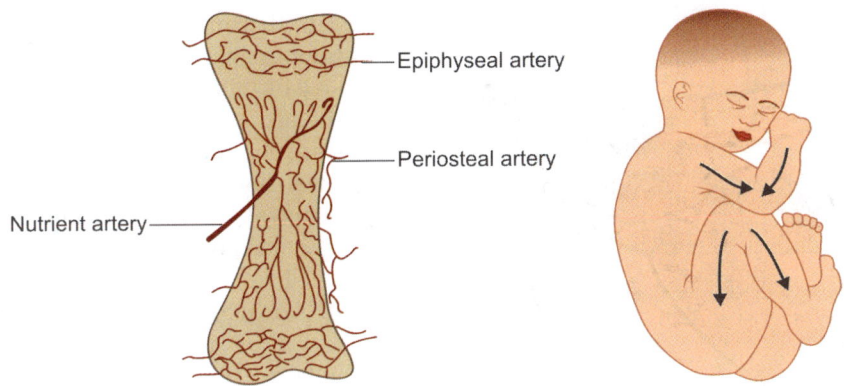

Fig. 9: Blood supply of long bone.

Applied Anatomy

- Avascular necrosis due to interruption of blood supply
- Hair pin bend of the metaphyseal arteries before fusion function as end arteries. It is the common site for osteomyelitis in children as the emboli or infection are trapped in the bends causing infarction
- The endosteal vessels are liable for injury during intramedullary nailing for fractures.

3. Karyotyping.

Refer Short Notes 40 – 2008.

4. Lesser sac.

Refer Short Notes 10 – 2005.

5. Thoracolumbar fascia.

- It is also called lumbar fascia
- It is the fascia enclosing the deep muscles of the back
- It is made up of 3 layers—posterior, middle and anterior
- The posterior layer is the thickest and the anterior layer is the thinnest.
- Attachments
  - **Posterior layer:**
    - Medial—tips of the lumbar and sacral spines and the supraspinous ligaments
    - Lateral—blends with the middle layer at the lateral border of erector spinae
    - Superior—fuses with deep fascia of thoracic region
    - Inferior—the outer lip of iliac crest.
  - **Middle layer:**
    - Medial—tips of the lumbar transverse processes and the inter transverse ligaments
    - Lateral—blends with the anterior layer at the lateral border of the quadratus lumborum
    - Superior—lower border of 12th rib and to the lumbocostal ligament
    - Inferior—intermediate area of the iliac crest.
  - **Anterior layer:**
    - Medial—to the anterior surfaces of the lumbar transverse processes
    - Lateral—blends with middle layer at the lateral border of the quadratus lumborum
    - Superior—lateral arcuate ligament from transverse process of 1st lumbar vertebra to 12th rib
    - Inferior—inner lip of the iliac crest and the iliolumbar ligament.
- **Muscles enclosed:**
  - Between posterior and middle: Erector spinae muscle
  - Between middle and anterior: Quadratus lumborum muscle
  - **Muscles taking origin from thoraco-lumbar fascia.**

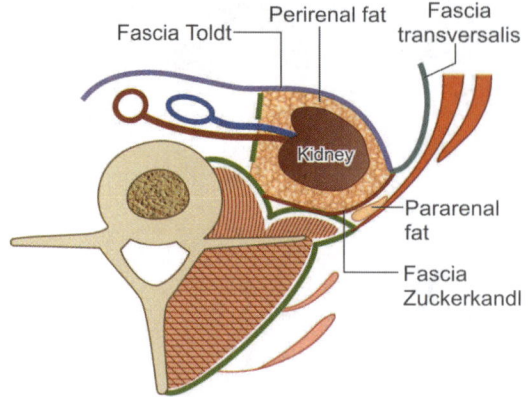

Fig. 10: Thoracolumbar fascia.

- From anterior layer—few fibers of diaphragm
- From fusion of anterior and middle layer—transverse abdominis and internal oblique
- From posterior layer—latissimus dorsi, serratus posterior inferior, gluteus maximus.

6. **Histology of duodenum.**

Refer Short Notes 9 – 2004.

7. **Axillary lymph nodes.**

- The axillary lymph nodes are about 20 to 30 in number
- Situated in the fat of the axilla
- They drain the entire upper limb, mammary gland, anterior abdominal wall above umbilicus
- They are grouped into five groups—anterior (pectoral), posterior (subscapular), central, lateral, and apical **(Fig. 11)**
- The apical is the terminal node.
  - **Lateral group:**
    - Four to six nodes
    - Situated along the axillary vein
    - They drain the entire upper limb except the lymph vessels accompanying cephalic vein
    - The efferent pass to apical, central axillary nodes and deep cervical nodes.
  - **Anterior group:**
    - Four to six nodes
    - Situated along the inferior border of pectoralis minor and related to lateral thoracic vessels
    - Receive lymph from the anterior wall of the trunk above umbilicus and breast
    - The efferent pass to the apical and central group of axillary nodes.
  - **Posterior group:**
    - Six to seven nodes
    - Lie along the posterior axillary wall and related to the subscapular vessels

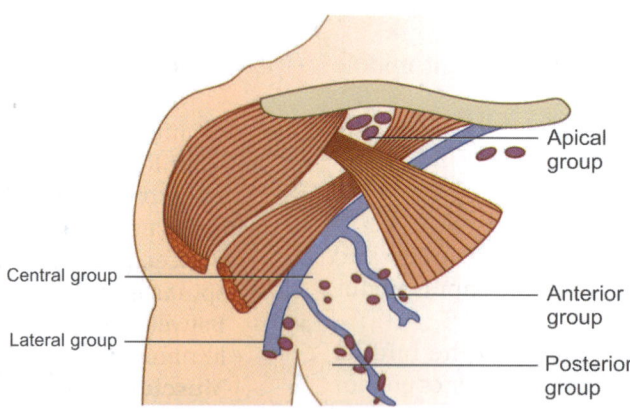

Fig. 11: Axillary lymph nodes.

- Receive lymph from the posterior part of neck, and dorsal surface of trunk up to iliac crest
- Efferent to the apical and central group of axillary nodes.
– **Central group:**
  - Includes about three to four nodes
  - Situated in the axillary fat
  - Receives afferent from the lateral, posterior, and anterior group axillary nodes
  - The efferent to apical node.
– **Apical group:**
  - Ten to twelve nodes
  - Situated behind and above the upper part of pectoralis minor
  - It is medial to axillary vein
  - Afferent from the other axillary group nodes, upper part of breast, lymph accompanying cephalic vein
  - Efferent unite to form subclavian trunk and drain to subclavian vein or jugular lymphatic trunk. Few pass to inferior deep cervical node.
– **Rotter's node:**
  - As per the surgeons it is included as another group
  - Situated between the pectoralis major and minor muscles.

Applied anatomy: Infections or malignancy in any part of the territory of drainage will cause enlargement of the axillary lymph nodes, hence examination of these lymph nodes is important in clinical practice.

8. **Popliteal fossa.**

- The popliteal fossa is a diamond-shaped depression felt at the back of the semi-flexed knee joint
- **Boundaries (Fig. 12A):**
  – **Superolaterally:** The biceps femoris
  – **Superomedially:** The semitendinosus and semimembranosus, supplemented by the gracilis
  – **Inferolaterally:** Lateral head of the gastrocnemius supplemented by the plantaris
  – **Inferomedially:** Medial head of the gastrocnemius.
- **Roof:**
  – The deep fascia or popliteal fascia forms the roof of the fossa
  – The fascia is pierced by sural nerve and short saphenous vein.
- **Floor:**
  – Formed from above downwards by:
  – The popliteal surface of the femur
  – The capsule of the knee joint and the oblique popliteal ligament

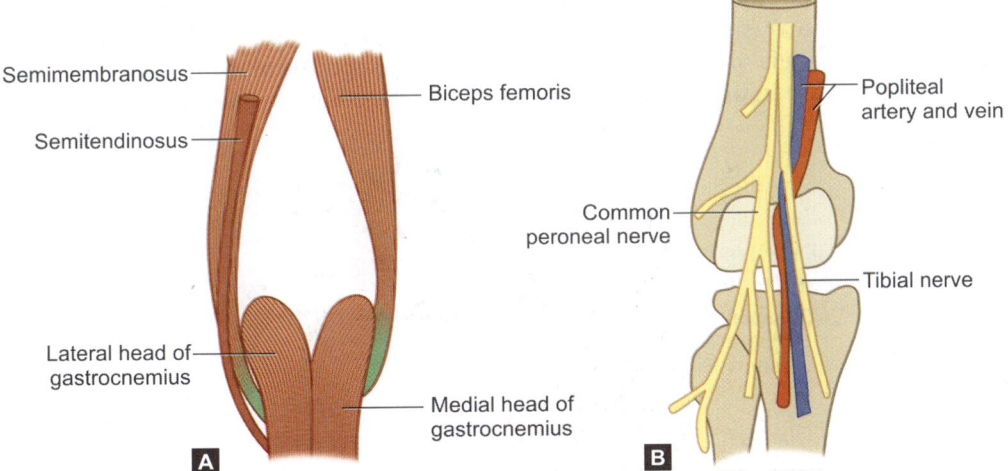

Figs. 12A and B: Popliteal fossa: (A) Boundaries; (B) Contents.

- The strong popliteal fascia covering the popliteus muscle.
- **Contents (Fig. 12B):**
  - Popliteal artery and its branches
  - Popliteal vein—the vein is posterolateral to artery in the upper part, then behind and medial in the lower part
  - Tibial nerve and its branches
  - Common peroneal nerve and its branches
  - Posterior cutaneous nerve of thigh
  - Genicular branch of the obturator nerve
  - Sural nerve
  - Short saphenous vein
  - Popliteal lymph nodes
  - Fat.
- **Applied anatomy:**
  - **Aneurysm of popliteal artery**—is dilatation of popliteal artery results in pulsatile swelling in midline of popliteal fossa
  - **Popliteal artery entrapment**—the contraction of medial head of gastrocnemius, can cause occlusion of the artery as it passes deep to the muscle
  - **Enlargement of popliteal node**—in inflammatory lesion of heel, lateral side of foot, and back of leg
  - **Baker's cyst**—protrusion of synovial membrane through the fibrous capsule of knee joint, or due to inflammation of semimembranosus bursa
  - Popliteal artery is used for **measuring blood pressure** in the lower limb.

9. Neural tube.
Refer Short Notes 20 – 2004.

10. Coeliac trunk.

- It is the artery of the foregut
- It is a ventral branch from abdominal aorta
- It supplies the structures derived from the foregut namely.
  - Lower part of esophagus
  - Stomach
  - Duodenum—1st and 2nd parts up to hepatopancreatic ampulla (major duodenal papilla)
  - Spleen
  - Pancreas
  - Liver
  - Gallbladder.
- **Origin:** From abdominal aorta at the level of T12 vertebra, just below the aortic orifice of diaphragm
- **Length:** 1.5 to 2 cm
- **Termination:** Divides into 3 branches namely.
  1. **Left gastric artery:** Ascends upwards and forms a loop to enter the lesser curvature of stomach
  2. **Common hepatic artery:** It gives off right gastric and gastroduodenal arteries and then continues as the hepatic artery proper
  3. **Splenic artery:** It is tortuous and is an end artery. It runs along the upper border of pancreas and divides into 5 segmental branches. It supplies pancreas, stomach and spleen.

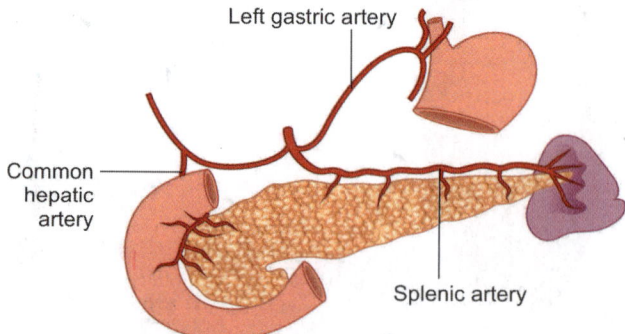

Fig. 13: Branches of celiac trunk.

- **Relations:**
  - Inferiorly—tuber omentale of pancreas, splenic vein
  - Anteriorly—lesser sac
  - Right—right celiac ganglion, left crus of diaphragm, caudate lobe of liver
  - Left—left celiac ganglion, right crus of diaphragm, cardiac end of stomach
  - It is surrounded by the celiac plexus of nerves.
- **Applied anatomy:**
  - Obstruction of the common hepatic artery proximal to right gastric artery establishes collateral circulation between gastric and gastroepiploic arteries. The blood supply to liver is restored
  - If the occlusion affects the hepatic artery proper, necrosis of liver is seen.

11. Femoral sheath.

Refer Short Notes 4 – 2005.

12. Subtalar joints.

- Joint between talus and the calcaneum on the anterior and posterior aspect is together called subtalar joint
- The posterior is called as talocalcaneal joint
- The anterior is called as talocalcaneonavicular joint.
  - **Type:** Modified multiaxial synovial joint.
  - **Bones taking part:**
    - Concave posterior articular facet along lower surface of body of talus
    - Convex posterior facet on the upper surface of calcaneum.
  - **Ligaments:**
    - Fibrous capsule is attached to articular margins and covers the joint
    - The lateral talocalcanean ligament—extends from lateral tubercle of talus to lateral surface of calcaneus
    - Medial talocalcanean ligament from medial tubercle of talus to the medial surface of calcaneus behind sustentaculum tali
    - The interosseous talocalcanean ligament—thick and very strong. It is the main ligament between the talus and the calcaneum. It extends from sulcus tali to calcaneus sulcus
    - The cervical ligament is lateral to the sinus tarsi. Extends from the superior surface of calcaneus to neck of talus.

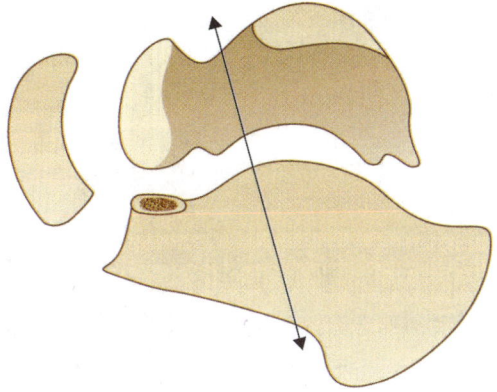

Fig. 14: Subtalar joint.

- **Nerve supply:** Posterior tibial nerve, sural nerve and medial plantar nerve
- **Movements:** The joint participates in the movements of inversion and eversion of the foot
- **Axis of movement:** The axis passes from posterior part of calcaneus through sinus tarsi, to the superomedial part of neck of talus
- **Muscles producing:**
  - **Inversion:** Tibialis anterior and tibialis posterior
  - **Eversion:** Peroneus longus and brevis.

13. Histology of spleen.

Refer Short Notes 3 – 2005.

14. Development of urinary bladder.

Refer Short Notes 10 – 2007.

15. Superficial perineal pouch.

- It is a triangular space in the perineum lying superficial to the perineal membrane.
- **Boundaries:**
  - Superficially: Colle's fascia
  - Deep: perineal membrane
  - On each side: Ischiopubic rami
  - Posteriorly: Closed by the fusion of perineal membrane with Colle's fascia

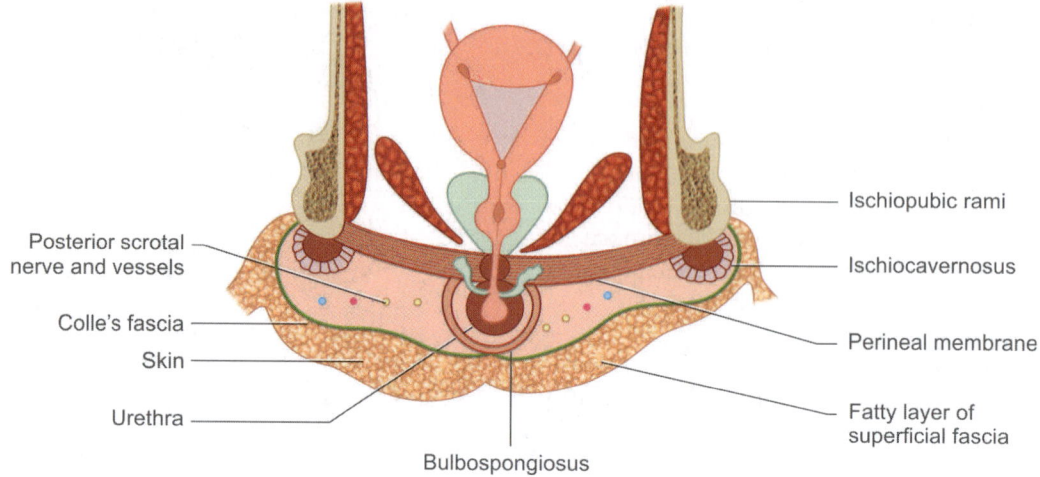

Fig. 15: Superficial perineal pouch.

- Anteriorly: In male, open and continuous with the spaces of scrotum, penis and anterior abdominal wall (superficial inguinal space)
- In female, open and continuous with the spaces of clitoris and the anterior abdominal wall.
- **Contents:**
  - 3 muscles: Ischiocavernous, transverse perineii superficialis, bulbospongiosus
  - 3 vessels: Two posterior scrotal or labial vessels, transverse perineal vessels
  - 3 nerves: Two posterior scrotal or labial branches of the perineal nerve, perineal branch of posterior femoral cutaneous nerve
  - 3 roots: Two Crura of penis or crura of clitoris, bulb of penis/vestibule
  - In male, urethra
  - In female, urethra and vagina and greater vestibular gland.
- **Applied anatomy:** In extravasation of urine, urine accumulates in this pouch, then ascends into the anterior abdominal wall in front of pubic symphysis.

16. Arteria profunda brachii.

- It is the larger branch of the brachial artery.
- **Origin:** It arises from brachial artery posteromedially
- **Level:** Arises just below the level of teres major

- **Course:**
  - It enters the lower triangular space along with the radial nerve between long and medial heads of triceps
  - Runs downwards and laterally in the spiral groove covered by the lateral head of triceps.
- **Termination:** In radial groove, terminates by dividing into anterior and posterior descending branches.
- **Branches:**
  - **Radial collateral (anterior descending) artery:** It is continuation of profunda brachii artery. It accompanies the radial nerve, pierces the lateral intermuscular septum and ends in front

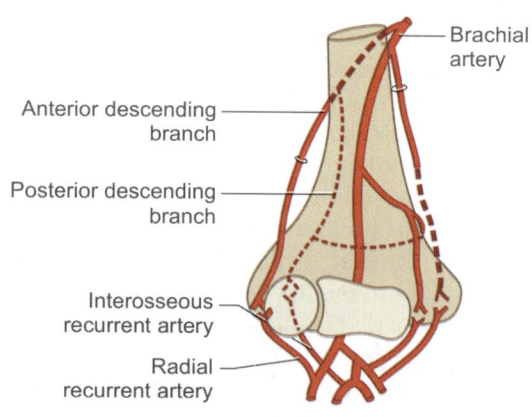

Fig. 16: Profunda brachii.

of the lateral epicondyle of humerus, by anastomosing with the radial recurrent artery branch of radial artery
- **Middle collateral (posterior descending) artery:** It descends downwards within the medial head of the triceps and ends behind the lateral epicondyle of humerus, by anastomosing with the interosseous recurrent artery
- **Muscular branches**
- **Nutrient branch** to humerus
- **Ascending branch (Deltoid branch):** Anastomose with branch from posterior circumflex humeral artery.

17. Turner's syndrome.

Refer Short Notes 28 – 2006.

18. Lesser sac.

Refer Short Notes 10 – 2005.

19. Popliteus muscle.

- It is one of the deep muscles of the posterior compartment of leg
- **Shape:** Triangular
- **Situation:** Forms the floor of the popliteal fossa.
- **Origin:**
  - Origin is intracapsular but extra synovial
  - The origin is tendinous in nature
  - The tendon is about 2.5 cm long

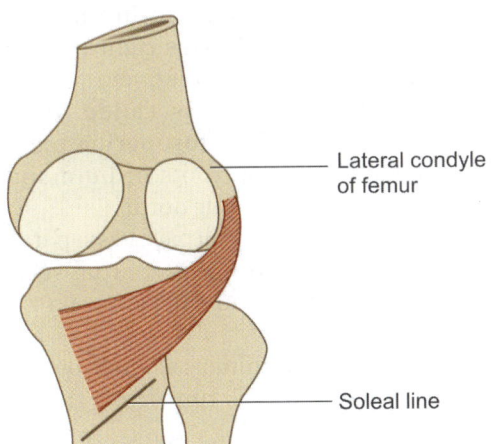

Fig. 17: Popliteus muscle.

  - From the popliteal groove on the lateral surface of lateral condyle of femur
  - Few fibers are attached to the posterior part of lateral meniscus
  - Few fibers arise from posterior surface of lateral tibial condyle, deep to popliteus are inserted to oblique popliteal ligament called **popliteus minor.**
- **Course of the tendon**
  - The tendon passes deep to fibular collateral ligament and pierces fibrous capsule of knee joint
  - Then it passes deep to inferior band of arcuate ligament (called popliteal foramen) and ends in fleshy fibers.
- **Insertion:**
  - Insertion is fleshy
  - Into the posterior surface of the shaft of tibia above the soleal line.
- **Nerve supply:**
  - Nerve to popliteus which is a branch from the tibial nerve
  - This nerve winds around the lower margin of the muscle and supplies on its anterior surface.
- **Blood supply:** By branches of popliteal artery.
- **Relations:** Posteriorly—fascia covering the muscle, gastrocnemius, plantaris, popliteal vessels, tibial nerve.
- **Action:**
  - It is the key muscle which unlocks the knee joint by lateral rotation of femur on tibia and initiates flexion in fully extended knee
  - Pulls the lateral meniscus backwards so that it is not crushed between the condyles of femur and tibia.
- **Peculiarities of the muscle:**
  - The origin is intracapsular
  - Origin is extra synovial
  - Origin is tendinous in nature
  - Insertion is fleshy
  - The nerve to the muscle winds around the lower border of the muscle to supply the anterior surface.

20. Dorsalis pedis artery.
Refer Short Notes 19 – 2008.

21. Development of face.
Refer Short Notes 22 – 2007.

22. Otic ganglion.
- It is a peripheral parasympathetic ganglion
- Anatomically related to the mandibular nerve, functionally to the glossopharyngeal nerve
- Situated in the infratemporal fossa below foramen ovale medial to trunk of mandibular nerve
- It is concerned with supply of secretomotor fibers to parotid gland
- **Relations**
  Laterally—lateral pterygoid muscle and trunk of mandibular nerve
  Medially—tensor palati muscle.
- **Roots (Fig. 18)**
  - *Parasympathetic root:* Inferior salivatory nucleus ⟶ glossopharyngeal nerve ⟶ tympanic branch and plexus ⟶ lesser petrosal nerve (relays) ⟶ otic ganglion (postganglionic fibers) ⟶ auriculotemporal nerve parotid gland
  - *Sympathetic root:* Postganglionic fibers from superior cervical ganglion passes through otic ganglion without relaying. It supplies vasomotor fibers to parotid gland.
  - *Sensory root:* Sensation from parotid gland is carried by auriculotemporal nerve.
- **Branches (Fig. 18)**
  - Branch to auriculotemporal nerve containing postganglionic fibers to the parotid gland
  - Nerve to tensor palati and tensor tympani pass through the ganglion without relaying
  - Communicating branch to chorda tympani nerve
  - Communicating branch to the nerve of pterygoid canal. Through this communication an additional pathway is made for the taste sensation from the anterior two-thirds of the tongue. It reaches the geniculate ganglion directly bypassing the tympanic cavity.

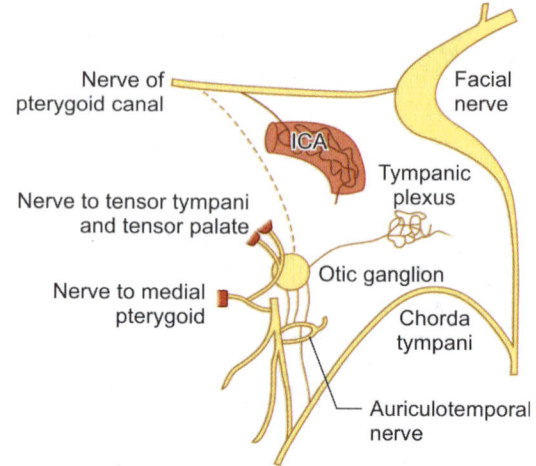

Fig. 18: Otic ganglion.

23. Cerebellar peduncles.
Refer Short Notes 20 – 2006.

24. Right atrium.
- **External features**
  - Right atrium contributes for sternocostal surface, right border and base (posterior surface) of heart
  - Sternocostal surface: It is separated from right ventricle by anterior part of coronary sulcus (atrioventricular sulcus), which lodges right coronary artery and small cardiac vein
  - A muscular process called auricle extend from anterosuperior part of atrium covering roots of pulmonary trunk and ascending aorta
  - Base: It forms a small part. It is separated from left atrium by inter atrial sulcus. The superior and inferior vena cava enter posteriorly
  - The sulcus terminalis extends between the SVC and IVC, runs along the right border.
- **Internal Features**
  Refer Essay 7 – 2006.

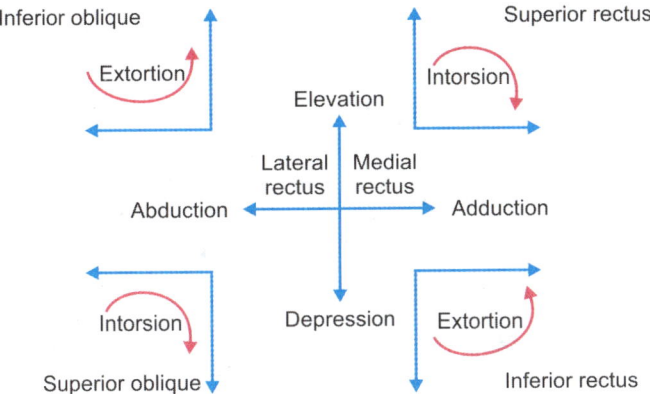

Fig. 19: Movements of extraocular muscles.

25. Extraocular muscles.

- Extraocular muscles are seven in number
- Four recti, two oblique muscles and levator palpabrae superioris
    - The **recti muscles** are strap muscles—superior, inferior, medial and lateral recti
    - Arises from common tendinous ring
    - Inserted to the sclera in front of equator
    - All the recti except lateral rectus is supplied by the oculomotor nerve
    - The lateral rectus by abducent nerve
    - The **oblique muscles** are:
        - The superior oblique is originates from roof and the inferior oblique from floor of the orbit
        - The oblique muscles are inserted to the sclera behind the equator
        - The superior oblique is supplied by trochlear nerve
        - The inferior by oculomotor nerve.
    - **Levator palpabrae superioris** arises from roof of the orbit. It is inserted to skin of upper eyelid, superior tarsal plate, lateral Whitnall's tubercle, medial palpabral ligament. It is supplied by oculomotor nerve.
- The actions of the muscle are **(Fig. 19)**:
    - Medial rectus—adduction
    - Lateral rectus—abduction
    - Superior rectus—elevation, adduction, intorsion
    - Inferior rectus—depression, adduction, extorsion
    - Superior oblique—abduction, depression and intorsion
    - Inferior oblique—abduction, elevation, extorsion
    - levator palpabrae superioris elevates the upper eyelid.

26. Palatine tonsil.

Refer Short Notes 32 – 2008.

27. Nerve supply of tongue.

Refer Essay on Q. No. 6 – 2007.

28. Tympanic membrane.

Refer Short Notes 26 – 2005.

29. Bronchopulmonary segments.

Refer Essay Q. No. 3 – 2004.

30. Ansa cervicalis.

Refer Short Notes 26 – 2008.

31. Ciliary ganglion.

- It is one of the peripheral parasympathetic ganglion
- It is concerned with supply of intraocular muscles namely iris (sphincter and dilator pupillae) and ciliaris
- It is functionally connected to oculomotor nerve and anatomically related to optic nerve
- **Situation (Fig. 20)**
    - In the orbit close to its apex
    - In between optic nerve and lateral rectus
    - Connected to nasociliary nerve
    - It is 1cm in front of medial end of superior orbital fissure

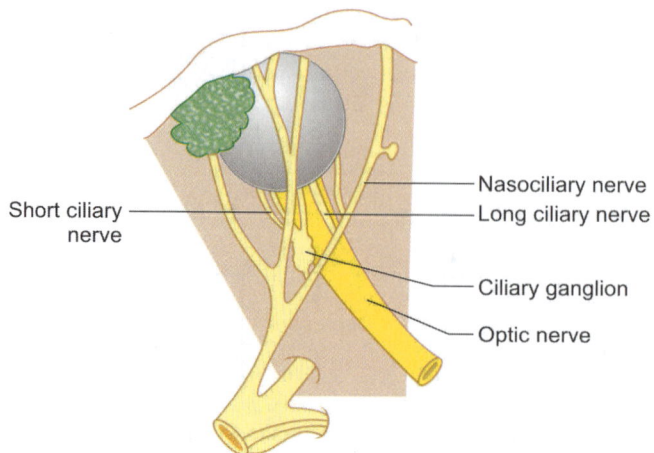

Fig. 20: Ciliary ganglion.

- The ophthalmic artery is medial to the ganglion.
- Size of pins head
- **Roots (Fig. 21)**
    - **Parasympathetic root**
    Preganglionic fibers arise from Edinger Westphal nucleus in midbrain ----- oculomotor nerve ----- inferior division ------ nerve to inferior oblique ------- ciliary ganglion --Synapse-- short ciliary nerve (post ganglionic fibers) ------- to sphincter pupillae and ciliaris. 95 % of the fibers are for ciliaris muscle.
    - **Sympathetic root**
    Postganglionic fibers from superior cervical ganglion --------- plexus around internal carotid artery ----- ophthalmic artery ------ ciliary ganglion (without relaying) --------- short ciliary nerves ---- dilator papillae and blood vessels of uveal tract.
    - **Sensory root**
    The sensation from cornea, ciliary body and iris is carried by short ciliary nerves ----- ciliary ganglion ------- communicates with long ciliary nerve--------- ophthalmic nerve.
- **Branches**
Short ciliary nerve about 5 – 8 branches surround the optic nerve. Each branch in turn divides and pierces the sclera around optic nerve.

32. Facial artery.
Refer Short Notes 26 – 2007.

33. Interpeduncular fossa.
- It is a depressed area situated in the base of brain.
- **Boundaries (Fig. 22):**
    - Anteriorly: Optic chiasma
    - Anterolaterally: Optic tracts
    - Posterolaterally: Crus cerebri
    - Posteriorly: Upper border of pons.
- **Contents:**
    - Tubercinerium: Situated between optic chiasma and mammillary bodies. It is an elevated structure made of gray matter. To this the infundibulum of pituitary is attached
    - Mammillary bodies: Smooth pea shaped eminences. It encloses the nuclei derived from fornix
    - Posterior perforated substance: Found between the two crura cerebri. The central branches of posterior cerebral arteries pierces it
    - Oculomotor nerve: Emerges medial to the crus cerebri, between posterior cerebral and superior cerebellar arteries.

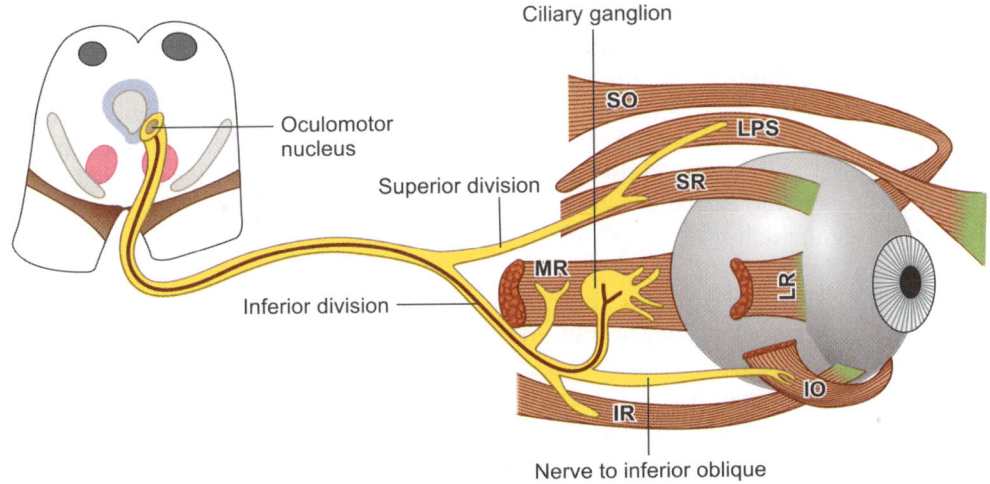

Fig. 21: Parasympathetic root of ciliary ganglion.

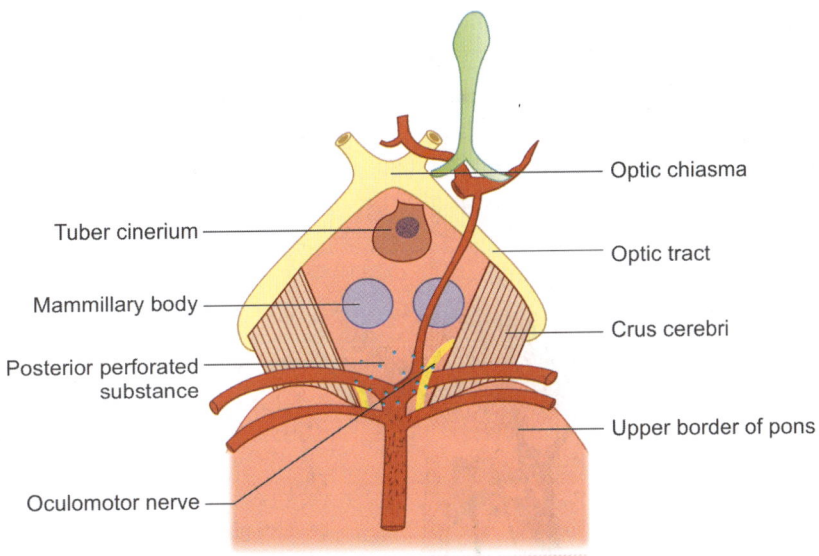

Fig. 22: Interpeduncular fossa.

- **Relations:** The interpeduncular cistern and circle of Willis
- **Applied anatomy:** Upward enlargement of pituitary gland may compress the structures found in relation to the fossa.

34. Midline structures of the neck.

The midline of neck extends from symphysis menti to suprasternal notch.
It is divided into suprahyoid and infrahyoid structures.

- Suprahyoid structures:
  – Below symphysis menti is the raphe formed by decussation of mylohyoid muscle fibers. It extends from symphysis menti to the hyoid bone
  – Body of hyoid bone.
- Infrahyoid structures:
  – Thyroid cartilage with laryngeal prominence
  – Thyrohyoid membrane between thyroid cartilage and hyoid bone

- Anterior arch of cricoid cartilage
- Anterior (median) cricothyroid ligament between the thyroid and cricoid cartilages
- The trachea
- Cricotracheal membrane between trachea and cricoid cartilage
- Anterior jugular ach
- Isthmus of thyroid gland
- Anastomosis of the superior thyroid arteries along upper border of thyroid gland
- Pyramidal lobe a glandular projection from isthmus sometimes present
- Levator glandulae thyroideae
- Inferior thyroid vein
- Suprasternal space of burns.

35. Histology of cornea.

- The cornea is made up of five layers, from anterior to posterior are: 1. Corneal epithelium, 2. Anterior limiting lamina (Bowman's layer), 3. Substantia propria (Corneal stroma), 4. Posterior limiting lamina (Descemet's membrane) and 5. Endothelium
- **Corneal epithelium**
  - 10% of the corneal thickness is contributed by the corneal epithelium
  - It is lined by non-keratinized stratified squamous epithelium
  - It is usually made of 5 – 6 layers of cells
  - The deepest cells are columnar
  - Middle 2 – 3 layers are made of polyhedral cells
  - The more superficial cells are flat
  - The surface cells are provided with finger-like microvilli which helps to retain the tear fluid.
- **Anterior limiting lamina (Bowman's layer)**
  - It contains bundles of collagen fibrils
  - It is like that of the substantia propria
  - But fibroblasts are absent.
- **Substantia propria (Corneal stroma)**
  - The substantia propria forms major part of the cornea
  - It is composed of 200 – 250 lamellae

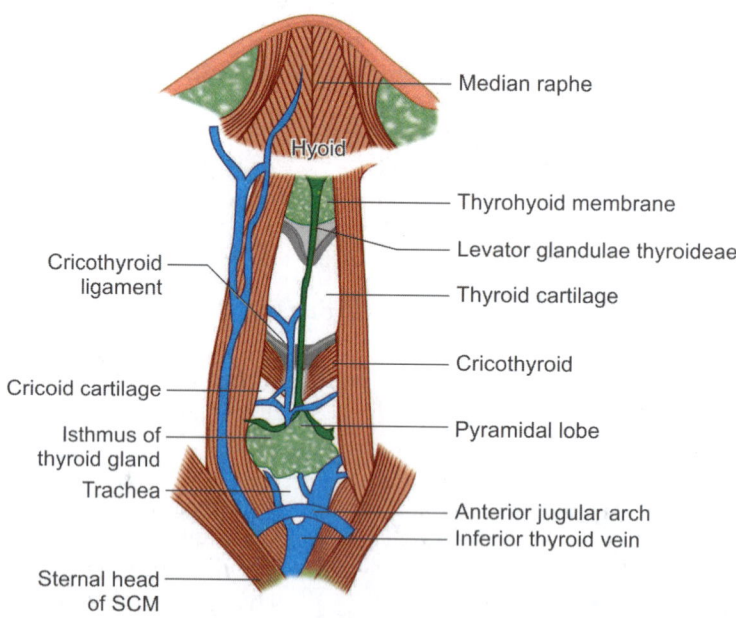

Fig. 23: Midline structures of neck.

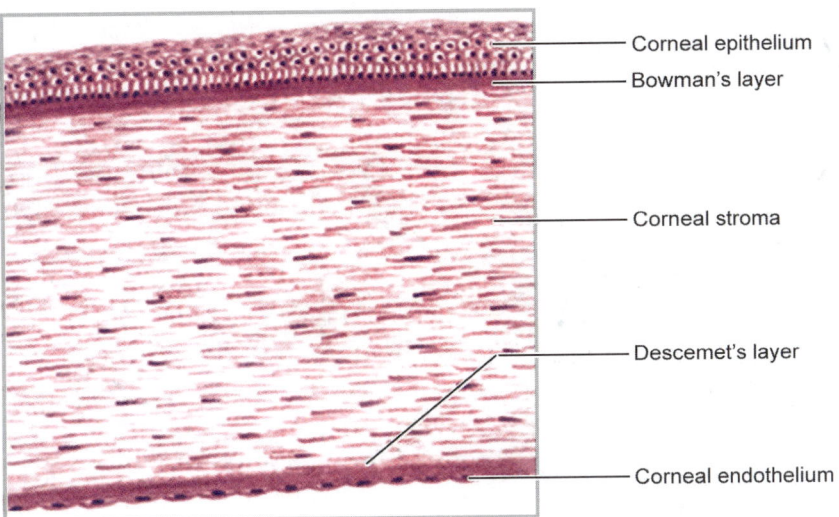

Fig. 24: Histology of cornea.

- Fine Type I collagen fibrils are present in the lamella
- The collagen fibers run parallel to each other
- Corneal corpuscles/keratocytes are flat dendritic interconnecting fibroblasts seen between the lamellae
- The regular arrangement of the collagen fibers are responsible for transparency.

- **Posterior limiting lamina (Descemet's layer)**
  - The posterior limiting lamina covers the substantia propria posteriorly
  - It is thin and similar to corneal stroma
  - It is considered as the basement membrane of the endothelium.
- **Endothelium**
  - The endothelium covers the posterior surface of the cornea
  - It is made of a simple squamous cells
  - It is in contact with aqueous humour
  - It helps for transport of ions by diffusion
  - Helps to pump out the excess fluid and helps for transparency.

36. Pleural recesses.
Refer Essay Q. No. 3 – 2003.

37. Development of thyroid gland.
Refer Essay on Q. No. 8 – 2007.

38. Lateral medullary syndrome.
- It is also known as **Wallenberg/PICA syndrome**
- It is due to vascular lesion of posterior inferior cerebellar artery branch of vertebral artery
- It may be due to thrombosis or hemorrhage of the vessel
- The artery supplies the lateral part of the medulla oblongata
- The **structures affected** are:
  - Spinal nucleus and tract of trigeminal
  - Nucleus ambiguous
  - Inferior cerebellar peduncle
  - Vestibular nuclei
  - Anterior spinocerebellar tract
  - Lateral spinothalamic tract.
- **Effect of lesion**
  - Due to lesion of vestibular nuclei: Vertigo, nausea, nystagmus
  - Due to lesion of nucleus ambiguus: Dysphagia, dysarthria as the muscles of palate, pharynx and larynx are paralyzed
  - Due to involvement of spinal nucleus and tract of trigeminal: Analgesia and

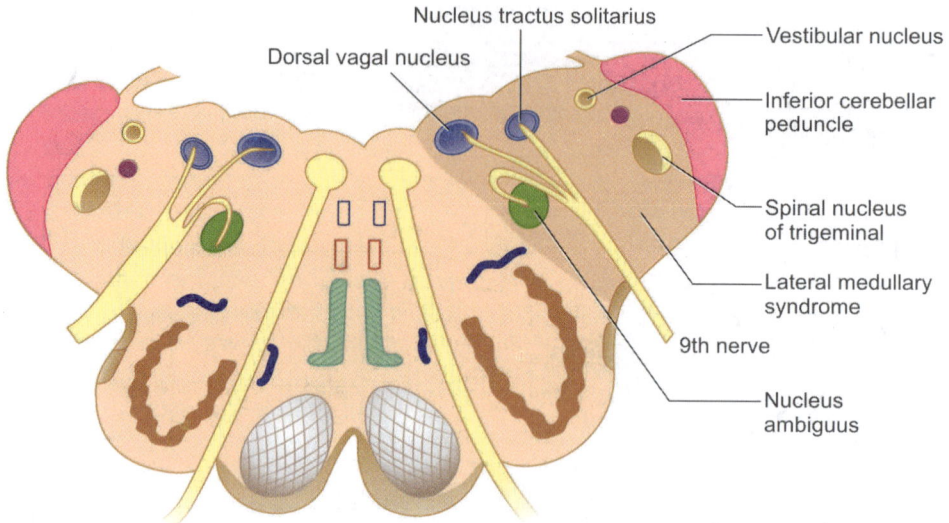

Fig. 25: Lateral medullary syndrome.

thermoanesthesia over the opposite side of face
- Due to spinothalamic tract involvement: Contralateral thermoanesthesia (loss of pain and temperature).

39. Subclavian triangle.

- The posterior triangle of neck is divided into two by the inferior belly of omohyoid muscle
- The inferior belly of omohyoid crosses the triangle, approximately 2.5 cm above the clavicle
- By that, the triangle is subdivided into occipital and subclavian triangles
- The subclavian triangle is the lower and smaller division of the posterior triangle
- It is also called as **supraclavicular or omoclavicular triangle**
- In the living the triangle is represented as hollow supraclavicular fossa
- **Boundaries**
  - Superiorly—inferior belly of omohyoid
  - Floor—the first rib, scalenus medius and the first digitation of serratus anterior
  - Anteriorly—posterior border of sternocleidomastoid
  - Posteriorly—anterior border of trapezius
  - Roof—skin, superficial fascia with platysma and investing layer of deep cervical fascia and crossed by the supraclavicular nerves.
- **Contents**
  - Third part of subclavian artery
  - Subclavian vein (sometimes)
  - Trunks of brachial plexus
  - Suprascapular artery and transverse cervical artery
    - Branches from thyrocervical trunk—1st part of subclavian artery
  - Terminal part of external jugular vein and its tributaries
  - Nerve to subclavius and suprascapular nerve
    - Branches from upper trunk (Erb's point)
  - Lymph nodes
- **Applied anatomy:** Brachial plexus block is done by injecting anesthetic drugs into the supraclavicular part of brachial plexus at the midpoint of the clavicle.

40. TS at the level of superior colliculus of midbrain.

- Interior of midbrain is divided by the cerebral aqueduct into a ventral part called cerebral peduncle and a dorsal part the tectum

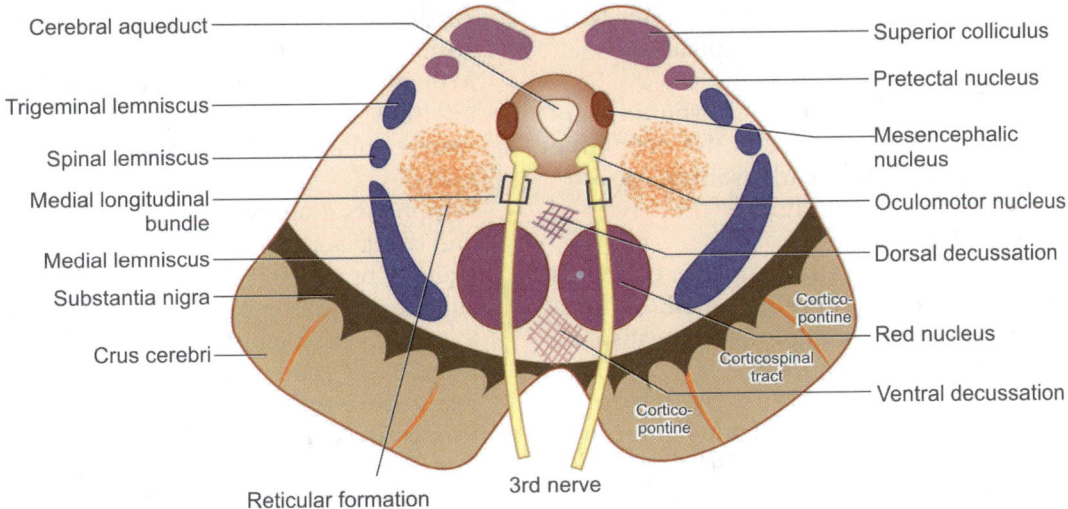

Fig. 26: Section of midbrain at superior colliculus.

- The cerebral peduncle includes—1. **crus cerebri** which is a divided part, 2. united **tegmental part** and 3. **substantia nigra** which is in between the two parts
- **Crus cerebri (basis pedunculi)**
  - Consists of bundles of corticospinal and corticobulbar fibers occupying middle two-third.
  - The corticobulbar fibers are for cranial nerve nuclei and corticospinal the pyramidal tract from motor area
  - Medial one-sixth frontopontine fibers
  - Lateral one-sixth by temporopontine and parieto, occipitopontine fibers
  - The pontine fibers arise from area 4, and 6 of cerebral cortex.
- **Tegmentum**
  - Gray matter
    - Periaqueductal gray matter is present.
    - The **oculomotor nucleus** is situated in it. The oculomotor nucleus contains motor nucleus to supply extraocular muscles and a parasympathetic component the Edinger-Westphal nucleus to supply intraocular muscles
    - The oculomotor nerve passes ventrally through red nucleus and emerges medial to the crus cerebri
    - **Mesencephalic nucleus of trigeminal is** dorsolateral in the gray matter.

It receives proprioceptive impulses from muscles of mastication, ocular and facial muscles
  - **Red nucleus** is situated dorsomedial to substantia nigra. Afferent connection: Dentatorubral and Corticorubral, pallidorubral fibers. Efferent connections: Rubrospinal and rubroreticular tracts
  - The fibers from red nucleus decussate ventrally forming **ventral decussation of Forel**.
  - White matter
    - **Decussation** of the tectospinal and tectobulbar fibers arising from superior colliculi form the **dorsal tegmental decussation of Meynert**
    - **Medial longitudinal fasciculus** is ventral to oculomotor nucleus
    - The **lemnisci**—medial, spinal, trigeminal are present. The medial lemniscus is crossed posterior column of spinal cord. The spinal lemniscus is crossed lateral spinothalamic tract and trigeminal lemniscus is crossed fibers carrying sensation from one half of face.
- **Substantia nigra** is connected to basal ganglia.

- It is divided into i) dorsal pars compacta and ii) ventral pars reticulate
- Dopamine is secreted by it
- Degeneration of the substantia nigra results in decrease in the dopamine level leading to Parkinson's diseases
- **Cerebral aqueduct** is the cavity of midbrain
- **Tectum:** Nucleus of superior colliculus is present. The efferent fibers from superior colliculus form the tectospinal and tectobulbar tracts
- Pretectal nucleus is situated superolateral to colliculus. It receives afferent fibers from optic tract and efferent to Edinger-Westphal nucleus. It is concerned with pupillary reflex and consensual light reflex.

III. SHORT ANSWER QUESTIONS

1. Enumerate the contents of spermatic cord.

- Vas deferens—passes along posterior part of cord. The tail of epididymis is continued as vas
- Pampiniform plexuses of veins—at superficial inguinal ring join to form four veins. In turn it forms two veins at deep inguinal ring. In abdomen continued as testicular vein. The right vein drains to IVC and left to left renal vein
- Testicular artery—branch of abdominal aorta
- Artery to vas—branch from superior/inferior vesical artery
- Artery to cremaster—from inferior epigastric artery
- Lymphatics draining the testis end in pre- and lateral aortic nodes
- Genital branch of genitofemoral nerve supplies cremaster muscle
- Sympathetic plexus—testicular plexus from T_{10} - T_{11} and pelvic plexus accompanying artery to vas
- Processus vaginalis persists as fibrous thread
- Accessory suprarenal cortical tissue sometimes present.

2. Enumerate the bare areas of liver.

- The bare area on the posterior surface of right lobe, bounded by superior, inferior coronary ligaments and groove for inferior vena cava
- Groove for inferior vena cava at the medial end of bare area
- Fossa for gallbladder, contains loose areolar tissue.

3. Name four tributaries of inferior vena cava.

- Pair of common iliac veins
- Pair of renal veins
- Pair of inferior phrenic veins
- Right gonadal vein

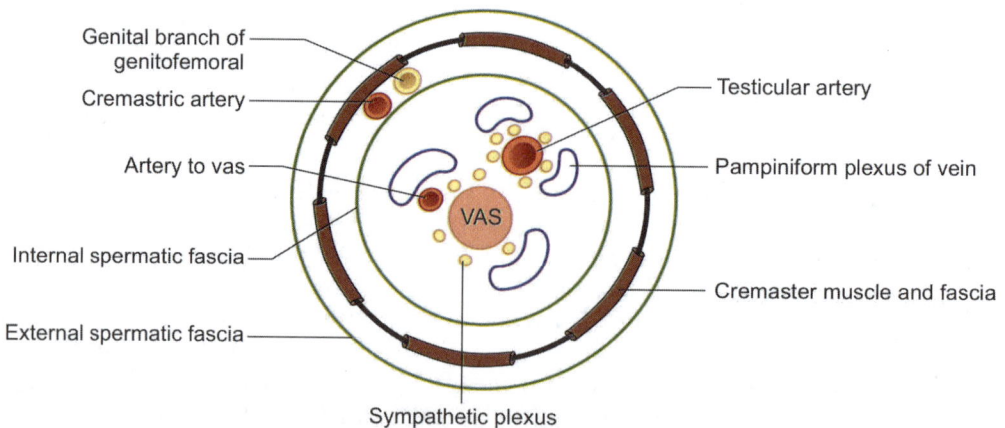

Fig. 27: Contents of spermatic cord.

- Right suprarenal vein
- Four pairs of lumbar veins
- Hepatic veins.

4. Nerve supply of the lumbricals of the hand.

- There are four lumbricals and are numbered from lateral to medial side.
  - 1st and 2nd are unipennate, 3rd and 4th are bipennate muscles
  - Lumbricals 1 and 2—from the tendons of flexor digitorum profundus for index and middle fingers along its lateral side
  - Lumbricals 3 and 4—from adjacent sides of tendons of flexor digitorum profundus for middle, ring and little fingers.
- **Nerve supply:**
  - First and second lumbricals by median nerve
  - Third and fourth lumbricals by deep branch of ulnar nerve.

5. Name the muscles supplied by the obturator nerve.

- Obturator nerve is a branch of the lumbar plexus
- It is formed by the **ventral divisions** of the anterior primary rami of L_2, L_3, L_4
- Within the obturator canal, the nerve divides into anterior and posterior divisions.
- Structures **supplied**:
  - **Anterior division**
    - **Muscular branches** to adductor longus, gracilis, pectineus, adductor brevis
    - **Articular branch** to hip joint
    - **Cutaneous branch** through sub sartorial plexus to skin of medial side of thigh
    - **Vascular branch** to femoral artery.
  - **Posterior division** supplies the following:
    - **Muscular branches** to obturator externus, adductor brevis, adductor magnus
    - **Articular branch** to knee joint (genicular branch)
    - **Vascular branch** to popliteal artery.

6. Erb's point.

- Erb's point is a point which is junction point of six nerves
- Six nerves are: Ventral rami of C_5 and C_6 join to form upper trunk of brachial plexus
- The upper trunk divides into anterior and posterior divisions
- The branches from upper trunk are suprascapular nerve and nerve to subclavius
- It is situated above the clavicle and a content of the subclavian triangle
- Applied anatomy: **Erb's palsy/Erb – Duchenne paralysis**
- **Causes of injury:** Birth injury—traction of arm, motor cycle accidents with outstretched hand and fall on the shoulder
- **Muscles paralyzed:** Mainly biceps brachii, deltoid, brachialis and short muscles of shoulder—supraspinatus, infraspinatus and supinator
- The deformity is known as **policeman receiving tip** or **waiter receiving tip**.

7. Name the contents of superficial perineal pouch.

- 3 muscles: Ischiocavernous, transverse perineii superficialis, bulbospongiosus
- 3 vessels: Two posterior scrotal or labial vessels, transverse perineal vessels
- 3 nerves: Two posterior scrotal or labial branches of the perineal nerve, perineal branch of posterior femoral cutaneous nerve
- 3 roots: Two crura of penis or crura of clitoris is, bulb of penis or vestibule
- Urethra in both sex
- In addition in female, vagina and greater vestibular gland.

8. Name the bones forming medial longitudinal arch of foot.

- Medial longitudinal arch is made of calcaneus, head of talus, navicular, three cuneiforms, first three metatarsal bones
- Anterior end—by heads of 1st, 2nd and 3rd metatarsals
- Posterior end—by medial tubercle of the calcaneum

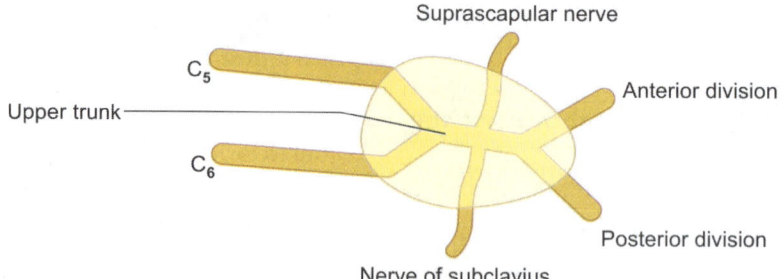

Fig. 28: Erb's point.

- Summit—by superior articular surface of body of talus.
- Pillars:
  - Anterior pillar is long and weak, formed by talus, navicular, the three cuneiform bones and the first 3 metatarsals
  - Posterior pillar is short and strong, formed by medial part of calcaneum.

9. Enumerate four structures related to the anterior surface of left kidney.

- Superior pole: Left suprarenal gland
- Left half: Spleen
- Central quadrilateral area: Pancreas and splenic vessels
- Above pancreas triangular area: Stomach
- Below pancreas along lateral border: Left colic flexure
- Medial area below pancreas: Coils of jejunum.

10. Name four derivatives of ectoderm.

- **Surface ectoderm** gives rise to:
  - Epidermis of skin
  - Epithelium of cornea and conjunctiva
  - Lens of eye
  - Enamel of tooth
  - Hair and nails
  - Arrector pilorum
  - Sebaceous and sweat glands
  - Anterior pituitary
  - Epithelium of cheek, gum, palate
  - Epithelium of external acoustic meatus
  - Lining of membranous labyrinth of the internal ear.
  - Secretory part and ducts lining the lacrimal, nasal, labial, oral and salivary glands.
- **Neuroectoderm** gives rise to:
  - Brain
  - Spinal cord

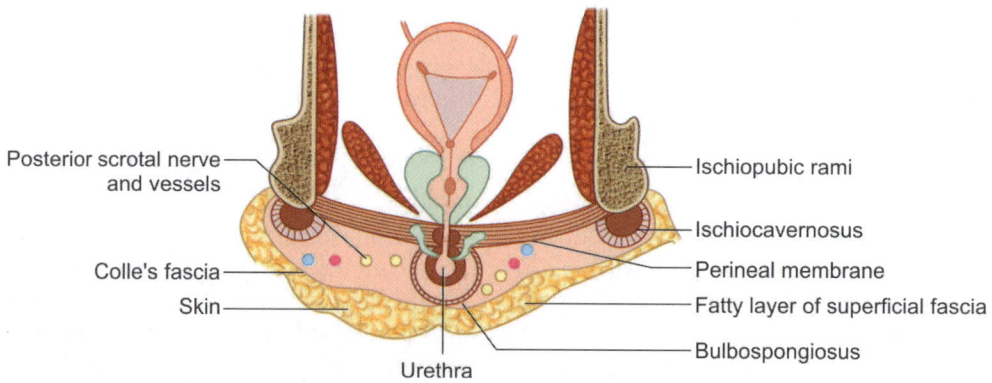

Fig. 29: Contents of superficial perineal pouch.

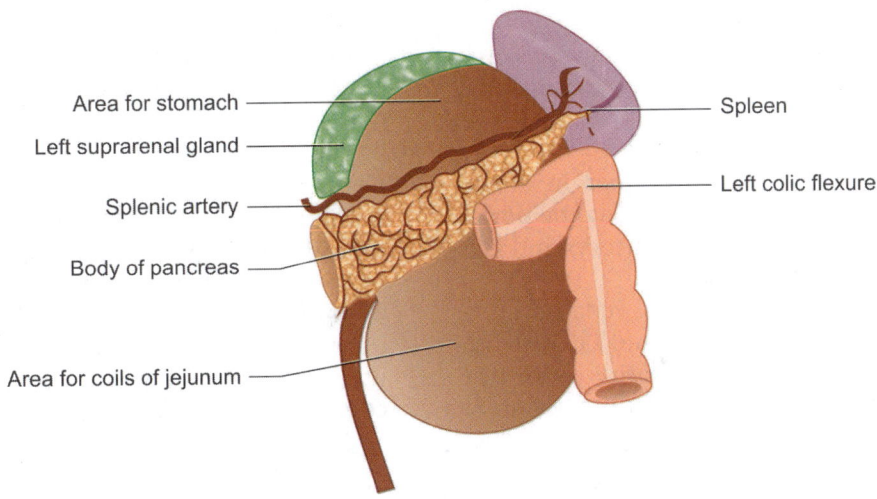

Fig. 30: Relations of anterior surface of left kidney.

- Neural crest derivatives—autonomic nervous system, melanocytes, adrenal medulla
- Posterior pituitary
- Muscles of iris—sphincter and dilator pupillae

(All the muscles of the body are developed from mesoderm except the muscles of iris and arrector pilorum of skin).

11. Name the structures piercing clavipectoral fascia.

- Clavipectoral fascia is a fibrous sheet
- Extends from pectoralis minor to clavicle
- Situated deep to the clavicular part of pectoralis major muscle
- Structures piercing: (CALL)
  - **C**ephalic vein
  - **A**cromiothoracic (Thoraco-acromial) artery
  - **L**ateral pectoral nerve
  - **L**ymphatics draining into the apical group of lymph node.

12. Give the action of lumbrical muscle.

- The lumbricals are attached to the tendons of flexor digitorum profundus
- The tendons of the lumbricals cross the radial side of metacarpophalangeal joints
- Insertion is through the dorsal digital expansion of the corresponding digit from second to fifth
- Inserted into the lateral side of dorsal surface of bases of middle and distal phalanges
- Actions
- Lumbricals flex the metacarpophalangeal joints and extend the interphalangeal joints.

13. Name the structures deep to flexor retinaculum of hand.

- Flexor retinaculum is a strong fibrous band bridging the anterior concavity of the carpal bones and converting it into a tunnel called the carpal tunnel
- It extends from pisiform bone, hook of the hamate medially to tubercle of the scaphoid, crest of the trapezium laterally
- **Structures passing deep** to flexor retinaculum:
  - Median nerve
  - Tendons of flexor digitorum superficialis
  - Tendons of flexor digitorum profundus
  - Tendon of flexor pollicis longus
  - Tendon of flexor carpi radialis
  - Ulnar bursa
  - Radial bursa.

14. Give the boundaries of epiploic foramen.

- It is also known as **foramen of Winslow**
- Epiploic foramen is **situated** behind the free border of lesser omentum

- **Level of situation:** T12 vertebra
- **Communication:** The greater sac communicates with the lesser sac through this foramen.
- **Boundaries:**
  - Anteriorly: Right free margin of the lesser omentum containing the portal vein, proper hepatic artery, and the common hepatic duct
  - Posteriorly: The inferior vena cava, the right suprarenal gland and T12 vertebra
  - Superiorly: Caudate process of the liver
  - Inferiorly: First part of the duodenum and the horizontal part of the hepatic artery.
- **Applied anatomy:**
  - Internal herniation—the loop of intestine herniates through epiploic foramen into the lesser sac
  - The collection of fluid in the hepatorenal pouch can enter the lesser sac through this foramen.

15. Give the significance of Douglas pouch.

- It is also known as **pouch of Douglas**
- In female peritoneum from rectum is reflected to the posterior wall of vagina forming this pouch
- Boundaries:
  - Anteriorly: Upper one-third of posterior wall of vagina, supra vaginal part of cervix
  - Posteriorly: Peritoneum covering upper two-third of anterior surface of rectum
  - Floor: It is 5.5 cm from anal orifice and 7.5 cm from orifice of vagina
  - Lateral walls: Rectouterine folds
- **Contents:** Sigmoid colon and coils of intestine
- **Significance:** The pus/blood collected in the pouch may be removed, without opening the anterior abdominal wall, by an incision or needling through posterior fornix of vagina called **posterior colpotomy**.

16. What is annular pancreas?

- Pancreas is endodermal in origin
- It is developed from the lower end of foregut which forms the second part of duodenum
- Developed in 2 parts—dorsal bud and ventral bud
  - Dorsal bud arises from dorsal wall of primitive duodenum. It is proximal to ventral bud
  - Ventral bud has two components and is from the bile duct which arises from junction of foregut and midgut. The two components fuse and then undergoes rotation
- **Annular pancreas:** The two components of the ventral pancreatic bud sometimes

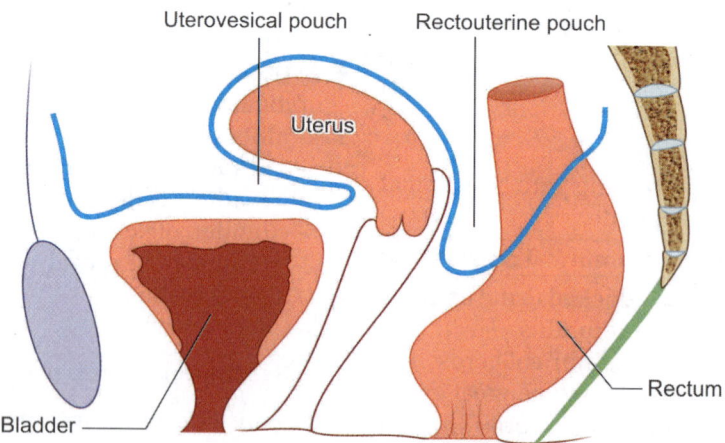

Fig. 31: Pouch of Douglas.

fail to fuse. In such conditions, these two components grow in opposite directions around the duodenum and meet the dorsal pancreatic bud. The annular pancreas thus formed produces duodenal obstruction.

17. Name the branches of external iliac artery.

- The external iliac is principally the artery of lower limb.
- Common iliac artery divides into external and internal iliac arteries at the level of sacroiliac joint
- The external iliac artery is continued as femoral artery from the level of midinguinal point
- The **branches** given by the external iliac are
    - **Inferior epigastric artery**
        - Arises posterior to inguinal ligament
        - Ascends up medial to the deep inguinal ring, deep to spermatic cord
        - It pierces the transversalis fascia and enters the rectus sheath
        - It produced an elevation in the parietal peritoneum called **lateral umbilical fold**
        - It anastomoses with the superior epigastric artery above umbilicus within the rectus sheath
        - It also anastomoses with lower six intercostal arteries deep to rectus abdominis
        - The **cremastric artery** is branch from inferior epigastric and supplies cremaster
        - **Pubic branch** given near femoral ring anastomose with pubic branch of obturator artery
        - The artery forms the lateral boundary for the Hesselbach triangle.
    - **Deep circumflex iliac artery**
        - Runs laterally behind inguinal ligament to anterior superior iliac spine
        - Anastomose with lateral circumflex artery.
- **Applied anatomy**:
    - The pubic branch from inferior epigastric is sometimes larger than obturator artery called **aberrant obturator artery**. If present will be related to the medial border of femoral ring may be injured during femoral hernial repair
    - Collateral circulation is established by the anastomosis between superior and inferior epigastric arteries.

18. Name the structures piercing oblique popliteal ligament.

- The oblique popliteal ligament is a ligament of knee joint
- The oblique popliteal ligament is a fibrous expansion from semimembranosus muscle
- It extends from tendon of the muscle to lateral condyle of femur and intercondylar line
- **Structures piercing are:**
    - Middle genicular artery branch from popliteal artery pierces the oblique popliteal ligament to supply the cruciate ligament and synovial membrane. It is given at mid-point of posterior surface of knee joint
    - Articular branch from posterior division of obturator nerve pierces the oblique popliteal ligament and supplies the fibrous capsule
    - Some lymph vessels which drain the knee joint and terminates to popliteal node.

19. Name the arteries forming trochanteric anastomosis.

- **Situation:**
    - Close to the trochanteric fossa of femur
    - Extracapsular arterial ring formed around the neck of femur
    - Anastomosis formed between internal iliac and profunda femoris.
- **Formation:**
    - Descending branch of superior gluteal artery branch from internal iliac artery

- Descending branch of inferior gluteal artery from anterior iliac artery
- Ascending branch of medial circumflex femoral artery branch of profunda femoris
- Branch of lateral circumflex femoral artery branch of profunda femoris
- First perforating branch of profunda femoris.
- **Function:**
  - From the arterial ring retinacular branches arise pass along the neck of femur
  - Supplies the head of femur.
- **Applied anatomy:** Intracapsular fracture neck of femur results in injury to these vessels, leading to avascular necrosis of head of femur.

20. Name the contents of subsartorial canal.
- Subsartorial canal is an intermuscular tunnel in the thigh region
- Situation: In distal ⅔ of medial side of thigh.
- Extent: From apex of femoral triangle to tendinous opening in adductor magnus
- Contents:
  - Femoral artery
  - Femoral vein is posterior to artery in the upper part and then it becomes lateral
  - Saphenous nerve crosses the artery from lateral to medial side
  - Nerve to vastus medialis
  - Descending genicular artery
  - Posterior division of obturator nerve.

21. Draw and label the histology of trachea.
Refer Short Notes 32 – 2005.

22. Name the structures present in the lateral wall of cavernous sinus.
- Cavernous sinus extends from apex of petrous part of temporal bone to medial end of superior orbital fissure
- It has a roof, floor, medial and lateral walls, anterior and posterior ends
- Structures present in the lateral wall are:
  - Oculomotor nerve—pierces the roof and runs forward and divides into two divisions
  - Trochlear nerve—runs forwards and laterally
  - Ophthalmic nerve—runs forwards and divides into 3 branches namely frontal, lacrimal and nasociliary nerves
  - Maxillary nerve—leaves the lateral wall to pass through foramen rotundum.

23. Nerve supply of larynx.
- Motor nerve supply:
  - **Somatomotor fibers**—all the intrinsic muscles of larynx are supplied by the recurrent laryngeal nerve except cricothyroid by the external laryngeal nerve

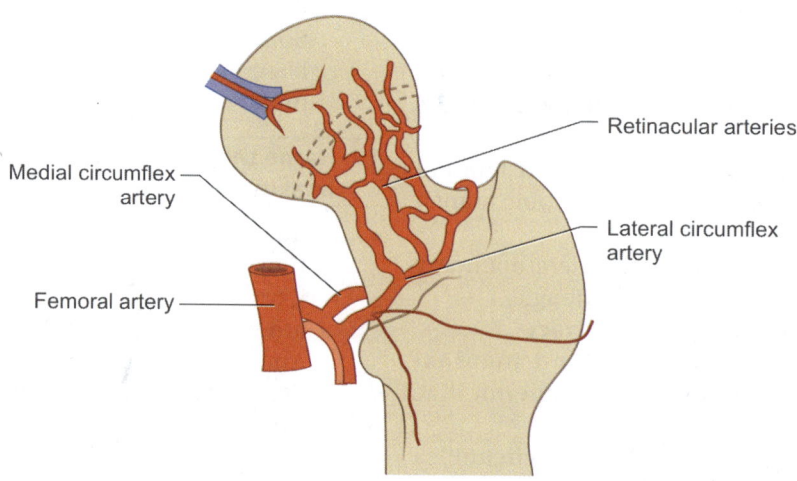

Fig. 32: Trochanteric anastomosis.

- **Secretomotor fibers** to the mucous glands of the larynx, supplied by the recurrent and internal laryngeal nerves
- **Vasomotor fibers** to the vessels of larynx by the postganglionic sympathetic fibers from superior and middle cervical ganglions.
- Sensory nerve supply:
  - The mucous membrane above vocal cord supplied by the internal laryngeal nerve
  - The mucous membrane below vocal cord by the recurrent laryngeal nerve.

24. Parts of corpus callosum.

- Corpus callosum forms the commissural fibers of white matter
- It is the largest commissural fiber of brain connecting the two cerebral hemispheres.
- It connects all the parts of cerebral hemispheres of two sides
- Shape: C shaped
- **Parts of corpus callosum**:
  - Rostrum
  - Genu
  - Body
  - Splenium.

25. Four derivatives of ectoderm.

Refer Short Answers 10 – 2009.

26. Enumerate four branches of 1st part of maxillary artery.

- The maxillary artery is the larger terminal branch of external carotid artery
- It is given posterior to the neck of mandible
- The maxillary artery passes medial to the neck of mandible and reaches the lower border of lateral pterygoid muscle
- Then it lies superficial to the muscle and dips into the pterygomaxillary fissure
- It enters the pterygopalatine fossa and terminates as sphenopalatine branches
- The lateral pterygoid muscle divides the artery into three parts
- The first part is from origin to lower border of lateral pterygoid muscle
- The branches from 1st part are:
  - **Anterior tympanic**—supply middle ear by passing through the petrotympanic fissure
  - **Deep auricular**—to external acoustic meatus
  - **Middle meningeal**—enters cranial cavity through foramen spinosum to supply meninges of middle and anterior cranial fossae
  - **Accessory meningeal**—passes through foramen ovale and supply meninges of middle cranial fossa
  - **Inferior alveolar**—enters mandibular foramen to supply lower jaw teeth.

27. Structures passing through the foramen ovale (MALE).

- Foramen ovale is in the greater wing of sphenoid bone
- It connects the middle cranial fossa with infratemporal fossa
- The structures passing are:
  - **M**andibular nerve—both sensory and motor roots
  - **A**ccessory meningeal artery
  - **L**esser petrosal nerve
  - **E**missary vein.

28. Tributaries of coronary sinus.

Refer Essay Q. No. 5 – 2005.

29. Name the bones forming the nasal septum.

Refer Short Notes 17 – 2003.

30. Name muscles of mastication.

- The muscles of mastication produce movement of the mandible at temporomandibular joint
- They are developed from 1st pharyngeal arch
- Supplied by mandibular nerve
- The muscles included are:
  - Masseter
  - Temporalis
  - Lateral pterygoid
  - Medial pterygoid.

31. What is ligamentum arteriosum?

- The sixth aortic arch proximal and distal parts behave differently on right and left side
- On the right side proximal part forms the right pulmonary artery and the dorsal part disappears
- On the left side the proximal part forms the left pulmonary artery and dorsal part persists as the ductus arteriosus in fetal life
- The ductus connects the left pulmonary artery to the arch of aorta
- Connection between left pulmonary artery to arch of aorta is distal to the left subclavian artery
- The duct gets obliterated soon after birth to form **ligamentum arteriosum**
- The duct is closed functionally by contraction of muscular wall of the artery
- Anatomical closure occurs 3 months after birth by proliferation of tunica intima
- The left recurrent laryngeal nerve passes lateral to the ligamentum arteriosum

Applied anatomy: Patent ductus arteriosus is failure of closure of the ductus arteriosus.

32. Significance of pyriform fossa.

- It is a fossa in the laryngopharynx
- It is situated on either side of inlet of larynx
- **Boundaries:**
  - Medially—aryepiglottic fold of mucous membrane
  - Laterally—thyroid cartilage and thyrohyoid membrane
  - Posteriorly—extends from lower part of C_3 to upper part of C_6.
- **Applied anatomy**
  - Acts as a catch point for foreign body. Fish bone or foreign body stuck in the floor of the fossa can damage the internal laryngeal nerve leading to hoarseness of voice
  - Sometimes the fossa is artificially deepened by smugglers to hide some materials.

33. Name the muscles of mastication.

Refer Short Notes 30 – 2009.

34. Give the subdivisions of mediastinum.

- **Subdivisions:**
  - The mediastinum is divided into **superior** mediastinum and **inferior** mediastinum by an imaginary line passing through the lower border of body of 4th thoracic vertebra behind and the sternal angle of Louis in front
  - The inferior is further subdivided into 3 by the pericardium:
    i. Anterior mediastinum—part in front of pericardium
    ii. Middle mediastinum—part enclosed within pericardium
    iii. Posterior mediastinum—part behind the pericardium.

35. What are Hassall's corpuscles?

- Thymus contains numerous Hassall's corpuscles in the medulla
- They are also known as thymic corpuscles
- Hassall's corpuscles start appearing before birth and increase in number throughout life
- They are round/oval in shape
- The corpuscles contain **degenerating centers** formed by cellular debris, degenerating thymocytes forming a homogenous eosinophilic mass encircled by concentrically (whorls) arranged flattened epitheliocytes
- The function of the corpuscles are unknown.

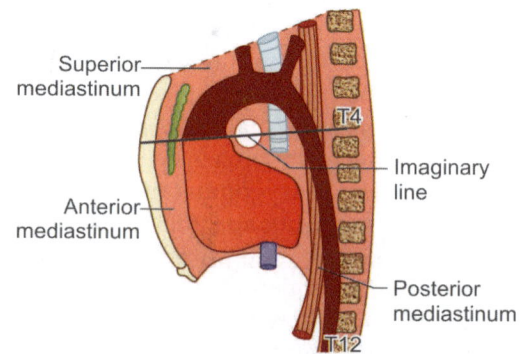

Fig. 33: Subdivisions of mediastinum.

36. Name the splanchnic nerves in the thoracic region.

- **Greater splanchnic nerve**
  - Formed by fusion of branches from fifth to ninth thoracic sympathetic ganglions
  - It is myelinated preganglionic fibers
  - It contains efferent and visceral afferent fibers
  - It supplies descending thoracic aorta
  - It pierces the crus of diaphragm
  - It ends in celiac ganglion, aortic renal ganglion, suprarenal gland.
- **Lesser splanchnic nerve**
  - From ninth and tenth ganglion
  - It pierces the crus of diaphragm and end in aorticorenal ganglion.
- **Least splanchnic nerve**
  - From twelfth thoracic ganglion and end in renal plexus
  - Enters the abdomen by passing deep to medial arcuate ligament.

37. What is danger area of face?

- The upper lip and the adjoining part of the nose form the dangerous area of face.
- The face is connected to cavernous sinus by two routes:
  1. **Direct route** connecting facial vein with cavernous sinus through superior ophthalmic vein
  2. **Indirect route** is the anterior facial vein connected to pterygoid venous plexus through deep facial vein which in turn is connected to cavernous sinus through emissary veins through foramen ovale and lacerum.
- The facial vein is devoid of valves and rests directly on the facial muscles
- The movement of facial muscles may facilitate the spread of septic emboli from the infected area of upper lip and lower part of the nose in retrograde direction and cause thrombosis of cavernous sinus.

38. Give the attachment of suprapleural membrane.

- Suprapleural membrane covers the cervical pleura over the apex of the lung
- The summit of the pleura is 3 to 4 cm above the 1st costal cartilage.
- It is covered by suprapleural membrane called **Sibson's fascia**
- It **extends** from tip of 7th cervical vertebra to the inner border of 1st rib

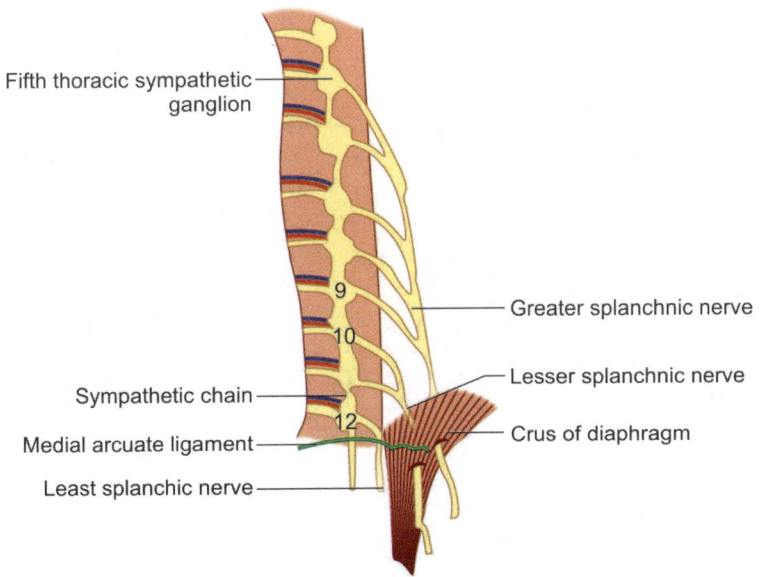

Fig. 34: Splanchnic nerves.

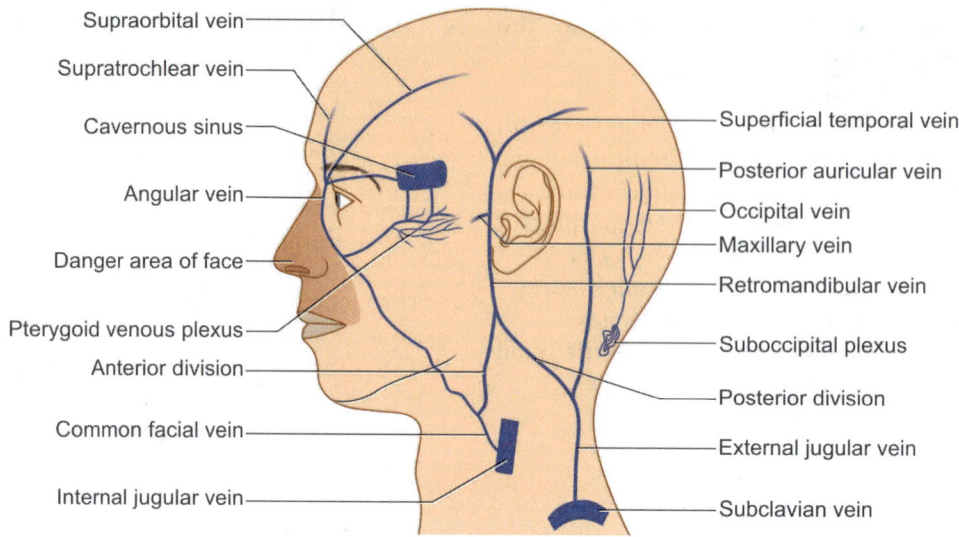

Fig. 35: Danger area of face.

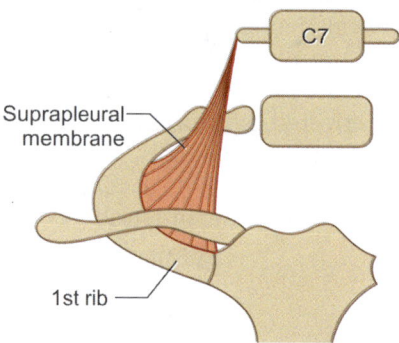

Fig. 36: Suprapleural membrane.

- It contains few muscle fibers derived from scalenus medius muscle known as **scalenus minimus**.

39. What is insula?

- Insula is the submerged cortex
- It is also known as **island of Reil**
- It is considered as **fifth lobe**
- Situated in the superolateral surface of cerebrum
- It lies deep to the posterior ramus of lateral sulcus
- It is covered by three opercula namely:
  1. Frontal operculum formed by pars opercularis of the inferior frontal gyrus
  2. Frontoparieto operculum by posterior part of inferior frontal gyrus, pre and post central gyri
  3. Temporal operculum by the superior temporal gyrus.
- It is surrounded by a circular sulcus, which is deficient anteriorly called **limen insuli**
- The insula is **divided** by a central insular sulcus into a larger anterior and smaller posterior part **(Fig. 37)**
- The anterior part is divided into three or four smaller gyri and posterior part has one long gyrus
- The middle cerebral artery is related to the insula
- **Deep to the insula** are claustrum, external capsule and lentiform nucleus **(Fig. 38)**.

40. What is visual stria?

- Visual cortex is characterized by the presence of outer band of Baillarger - **stria of Gennari**

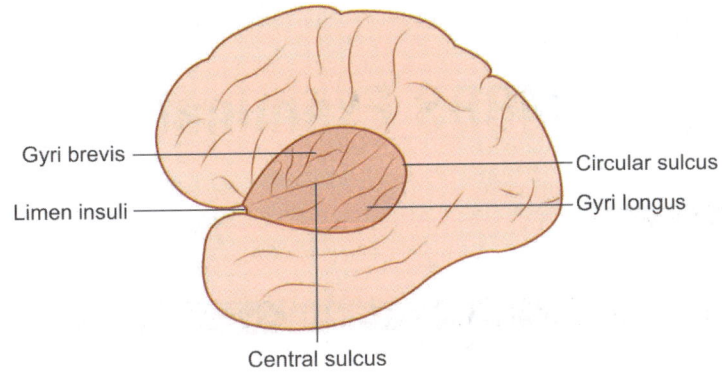

Fig. 37: Insula.

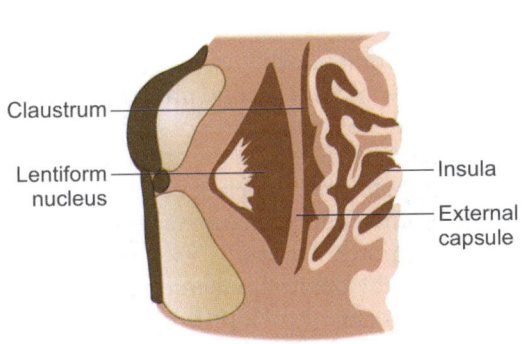

Fig. 38: Structures deep to insula.

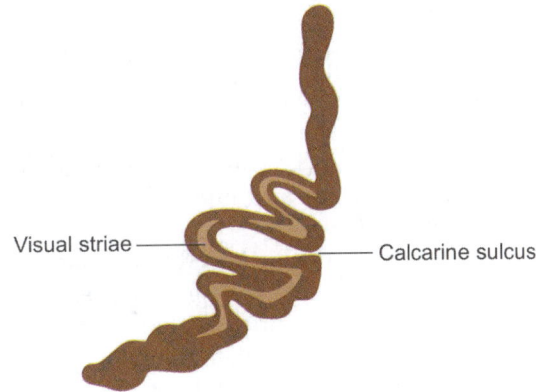

Fig. 39: Visual striae.

- It is a prominent white line within the gray matter of visual cortex
- It is present in the layer 4 of cerebral cortex.
- The visual cortex is granular
- The layer 4 is subdivided into three layers— from superficial to deep are IVa, IVb, IVc

- IVc contains more neurons and is further divided into superficial and deep layers
- The stria is present in IVb
- IVb contains less cells and more non-pyramidal neurons
- The fibers from lateral geniculate body mainly end in IVa and IVc.

MBBS Examination 2010

ANSWER ALL QUESTIONS

I. Essay questions (15/10 Marks)

1. Describe the stomach under the following headings: Parts, relations, blood supply, lymphatic drainage and applied aspects.
2. Describe the formation, course, relations, branches and distribution of radial nerve and effects of injury of radial nerve.
3. Describe the urinary bladder under the following headings surfaces and borders, relations, blood supply, histology and applied aspects.
4. Describe the shoulder joint under articular surfaces, capsule, ligaments, movements and muscles causing them, applied aspects.
5. Describe the parotid gland under the following headings: (a) Location and parts, (b) Relations, (c) Covering, (d) Nerve Supply and (e) Applied anatomy.
6. Describe in detail congenital anomalies of the heart.
7. Describe the superolateral surface of the cerebral hemisphere under the following headings: Sulci and gyri, functional areas and arterial supply.
8. Describe the arch of aorta under the following headings: Extent, relations, branches and microscopic anatomy.

II. Short notes (5/4 Marks)

1. Cubital fossa.
2. Cartilaginous joints.
3. Microscopic structure of suprarenal gland.
4. Inguinal canal.
5. Ligaments around the hip joint.
6. Turner's syndrome.
7. Microscopic structure of hyaline cartilage.
8. Omental bursa.
9. Derivatives of second pharyngeal arch.
10. Peroneal retinacula.
11. Carpal tunnel.
12. Hepatorenal pouch
13. Microscopic structure of testis.
14. Supports of uterus.
15. Medial longitudinal arch of foot.
16. Blood supply of long bone.
17. Obturator nerve.
18. Epiploic foramen.
19. Klinefelter's syndrome.
20. Menisci of knee joint.
21. Development of tongue.
22. Facial artery.
23. Nerve supply of lacrimal gland.
24. Histology of pituitary gland.
25. Atlantoaxial joints.
26. Hyoglossus muscle.
27. Cardiac plexuses.
28. Right coronary artery.
29. Mediastinal surface of left lung.
30. Klinefelter syndrome.
31. Vocal cord.
32. Hilum of right lung.
33. Styloid apparatus.
34. Histology of parathyroid gland.
35. Development of interatrial septum.
36. Parotid duct.
37. Blood supply of spinal cord.
38. Venous drainage of face.
39. Middle meatus of nose.
40. Carotid sheath.

III. Short answer questions (3/2 Marks)

1. Name the arteries supplying transverse colon.
2. Name the muscles forming rotator cuff around shoulder joint.
3. Name the Hamstring muscles.
4. Name the muscles within the rectus sheath.
5. Name the branches arising from lateral cord of brachial plexus.
6. Name the ligaments present within the knee joint.
7. Popliteus muscle.
8. Name the coverings of testis.
9. Name the muscles of I layer of sole of the foot.
10. Name the muscles causing lateral rotation at hip joint.
11. Name any two tarsal bones of the foot.
12. Name the muscles causing abduction at wrist joint.
13. Name the terminal branches of sciatic nerve.
14. Name the arteries supplying transverse colon
15. Name the branches arising from posterior cord of the brachial plexus.
16. Name the muscles present within the deep perineal pouch.
17. Name the parts of the uterine tube.
18. Name the coverings of kidney.
19. Name the two most common positions of appendix.
20. Name the structures piercing the clavipectoral fascia.
21. Mention different parts of diencephalon.
22. Emissary veins.
23. Lacus lacrimalis.
24. Lymphatic drainage of the face.
25. Horner's syndrome.
26. Histology of skeletal muscle.
27. Triangle of Koch.
28. Barr body.
29. Types of chromosomes.
30. Bones derived from 1st pharyngeal arch.
31. Name the bones taking part in the formation of nasal septum.
32. Name the structures passing through foramen spinosum.
33. Name any two nerves emerging from medulla oblongata.
34. Name any two structures in relation to mediastinal surface of left lung.
35. Name the parts of lacrimal apparatus.
36. Name the arteries which supply the heart.
37. Name the infrahyoid muscles of the neck.
38. Name the muscles of mastication.
39. Name the terminal branches of facial nerve.
40. Name the unpaired cartilages of the larynx.

I. ESSAY QUESTIONS

1. **Describe the stomach under the following headings: Parts, relations, blood supply, lymphatic drainage and applied aspects.**

Parts, relations, blood supply, applied anatomy - Refer Essay Q. No. 2 – 2007.
Lymphatic drainage – Refer Short Notes 6 – 2007.

2. **Describe the formation, course, relations, branches and distribution of radial nerve and effects of injury of radial nerve.**

- It is the largest branch of the posterior cord of the brachial plexus
- It is a nerve of extensor compartment of arm and forearm
- It supplies the muscles of the posterior compartment of arm and forearm.

Formation (Root Value)

It is a branch from the posterior cord with a root value of C5-C8, T1.

Course

- **In the axilla**: It runs posterior to the 3rd part of axillary artery. It leaves the axilla by passing posteriorly accompanied by profunda brachii through lower triangular space.

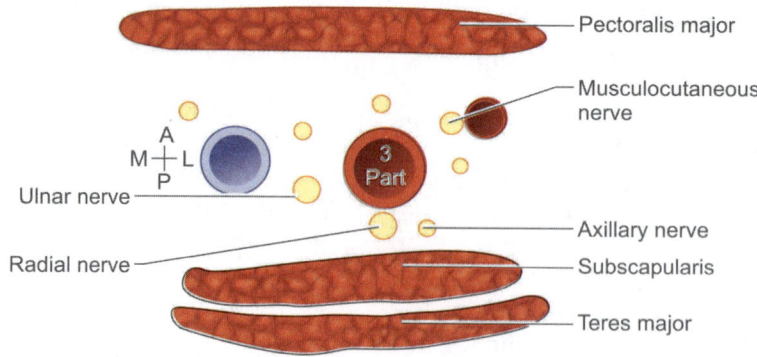

Fig. 1: Relation in axilla.

- **In the spiral groove:**
  - By passing through the lower triangular space the radial nerve reaches the radial groove (spiral groove) on the back of the humerus
  - In the spiral groove, it runs downwards and laterally
  - Pierces the lateral intermuscular septum to enter front of arm.
- **In the anterior compartment of arm**
  - It passes in the groove between the brachialis and laterally brachioradialis and extensor carpi radialis longus
  - In the cubital fossa, it terminates by dividing into a superficial and a deep branch at the level of lateral epicondyle of humerus.

Relations

- **In the axilla (Fig. 1):**
  - Anterior—3rd part of axillary artery
  - Posterior—subscapularis, latissimus dorsi, teres major
  - Medial—axillary vein
  - Lateral—axillary nerve and coracobrachialis.
- **In the upper part of arm:**
  - Anterior: Brachial artery
  - In lower triangular space
    - Above—teres major
    - Medial—long head of triceps brachii
    - Lateral—humerus.
- **In radial groove:** Anterior: Spiral groove of humerus, separated from bone by the medial head of triceps

- **In anterior compartment of arm:**
  - Medial: Brachialis
  - Lateral: Brachioradialis above, and extensor carpi radialis longus below.

Branches and Distribution

- **In the axilla (Fig. 2):**
  - **Muscular branches**
    - Branch to the long head of triceps
    - Branch to the medial head of triceps – the branch is long and lies close to ulnar nerve extends up to distal third of arm, hence called as **ulnar collateral nerve.**
  - **Cutaneous branch:** Posterior cutaneous nerve of arm supplies the skin on the posterior surface of arm
  - **Articular branch:** The ulnar collateral branch supply the elbow joint.
- **In the spiral groove (Fig. 2):**
  - **Muscular branches**
    - Branch to lateral head of triceps
    - Branch to medial head of triceps
    - Branch to anconeus given in spiral groove descends within the medial head of triceps and terminate by supplying the muscle
  - **Cutaneous branches**
    - Lower lateral cutaneous nerve of arm supplies the skin of lower half of lateral part of arm
    - Posterior cutaneous nerve of forearm supplies dorsum of forearm

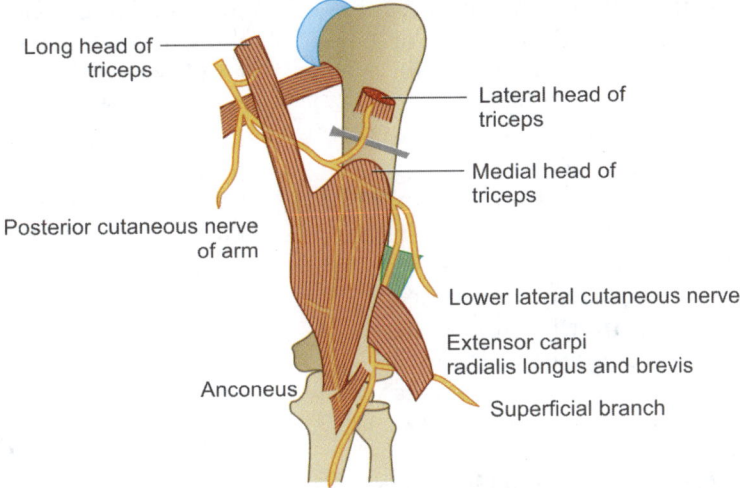

Fig. 2: Radial nerve in spiral groove.

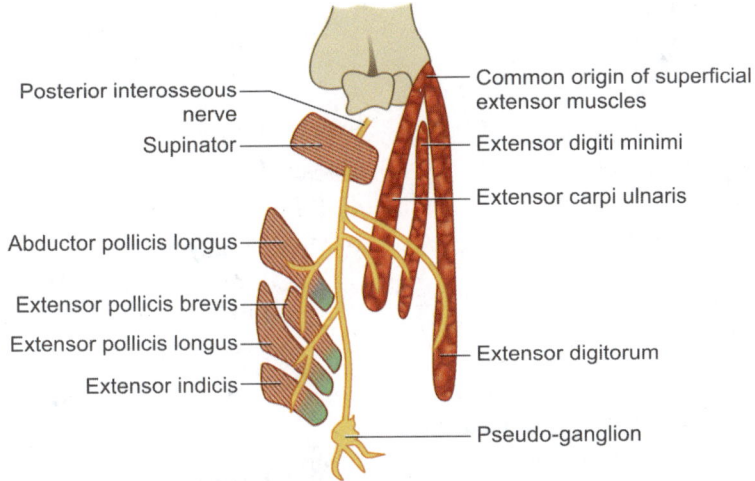

Fig. 3: Posterior interosseous nerve.

- Articular branch: To elbow joint. Nerve to anconeus supplies the elbow joint.
- **In the anterior compartment of arm:**
  - **Muscular branches to:**
    - Brachioradialis
    - Extensor carpi radialis longus
    - Lateral part of brachialis.
  - **Terminal branches**
    - Deep branch (posterior interosseous nerve)
    - Superficial branch.

- **Posterior interosseous nerve (Fig. 3):**
  - Course:
    - It enters the extensor (posterior) compartment of forearm by passing between the superficial and deep heads of supinator
    - The nerve lies between superficial and deep group of muscles
    - In the distal part it passes deep to extensor pollicis longus
    - It thins out and lies on the interosseous membrane

- It passes through fourth compartment of extensor retinaculum of wrist along with extensor digitorum longus, and extensor indicis
- It terminates as pseudoganglion dorsal to carpal bone
- It is accompanied by anterior interosseous artery.
- **Branches**
  - Muscular branches: It supplies the muscles in the posterior compartment of forearm namely
    * Extensor carpi radialis brevis given before it enters supinator muscle
    * Supinator—supplies before and while passing through two heads.
    * Extensor digitorum
    * Extensor digiti minimi
    * Extensor carpi ulnaris
    * Abductor pollicis longus
    * Extensor pollicis brevis
    * Extensor pollicis longus
    * Extensor indicis.
  - Articular branch
    * Distal radioulnar joint
    * Intercarpal joints
    * Intermetacarpal joints.
- **Superficial branch**
  - Course:
    - In the upper third of forearm it lies on supinator, lateral to radial artery, and behind brachioradialis

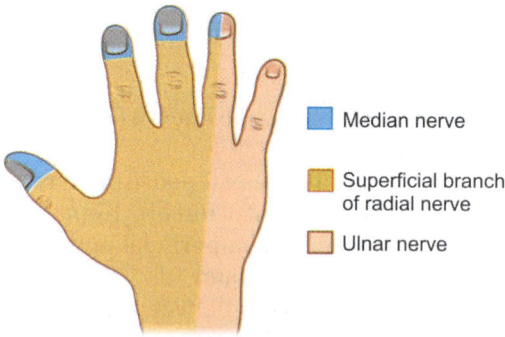

Fig. 4: Cutaneous innervation—superficial branch of radial nerve.

- In the middle third it lies on pronator teres, flexor digitorum superficialis, and flexor pollicis longus
- About 7 cm proximal to wrist it deviates away from radial artery, deep to brachioradialis tendon
- Winds around the lateral side of radius
- Pierces deep fascia and terminates into four or five dorsal digital branches.
- **Branches (Fig. 4):**
  - **Cutaneous branch:** It supplies the skin of the lateral half of dorsum of hand, proximal parts of dorsal surface of thumb, index finger and lateral half of middle finger (three and a half fingers)
  - **Articular branch:** Metacarpo phalangeal joints, proximal interphalangeal joints.

Effects of Injury

Levels

Axilla

- **Crutch palsy:**
  - Compression of radial nerve in axilla
  - All the muscles supplied by the radial nerve are paralyzed.
- **Effect:**
  - Loss of extension at elbow
  - Loss of extension at wrist (wrist drop).
- **Wrist drop features:**
  - Wrist drops due to paralysis of extensor carpi radialis longus and brevis and extensor carpi ulnaris
  - Hand drops due to paralysis of extensor digitorum and so there is loss of extension at metacarpophalangeal joints of fingers.
- Thumb drops due to paralysis of extensor pollicis longus and brevis
  - Loss of extension at metacarpophalangeal joint (finger drop)
  - Loss of sensation at the dorsum of hand (base of thumb).

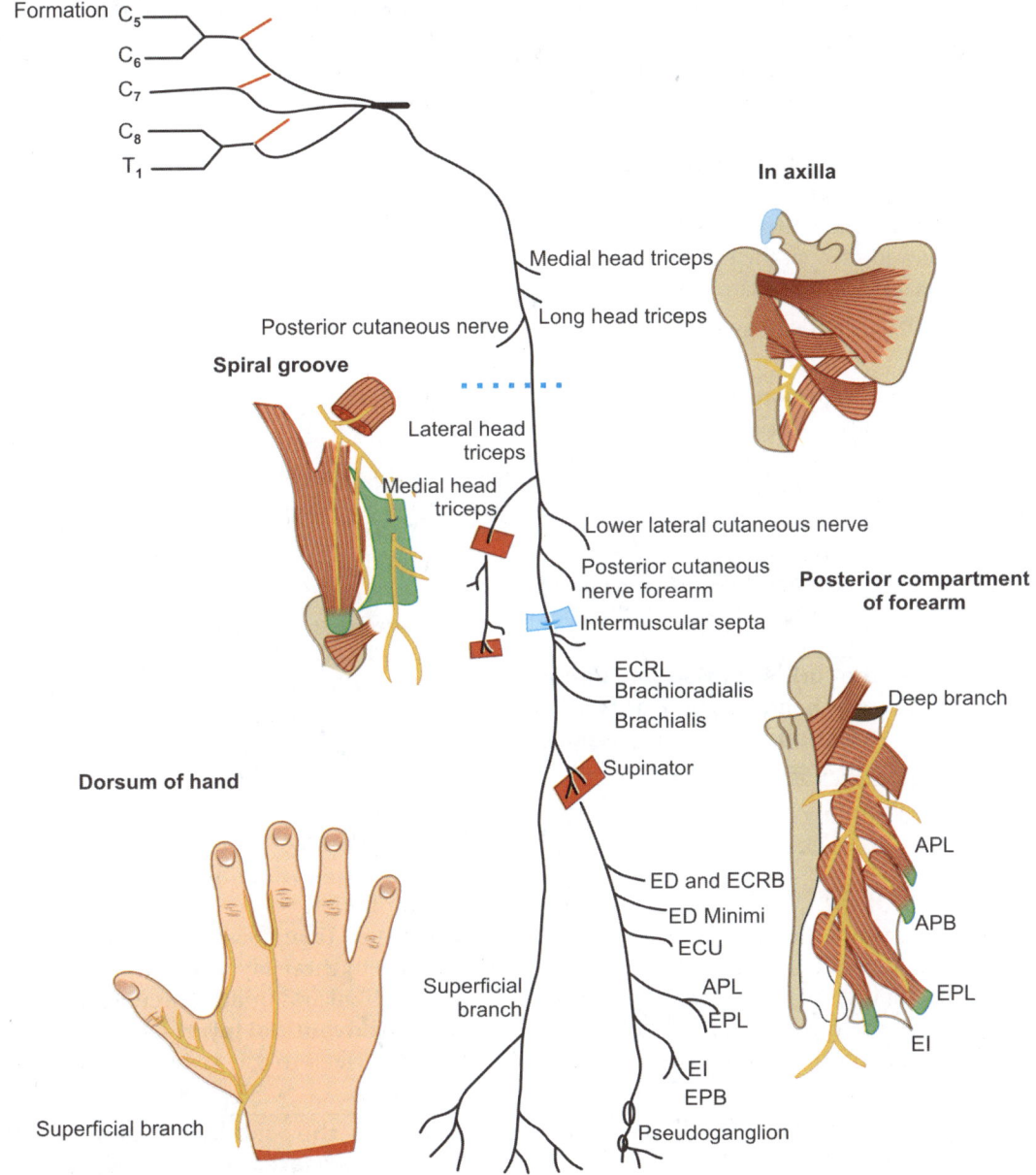

Fig. 5: Course and branches of radial nerve.

(ED: extensor digitorum; ECRB: extensor carpi radialis brevis; ED minimi: extensor digiti minimi; ECU: extensor carpi ulnaris; APL: abductor pollicis longus; EPL: extensor pollicis longus; EI: extensor indicis; EPB: extensor pollicis brevis; ECRL: extensor carpi radialis longus)

Middle of arm: Saturday night palsy

- Compression of radial nerve in the spiral groove
- Long head of triceps is spared as the branch arises at the level of axilla.

Elbow: Radial tunnel syndrome

- Due to compression of the radial nerve near the elbow
- Four structures can cause compression of the nerve. (i) The nerve is attached

by fibrous bands to humeroradial joint, (ii) medial border of extensor carpi radialis brevis which is tendinous (iii) branches from the radial recurrent artery, (iv) the arcade of Frohse, is the proximal edge of the superficial part of supinator which is aponeurotic
- The person will complain of pain distal to the elbow joint, over the extensor muscles. There is no loss of sensation or motor loss.

Forearm: Posterior interosseous nerve palsy
- The causes of posterior interosseous nerve palsy are trauma and inflammatory swellings, entrapment in radial tunnel syndrome. Pain is over the extensor compartment and is later followed by weakness and paralysis
- There is no sensory loss as the dorsal branch arises at a higher level.

3. **Describe the urinary bladder under the following headings surfaces and borders, relations, blood supply, histology and applied aspects.**

Surfaces and borders, relations, and applied aspects Refer Essay Q. No. 2 – 2003.

Blood Supply of Bladder
- **Arterial supply**
  - Superior vesical artery—branch from anterior division of internal iliac artery supply the fundus of the bladder. Its proximal portion represents the patent umbilical artery
  - Inferior vesical artery—branch from anterior division of internal iliac or middle rectal artery supply the base of bladder
  - Obturator artery—vesical branch from it supplies the bladder. Sometimes this branch replaces the inferior vesical artery
  - Inferior gluteal artery—branch of anterior division of internal iliac supply the bladder
  - Uterine artery and vaginal artery in female—replaces the inferior vesical artery.
- **Venous drainage**
  - Plexus of veins in the inferolateral surface of bladder in the space of Retzius
  - They unite and pass along the lateral ligament
  - Drain to the internal iliac vein
  - They communicate with internal vertebral venous plexus.

Histology (Fig. 6)
The mucous membrane of bladder is has many folds except at trigone.
It is made of four layers from inner to outer are as follows:
- **Mucous layer**
  - The epithelium is urothelium (transitional epithelium). The basal layer lined by cuboidal cells resting on basement membrane, the intermediate layer by polygonal cells and top layer by umbrella shaped cells
  - Lamina propria (submucosa): Made of connective tissue with elastic fibers and few smooth muscle fibers. It is rich with capillaries, nerve endings and lymphatics.
- **Muscular layer:** Made of ill-defined bundles in three layers—inner and outer longitudinal and middle circular layer
- **Serous/adventitial layer:** Layer of mesothelium. Deep to this layer adipose tissue is seen.

4. **Describe the shoulder joint under articular surfaces, capsule, ligaments, movements and muscles causing them, applied aspects.**

Refer Essay Q. No. 2 – 2006.

5. **Describe the parotid gland under the following headings: (a) Location and parts (b) Relations (c) Covering (d) Nerve Supply (e) Applied anatomy.**

Refer Essay Q. No. 4 – 2004.

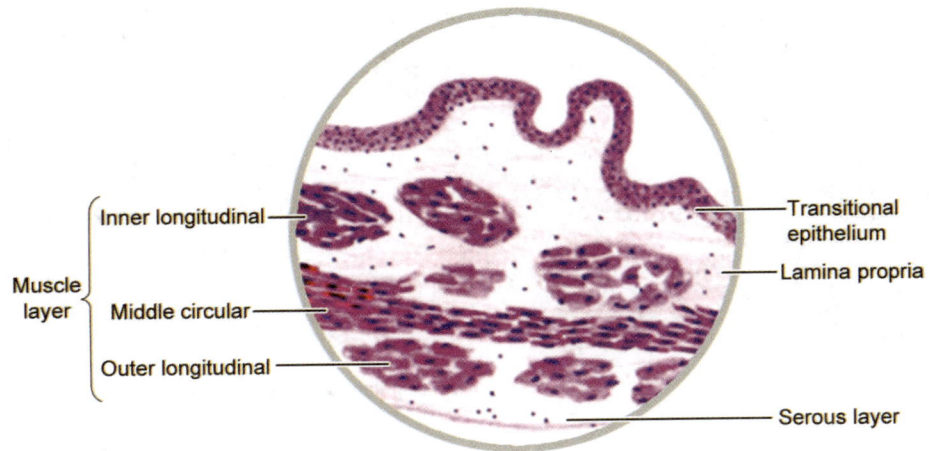

Fig. 6: Histology of urinary bladder.

6. Describe in detail congenital anomalies of the heart.

Normal Development of Heart

- The heart is developed from heart tubes
- The heart tube elongates and form four sacculations called sinus venosus, primitive atrium, primitive ventricle and bulbus cordis
- On 23rd day the tube begins looping to the right side and is completed by 28th day
- Sinus venosus gives rise to posterior smooth part of right atrium
- From atrial portion common atrium is developed
- Primitive ventricle form primitive left ventricle
- The bulbus cordis is divided into three parts. The proximal part forms the rough part of right ventricle, the middle part the conus cordis form the outflow portion of both ventricles, the distal part the truncus arteriosus
- The conotruncal part of the heart tube initially on the right side shifts gradually medial side
- This results in formation of transverse dilatations of the atrium.
- **Septation** starts in:
  - Septation of common atrium by interatrial septum by end of 4th week
  - Septation of atrioventricular canal by end of 4th week
  - Septation of ventricles by interventricular septum by end of 4th week
  - Septation of truncus arteriosus into aortic and pulmonary channel.

Congenital Anomalies of Heart

- The heart defects are reported about 1% in the live born infants
- 33% of babies with chromosomal abnormalities have cardiac defect.
- 2% of the defect are due to environmental effect—diabetic mother, drug induced, rubella virus
- Newborn babies with congenital heart disease may present with rapid heart rate, cyanosis, difficulty in feeding.
- **Depending on position:**
  - **Dextrocardia**
    - The heart lies on the right side of the thorax
    - It occurs when the heart loops to the left instead of to right side
    - Total reversal of the chambers of the heart with blood vessels
    - Left ventricle and arch of aorta are on the right side
    - It usually occurs with situs inversus
    - Commonly seen in Kartagener's syndrome.

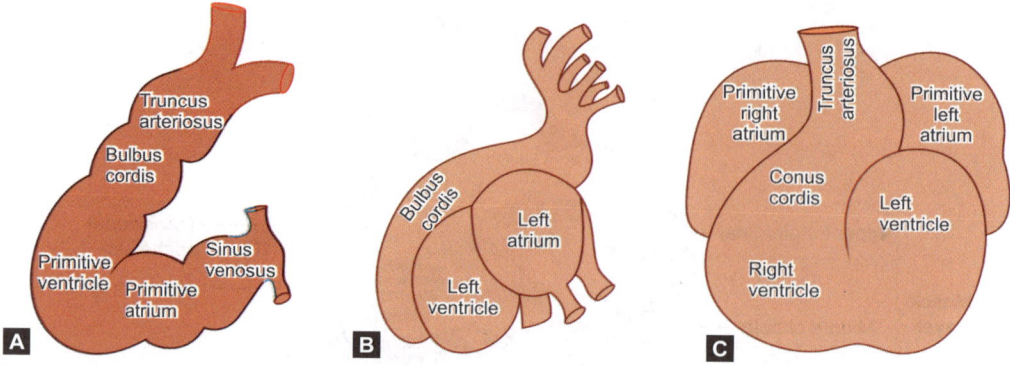

Figs. 7A to C: Normal development of heart.

- **Ectopia cordis**
  - The heart is exposed
  - It lies on the chest
  - There is failure of formation of anterior body wall.
- **Depending on septal formation**
  - **Ventricular septal defect (VSD) (Fig. 8):**
    - Commonest congenital anomaly of the heart
    - The defect commonly involves the membranous part of the interventricular septum
    - It is due to defect in partition of conotruncal region
    - Interventricular septal defect in the muscular part is not common.
  - **Fallot's tetralogy (Fig. 9):**
    - Tetralogy of Fallot is a commonly occurring abnormality of the conotruncal region
    - It is due to unequal division of the conus resulting from anterior displacement of the conotruncal septum
    - During fifth week, division of the truncus into aortic and pulmonary vessels starts under the influence of the neural crest
    - The septation starts with the formation of the ridges along the walls of the truncus. The septum is called as **aorticopulmonary/spiral septum**

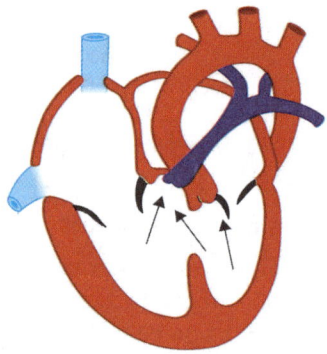

Fig. 8: Ventricular septal defect.

  - Meanwhile the two conal cushions along conus cordis fuse with each other and unite with the spiral septum
  - Proliferation of these conal cushions along with the anterior endocardial cushions close the interventricular foramen and forms the membranous portion of the interventricular septum
  - Abnormal migration of neural crest cells results in defective development of the spiral septum leading to congenital malformations
  - The components of Fallot's are
    * Pulmonary infundibular stenosis: Due to unequal division of conus resulting in a narrow right ventricular orifice

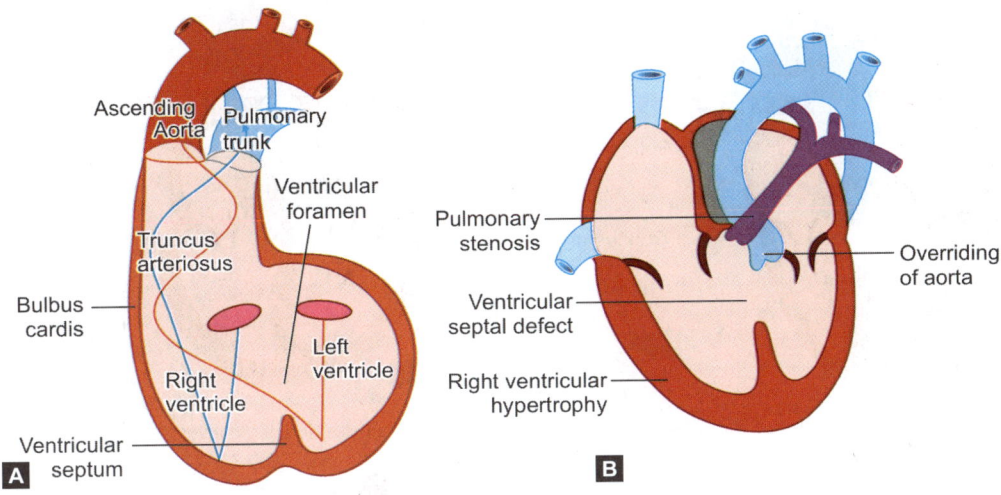

Figs. 9A and B: Fallot's tetrology.

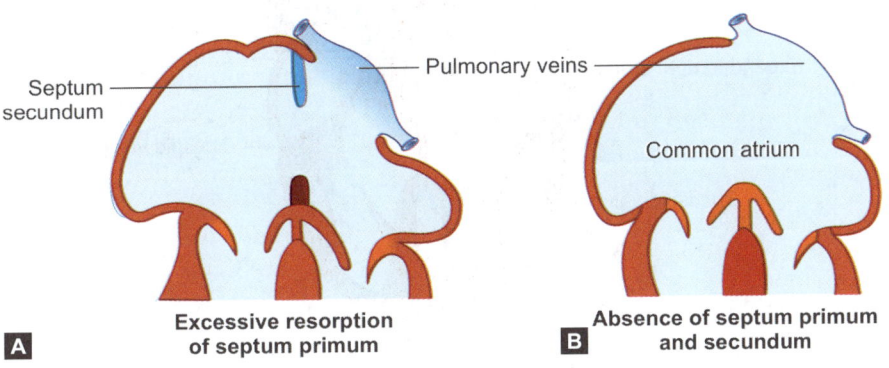

Figs. 10A and B: Atrial septal defects.

* Right ventricular hypertrophy: Due to increase in pressure on right side
* Large ventricular septal defect: Failure of fusion of bulbar septum
* Overriding of aorta: Because of ventricular septal defect and aorta arises directly above the defect: The defect may be cyanotic or acyanotic if the shunt is from left to right. If Fallot's is associated with ASD then it is called as **pentalogy**.
- Atrial septal defect (ASD) (Fig. 10)
  - It is one of the congenital abnormality
  - More common in female than male (2: 1)
  - Its types are:
    - Ostium primum—failure of fusion of endocardial cushions of the AV canal
    - Ostium secundum defect—resorption of septum primum is more or inadequate septum secundum.
  - Patent foramen ovale
  - Probe patency of the foramen ovale
  - Cor triloculare and biventriculare—complete absence of atrial septum
  - Premature closure of foramen ovale
- **Persistent truncus arteriosus (Fig. 11A):** It is due to failure of formation of conotruncal ridges resulting in undivided outflow tract.

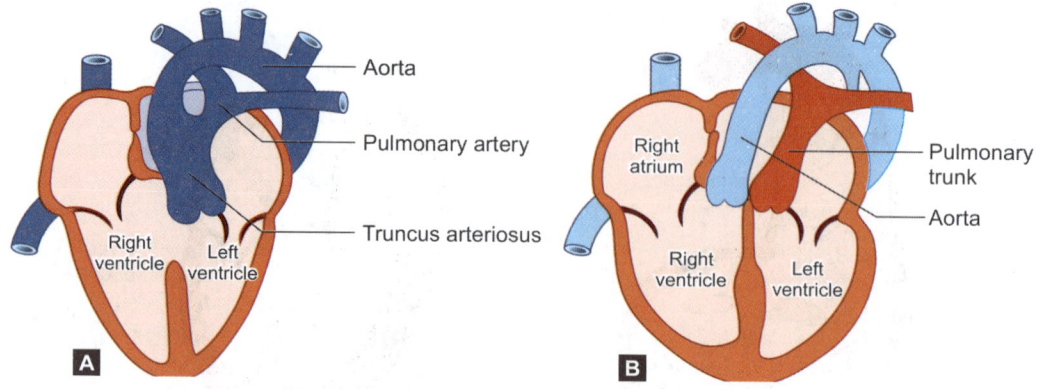

Figs. 11A and B: (A) Persistent truncus arteriosus; (B) Transposition of great vessels.

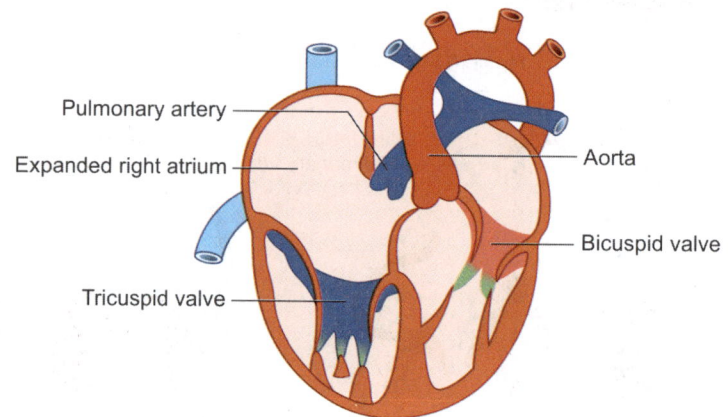

Fig. 12: Ebstein anomaly.

- **Transposition of great arteries (Fig. 11B)**
  - This cyanotic disease of the heart mostly occurs due to transposition of great vessels
  - It is due to failure of the aortopulmonary septum (spiral/conotruncal septum) to follow its normal spiral course
  - The aorta originates from right ventricle and pulmonary trunk from left ventricle.
- **Depending on cyanosis**
  - **Cyanotic:** In cyanotic type of congenital anomalies of the heart. The shunt is from right to left
    - Tetralogy of Fallot
    - Transposition of great arteries.
  - **Acyanotic:** The shunt is left to right
    - Atrial septal defect
    - Ventricular septal defect
    - Aortic stenosis.
- **Valvular defects**
  - **Ebstein anomaly:** The tricuspid leaflet is large and abnormally placed, resulting in hypertrophy of the right atrium and small right ventricle (Fig. 12)
  - **Valvular stenosis:** The semilunar valves of aorta or pulmonary trunk are stenosed resulting in narrowing of the lumen of the vessels.

7. **Describe the superolateral surface of the cerebral hemisphere under the following headings: Sulci and Gyri, functional areas and arterial supply.**

Sulci, gyri, functional areas - Refer Essay Q. No. 7 – 2007.

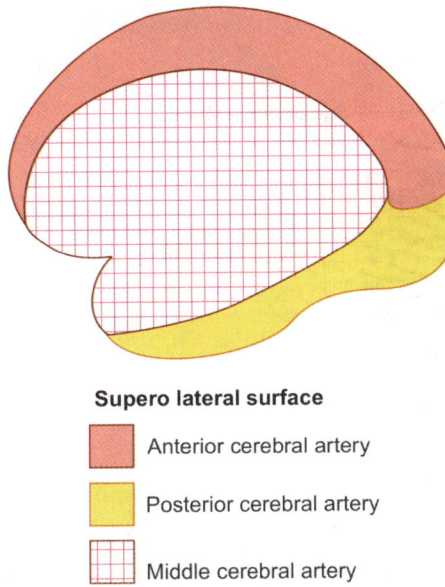

Supero lateral surface

▨ Anterior cerebral artery

▨ Posterior cerebral artery

▨ Middle cerebral artery

Fig. 13: Arterial supply of superolateral surface.

- **Arterial supply (Fig. 13)**
  - The cerebral cortex is supplied by the **cortical branches** of the anterior, middle and posterior cerebral arteries
  - **The superolateral surface** of the hemisphere
    - The surface is supplied by all three cerebral arteries
    - It is mainly supplied by the middle cerebral artery
    - The middle cerebral supplies the motor and somatosensory areas, the auditory cortex and speech areas
    - The anterior cerebral artery supplies a strip close to the superomedial border of the hemisphere
    - The occipital pole and most of the inferior temporal gyrus are supplied by the posterior cerebral artery.
- **Central branches** perforate the white matter and supply thalamus, the corpus striatum and internal capsule. They are from **circle of Willis**/circulus arteriosus (Refer Short Notes 24 – 2005).

8. Describe the arch of aorta under the following headings: Extent, relations, branches and microscopic anatomy.

Extent, Relations, Branches - Refer Short Notes 11 – 2004.

Microscopic anatomy

- It is also called as elastic artery
- Is made up of three layers from inner to outer are tunica intima, tunica media and tunica adventitia
- **Tunica intima** is made of
  - Endothelium—lined by simple squamous epithelium
  - Subendothelial layer (lamina propria)—is made of elastic fibers and collagen fibers type I, fibroblasts and smooth muscle fibers
  - Inner elastic lamina is ill defined.
- **Tunica media**
  - It contributes for more than half of the thickness of the wall of the artery
  - Mainly made of collagen and elastic fibers
  - The smooth muscle fibers are less
  - The elastic fibers anastomose with each other and are arranged circularly in the form of lamellae
  - The layers of elastic lamellae alternate with smooth muscle fibers, collagen and fine elastic fibers
  - The layers are regularly arranged
  - About 52 lamellar layers are seen in the human aorta
  - The outer elastic lamina is also not seen as it merges with the elastic fibers of media.
- **Tunica adventitia**
  - Is formed of connective tissue, containing bundles of collagen fiber of varying thickness
  - The adventitia is well developed
  - Fibroblasts macrophages and mast cells, nerve bundles and lymphatic vessels are present in addition to collagen and elastic fibers

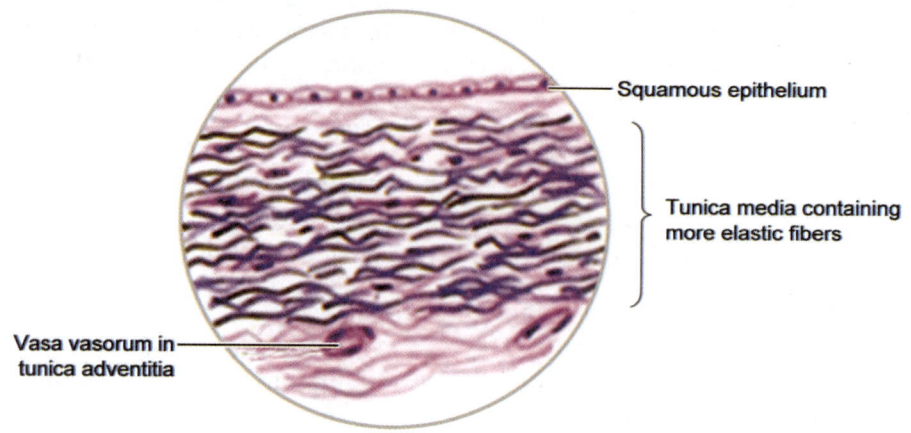

Fig. 14: Histology of aorta.

- The vasa vasorum are present in the adventitia.
- Applied anatomy:
  - Aortic aneurysm (dilatation)
  - Dissecting aneurysm
  - Coarctation of aorta: Due to congenital stenosis or atresia of the arch of aorta distal to the origin of the left subclavian artery maybe preductal or postductal
  - Angiogram (diagnostic procedure to visualize the aorta and the coronary arteries by injecting a radio opaque dye through the catheter into the aortic sinuses).

II. SHORT NOTES

1. Cubital fossa.

Refer Short Notes 16 – 2008.

2. Cartilaginous joints.

- The cartilaginous joint is one of the subdivision of synarthrosis
- The movement in this joint is restricted
- In this type of joint the bones are joined to each other by cartilage
- It is classified into primary (synchondrosis), and secondary (symphysis) depending on the type of cartilage intervening
- The synchondrosis are temporary concerned with growth, and the symphysis are permanent joints concerned with movements
- These joints are less rigid
- **Primary cartilaginous joint** (synchondrosis) **(Fig. 15)**
  - The bones are united by a plate of hyaline cartilage
  - These joints are temporary in nature
  - The property of hyaline cartilage is to ossify, in advancement of age, the synchondrosis tend to ossify when the growth is completed
  - The ossified bone is synostosis
  - Example: Joint between epiphysis and diaphysis of a growing long bone (growth plate), spheno-occipital synchondrosis.
- **Secondary cartilaginous joint** (symphysis) **(Fig. 16)**
  - A thin layer of hyaline cartilage covers the articular surfaces and united by a plate of fibrocartilage
  - These joints are permanent and persist throughout life
  - They occur in the median plane of the body
  - These joints withstand compression, tension and torsion
  - The movement is restricted

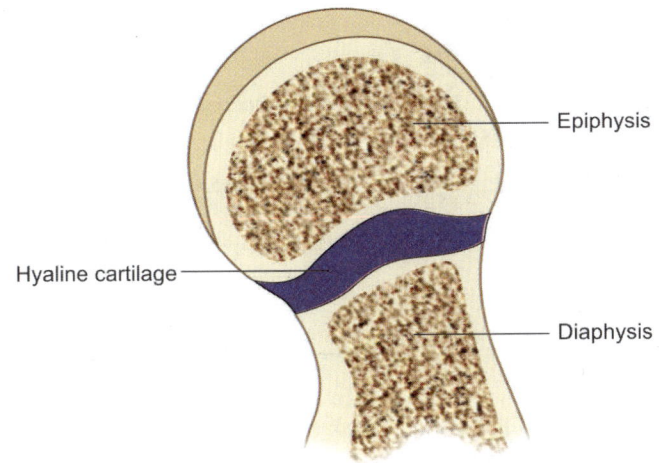

Fig. 15: Primary cartilaginous joint.

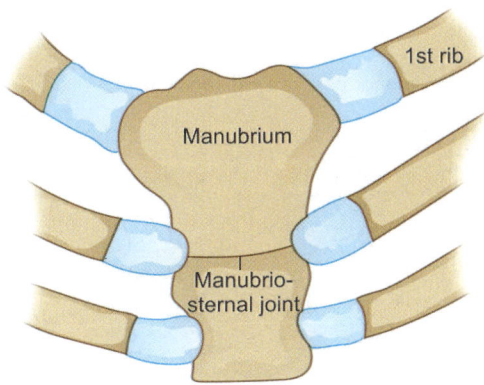

Fig. 16: Secondary cartilaginous joint.

- Example: Pubic symphysis, manubriosternal, intervertebral disc, symphysis menti.
- **Applied anatomy:** The joints between the epiphysis and diaphysis allows the growth of long bone, and hence it is called as growth plate. Damage to the epiphyseal plate at the growing end in child may lead to shortening of the limb.

3. **Microscopic structure of suprarenal gland.**

- The adrenal/suprarenal gland is made up of outer cortex and inner medulla. The medulla is completely covered by cortex except at hilum
- **Cortex**—arranged as 3 zones
  1. **Zona glomerulosa**: Columnar cells arrange in arched or rounded cluster pattern. The cells contain abundant smooth endoplasmic reticulum. Secretes mineralocorticoids
  2. **Zona fasciculata**: Polyhedral cells arranged as straight cords of two cells separated by fenestrated sinusoids. Lipid droplets and smooth endoplasmic reticulum are present in the cytoplasm. Secretes glucocorticoids
  3. **Zona reticularis**: Cells are round. Columnar cells arranged irregularly, branching interconnected columns of cells. The cells contain more lysosomes, and brown lipofuscin pigment, which increase as age advances. Secretes sex hormones.
- **Medulla**: Forms one tenth of gland. Consists of chromaffin cells, ganglion cells, sinusoids lined by fenestrated endothelium
- Fetal cortex is larger and forms foeto placental unit for the synthesis of placental estrogen.

4. **Inguinal canal.**

Refer Short Notes 20 – 2008.

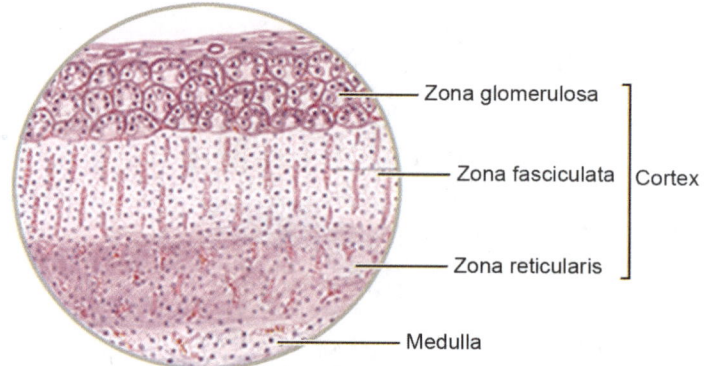

Fig. 17: Histology of suprarenal gland.

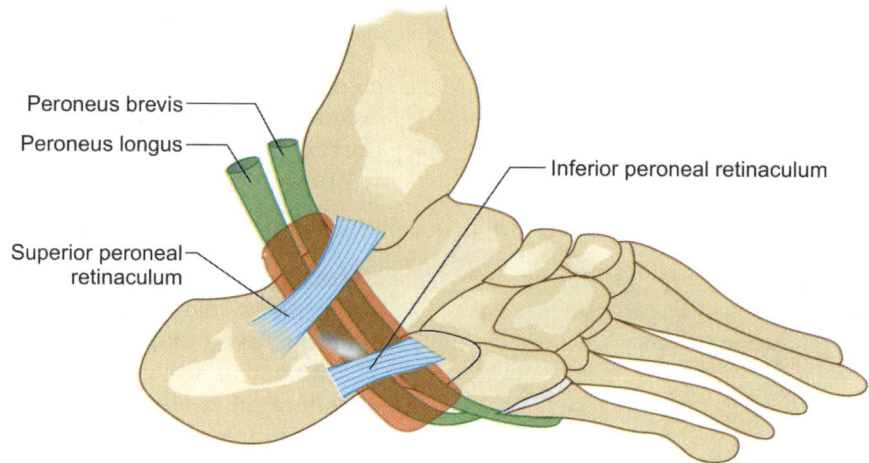

Fig. 18: Peroneal retinaculum.

5. **Ligaments around the hip joint.**
Refer Essay Q. No. 1 – 2004.

6. **Turner's syndrome.**
Refer Short Notes 28 – 2006.

7. **Microscopic structure of hyaline cartilage.**
Refer Short Notes 1 – 2006.

8. **Omental bursa.**
Refer Short Notes 10 – 2005.

9. **Derivatives of second pharyngeal arch.**
Refer Short Notes 27 – 2005.

10. **Peroneal retinacula.**
- These are thickenings of deep fascia
- Situation: Lateral aspect of ankle joint
- They hold the peroneus longus and brevis tendons
- They are 2 in number—superior and inferior peroneal retinaculum.
    i. **Superior peroneal retinaculum:**
    - Attachment:
        - Anteriorly to the posterior margin of lateral malleolus
        - Posteriorly to the lateral surface of the calcaneus and deep fascia of leg.
    ii. **Inferior peroneal retinaculum:**
    - Attachment:
        - Anteriorly continuous with the stem of the inferior extensor retinaculum

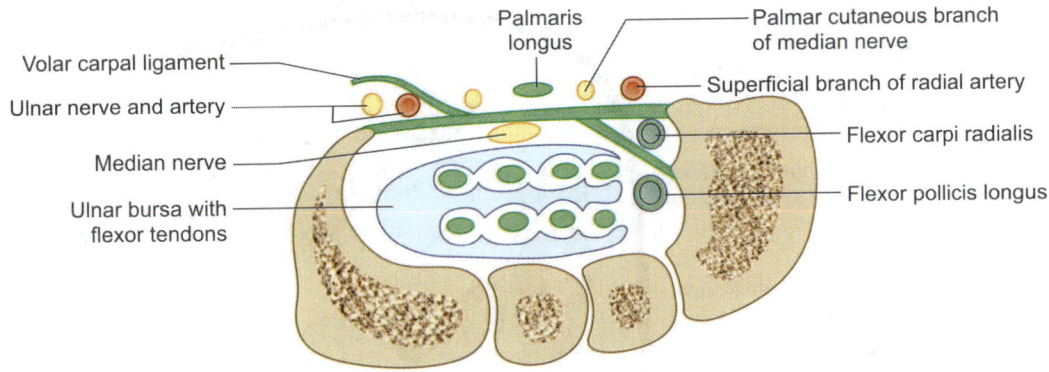

Fig. 19: Carpal tunnel.

- Posteriorly to the lateral surface of calcaneus
- A septum from the retinaculum, passes between peroneus longus and brevis, and is attached to the peroneal tubercle.
- **Structures passing deep:** Tendon of peroneus longus, peroneus brevis
- **Applied anatomy:** Injury to retinaculum results in instability of lateral muscles.

11. Carpal tunnel.

- **Formation of tunnel:** The anterior concave surface of carpal bones is converted into an osseo-fibrous tunnel by the flexor retinaculum, known as carpal tunnel.
- **Attachment of retinaculum:** Medial: Pisiform bone, hook of the hamate
  - Lateral: Tubercle of the scaphoid, crest of the trapezium
  - Proximally: It blends with the antebrachial fascia
  - Distally: It is continuous with palmar aponeurosis and gives attachment to thenar and hypothenar muscles.
- **Contents (Fig. 19)**
  - Digital flexor tendons of flexor digitorum superficialis
  - Digital flexor tendons of flexor digitorum profundus
  - Tendon of flexor pollicis longus
  - Tendon of flexor carpi radialis with a separate synovial sheath
- Median nerve
  - **Radial bursa:** The synovial sheaths around the flexor pollicis longus
  - **Ulnar bursa:** Synovial sheath surrounding the flexor digitorum tendons.
- **Carpal tunnel syndrome:** Ref Essay Q. No. 1 – 2008

12. Hepatorenal pouch.

- It is the right subhepatic space
- It is part of greater sac
- It is between right lobe of liver and right kidney
- It is known as **Morrison's pouch**
- **Boundaries (Fig. 20):**
  - Posteriorly—anterior surface of upper part of right kidney
  - Anteriorly—right lobe of liver
  - Medially—second part of duodenum, right colic flexure, transverse mesocolon, head of pancreas
  - Laterally—lateral abdominal wall on right side
  - Superiorly—the inferior layer of the coronary ligament
  - Inferiorly—open.
- Communicates with right paracolic gutter and with lesser sac through epiploic foramen
- **Applied anatomy:** Fluid collection after surgery is more common in this space than paracolic gutter as this space is more dependent in supine position.

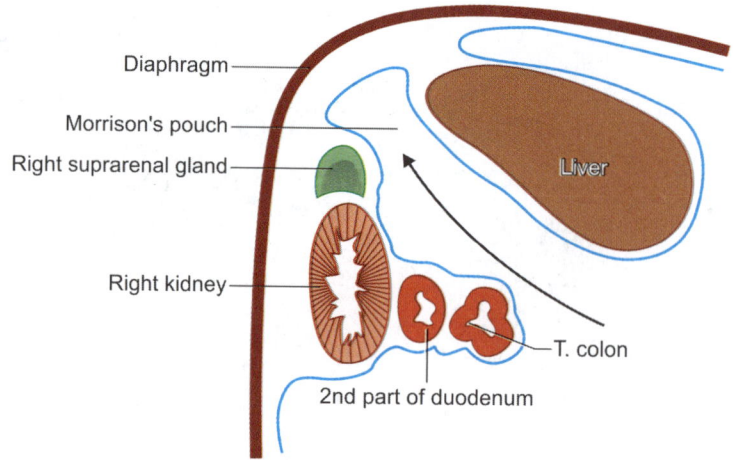

Fig. 20: Hepatorenal pouch.

13. Microscopic structure of testis.

- Testis has an outer fibrous layer the tunica albuginea
- The tunica albuginea expands posteriorly to form mediastinum testis
- Numerous septae extends from mediastinum testis and divides the substance of testis into many lobules
- Each lobule contains one or more coiled seminiferous tubules
- Deep to tunica albuginea sections of seminiferous tubules are present
- Each tubule is lined by several layers of cells
- Two types of cells are present in the tubules
  i. Spermatogenic cells
  ii. Sustentacular cells
- **Spermatogenic cells** produce spermatozoa. Hence they are called as germ cells
  - Spermatogenic cells represent various stages in the formation of spermatozoa.
  - They are spermatogonia, primary and secondary spermatocytes, spermatids and spermatozoa
  - Spermatogonia: The stem cells are named as spermatogonia. They lie near the basal lamina. They undergo several mitotic divisions
  - Primary spermatocyte: They are situated in the middle region of the tubule. They undergo meiosis to form secondary spermatocyte
  - Secondary spermatocyte: They are smaller than primary cell. Each cell has haploid number of chromosomes. It divides to form two spermatids
  - Spermatids: Rounded cells with spherical nucleus. They undergo changes in shape to form spermatozoa.
- **Sustentacular (Sertoli) cell**
  - Are tall pyramidal in shape
  - They extend from base to lumen of the tubule
  - Recesses are present at the sides and apex of the cell
  - The recesses are occupied by the spermatogonia, spermatocytes, spermatids
  - These cells provide support to germ cells
  - The fluid secreted by it helps to move spermatozoa along the tubule
  - The cells produce Mullerian inhibitory substance in the fetal life which suppresses the development of paramesonephric duct
  - In adult, it produces androgen binding protein which binds to testosterone

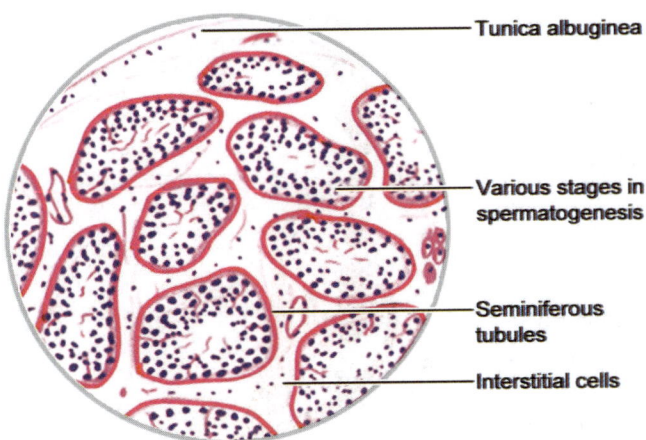

Fig. 21: Histology of testis.

- Inhibin produced by the Sertoli cells inhibits the production of FSH.
- **The interstitial cells of Leydig**
  - Are large polyhedral cells
  - Seen in the connective tissue between the seminiferous tubules
  - They secrete male hormone—testicular androgens
  - Some interstitial cells are present in mediastinum testis, epididymis.
- The interstitial tissue contains collagen fibers, macrophages, fibroblast, mast cells, blood vessels, and lymphatics.

14. Supports of uterus.
Refer Essay Q. No. 2 – 2004.

15. Medial longitudinal arch of foot.
Refer Essay Q. No. 1 – 2003.

16. Blood supply of long bone.
Refer Short Notes 2 – 2009.

17. Obturator nerve.
- The obturator nerve is the chief nerve of the adductor/medial compartment of the thigh. Supplies the adductor group of muscles **(Fig. 22)**
- **Origin and root value:**
  - It is a branch of the lumbar plexus
  - It is formed by the **ventral divisions** of the anterior primary rami of L_2, L_3, L_4.
- **Course and relations in pelvis:**
  - Emerges along the medial border of psoas major
  - Crosses the anterolateral angle of ala of sacrum
  - It is behind the common iliac and lateral to internal iliac arteries at the brim of pelvis
  - Runs downwards and forwards in the lateral wall of pelvis
  - In the lateral wall of pelvis in female related to ovary and it forms floor of the ovarian fossa
  - Here it lies on obturator internus, and related to obturator vessels
  - Leaves the pelvic cavity through obturator canal.
- **Course and relations in thigh**
  - Within the obturator canal, the nerve divides into anterior and posterior divisions
  - The anterior division descends in front of obturator externus and adductor brevis and behind the pectineus and adductor longus
  - The posterior division pierces obturator externus, passes in front of adductor magnus and behind adductor brevis.

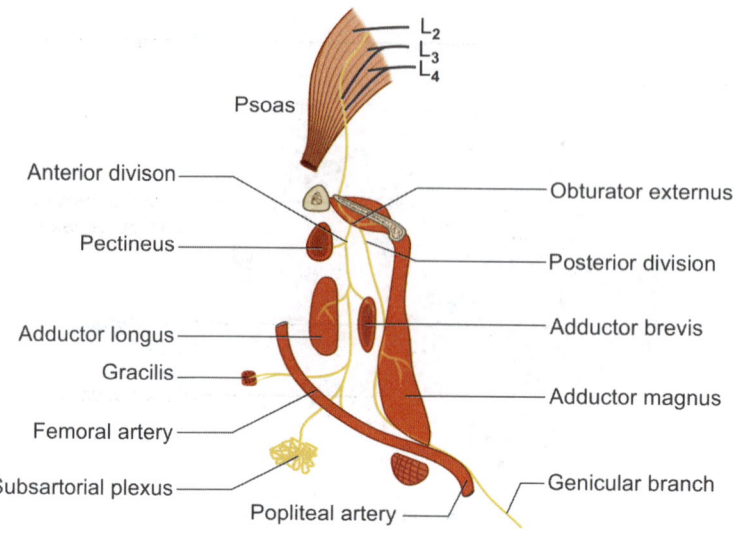

Fig. 22: Obturator nerve.

- **Distribution**
  - Anterior division
    - Muscular branches to adductor longus, gracilis, pectineus, adductor brevis
    - Articular branch to hip joint
    - Cutaneous branch through sub sartorial plexus to skin of medial side of thigh
    - Vascular branch to femoral artery
  - Posterior division supplies the following:
    - Muscular branches to obturator externus, adductor brevis, adductor magnus
    - Articular branch to knee joint (genicular branch)
    - Vascular branch to popliteal artery.
- **Applied anatomy**
  - The common nerve supply of hip and knee joint by the obturator nerve results in referred pain to knee when there is any disease in the hip joint
  - Any inflammation of ovary, results in irritation of obturator nerve, and the elderly female patient complains of persistent pain along the medial side of thigh, which is supplied by the obturator nerve.

18. Epiploic foramen.
Refer Short Answer Q. No. 14 – 2009.

19. Klinefelter's Syndrome.
Refer Short Notes 39 – 2005.

20. Menisci of knee joint.
- The menisci are two semilunar discs
- **Nature** fibrocartilaginous discs
- They are intracapsular situated on the tibial condyles
- They deepen the articular surfaces of the condyles of the tibia
- Partly divide the joint cavity into upper and lower compartments
- Each meniscus has the following parts
  - **Two ends/horns:** Both of which are attached to the tibia
  - **Two borders:** The **outer border** is thick, convex and attached to the fibrous capsule and margins of tibial condyles through coronary ligaments; while the **inner border** is thin, concave and free
  - **Two surfaces:** The **upper surface** is concave to articulate with the femur condyles. The **lower surface** is flat and rests on the peripheral two-thirds of the superior surface of condyles of tibia.

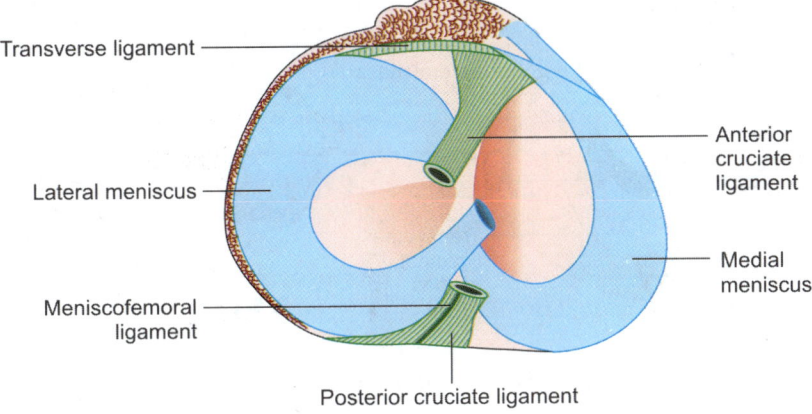

Fig. 23: Menisci of knee joint.

- **Medial meniscus**
  - It is elongated anterolaterally nearly 'C'/semicircular in **shape.** It is wider behind than in front
  - Attachment: Anterior horn to anterior part of intercondylar area of tibia. Posterior horn to intercondylar area between lateral meniscus and posterior cruciate ligament. The outer border in addition is attached to the tibial collateral ligament.
- **Lateral meniscus**
  - It is nearly circular
  - Attachment: The anterior horn to the intercondylar area of tibia between anterior cruciate ligament and intercondylar tubercle. Posterior horn behind the intercondylar tubercle. In addition the posterior end of the meniscus is attached to the femur through two meniscofemoral ligaments.
- **Functions:**
  - They help in making the articular surfaces more congruent
  - The menisci serve as shock absorbers
  - They help in lubrication of the joint cavity.
- **Applied anatomy:**
  - **Bucket handle tear**:
    - **Reason**: The medial meniscus is torn
    - The menisci may be torn/injured due to twisting strain applied to the flexed knee
    - It is common in football players
    - The medial meniscus is more affected because of its attachment to the tibial collateral ligament and the rotatory movement is more than the lateral
    - **Cause of lesion:** The medial rotation of thigh in semiflexed position of knee, induces forced abduction of tibia on the femur
    - **Effect of lesion**: The detached portion may get displaced to the centre of the joint, restricting all the movements.

21. Development of tongue.
Refer Short Notes 20 – 2003.

22. Facial artery.
Refer Short Notes 26 – 2007.

23. Nerve supply of lacrimal gland.
Refer Short Notes 27 – 2006.

24. Histology of pituitary gland.
Refer Short Notes 23 – 2005.

25. Atlantoaxial joints.
- Three synovial joints are formed by the articulation of atlas with the axis
  - A pair of joints between the lateral masses

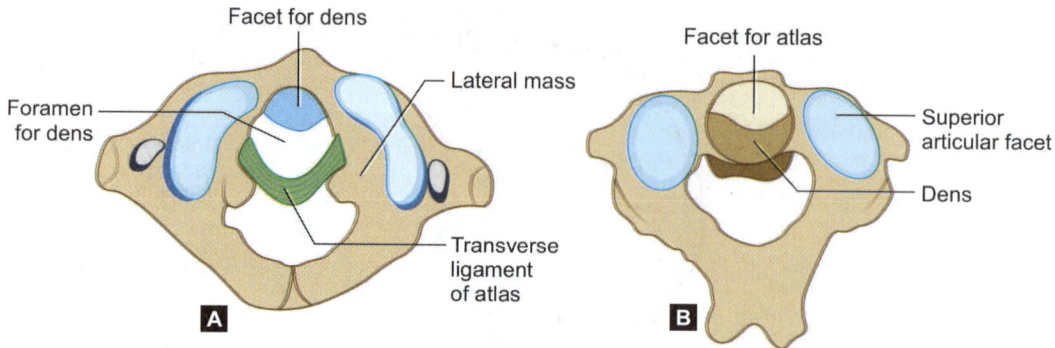

Figs. 24A and B: Atlantoaxial joint: (A) Atlas; (B) Axis.

- A median joint between the dens of the axis and the anterior arch and transverse ligament of the atlas.
- Lateral atlantoaxial joint
- Type of joint: Synovial, plane variety
- Articular surfaces
  - The circular inferior articular facet of the lateral mass of atlas
  - Ovoid articular facets are at the junction of the body and neural arch.
- **Ligaments**
  - Fibrous capsule is thin and lax, attached to the articular margins
  - Anterior longitudinal ligament
  - Ligamenta flava posteriorly.
- Median atlantoaxial joint
- Type of joint: Pivot variety
- Articular surfaces
  - The vertically facet on the anterior surface of dens, is oval in shape
  - A facet on the posterior aspect of the anterior arch of atlas
  - An osseofibrous ring is formed by the transverse ligament of the atlas.
- Ligaments
  - Transverse ligament
  - The transverse ligament lies behind the dens, and is broad and strong
  - It is attached laterally to tubercle on the side of lateral mass of atlas
  - A thin layer of articular cartilage covers the ligament anteriorly
  - A longitudinal band arises from middle of upper and lower margins and get attached to the basilar part of the occipital bone and posterior surface of axis correspondingly
  - **The cruciform ligament** is formed by the transverse and longitudinal components
  - The ring of the atlas is divided into unequal parts by the transverse ligament
  - The posterior two-thirds surrounds the spinal cord and meninges
  - The anterior third contains the dens
  - The dens is held in position by the transverse ligament, even when all other ligaments are divided.
- **Nerve supply:** Ventral ramus of the second cervical spinal nerve
- **Blood supply:** Branches of the deep cervical, occipital and vertebral arteries
- **Movements** (say **No**- rotating head/ No movement)
  - Rotation around axis
  - The normal range of atlantoaxial rotation is about 40°
  - The muscles producing the movement are obliquus capitis inferior, rectus capitis posterior major and splenius capitis of one side.

26. Hyoglossus muscle.
Refer Short Notes 15 – 2004.

27. Cardiac plexuses.
Refer Short Notes 17 – 2007.

28. Right coronary artery.
Refer Essay Q. No. 5 – 2005.

29. Mediastinal surface of left lung.

Refer Essay Q. No. 3 – 2004.

30. Klinefelter syndrome.

Refer Short Notes 39 – 2005.

31. Vocal cord.

Refer Short Notes 33 – 2005.

32. Hilum of right lung.

Refer Essay Q. No. 3 – 2004.

33. Styloid apparatus.

Refer Short Notes 38 – 2005.

34. Histology of parathyroid gland.

- Each parathyroid gland is covered by a thin connective tissue capsule
- Septae extends into the gland from the capsule
- The gland is not divided into definite lobules
- Parathyroid contains two types of cells— (1) chief cells (2) oxyphil cells
    1. **Chief cells:** Depending on the level of activity the structure of chief cells differ
        - **Active cells** are provided with large Golgi complexes with numerous vesicles and small membrane-bound granules
        - **Inactive cells** are called as **clear cells,** have abundant glycogen granules and they appear clear as the cytoplasmic features of secretory activity are less
        - In human parathyroid glands, inactive chief cells more than active cells in a ratio of 3 to 5: 1.
    2. **Oxyphil cells** (eosinophil)
        - The oxyphil cell, appears just before puberty
        - Number of cells increases with age
        - Oxyphil cells are larger than chief cells and rich with cytoplasm
        - The nucleus is smaller and more darkly stained
        - The cytoplasm contains more mitochondria
        - The function of oxyphil cells are not known.

35. Development of interatrial septum.

Refer Short Notes 25 – 2006.

36. Parotid duct.

Refer Essay Q. No. 4 – 2004.

37. Blood supply of spinal cord.

Refer Short Notes 27 – 2008.

38. Venous drainage of face.

- The veins accompany the branches of the arteries supplying the face
- **Supratrochlear vein** joins with **supraorbital vein** at the medial angle of eye to form **angular vein**

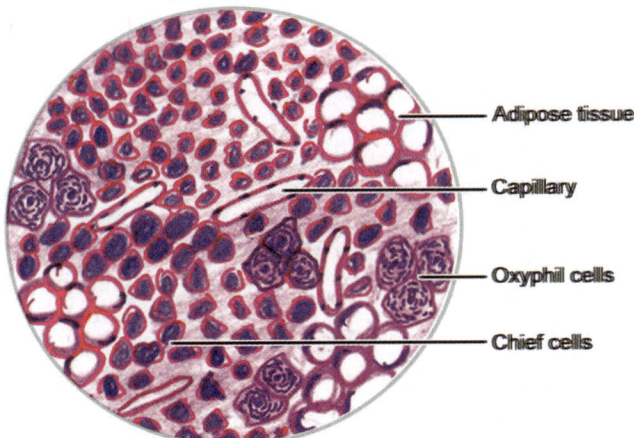

Fig. 25: Histology of parathyroid gland.

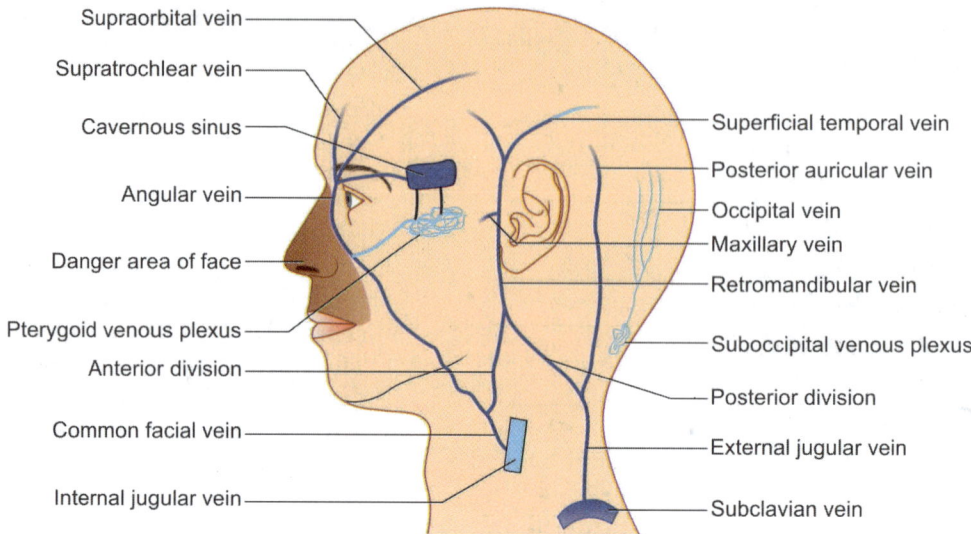

Fig. 26: Venous drainage of face.

- **Superficial temporal vein** joins with **maxillary vein** to form **retromandibular vein** which in turn divides into anterior and posterior divisions
- Anterior division of retromandibular vein joins with **anterior facial vein** to form **common facial vein** which drains to internal jugular vein
- Posterior division of retromandibular vein joins with **posterior auricular vein** to form external jugular vein which end in subclavian vein
- Face is **connected to cavernous sinus** by two routes—direct and indirect
    1. **Direct route** is angular vein connected to ophthalmic vein which drains to cavernous sinus
    2. **Indirect route** is the anterior facial vein is connected to pterygoid venous plexus through deep facial vein, which in turn is connected to cavernous sinus by emissary veins.

Applied Anatomy

Danger area of face: The upper lip and the adjoining part of the nose lying between the angular and deep facial veins form the dangerous area of face. The facial vein is devoid of valves and rests directly on the facial muscles. The movement of facial muscles may facilitate the spread of septic emboli from the infected area of upper lip and lower part of the nose in reverse direction and cause thrombosis of cavernous sinus.

39. Middle meatus of nose.
Refer Short Notes 16 – 2004.

40. Carotid sheath.
- The carotid sheath contributed by all the three layers of deep cervical fascia
- **Extent:** It extends from root of neck to the base of skull. The carotid sheath is **formed** anterolaterally by portions of the investing and pretracheal layer of deep cervical fascia, and posteriorly the prevertebral fascia **(Fig. 27)**.
- **Contents (Fig. 28)**
    - The common carotid artery (CCA) up to upper border of thyroid cartilage
    - Internal carotid artery (ICA) from upper border of thyroid cartilage to carotid canal
    - The internal jugular vein (IJV) lateral to the arteries from jugular foramen to root of neck
    - The vagus nerve – posterior to vessels entire length of the sheath.

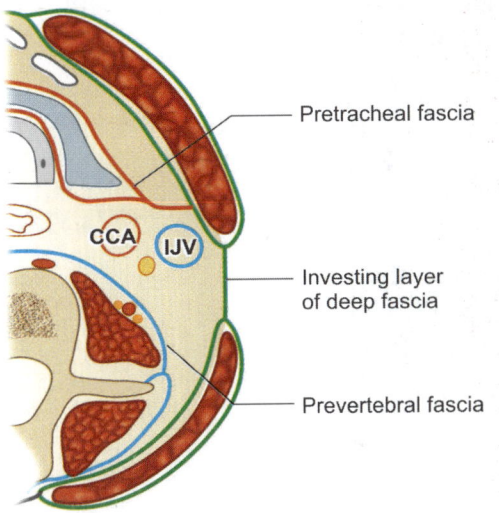

Fig. 27: Formation of carotid sheath.

- **Nature**
  - The sheath thicker around the arteries than the vein, for the vein to expand
  - Externally the loose areolar tissue connect the carotid sheath with adjacent fascial layers.
- **Relation**
  - The cervical sympathetic trunk lies behind the carotid sheath
  - The deep cervical lymphatic nodes lie alongside the carotid sheath
  - The carotid sheath is deep to sternocleidomastoid muscle

  - The ansa cervicalis is embedded in the anterior wall of carotid sheath.
- **Structures piercing (Fig. 29)**
  - External carotid artery
  - Tributaries of internal jugular vein – facial, lingual, pharyngeal veins
  - Pharyngeal and laryngeal branches of vagus
  - 9th, 11th, 12th cranial nerves pierce at various levels.
- **Carotid space**: A potential space is enclosed within the carotid space
- **Applied anatomy**
  - Infection that spreads into the parapharyngeal space may involve the carotid sheath and results in thrombosis of the internal jugular vein
  - Carotid space syndrome is due to infections from the visceral spaces may enter into the carotid space. It is restricted to this space by the hyoid bone above and root of the neck below.

III. SHORT ANSWER QUESTIONS

1. **Name the arteries supplying transverse colon.**

- The transverse colon is developed from mid and hind gut
- The arteries supplying transverse colon are middle colic branch of superior mesenteric artery and left colic branch of inferior mesenteric artery

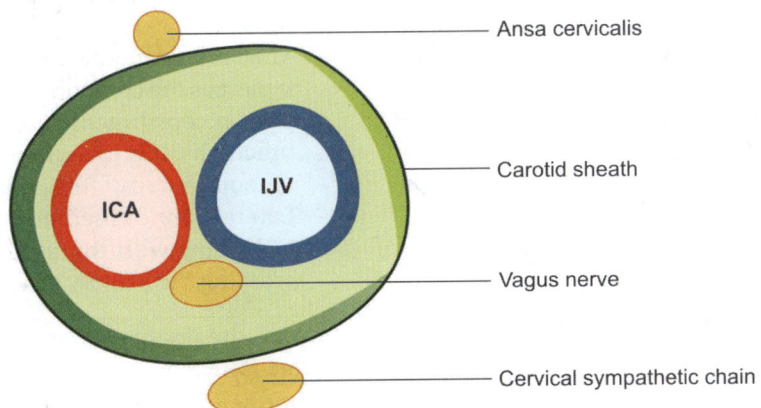

Fig. 28: Contents of carotid sheath.

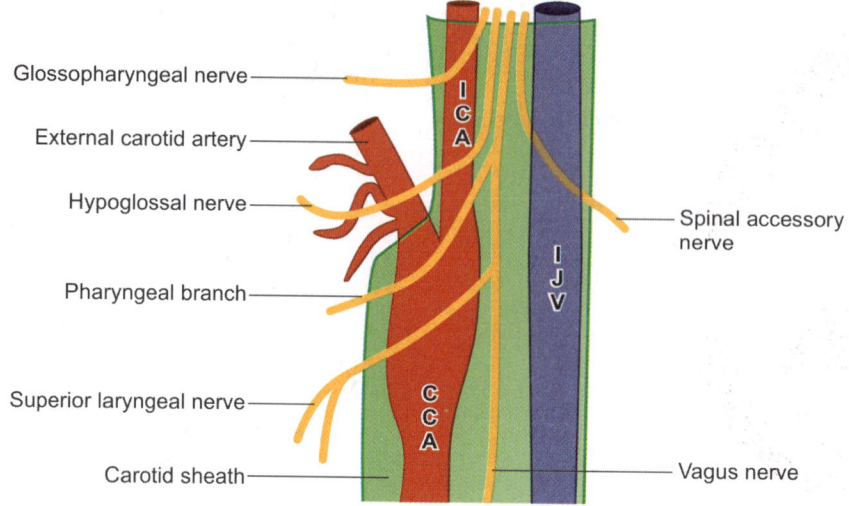

Fig. 29: Structures piercing.

- The middle colic supplies right ⅔ of transverse colon
- The left colic supplies left ⅓ of transverse colon.

2. Name the muscles forming rotator cuff around shoulder joint.

Refer Short Notes 4 – 2003.

3. Name the Hamstring muscles.

- The muscles of the back of thigh are known as hamstring
- The **features** of it are:
  - **Origin** is from ischial tuberosity
  - **Inserted** to any bone of leg
  - **Nerve supply** is by tibial component of sciatic nerve
  - **Action** is flexors of knee and extensors of hip.
- The hamstring muscles are semitendinosus, semimembranosus, long head of biceps, hamstring part of adductor magnus.

4. Name the muscles within the rectus sheath.

Two muscles within the sheath are:
  i. Rectus abdominis
  ii. Pyramidalis.

5. Name the branches arising from lateral cord of brachial plexus.

- The anterior primary rami of C5, C6, C7, C8 and T1 contribute for brachial plexus
- Roots C5 and C6 join to form the upper trunk. Root C7 forms the middle trunk. Roots C8 and T1 join to form the lower trunk
- Each trunk divides into ventral and dorsal divisions
- **Lateral cord** is formed by the union of the ventral divisions of upper and middle trunks
- Branches of lateral cords:
  - Lateral pectoral nerve (C5, C6, C7): It pierces the clavipectoral fascia and supplies pectoralis major and minor muscles
  - Musculocutaneous nerve (C5, C6, C7): It pierces the coracobrachialis and supplies biceps brachii, coracobrachialis, brachialis. It is continued as lateral cutaneous nerve of forearm
  - Lateral root of median nerve (C5, C6, C7): Joins with the medial root, after crossing the axillary artery.

6. Name the ligaments present within the knee joint.

- Anterior cruciate ligament
- Posterior cruciate ligament
- Anterior meniscofemoral ligament

- Posterior meniscofemoral ligament
- Medial menisci
- Lateral menisci.

7. Popliteus muscle.

Refer Short Notes 19 – 2009.

8. Name the coverings of testis (Fig. 30).

- **Intrinsic covering**: Formed by three layers from outer to inner are as follows:
  - **i. Tunica vaginalis**:
    - During fetal life the testis descends from abdomen to scrotum
    - As it descends it pulls the peritoneum called processus vaginalis
    - After testis enters into the scrotum, the proximal part of the processus gets obliterated
    - Lower end of the processus vaginalis persists and covers the testis and is reflected on to inner surface of scrotum
    - The layer covering the testis is the visceral layer of tunica vaginalis.
  - **ii. Tunica albuginea**:
    - It is a thick fibrous covering made of collagen fibers.
    - From it at posterior border incomplete septum extend and form mediastinum testis through which the blood vessels pass
    - It sends septae dividing the testis into lobules.
  - **iii. Tunica vasculosa**: It contains connective tissue and plexus of blood vessels pass covering the septae.
- **Extrinsic coverings**: Formed by six layers which constitute the layers of scrotum. From outer to inner are (**S**ome **D**ame **E**nglish **C**alled **I**t **T**estis):
  - **S**kin
  - **D**artos muscle—subcutaneous muscle
  - **E**xternal spermatic fascia—continuation of aponeurosis of external oblique
  - **C**remaster muscle and fascia—from internal oblique and transversus abdominis
  - **I**nternal spermatic fascia—continuation of transversalis fascia
  - **T**unica vaginalis (parietal layer).

9. Name the muscles of I layer of sole of the foot.

S. No.	Layers	Muscles	Nerve supply
1	First	Abductor hallucis	Medial plantar
		Abductor digiti minimi	Lateral plantar
		Flexor digitorum brevis	Medial plantar

10. Name the muscles causing lateral rotation at hip joint.

- Rotation occurs around vertical axis passing through the center of head of femur

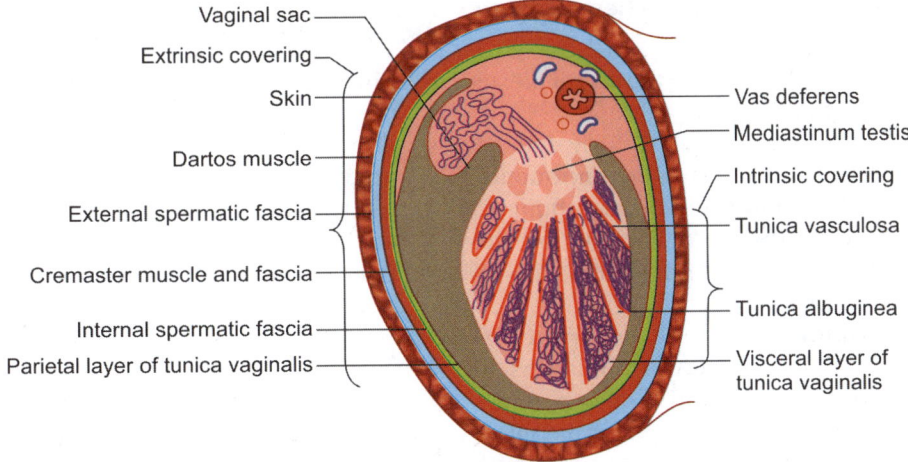

Fig. 30: Coverings of testis.

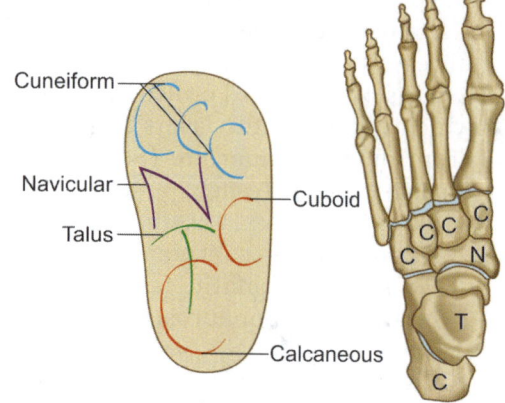

Fig. 31: Tarsal bones.

- **Muscles producing** lateral rotation: Gluteus maximus, and short lateral rotators namely piriformis, obturator externus, obturator internus and two gemelli.

11. Name any two tarsal bones of the foot.
- Calcaneus
- Talus
- Navicular
- Medial cuneiform
- Intermediate cuneiform
- Lateral cuneiform
- Cuboid.

12. Name the muscles causing abduction at wrist joint.
Refer Short Answer Q. No. 3 – 2008.

13. Name the terminal branches of sciatic nerve.
- It is the largest branch of the sacral plexus formed in the pelvis
- Root value: L_4, L_5, S_1, S_2, S_3
- The nerve is made up of 2 components: Tibial and common peroneal components
  - **Tibial component**: Formed by the ventral divisions of anterior primary rami of L_4, L_5, S_1, S_2, S_3
  - **Common peroneal component**: Formed by the dorsal divisions of anterior primary rami of L_4, L_5, S_1, S_2.
- It terminates in the superior angle of popliteal fossa into tibial and common peroneal nerves.

14. Name the arteries supplying transverse colon.
Refer Short Answer Q. No. 1 – 2010.

15. Name the branches arising from posterior cord of the brachial plexus.
Refer Short Answer Q. No. 4 – 2008.

16. Name the muscles present within the deep perineal pouch.
- Sphincter urethrae is part of levator ani muscle. It surrounds membranous part of the urethra in male. In female, it surrounds the urethra at the junction of middle and lower third of urethra
- Deep transversus perineii muscle extends from ischiopubic rami. The fibers decussate with opposite side and are attached to the perineal body.

17. Name the parts of the uterine tube.
From medial to lateral are:
- Intramural part which is inside the myometrium—1 cm in length
- Isthmus the narrowest, muscular and firm part—3 cm long
- Ampulla dilated tortuous part where fertilization occurs—5 cm long
- Infundibulum expanded funnel shaped part
- Fimbriae are finger like folds attached to infundibulum
- Two openings—uterine and abdominal os.

18. Name the coverings of kidney.
- **Fibrous capsule**: It covers the entire organ and lines the walls of renal sinus, minor and major calyces and pelvis of ureter. The capsule is made of connective tissue with more collagen fibers, elastic and few smooth muscle fibers
- **Perirenal fascia**: It is seen between false and true capsules. It is more along the borders of kidney and is a content of renal pelvis
- **Renal fascia (Gerota's fascia) (Fig. 32A)**:
  - Formed by condensation of extra-peritoneal connective tissue containing dense elastic fibers

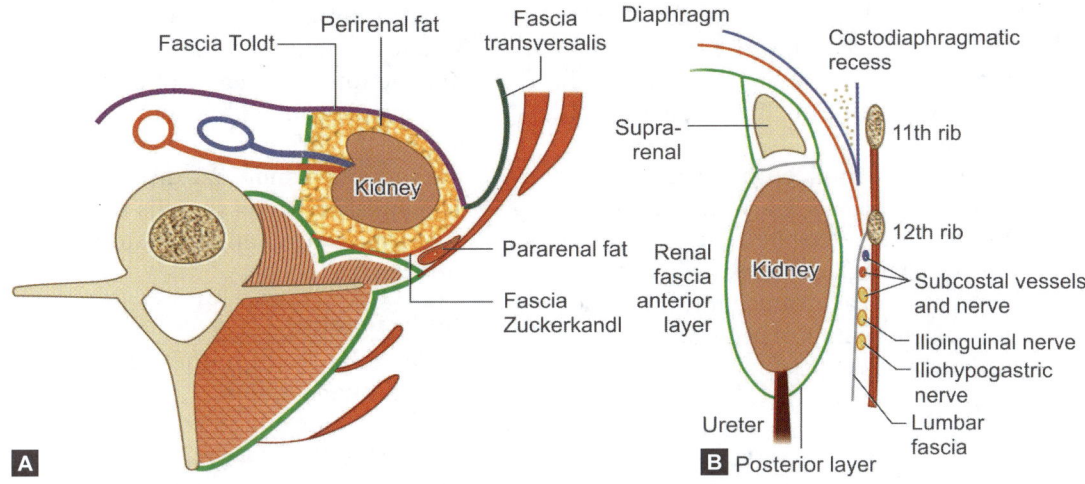

Figs. 32A and B: Renal fascia.

- It is seen as anterior layer (**fascia of Toldt**) and posterior layer (**fascia of Zuckerkandl**)
- The posterior layer is attached to fascia covering psoas major and quadratus lumborum
- Above, it encloses suprarenal gland and is continuous with diaphragmatic fascia (**Fig. 32B**)
- Laterally the two layers fuse to form lateral conal fascia and fuses with parietal peritoneum
- Below both layers fuse and attach with fascia of iliac vessels and with periureteric connective tissue
- Medially anterior layer is continuous with that of opposite side at the level of L3 – L5. Above L3 the two layers fuse.
- **Pararenal fat**: It is abundant on the posterior surface of the lower part of kidney.

19. Name the two most common positions of appendix.

Refer Short Answer on Q. No. 6 – 2008.

20. Name the structures piercing the clavipectoral fascia.

Refer Short Answer on Q. No. 11 – 2009.

21. Mention different parts of diencephalon.

- **Dorsal diencephalon** consists of
  - Thalamus
  - Meta thalamus—medial and lateral geniculate bodies
  - Epithalamus—pineal gland, posterior commissure, habenular nucleus and commissure, stria medullaris thalami.
- **Ventral diencephalon** consists of:
  - Hypothalamus
  - Subthalamus.

22. Emissary veins.

- Emissary veins **pass** through cranial openings
- **Connect** intracranial veins or venous sinuses with extracranial veins
- They are **not constant**
- **Valves** are absent
- By these connections the infection spreads from extracranial foci to venous sinuses
- They **help** to maintain the intracranial pressure
- **Examples** are:
  - The sigmoid sinus is connected with the posterior auricular or occipital veins by mastoid emissary vein, passes through the mastoid foramen
  - The veins of the scalp are connected with the superior sagittal sinus by the parietal emissary vein in the parietal foramen
  - The venous plexus of the hypoglossal canal, connects the sigmoid sinus and the internal jugular vein

- A (posterior) condylar emissary vein passing through the (posterior) condylar canal connects the sigmoid sinus and veins in the suboccipital triangle
- Cavernous sinus connected to the pterygoid plexus by emissary vein through foramen ovale
- Veins through foramen lacerum, connect the cavernous sinus and the pharyngeal veins and pterygoid plexus
- Emissary vein through sphenoidal foramen (of Vesalius) connects the cavernous sinus with the pharyngeal veins and pterygoid plexus
- Through the carotid canal the venous plexus around internal carotid passes, connecting the cavernous sinus and the internal jugular vein
- The external jugular vein is connected to the transverse sinus through petrosquamous sinus
- Through the foramen cecum veins pass, connecting nasal veins with the superior sagittal sinus
- The confluence of sinuses with the occipital vein through occipital emissary vein
- The ophthalmic veins are considered as emissary, because they connect intracranial to extracranial veins.

- **Applied anatomy**
  - When the jugular vein is blocked or tied, venous drainage can be through the occipital sinus that connects veins around the foramen magnum and with the vertebral venous plexuses
  - The emissary veins spreads the infection from extracranial foci to venous sinuses.

23. Lacus lacrimalis.

- It is triangular space in the conjunctival sac at the inner canthus
- The medial canthus is separated from eyeball by the lacus lacrimalis
- It is also called lacrimal lake
- Boundaries: Laterally crescent shaped fold of conjunctiva
  - Above and below by lacrimal part of eyelid
- The lacrimal caruncle is a reddish body situated in this.

24. Lymphatic drainage of the face.

- The lymphatic drainage of face is divided into three regions
  i. Upper area
     - Areas include lateral part of forehead, temple, lateral half of eyelids, conjunctiva, lateral part of cheek, parotid region

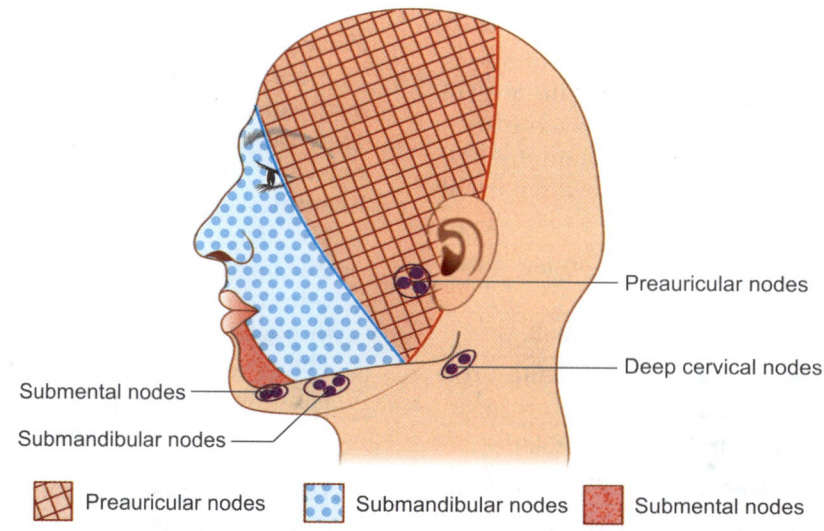

Fig. 33: Lymphatic drainage of face.

- The lymph node draining is pre-auricular nodes.
ii. Intermediate area
   - Areas include central part of forehead, medial half of eyelids, nose, upper lip, medial part of cheek, greater part of lower jaw, frontal and maxillary sinuses
   - Drains into submandibular node.
iii. Lower area
   - Areas include central part of lower lip and chin
   - Drains into submental nodes.

25. Horner's syndrome.

- Any injury to the sympathetic trunk ascending from thorax to the face results in Horner's syndrome
- This occurs in
  - Bronchial carcinoma invading sympathetic
  - Pancoast tumor
  - Radical neck dissection
  - Post cervical sympathectomy surgery complication
  - Avulsion of T_1 nerve from spinal cord.
- Features on the affected side
  - Ptosis—drooping of upper eyelid
  - Enophthalmos—sunken eyes
  - Meiosis—constriction of pupil
  - Narrow palpabral fissure
  - Vasodilatation
  - Anhydrosis—loss of sweat.

26. Histology of skeletal muscle.

- Skeletal muscles are striated muscle
- The muscle fibers are long, cylindrical in shape
- The cytoplasm of each fiber, is known as **sarcoplasm**
- It is surrounded by a plasma membrane called the **sarcolemma**
- Sarcoplasm contains the contractile unit the **myofibrils**, which form the bulk
- The other cell organelles are present in the cytoplasm.

Longitudinal section

- Each muscle fiber is a syncytium with multiple nucleus
- Numerous oval nuclei usually occupy periphery of sarcoplasm between the myofibrils and the sarcolemma
- In high power, myofibrils are seen to consist of two types of filament, thick and thin
- The myofibrils are long filaments and extend along the length of the fiber
- The thick filaments, are mainly made of **myosin**
- The thin filaments, are formed by **actin**
- The cross-striations are present, and they are represented as alternating dark and light bands
- The darker, anisotropic or A-bands, the lighter, isotropic or I-bands
- The Z-lines/Z-discs are transverse lines interrupt at regular intervals and are densely stained lines
- The A-band is formed by the interdigitation of thick filaments myosin and the thin filaments the actin, and at either end actin overlaps the thick filaments. The central,

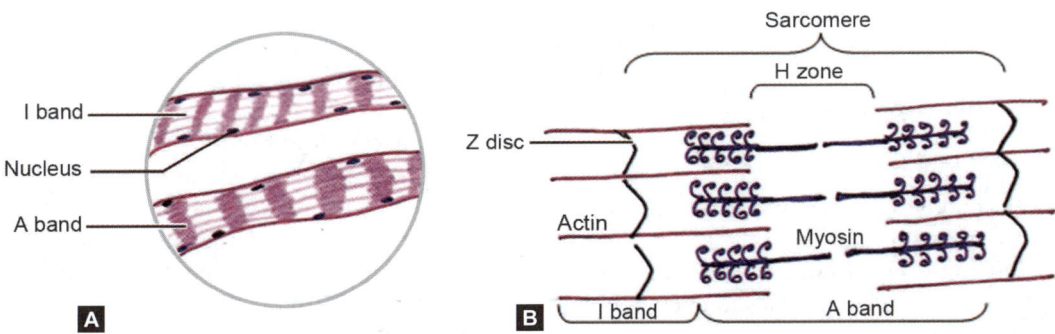

Figs. 34A and B: Histology of skeletal muscle.

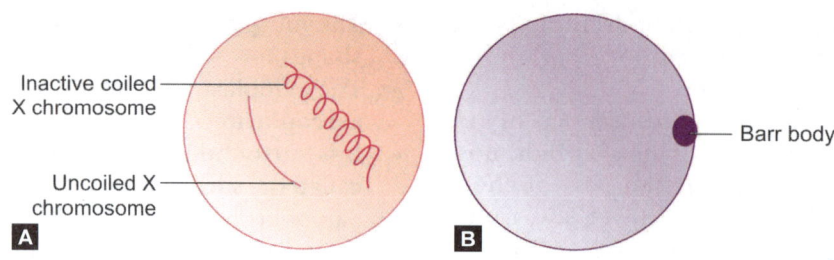

Figs. 35A and B: Barr body.

paler region of the A-band, where the thin filaments are absent, is called the H-zone. At the center of H-zone, the thick filaments are linked together transversely called the M-line
- I-band is the adjacent portions of two neighboring sarcomeres in which the thin filaments are present. The Z-disc, bisects the I-band.

Transverse section: The section shows
- Each muscle bundle is surrounded by connective tissue called **epimysium**
- Individual muscle fasciculus is surrounded by **perimysium**
- Individual muscle fiber is surrounded by **endomysium**.

27. Triangle of Koch.
- Triangle of Koch is related to anteroinferior part of interatrial septum
- **Boundaries:**
  - Septal leaflet of tricuspid valve guarding the right AV orifice
  - Tendon of Todaro—is a sub endocardial ridge extending dorsally from the central fibrous body to the left horn of the valve of the inferior vena cava
  - Coronary sinus opening—situated between the opening of the inferior vena cava and the right atrioventricular orifice.
- **Content:** AV node is situated in it.

28. Barr body.
- Barr body is the inactive X-chromosome in a female somatic cell
- During embryonic development one of the two X chromosomes in each cell does not uncoil into chromatin
- The coiled genetically inactive X chromosome is seen as a heterochromatic body called **sex chromatin (Fig. 35A)**
- The X chromosome remains inactive, coiled as a dark body is also known as **Barr body**
- It is named after the discoverer, Murray Barr **(Fig. 35B)**
- Barr bodies can be seen on the nucleus of the neutrophils as a knob known as drumstick
- In neuron it appears as a small dark body opposite to nucleolus
- Normal number:
  - Normal female has one Barr body per somatic cell
  - A normal male does not possess Barr body.
- Abnormal number:
  - The presence of Barr body in male is called Kleinefelter's syndrome
  - Turner's syndrome is absence of Barr body in female
  - In triple X syndrome two barr bodies.
- Cells used for detecting Barr bodies from:
  - Skin
  - Oral mucosa—mostly used
  - Vagina
  - Urethral epithelium
  - Blood.

29. Types of chromosomes.
- **Types of Chromosomes:**
  - The **autosomes** are the general chromosomes that carry the information to make a human being. They all come in pairs. Humans can have only 22 pairs of chromosomes

- The **sex chromosomes** also come in pairs, but come in two types—X and Y.
- Chromosome are of 4 types based on their **position of centromeres (Fig. 36A to D)**
  1. Telocentric—centromere is at one end, so only long limb is present
  2. Acrocentric—centromere very near the end, so that one arm is very small and the other very long
  3. Submetacentric—centromere is slightly away from the centre, one arm is short and the other arm is long
  4. Metacentric—centromere near the center.
- According to **banding techniques**: Each arm is divided into regions 1, 2, so on beginning from centromere
- According to the **descending length of the chromosomes**:
  According to **Denver classification** the chromosomes are grouped according to descending length of chromosomes into 7 groups—A to G groups
  - *A group*: Chromosomes 1,2,3 are included and all are metacentric
  - *B group*: Chromosomes 4 and 5. They are submetacentric
  - *C group*: Chromosomes 6 – 12 and X chromosomes are included in this type. They belong to submetacentric type. In male 15 number and female 16 number of chromosomes are present
  - *D group*: Chromosomes 13 to 15 and they belong to acrocentric group
  - *E group*: Chromosomes 16, 17, 18 are included and are submetacentric type
  - *F group*: Chromosomes 19 and 20 are included and are metacentric type
  - *G group*: Chromosomes 21, 22 and Y chromosome. In male 5 numbers and female 4 numbers of chromosome are present. They belong to acrocentric type.

30. Bones derived from 1st pharyngeal arch.
Refer Short Notes 24 – 2007.

31. Name the bones taking part in the formation of nasal septum.
Refer Short Notes 17 – 2003.

32. Name the structures passing through foramen spinosum.
- Foramen spinosum is present in the greater wing of sphenoid bone
- It opens into infratemporal fossa
- It connects the middle cranial fossa with infratemporal fossa
- Structures passing are:
  - Middle meningeal artery
  - Nervus spinosus/meningeal branch of mandibular nerve.

33. Name any two nerves emerging from medulla oblongata.
- Anterolateral sulcus between pyramid and olive—hypoglossal nerve
- Posterolateral sulcus lateral to olive—from above downwards glossopharyngeal, vagus, and cranial accessory nerves.

34. Name any two structures in relation to mediastinal surface of left lung.
Refer Essay Q. No. 3 – 2004.

35. Name the parts of lacrimal apparatus.
Refer Short Notes 27 – 2006.

36. Name the arteries which supply the heart.
The myocardium is supplied by the **two coronary arteries**—the right and the left.
- They anastomose with each other
- But they function as end arteries

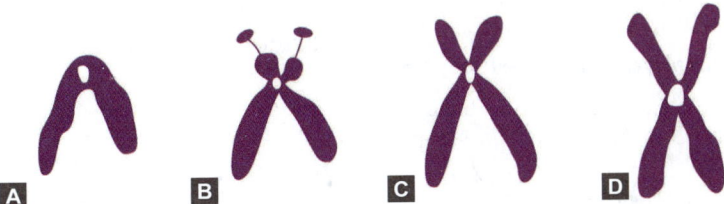

Figs. 36A to D: (A) Telocentric; (B) Acrocentric; (C) Submetacentric (D) Metacentric.

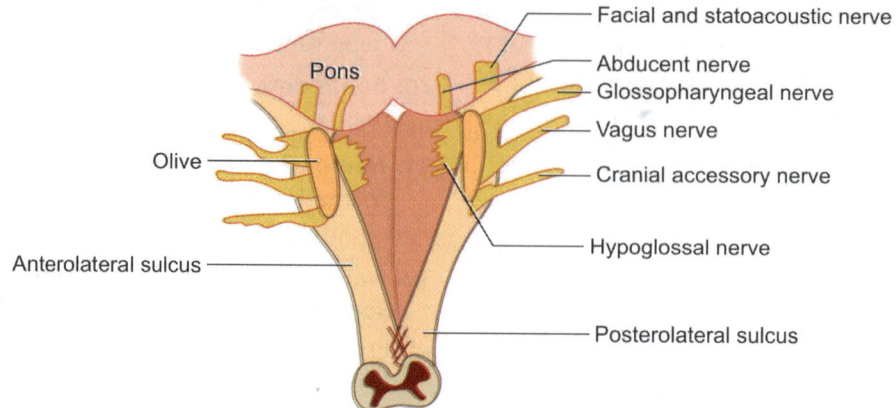

Fig. 37: Nerves emerging from medulla oblongata.

- **Right coronary** arises from anterior aortic sinus of the ascending aorta
- **Areas supplied**
  - Right atrium
  - Greater part of right ventricle except the part along the anterior interventricular groove
  - Smaller part of left ventricle along the posterior interventricular groove
  - Posterior one-third of interventricular septum
  - Whole of conducting system of heart except a part of the left branch of AV bundle.
- **Left coronary** from the left posterior aortic sinus of ascending aorta
- **Areas supplied**
  - Left atrium
  - Greater part of left ventricle except the region along the posterior interventricular groove
  - Smaller part of right ventricle along the anterior interventricular groove
  - Anterior two-third of interventricular septum
  - A part of left branch of AV bundle.

37. Name the infrahyoid muscles of the neck.

- Infrahyoid muscles are called as strap/ribbon muscles
- Situated below the hyoid bone.
- They are four in number:
  i. Sternohyoid
  ii. Sternothyroid
  iii. Thyrohyoid
  iv. Omohyoid—superior and inferior belly
- Innervation: The thyrohyoid muscle is supplied by C1 fibers through hypoglossal nerve. The other muscles by ansa cervicalis.

38. Name the muscles of mastication.

Refer Short Answer 33 – 2009.

39. Name the terminal branches of facial nerve.

- Temporal
- Zygomatic
- Buccal
- Marginal mandibular
- Cervical.

40. Name the unpaired cartilages of the larynx.

- Epiglottis—made of elastic cartilage
- Thyroid cartilage—made of hyaline cartilage
- Cricoid cartilage—made of hyaline cartilage.

MBBS Examination 2011

ANSWER ALL QUESTIONS

I. Essay questions (15/10 Marks)

1. Describe brachial plexus in detail under the following headings: Formation, branches and applied anatomy.
2. Describe male urethra in detail under the following headings: Extent, parts, sphincters and blood vessels.
3. Describe arches of foot in detail.
4. Describe relations, ligaments, nerve supply, histology and applied anatomy of urinary bladder.
5. Describe in detail about blood supply of brain.
6. Describe submandibular salivary gland under following heading: Parts, relations, blood supply, nerve supply, lymphatic drainage and clinical anatomy.
7. Describe cerebellum as: Classification, connections, nuclei, blood supply and clinical anatomy.
8. Describe boundaries, contents and clinical anatomy of carotid triangle.

II. Short notes (5/4 Marks)

1. Dorsal spaces in hand.
2. Branches of axillary artery in detail.
3. Histology of kidney.
4. Locking and unlocking of knee joint.
5. Femoral nerve.
6. Formation of blastocyst.
7. Sacral plexus.
8. Second part of duodenum.
9. Internal oblique muscle.
10. Portacaval anastomosis.
11. Descent of testis.
12. Klinefelter's syndrome.
13. Omental bursa.
14. Histology of suprarenal gland.
15. Blood supply of stomach.
16. Boundaries and contents of axilla.
17. Brachialis muscle.
18. Adductor canal.
19. Extensor retinacula of leg.
20. Histology of skin.
21. Azygos vein.
22. Relations of arch of aorta.
23. Left coronary artery.
24. Histology of cerebral cortex.
25. Corpus callosum.
26. Horns of lateral ventricle.
27. Contents of posterior triangle.
28. Extrinsic muscles of tongue.
29. Brachiocephalic vein.
30. Development of atria.
31. Histology of parotid gland.
32. Histology of cornea.
33. Development of lung.
34. Internal capsule.
35. Typical intercostal nerve.
36. Cavernous sinus.
37. Connections of basal ganglia.
38. Blood supply of thyroid gland.
39. Lymphatic drainage of tongue.
40. Maxillary air sinus.

III. Short answer questions (3/2 Marks)

1. Buttonhole deformity.
2. Brachioradialis muscle.
3. Muscle responsible for lateral rotation movement of shoulder joint.
4. Formation of superficial palmar arch.
5. Histology of layers of aorta.
6. Palthi posture.
7. Gracilis muscles.

8. Long saphenous vein.
9. Allantois.
10. Histology of cardiac muscle.
11. Transpyloric plane.
12. Branches of superior mesenteric artery.
13. Relations of inferior surface of liver.
14. Perineal body.
15. Anal fissure.
16. Muscles attached to extensor expansion of hand.
17. Name the structures piercing clavipectoral fascia.
18. Remnants of notochord.
19. Histological features of lymph node.
20. Contents of broad ligament.
21. Lateral rotation of hip joint.
22. Name the PIN structures.
23. Name the ligaments related to spleen.
24. Contents of pudendal canal.
25. Boundaries of auscultation triangle.
26. Interventricular septum.
27. Costodiaphragmatic recess.
28. Tricuspid valve.
29. Oblique fissure of lung.
30. Demilunes.
31. Falx cerebelli.
32. Substantia nigra.
33. List special somatic afferent nuclei.
34. Functional areas of superior temporal gyrus.
35. Waldeyer's ring.
36. Middle cervical ganglion.
37. Parotid duct.
38. Fenestra vestibule.
39. Epicranial aponeurosis.
40. Derivatives of third aortic arch.
41. Enumerate the muscles of palate.
42. Two features of nasopharynx.
43. Congenital anomalies of ventricles of heart.
44. Derivatives of second pharyngeal arch.
45. Arteries supplying the spinal cord.
46. Boundaries of submental triangle.
47. Structures present at hilum of left lung.
48. Name the unpaired dural venous sinuses.
49. Intrinsic muscles of larynx.

I. ESSAY QUESTIONS

1. **Describe brachial plexus in detail under the following headings: Formation, branches and applied anatomy.**

Refer Essay Q. No. 3 – 2005.

2. **Describe male urethra in detail under the following headings: Extent, parts, sphincters and blood vessels.**

Length: Male urethra is 18 – 20 cm long. Posterior part is about 4 cm longer than the anterior part

Extends from the internal urethral orifice in the urinary bladder to the external opening (meatus) at the end of the penis.

Parts (Fig. 1)

i. Preprostatic part
ii. Prostatic part   } Posterior part
iii. Membranous part
iv. Bulbar part
v. Penile part   } Anterior part

- **Preprostatic part**: Extends from base of bladder to the prostate. It is about 1cm in length
- **Prostatic part**
  Refer Short Notes 2 – 2006.

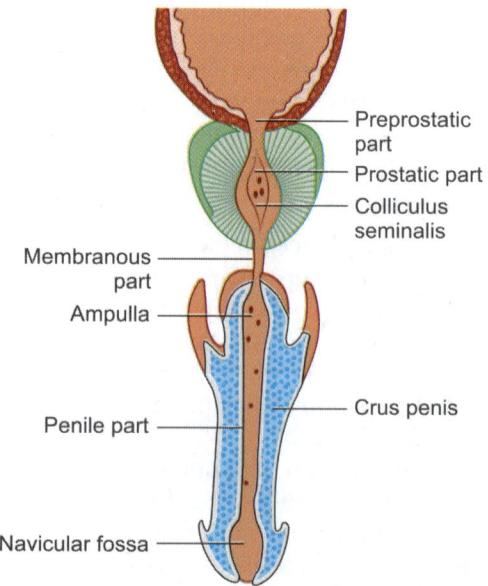

Fig. 1: Male urethra.

- **Membranous part**
  - It is narrower and shortest part of urethra
  - It extends from prostate to bulb of penis
  - It pierces the perineal membrane
  - It is a content of deep perineal pouch
  - It is 2.5 cm behind pubic symphysis
  - This part is surrounded by sphincter
  - Bulbourethral glands are situated on either side.
- **Bulbar part**
  - Widest part of the urethra
  - The ducts of bulbourethral glands open into it about 2.5 cm below perineal membrane
  - It is continued as penile urethra.
- **Penile part**
  - A dilatation is seen at glans penis called navicular fossa
  - At external os seen as a vertical slit, which is the narrowest part of urethra.

Part		Length	Shape of lumen on cross section	Epithelium	Development
Posterior part	Preprostatic part	1 cm	Stellate	Transitional epithelium	From mesonephric duct
	Prostatic part	3 – 4 cm	Crescent	Above colliculus seminalis—transitional epithelium; Below colliculus seminalis—pseudostratified or stratified columnar	Above colliculus seminalis—from mesonephric duct; Below colliculus—from endoderm of urogenital sinus
	Membranous part	2 cm	Stellate/irregular	Stratified columnar	Endoderm – urogenital sinus
Anterior part (spongiose part)	Bulbar part; Penile part a. Body of penis b. Base of glans penis c. At external orifice	15 cm	Transverse slit; Transverse slit; Inverted shape; Vertical slit	Stratified columnar; Nonkeratinized stratified squamous epithelium	Endoderm—urogenital sinus; From ectoderm

Sphincters
- External sphincter—surrounding the membranous part formed by pubourethral part of levator ani
- Internal sphincter—surrounding bladder neck and preprostatic part.

Blood Supply
- Arteries:
  - Urethral artery arises from internal pudendal artery
  - Dorsal penile artery via circumflex branches on each side.
- Veins:
  - Anterior part of urethra—dorsal vein of penis - internal pudendal vein which drains into prostatic venous plexus
  - Posterior part of urethra—prostatic and vesical venous plexus—internal iliac veins.

Applied Anatomy
- Rupture of the bulbar part of the male urethra which is a content of superficial perineal pouch results in collection of urine in the superficial perineal pouch leading to extravasation of urine
- Rupture of membranous part results in collection of urine in deep perineal pouch
- Following anatomy of urethra should be remembered during catheterization:
  - External urethral meatus is the narrowest part
  - Lacuna magna in the roof of navicular fossa.

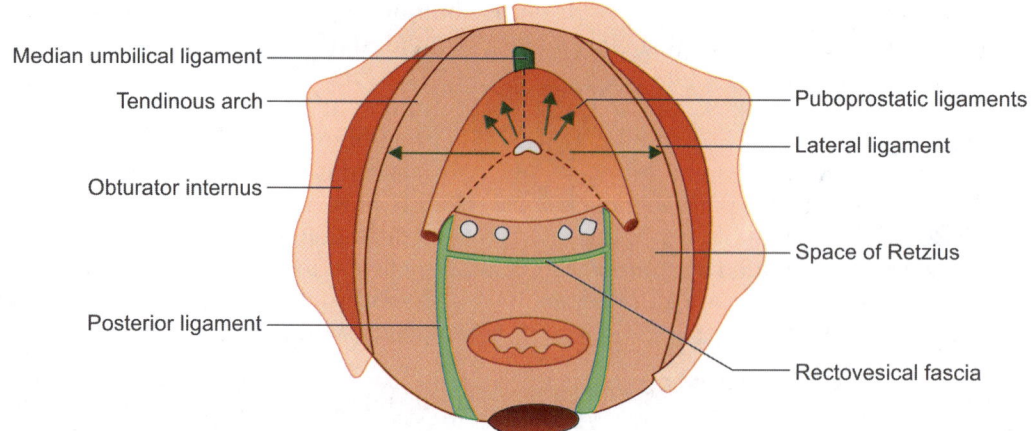

Fig. 2: Ligaments of urinary bladder.

3. Describe arches of foot in detail.
Refer Essay Q. No. 1 – 2003.

4. Describe the relations, ligaments, nerve supply, histology and applied anatomy of urinary bladder.
Relations, nerve supply and applied aspects refer essay Q. No. 2 – 2003.
Histology refer Essay Q. No. 3 – 2010.

Ligaments
- Pubovesical ligament: It extends from neck of bladder to inferior aspect of pubic bone. It lies one on either side of midline. They are derived from detrusor muscle. In female it is extended as pubourethral ligament. In male anteriorly it is continued as puboprostatic ligament
- Median umbilical ligament: It extends from apex to the umbilicus
- Posterior and lateral vesical ligaments: They formed by reflection of the peritoneum with condensation of connective tissue.

5. Describe in detail about blood supply of brain.

- **Arterial supply:** The brain is supplied by two systems of arteries—carotid and vertebrobasilar system
- **Carotid system:**
  - ICA pierces the roof of cavernous sinus and emerges lateral to optic chiasma.
  - Related to anterior perforated substance
  - Terminates by dividing into anterior and middle cerebral artery.
  - The following **branches** supply the brain:
    - Anterior cerebral artery
    - Middle cerebral artery
    - Anterior choroidal artery
    - Posterior communicating artery.
- **Vertebrobasilar system**:
  - Vertebral artery enters the cranial cavity through foramen magnum
  - Joins with the opposite artery to form basilar artery.
- **Branches from the vertebral artery** are:
  - Anterior spinal
  - Posterior spinal
  - Posterior inferior cerebellar
  - Medullary branches
- **Branches from basilar artery** are:
  - Superior cerebellar
  - Anterior inferior cerebellar
  - Pontine branches
  - Posterior cerebral arteries
- The **circle of Willis:**
  - It is an arterial circle

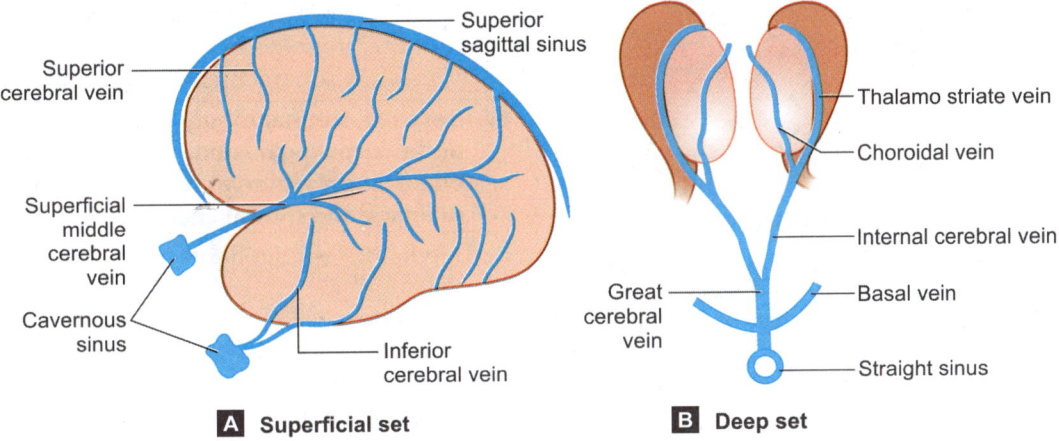

Figs. 3A and B: Venous drainage of cerebrum.

- Situated in the base of brain
- Related to interpeduncular fossa
- A communication is established between carotid and vertebrobasilar systems.
- **Formation:**
  - Anteriorly—anterior communicating arteries from anterior cerebral
  - Anterolaterally—anterior cerebral arteries from internal carotid
  - Laterally—terminal part of internal carotid arteries
  - Posterolaterally—posterior communicating arteries from internal carotid
  - Posteriorly—posterior cerebral arteries from basilar
  - Branches are central branches.
- **Areas supplied:**
  - **Medulla oblongata:** The medulla oblongata is supplied by the branches of the vertebral, anterior and posterior spinal, posterior inferior cerebellar and basilar arteries
  - **Pons:** The pons is supplied by the basilar artery and the anterior inferior and superior cerebellar arteries. Direct branches from the basilar artery enter the pons
  - **Midbrain:** The midbrain is supplied by the posterior cerebral, superior cerebellar and basilar arteries.
  - **Cerebellum:** The cerebellum is supplied by the posterior inferior, anterior inferior and superior cerebellar arteries.
  - **Cerebrum and medial surface:** Superolateral surface—Refer Essay Q. No. 7 – 2010.

  Medial surface of the hemisphere
  - Supplied by the anterior, middle and posterior cerebral arteries
  - The area supplied by the anterior cerebral artery is sensory and motor areas of lower limb and extending up to parieto-occipital sulcus
  - The posterior cerebral supplies visual area, cuneus
  - The middle cerebral supplies the temporal pole.

  Inferior surface
  - The medial part of orbital surface by anterior cerebral artery
  - The lateral part of the orbital surface and the temporal pole are supplied by the middle cerebral artery
  - The remaining inferior surfaces are supplied by the posterior cerebral artery.
- **Venous drainage:**
  - **Cerebrum:** The veins are seen as superficial and deep set
  - **Superficial set of cerebral veins** are divided into superior, middle and inferior cerebral veins

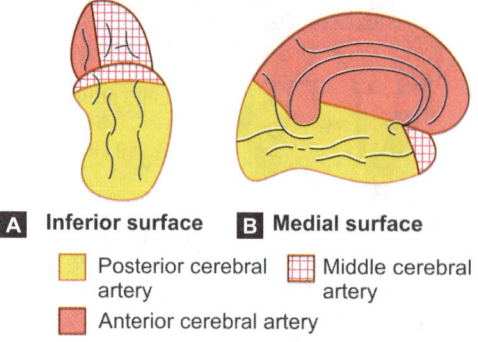

Figs. 4A and B: Arterial supply of cerebrum.

- The superior cerebral veins end in superior sagittal sinus
- The superficial middle cerebral and inferior cerebral veins end in cavernous sinus
- The deep middle cerebral vein joins with anterior cerebral vein to form basal vein which drains to great cerebral vein.
- **Deep set:**
  - The thalamostriate vein joins with choroidal veins to form the internal cerebral vein
  - The two internal cerebral veins join to form great cerebral vein which drains to straight sinus.
- **Cerebellum:** The veins of the cerebellum drain into adjacent sinuses
- **Midbrain** veins to basal vein
- **Pons** to basal vein and transverse sinuses
- **Medulla oblongata** to basilar venous plexus.
- **Applied anatomy:**
  - Lesion of lenticulostriate branches leads to contralateral hemiplegia
  - Lateral medullary/Wallenberg syndrome lesion of posterior inferior cerebellar artery

- Rupture of Berry aneurysm in any one of the branches of circle of Willis may result in subarachnoid hemorrhage.

6. **Describe submandibular salivary gland under following heading: Parts, relations, blood supply, nerve supply, lymphatic drainage and clinical anatomy.**

Parts, relations—Refer Short Notes on Q. No. 14 – 2003.

- **Blood supply:**
  - Facial artery
  - Lingual artery
  - Veins drain into common facial or lingual vein.
- **Nerve supply:**
  - Secretomotor **(Fig. 5)** (parasympathetic)
    - Superior salivatory nucleus---------- facial nerve ---------- chorda tympani _Joins_ Lingual nerves _to the_ submandibular ganglion _postganglionic fibers_ gland
  - Sympathetic
    - Postganglionic fibers from superior cervical ganglion ---------- plexus around facial artery -------------- gland
- **Lymphatic drainage:** Lymph passes to jugulo omohyoid nodes interrupted by submandibular nodes
- **Clinical anatomy:** Duct of submandibular gland impacted by small stone, are due to stasis of secretion of the gland. Gland is felt as a swelling during eating as it increases in size
  - Sialography—radiographic procedure in which dye is injected to study the duct pattern.

7. **Describe cerebellum as: Classification, connections, nuclei, blood supply and clinical anatomy.**

Cerebellum has two hemispheres united in the middle by vermis.

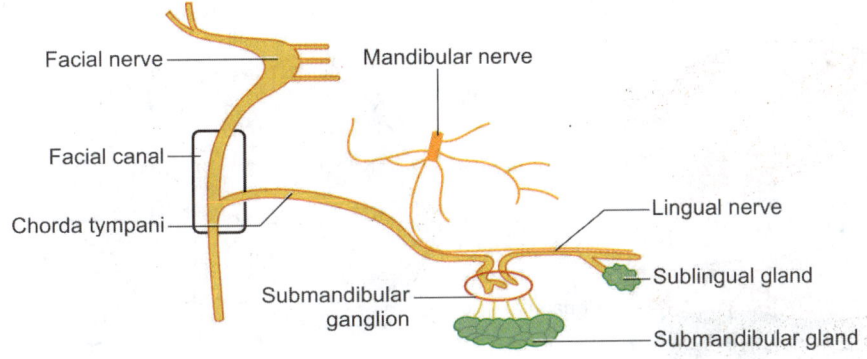

Fig. 5: Secretomotor pathway of submandibular gland.

Classification

- **Larsell's classification (Fig. 6):**

Parts of vermis	Subdivisions of cerebellar hemisphere
– Lingula	....
– Central lobule	.... ala of central lobule
– Culmen	.... quadrangular lobule
– Declive	.... lobules simplex
– Folium	.... superior semilunar lobule
– Tuber	.... inferior semilunar lobule
– Pyramid	.... biventral lobule
– Uvula	.... tonsil
– Nodule	.... flocculus connected by flocculonodular peduncle

- **Anatomical subdivision:**
  - Divided into:
    - Flocculonodular lobe
    - Corpus cerebellum which is further divided into:
      * Anterior lobe – separated from posterior lobe by the fissure prima
      * Posterior lobe – separated from the flocculonodular lobe by the posterolateral fissure.
- **Morphological divisions** of cerebellum:
  - **Archi cerebellum (Fig. 7):**
    - Phylogenetically it is the oldest part. It is made up of flocculonodular lobe and the lingula
    - Its connection are vestibulocerebellar
    - It controls the axial musculature and the bilateral movements used for locomotion and maintenance of equilibrium.
  - **Paleocerebellum:**
    - Made up of the anterior lobe except lingula and the pyramid and uvula of inferior vermis
    - Its connections are chiefly spinocerebellar
    - It controls tone, posture and crude movements of the limbs.
  - **Neocerebellum:**
    - It is the recent part to develop
    - It is made up of posterior lobe except pyramid and uvula
    - Its connections are corticopontine
    - It is mainly concerned with the regulation of fine movements of the body.
- **Functional divisions** of cerebellum: Functionally the anterior and posterior lobes are organized into 3 longitudinal zones (Fig. 7):
  1. Lateral zone: Connected with association areas of brain; it is involved in planning and programming of muscle activities
  2. Intermediate (paravermal) zone: Concerned with control of muscles of hands, fingers, feet and toes
  3. Vermal zone: Concerned with muscles of trunk, neck, shoulders and hip.

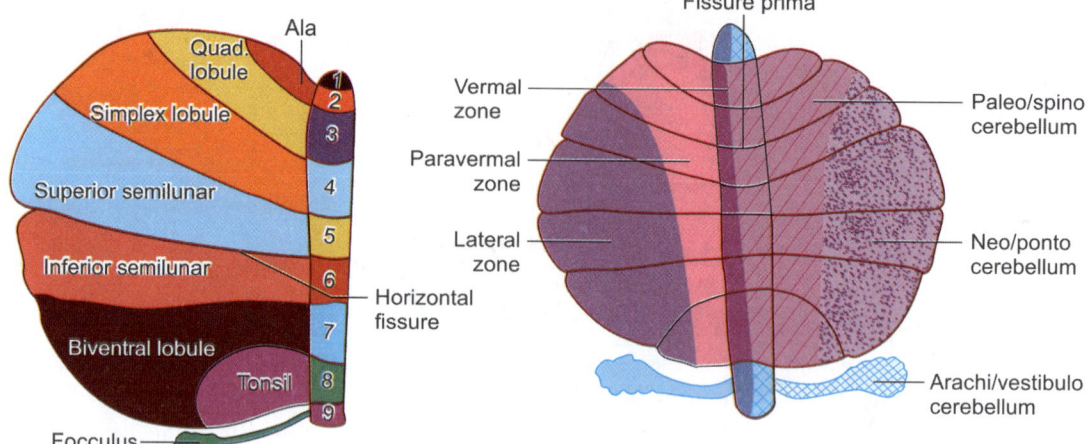

Fig. 6: 1. Lingual 2. Central lobule 3. Culmen 4. Declive 5. Folium 6. Tuber 7. Pyramid 8. Uvula 9. Nodule.

Fig. 7: Functional and morphological divisions.

Connections

Refer Short Notes 20 – 2006.

Nuclei

Nuclei: From lateral to medial (Doctors **E**at **G**ood **F**ood) **(Fig. 8)**

- **D**entate nucleus—neocerebellum
- **E**mboliform nucleus—paleo- cerebellum
- **G**lobosus nucleus—paleo- cerebellum
- **F**astigial nucleus—archicerebellum.

Blood Supply

Arterial Supply (Fig. 9)

The cerebellum is supplied by three cerebellar arteries.

1. **Posterior inferior cerebellar artery**
   - It is a branch from the 4th part of vertebral artery
   - It is given off at the lower end of olive of medulla oblongata
   - It ascends laterally and reaches the lower border of pons
   - Then descends downwards along the inferolateral boundary of the fourth ventricle
   - It turns laterally to reach the vallecula and terminates into medial and lateral branches
   - It supplies the posterior part of inferior surface of cerebellum
   - It anastomoses with superior and anterior inferior cerebellar arteries.

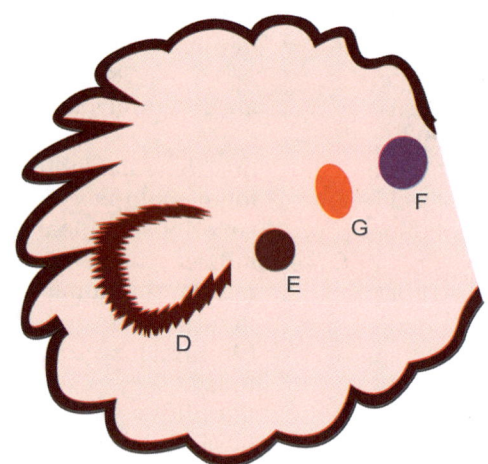

Fig. 8: Deep nuclei of cerebellum.

2. **Anterior inferior cerebellar artery**
   - It is a branch from basilar artery
   - It arises from the lower part of basilar artery
   - It runs laterally along the lower border of pons separated from labyrinthine artery by 6th, 7th and 8th nerves
   - It supplies the anterior part of inferior surface of cerebellum.

3. **Superior cerebellar artery**
   - It is a branch from the basilar artery
   - It arises from the distal part of basilar artery
   - It runs laterally along the upper border of pons and is parallel to the posterior

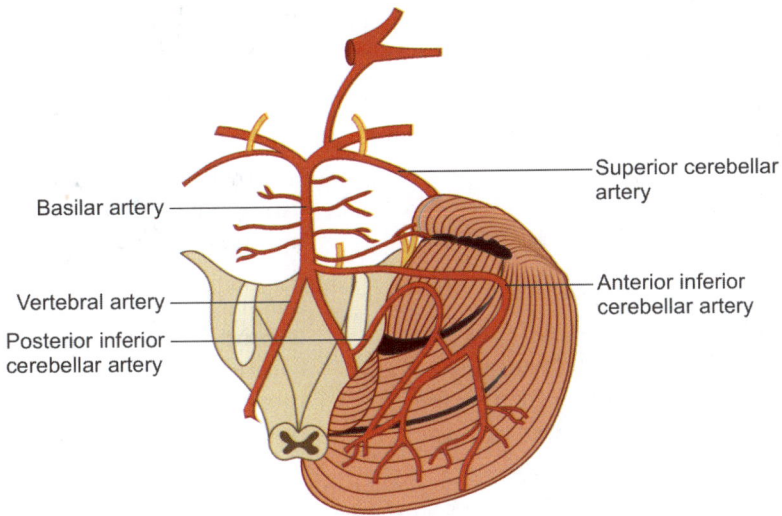

Fig. 9: Arterial supply of cerebellum.

cerebral artery separated by the oculomotor nerve
- It curves around the cerebral peduncles and reaches the superior surface of cerebellum
- It anastomoses with the inferior cerebellar arteries.

Venous Drainage
The veins of the cerebellum drain into adjacent sinuses.

Clinical Anatomy
- Unilateral lesions in the cerebellar hemispheres leads to:
  - Nystagmus
  - Incoordination of the same side upper limb as in the finger-nose test
  - The movements are inaccurate (dysmetria)
  - The limb swings to and fro, intention tremor
  - There is failure of cooperation between muscles controlling the joints of the upper limb (asynergia)
  - Alternating hand movements are awkward (dysdiadochokinesia)
  - Marked rebound of the limb, when the arm is outstretched.
- Bilateral lesions of the cerebellar hemisphere lead to:
  - Nystagmus
  - Dysarthria in which the syllables are extended (scanning speech)
  - The gait is wide based, reeling, and incoordinate (ataxia)
  - On eye closure, the ataxia is same as in eye opened (negative Romberg's sign).

8. Describe boundaries, contents and clinical anatomy of carotid triangle.

Carotid triangle: It is one of the anterior triangles of neck.

Boundaries (Fig. 10)
- Posteriorly: Anterior border of sternocleidomastoid muscle
- Anterosuperiorly: Posterior belly of digastric and stylohyoid
- Anteroinferiorly: Superior belly of omohyoid
- Roof: Skin, superficial fascia with platysma, cervical branch of facial nerve, investing layer of deep cervical fascia, transverse cutaneous nerve of the neck
- Floor: Anterior part of floor: Part of hyoglossus and thyrohyoid.

- Posterior part of floor: Middle and inferior constrictors of pharynx.
- Anterior angle—hyoid bone.

Contents (Fig. 11)

- **Common carotid artery**
  - Origin:
    - Right side—from brachiocephalic trunk
    - Left side—from arch of aorta.
- **Termination:**
  - Divides into external carotid artery (ECA) and internal carotid arteries (ICA) at the level of upper border of thyroid cartilage
  - The vertebral level disc between C_3 and C_4.
  - At the level of termination, a dilation is present extending to origin of internal carotid artery termed **carotid sinus** where the tunica media is thin and tunica adventitia is thick. It is supplied by sinus branches of IX and X cranial nerves and sympathetic chain and acts as a baroreceptor
  - Behind the termination of common carotid, a Small, oval, reddish-brown body is situated known as **carotid body**. It acts as chemoreceptor

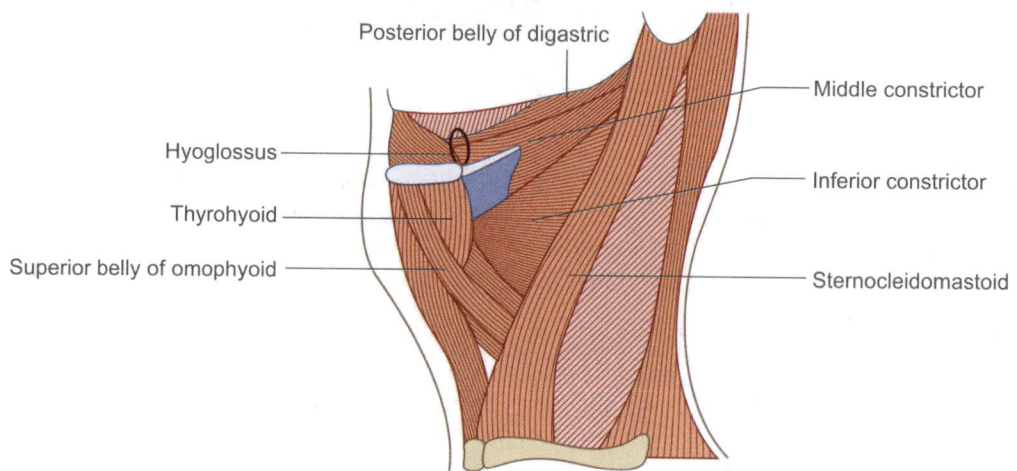

Fig. 10: Boundaries of carotid triangle.

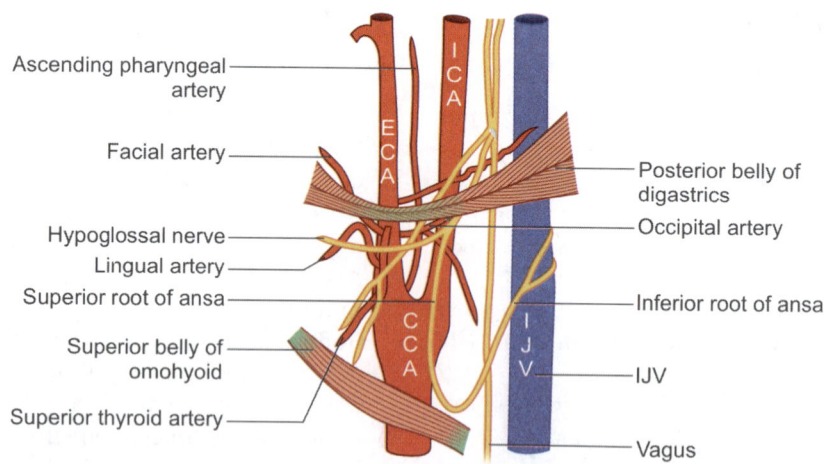

Fig. 11: Contents of carotid triangle.

- **Internal carotid artery:** It is one of the terminal branch of common carotid artery given at the level of upper border of thyroid cartilage. It ascends upwards and enters the cranial cavity through carotid canal. No branch is given by this artery in the neck.
- **External carotid artery:**
    - **Origin**
        - It arises at the level of upper border of thyroid cartilage or intervertebral disc between C3 and C4
        - It is initially anteromedial and then becomes anterior to the internal carotid artery.
    - **Termination**
        - Behind the neck of mandible by dividing into maxillary and superficial temporal arteries
        - Branches in carotid triangle:
            * Superior thyroid artery
            * Lingual artery
            * Facial artery
            * Ascending pharyngeal artery
            * Occipital artery.
- **Internal jugular vein**
    - Extends from base of skull to root of neck
    - Collects blood from brain, superficial part of the face and the neck
    - Formation: Continuation of sigmoid sinus
    - Vein lies lateral to internal and common carotid arteries inside the carotid sheath
    - Termination: Joins with subclavian vein to form brachiocephalic vein
    - Tributaries in carotid triangle are.
        - Pharyngeal veins
        - Common facial vein
        - Lingual vein
        - Superior thyroid vein
        - Middle thyroid vein
        - Occipital vein
    - Common carotid artery (CCA), internal carotid artery, internal jugular vein and vagus nerve are enclosed in a fascial sheath—**carotid sheath.**
- **Vagus nerve:** Descends downwards within the carotid sheath between internal carotid artery and internal jugular vein. The branches given in this triangle are the internal laryngeal nerve and, below it, the external laryngeal nerve, lie medial to the external carotid artery below the hyoid bone
- **Spinal accessory nerve:** Seen in the upper angle of triangle and leaves the triangle by passing deep to the sternocleidomastoid muscle
- **Hypoglossal nerve:** The hypoglossal nerve crosses the external and internal carotid arteries. It curves around the origin of the lower sternocleidomastoid branch of the occipital artery, and at this point the superior root of the ansa cervicalis leaves it to descend anteriorly in the carotid sheath. It crosses the loop of lingual artery
- **Ansa cervicalis:** It is a nerve loop to supply infrahyoid muscles.
    - Location: Situated on anterior surface of carotid sheath
    - Formation by union of:
        - Descendens cervicalis (inferior root of ansa)—C_2, C_3 fibers
        - Descendens hypoglossi (superior root of ansa)—C_1 fibers travelling via hypoglossal nerve.
- **Cervical sympathetic chain:** Situated behind the carotid sheath
- **Deep cervical nodes:** Vertical chain along the IJV. Jugulo-digastric group lie above the posterior belly of the digastric muscle, and Jugulo-omohyoid group below the muscle.

Applied Anatomy

- In the carotid triangle carotid pulse is felt just lateral to the upper margin of thyroid cartilage
- The enlargement of deep cervical lymph nodes due to tuberculosis are painless, seen along the internal jugular vein. Sometimes they degenerate and result in cold abscess.

II. SHORT NOTES

1. Dorsal spaces in hand.

- **Dorsal subcutaneous space:**
  - It lies immediately deep to the loose skin of the dorsum of the hand
  - It contains loose areolar tissue and lymphatics
  - In subcutaneous infections, the pus points through the skin and can be drained at the pointing site.
- **Dorsal subtendinous/subaponeurotic space:**
  - This space lies between the metacarpal bones and the extensor tendons which are united to one another by a thin aponeurosis
  - In subtendinous infection, the pus points either at the webs or at the borders of the hand and can be drained accordingly.
- **Posterior interosseous space:**
  - It is a closed space between the first dorsal interosseous muscle and the fascia covering it
  - The infection from subaponeurotic space can spread to this space along the radial artery.

2. Branches of axillary artery in detail.
Refer Essay Q. No. 4 – 2007.

3. Histology of kidney.
Refer Short Notes 3 – 2007.

4. Locking and unlocking of knee joint.

- The knee joint is a modified hinge variety with three joints—two condylar joints between the femur tibia and saddle joint between the femur and patella
- Locking and unlocking movements are the movements of knee joint
- In addition to flexion and extension, there is small amount of rotation of leg is possible in flexed position of knee
- **Locking of the knee joint**
  - **Definition:**
    - Locking is a mechanism in which the knee remains in the position of full extension as in standing with less muscular effort
    - This is described as **screw home movement**.
  - **Stages of action:**
    - During extension, the smaller and more rounded lateral femoral and tibial condyles are completely used
    - The medial condyle of femur is larger and the medial meniscus is elongated anteroposteriorly. The left over 30° of medial femoral and tibial condyles is used to complete full extension
    - At this stage the anterior cruciate ligament is taut and prevents further backward displacement of femur
    - With tight anterior cruciate ligament as an axis, the femur rotates medially passively
    - As a result, the lateral condyle of femur moves forwards and medial condyle moves backwards
    - The extra portions of medial femoral and tibial condyles are now completely used
    - The medial collateral ligament directed downwards and forwards becomes taut
    - The fibular collateral ligament directed downwards and backwards becomes taut
    - Then oblique popliteal ligament directed upwards and laterally also becomes taut
    - With all the ligaments being taut, the joint is stable and gets locked.
- **Muscles that lock the knee joint:** Quadriceps femoris and tensor fascia lata keep the knee in locked position.
- **Unlocking of the knee joint**
  - **Definition:**
    - Unlocking is the lateral rotation of the femur on tibia during flexion of the locked knee.
  - **Mechanism:**
    - Before flexion, the locked knee has to be unlocked first by lateral rotation of femur
    - The medially rotated femur during the extremes of extension is passively

rotated laterally by popliteus muscle which unlocks the knee
  - Unlocked knee can be flexed now.
- **Muscle that unlocks the knee joint:** Unlocking is done by **popliteus.**

5. Femoral nerve.

- The femoral nerve is the largest branch of the lumbar plexus
- It is a nerve of extensor compartment of thigh
- **Root value:** From dorsal branches of ventral rami of L_2, L_3, L_4
- **Course:**
  - **Abdominal course**:
    - Formed within the substance of the psoas major
    - Emerges along the lateral margin of the psoas major
    - Passes deep to the inguinal ligament and enters the thigh.
  - **In the thigh**:
    - Appears in between psoas major and iliacus
    - Enters the femoral triangle behind the inguinal ligament
    - It is situated lateral to the femoral artery and outside the femoral sheath
    - The lateral circumflex femoral artery passes between anterior and posterior divisions.
- **Branches and distribution:**
  - From trunk:
    - Muscular branch: Branch to iliacus, pectineus
    - Vascular branch: To femoral artery.
  - From anterior division:
    - Cutaneous branch:
    - Intermediate cutaneous branch of thigh.
      * Medial cutaneous branch of thigh
    - Muscular branch: to sartorius
- **From posterior division:**
  - Cutaneous branch: Saphenous nerve
  - Muscular branches: To quadriceps femoris—rectus femoris, vastus medialis, lateralis, intermedius
  - Articular branches: To hip and knee joints.
- **Applied anatomy:**
  - In psoas abscess the nerve may be compressed resulting in loss of knee jerk
  - Saphenous nerve is used for grafting as it is superficially situated
  - Femoral nerve block can be given below the mid inguinal point, about

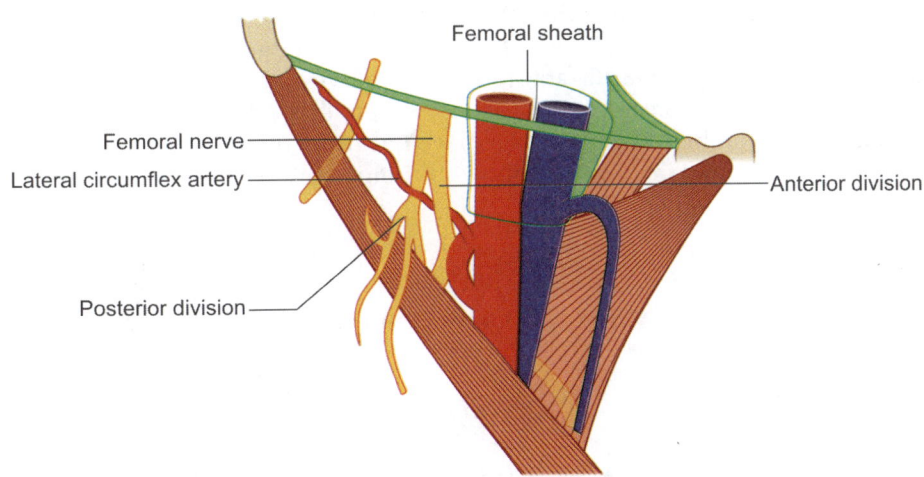

Fig. 12: Femoral nerve.

1.5 cm lateral to the pulsation of femoral artery.

6. Formation of blastocyst.

- Fertilization of ova occurs in ampulla of fallopian tube and zygote is formed
- The zygote undergoes cleavage
- Segmentation of zygote occurs within the zona pellucida
- The small cells formed are known as blastomeres **(Fig. 13A)**
- **Stages of cleavage**: 2 cell ------3 cell ------ 4 cell -----12 cell ------16 cell stage called the **morula**
- 12 – 16 cells stage (morula) enters the uterine cavity 72 hrs after fertilization
- The cells are differentiated into **inner cell mass** seen in the center of morula giving rise to the embryo proper and **outer cell mass (Fig. 13B)** which forms the protective and nutritive covering of the embryo
- When the cells of morula divide, fluid from uterine cavity enters the zygote and a cavity is formed. The cavity is called **blastocele** and the stage is known as **blastocyst** stage. **(Fig. 12C)**
- The inner cell mass pushed to one pole is called **embryoblast**
- The cells of the outer cell mass form the wall of blastocyst called **trophoblast**
- The trophoblast covering the embryonic pole is called polar trophoblast, the rest is known as mural trophoblast. This stage occurs by 4th - 5th day after fertilization
- 107 cells are present in blastocyst stage. 8 cells alone form embryoblast, 30 polar trophoblast and 69 mural trophoblast cells
- By 5th day the zona pellucida disappears
- The blastocyst gets **implanted** by 6th to 7th day by eroding into the decidua compactum and spongiosum of endometrium
- The implantation is in the uterus at the junction of fundus and posterior wall
- The side of the pole where the blastocyst gets implanted and the inner cell mass is attached is called **embryonic pole**
- The other end forms the **abembryonic pole** surrounded by mural trophoblast.

7. Sacral plexus.

- **Formation:**
  - It is formed by the ventral rami of part of L4, L5, S1, S2, S3 and part of S4. These divide into ventral and dorsal divisions
  - The lumbosacral trunk joins with the VR S1 – S4 to form the sacral plexus on the piriformis
  - The lumbosacral trunk is formed by the entire VR of fifth lumbar and the descending part of fourth lumbar nerve
  - VR of S1 – S4 emerge through the pelvic sacral foramina
  - The first and second rami are large, the other nerves diminish.
  - The S5 and coccygeal nerves emerge after piercing the sacrospinous ligament and coccygeus
  - All these nerves converge on the lower part of greater sciatic foramen
  - After formation, the plexus divides into a larger lateral branch the sciatic nerve and a smaller medial branch the pudendal nerve.
- **Location:** In the posterior wall of pelvis in front of piriformis.

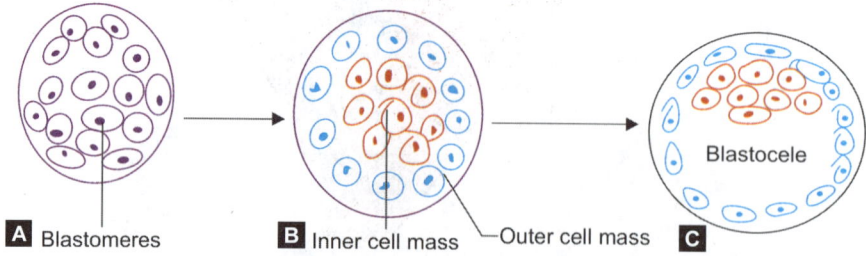

Figs. 13A to C: Formation of blastocyst.

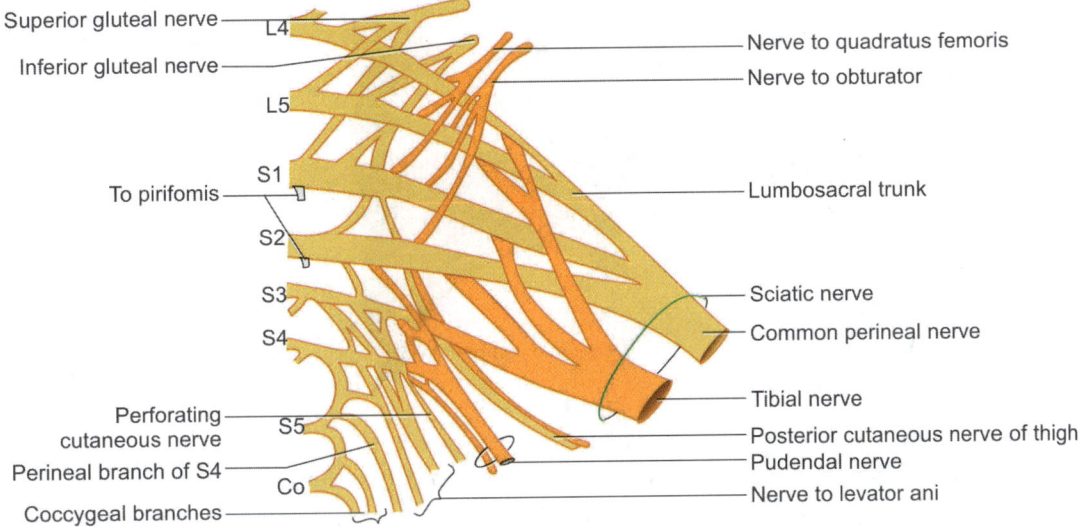

Fig. 14: Sacral plexus.

- **Relations:**
  - Anterior: Internal iliac vessels, ureter, sigmoid colon on the left side
  - Posterior: Piriformis.
- **Branches** are **classified** as i) branches from root, ii) terminal branches of the plexus, iii) branches arising from pelvic surface of plexus, iv) branches arising from dorsal surface of plexus
  - **Branches from roots:**
    - To piriformis from S1, S2
    - Branches to levator ani from S3, S4
    - Branches to coccygeus from S5, Co nerve
    - Pelvic splanchnic nerve from S2, S3, S4 containing preganglionic parasympathetic fibers.
  - **Terminal branches:**
    - Pudendal nerve smaller medial terminal branch. It is from S2,3,4
    - Sciatic nerve larger lateral terminal branch. Its root value is L4,5; S1,2,3.
  - **Branches from pelvic surface of plexus:**
    - Nerve to quadratus femoris (L 4,5; S1)
    - Nerve to obturator internus (L5:S1,2).
  - **Branches from dorsal surface of plexus:**
    - Superior gluteal nerve (L4,5; S1)
    - Inferior gluteal nerve (L5; S1,2)
    - Posterior cutaneous nerve of thigh (L5; S1,2)
    - Perforating cutaneous nerve (S2,3)
    - Perineal branch of S4.
- **Communication:**
  Gray rami communicans—all the ventral rami receive gray rami communicans from the sympathetic trunk
- **Applied anatomy:** In the infiltration of malignant tumor of the pelvis, there is severe pain in the distribution of the branches of the plexus.

8. Second part of duodenum.
Refer Short Notes 13 – 2006.

9. Internal oblique muscle.
Origin: The muscle arises from:
- The lateral two-third of the inguinal ligament.
- The anterior two-third of the intermediate area of the iliac crest
- The thoracolumbar fascia.

Insertion:
- The fibers from posterior part of iliac crest are inserted directly into the lower three or four ribs and their cartilages
- The greater part of the muscle ends in an aponeurosis through which it is inserted

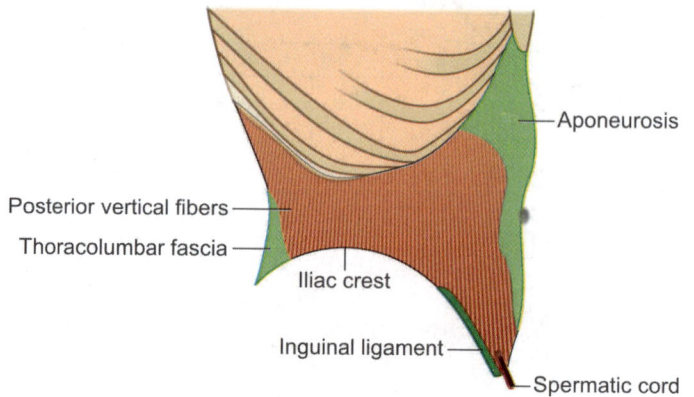

Fig. 15: Internal oblique muscle.

into the seventh, eighth, and ninth costal cartilages, xiphoid process, linea alba, pubic crest and pectineal line of the pubis
- The aponeurosis takes part in the **formation of rectus sheath**
- The fibers from inguinal ligament along with transversus abdominis form **conjoint tendon** (Falx inguinalis) and is attached to pubic crest and pectineal line
- Arched fibers of internal oblique form the **cremaster muscle** forming number of loops around the spermatic cord.

Nerve supply: Lower six thoracic nerves and the first lumbar nerve.

Action:
- Support the abdominal viscera along with the other anterior abdominal muscles
- Contraction of the muscle increases the intra-abdominal pressure
- Contraction of cremaster muscle pulls the testis upwards.

10. Portacaval anastomosis.
Refer Short Notes 6 – 2004.

11. Descent of testis.
Refer Short Notes 8 – 2007

12. Klinefelter's syndrome.
Refer Short Notes 39 – 2005.

13. Omental bursa.
Refer Short Notes 10 – 2005.

14. Histology of suprarenal gland.
Refer Short Notes 3 – 2010.

15. Blood supply of stomach.
Refer Essay Q. No. 2 – 2007.

16. Boundaries and contents of axilla.
Axilla is pyramidal space with four-sides situated between the upper part of the arm and chest wall.
- **Boundaries**
  - **Apex:** Directed upwards and medially. It forms the inlet of axilla which is a triangular interval called cervicoaxillary canal. The **cervicoaxillary canal** is formed:
    Anteriorly—clavicle
    Posteriorly—superior border of scapula
    Medially—outer border of first rib
  - **Base:** Formed by skin, superficial fascia and axillary fascia in between anterior axillary fold (by pectoralis major) and posterior axillary fold (by latissimus dorsi).
- Anterior wall: Pectoralis major and minor, and clavipectoral fascia
- Posterior wall: Subscapularis above and teres major and latissimus dorsi below
- Medial wall: First four ribs, intercostal spaces with corresponding muscles, and upper digitations of serratus anterior
- Lateral wall: It is narrow, anterior and posterior walls converge and consists of

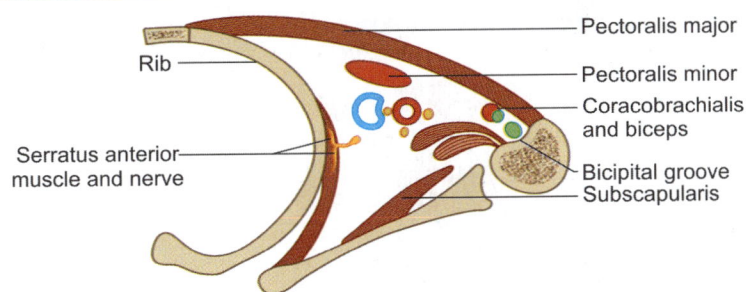

Fig. 16: Boundaries of axilla.

the bicipital groove. It lodges the coracobrachialis and biceps.
- **Contents:**
  - Axillary artery and its branches
  - Axillary vein and its tributaries
  - Infraclavicular part of brachial plexus (cords and branches)
  - Axillary lymph nodes and the associated lymphatics
  - Long thoracic and intercostobrachial nerves.
  - Lateral branches of intercostal nerves
  - Loose areolar tissue
  - Axillary tail of the breast (tail of Spence).
- **Applied anatomy: In axillary abscess**
  - The incision should be made through the base
  - It should be midway between the anterior and posterior walls
  - The knife should point towards the medial wall as there is no large vessel on the medial wall. The long thoracic nerve descends on serratus anterior
  - By this injury to the lateral thoracic, subscapular and axillary vessels on the anterior, posterior and lateral walls are avoided.

- **Origin:**
  - Lower half of front of the humerus
  - From anterolateral and anteromedial surfaces of humerus and
  - Anterior border of humerus
  - Medial and lateral intermuscular septa.
- **Insertion:** Rough anterior surface of the coronoid process of ulna.
- **Relations:**
  - Anterior—biceps brachii, brachial artery, musculocutaneous nerve and median nerve
  - Posterior—shaft of humerus and elbow joint
  - Medial—pronator teres
  - Lateral—radial nerve, brachioradialis.
- **Nerve supply:**
  - Musculocutaneous nerve
  - Radial nerve carries proprioceptive impulses.
- **Action:**
  - Flexes forearm at the elbow joint in all positions not affected by pronation or supination
  - It helps for sustained flexed position
  - Because of its constant and important role, it is called as **workhorse of flexors** of elbow.

17. Brachialis muscle.

- It is a hybrid muscle supplied by two nerves
- It is a fusiform muscle
- It is the main flexor of forearm, producing greatest amount of flexion force
- Situated deep to biceps brachii.

18. Adductor canal.

Refer Short Notes 3 – 2006.

19. Extensor retinacula of leg.

Extensor retinacula are thickened bands of deep fascia seen in front of lower part of leg.

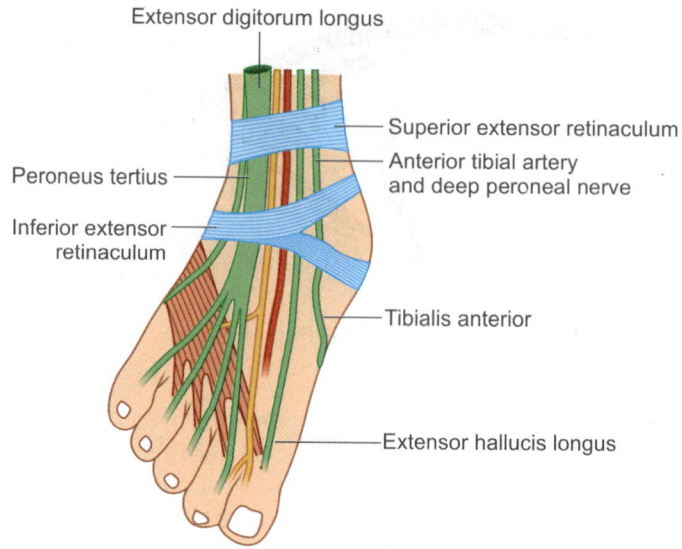

Fig. 17: Extensor retinaculum.

There are two retinacula.
1. Superior extensor retinaculum
2. Inferior extensor retinaculum.

Superior extensor retinaculum:
Attachments:
- Medially: Lower part of anterior border of tibia
- Laterally: Lower part of anterior border of fibula
- Proximally: Continuous with fascia of leg
- Distally: Connected to the inferior extensor retinaculum by connective tissue.

Inferior extensor retinaculum:
- Y-shaped band of deep fascia
- Situated in front of the ankle joint and over the posterior part of dorsum of the foot
- Stem of Y lies laterally and limbs lie medially
- Stem—attached to anterior non-articular part of superior surface of calcaneum in front of sulcus calcanei
- Upper limb—has two layers. Attached to anterior border of medial malleolus
- Lower limb—blends with plantar aponeurosis.

Structures passing under extensor retinacula (medial to lateral):
(**T**endulkar **H**ad **A N**ice **D**ay **T**oday)
- **T**ibialis anterior covered with synovial sheath till superior extensor retinaculum
- **E**xtensor hallucis longus covered with synovial sheath related to inferior extensor retinaculum
- **A**nterior tibial vessels
- **D**eep peroneal nerve
- **E**xtensor digitorum longus covered with synovial sheath related to inferior extensor retinaculum
- **P**eroneus tertius.

Structure passing superficially:
Superficial peroneal nerve
Function: Prevent bowstringing of the under lying tendons.

20. Histology of skin.

- There are two types of skin—thin and thick skin
- The thin skin is provided with hair follicle and sebaceous glands, whereas thick skin is devoid of hair follicles and the sebaceous glands
- The skin is divided into an outer epidermis and inner dermis
- **The epidermis** can be divided into a number of layers from deep to superficial as follows:

1. Basal layer (stratum basale), 2. Spinous or prickle cell layer (stratum spinosum), 3. Granular layer (stratum granulosum), 4. Clear layer (stratum lucidum) and

5. Cornified layer (stratum corneum). The first three layers change their form, and continue to differentiate, as they are metabolically active. Keratinization is seen in the cells of superficial layers.
1. **Stratum basale:** In hairless skin this layer is thick, as the dermal papillae (rete ridges) project superficially into the epidermal region. The basal layer cells are columnar to cuboidal in shape. The cells serve as stem cells. Melanocytes, occasional Langerhans cells and Merkel cells are present among the basal keratinocytes
2. **Stratum spinosum:** The prickle cell layer consists of several layers of closely packed keratinocytes and the surface projections of the cells interdigitate with neighboring cells
3. **Stratum granulosum:** Made of three to four layers of flattened cells
4. **Stratum lucidum:** The clear layer is only found in thick palmar or plantar skin. It is made up of clear non-nucleated cells
5. **Stratum corneum:** It consists of dead, flattened polyhedral squamous cells. Lateral margins of these cells overlap and connect with one another. Nucleus is not present and contains keratin filaments embedded in the cytoplasm.

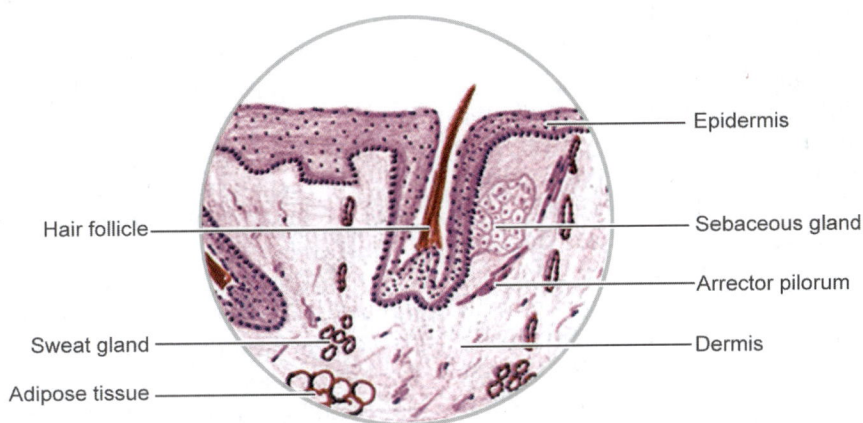

Fig. 18: Histology of thin skin.

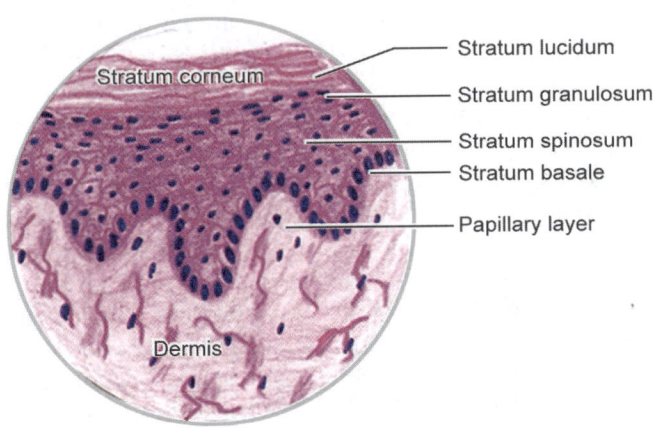

Fig. 19: Histology of thick skin.

- **Dermis** can be divided into two zones, narrow superficial **papillary layer** and deeper **reticular layer**.
  1. The papillary layer is immediately deep to the epidermis. It provides mechanical and metabolic support. It contains sensory nerve endings and blood vessels. The superficial surface of the dermis is shaped into numerous papillae or rete ridges, which interdigitate with evagination of the epidermis
  2. The reticular layer merges with the deep aspect of the papillary layer. Bundles of type I collagen fibers are present. It is thicker than those in the papillary layer and mingle with them.
- The **pilosebaceous unit** is made of the hair and its follicle, arrector pili muscle, sebaceous gland
- The hair follicle contains inner and outer root sheath and a centrally placed hair shaft. A fully developed **hair shaft** consists of cuticle, cortex and medulla
- The **arrector pili muscles** are made of smooth muscle strips
- **Sebaceous glands** are present over the whole body except the thick hairless skin of the palm, soles and flexor surfaces of digits. They are connected to hair follicles. They belong to holocrine type of gland.

21. Azygos vein.

- Drains the thoracic wall and the upper lumbar region
- Term azygos means unpaired
- It is a content of posterior mediastinum and arch is situated in superior mediastinum
- It starts from posterior aspect inferior vena cava or below renal vein.
- **Formation:**
  - The azygos vein is formed by the union of the lumbar azygos, right subcostal and ascending lumbar veins
  - The lumbar azygos vein is regarded as the abdominal part of the azygos vein. Its lower end communicates with the inferior vena cava
  - The ascending lumbar vein is formed by a vertical anastomosis that connects the lumbar veins.
- **Course:**
  - The azygos vein enters the thorax either by piercing the right crus of the diaphragm or passing deep to it or by passing through the aortic opening
  - The azygos vein ascends up to T4 vertebra where it arches forward over the root of the right lung.
- **Termination:** Ends by joining the posterior aspect of superior vena cava just before the superior vena cava pierces the pericardium.
- **Relations:**
  - Anteriorly: Right crus of diaphragm
  - Posteriorly:
    - Lower eight thoracic vertebrae and anterior longitudinal ligaments
    - Right posterior intercostal arteries.
  - Right lateral:
    - Right lung and pleura.
    - Greater splanchnic nerve.
  - Left lateral:
    - Thoracic duct and aorta in lower part
    - Esophagus, trachea and right vagus in upper part.
- **Tributaries:**
  - Right superior intercostal vein—the second, third and fourth posterior intercostal veins unite to form the superior intercostal vein. It drains to arch of azygos
  - Fifth to eleventh right posterior intercostal veins
  - Hemiazygos vein at the level of eighth thoracic vertebra draining left 8 – 11 posterior intercostal veins
  - Right bronchial vein near the terminal end of the azygos vein
  - Accessory hemiazygos vein at the level of the eighth thoracic vertebra draining left 5 – 7 posterior intercostal veins
  - Several esophageal, mediastinal and pericardial veins.
- **Applied anatomy:** Collateral circulation is established through the tributaries of

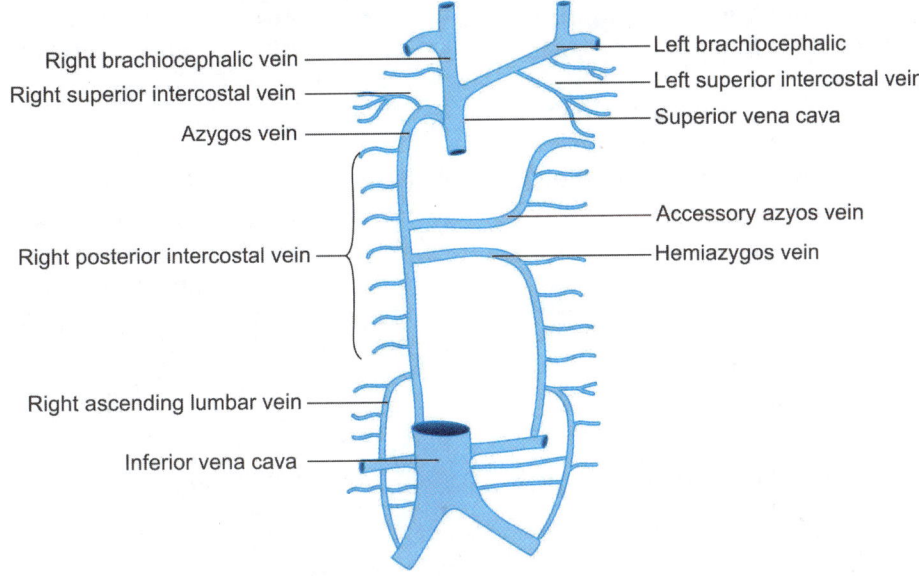

Fig. 20: Azygos vein.

azygos vein with IVC in case of blockage of SVC below the level of opening of azygos vein.

22. Relations of arch of aorta.
Refer Essay Q. No. 8 – 2010.

23. Left coronary artery.
Refer Essay Q. No. 5 – 2005.

24. Histology of cerebral cortex.
Refer Short Notes Q. No. 18 – 2003.

25. Corpus callosum.
- It forms the commissural fibers of white matter
- It is the largest commissural fiber of brain connecting the two cerebral hemispheres
- It connects all the parts of cerebral hemispheres of two sides
- Length: 10 cm in length
- Shape: C shaped
- It is situated more in front than behind about 4 cm from frontal pole and 6 cm from occipital pole.

Parts of Corpus Callosum (Fig. 21)
- Rostrum
- Genu
- Body
- Splenium.

Relations

Rostrum
- Thin and extends from genu to lamina terminalis
- Directed downwards and backwards
- Forms floor of anterior horn of lateral ventricle.

Genu
- It is the bend part
- Anterior end forms anterior limit of the lateral ventricle
- Related: Posteriorly to anterior horn of the lateral ventricle and septum pellucidum
- Anteriorly to anterior cerebral artery.

Body/Trunk
- It curves upwards and backwards with convexity above
- It forms floor of median longitudinal fissure of cerebral hemispheres
- Relation:
  - Superiorly:
    - Falx cerebri, anterior cerebral vessels, inferior sagittal sinus.
    - It is overlapped by cingular gyrus separated by callosal sulcus
    - It is covered by a layer of gray matter called inducium griseum and the

medial and lateral longitudinal striae are embedded in it.
- Inferiorly:
  - Gives attachment for septum pellucidum
  - Forms roof of central part of lateral ventricle
  - Lined by ependyma.

Splenium
- It is the posterior thickest part of corpus callosum
- Posteriorly related to great cerebral vein, straight sinus and free margin of tentorium cerebelli.

Fibers of Corpus Callosum (Fig. 22)
- Rostrum—connects orbital surface of frontal lobes
- Forceps minor—fibers from genu passes forwards connecting lateral and medial surfaces of frontal lobe
- Fibers from trunk:
  - Intersect with corona radiata
  - Tapetal fibers from trunk and splenium forms boundaries for lateral ventricle.
- Forceps major from splenium to occipital lobe.

Functional Significance
- The corpus callosum possibly helps in coordination of the activities of the two cerebral hemispheres
- It helps for transfer of learning process
- Its congenital absence does not cause much functional disturbance.

26. Horns of lateral ventricle.

Anterior (Frontal) Horn (Fig. 23):
- This is the part of the ventricle which lies anterior to the interventricular foramen. It forms the anterior limit of lateral ventricle.
- Shape: Triangular in cross section
- Boundaries:
  - Roof: Anterior most part of trunk of the corpus callosum.
  - Floor:
    - Head of caudate nucleus
    - Upper surface of rostrum of corpus callosum.
  - Medial wall:
    - Septum pellucidum
    - Column of fornix
      * The tela choroidea and choroid plexuses do not extend into the anterior horn.

Posterior (Occipital) Horn (Fig. 24):
- It is an extension of the cavity into the occipital lobe
- Directions: Backwards and medially
- Shape: Triangular in cross section
- Boundaries:
  - Roof—tepetum of corpus callosum

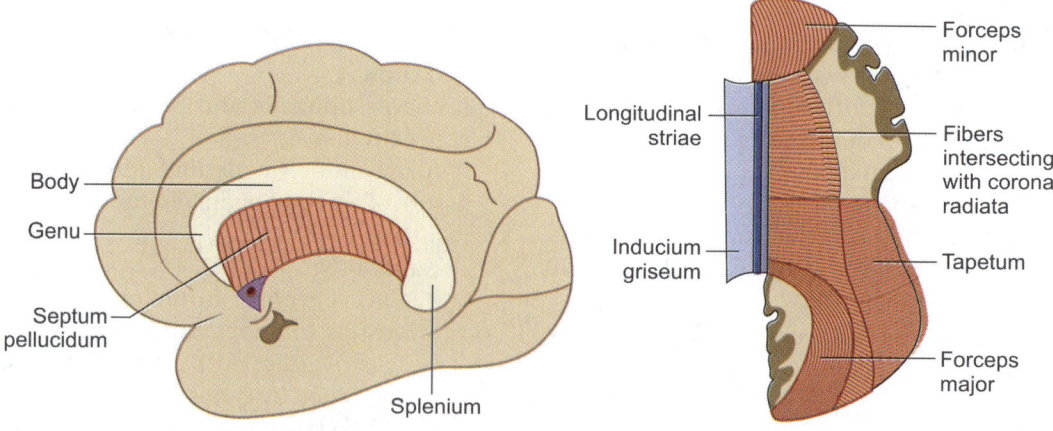

Fig. 21: Corpus callosum.

Fig. 22: Fibers of corpus callosum.

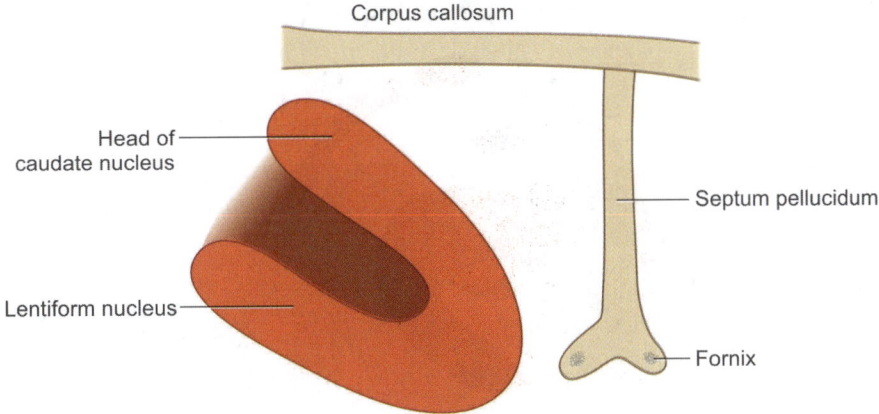

Fig. 23: Anterior horn.

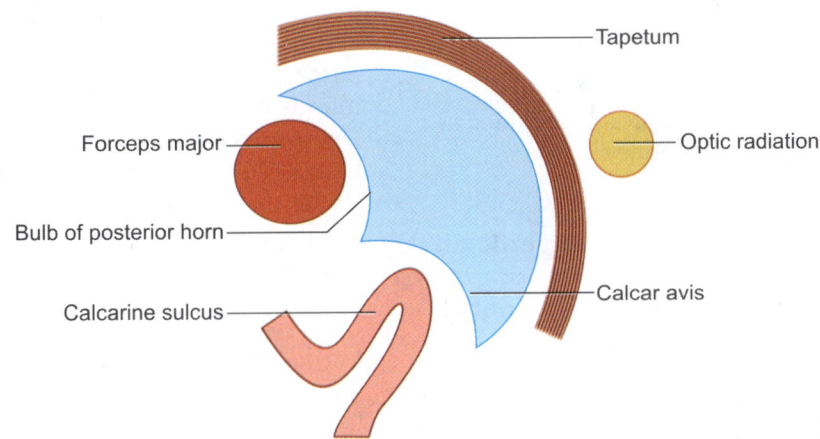

Fig. 24: Posterior horn.

- Lateral walls by tapetal fibers of corpus callosum separates it from the optic radiation
- Medial wall shows two elevations:
1. Upper is produced by fibers of the forceps major as they run backward from the splenium of the corpus callosum called **bulb of posterior horn**
2. Anterior part of calcarine sulcus which is a complete sulcus produces the lower elevation called **calcar avis**.

Inferior (temporal) horn (Fig. 25):

- It is the largest of all the horns
- It is in level with superior temporal sulcus
- It is 2.5 cm from temporal pole

- The choroid plexus extends into the inferior horn
  - Direction: It is directed downwards, laterally and forwards
- Boundaries:
  - Roof: Tapetal fibers, tail of caudate nucleus, stria terminalis, amygdaloid body
  - Floor: Two elevations are seen:
    1. **Collateral trigone** produced by collateral sulcus which is a complete sulcus
    2. The elevation called **pes hippocampus** formed by hippocampal gyrus. The pes hippocampus is covered by alveus. Alveus is continued as

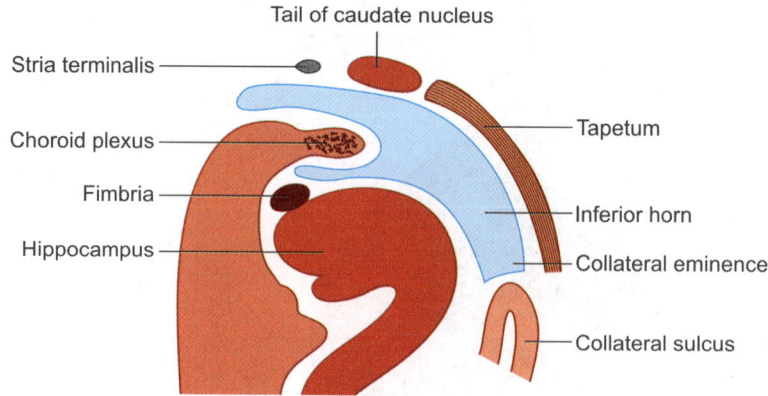

Fig. 25: Inferior horn.

fimbria and crux fornix. Below the alveus is the dentate gyrus.

27. Contents of posterior triangle.

Contents of posterior triangle are classified as nerve, vessel and lymph node contents.

Nerves

They may be classified as superficial, intermediate and deep group of nerves:

- **Superficial group**—are cutaneous branches lie in the roof (investing layer of deep fascia) of the triangle
  - Great auricular nerve (VR C2, C3) emerges along the posterior border of sternocleidomastoid muscle and reaches parotid gland
  - Lesser occipital nerve (VR C2) ascends upwards and winds around spinal accessory nerve
  - Transverse cervical nerve of neck (VR C2, C3) crosses the sternocleidomastoid muscle to supply skin of anterior triangle
  - Supraclavicular nerves (VR C3, C4) it descends downwards and divides into medial, intermediate and lateral supraclavicular nerves.
- **Intermediate group**—lies between roof and floor of the triangle (investing layer and prevertebral layer)

The spinal accessory nerve lies on levator scapulae. It is hooked by the lesser occipital nerve and passes downwards and backwards. It leaves the triangle by passing deep to the sternocleidomastoid muscle

- **Deep group**—lies deep to floor of the triangle (deep to prevertebral layer)
- Upper, middle and lower trunks of brachial plexus.
  - Suprascapular nerve
  - Nerve to subclavius
  - Nerve to sternocleidomastoid and trapezius.

Arteries

- Third part of subclavian artery. No branch is given by it
- Transverse cervical artery
- Suprascapular artery.

Veins

- Subclavian vein
- External jugular vein and its tributaries – anterior jugular, suprascapular, and transverse cervical veins.

Lymph Nodes

- Deep cervical nodes along spinal accessory nerve
- Supraclavicular nodes – Virchow's node

Applied Anatomy

- Injury to spinal accessory nerve results in wry neck or torticollis, due to paralysis of sternocleidomastoid muscle.

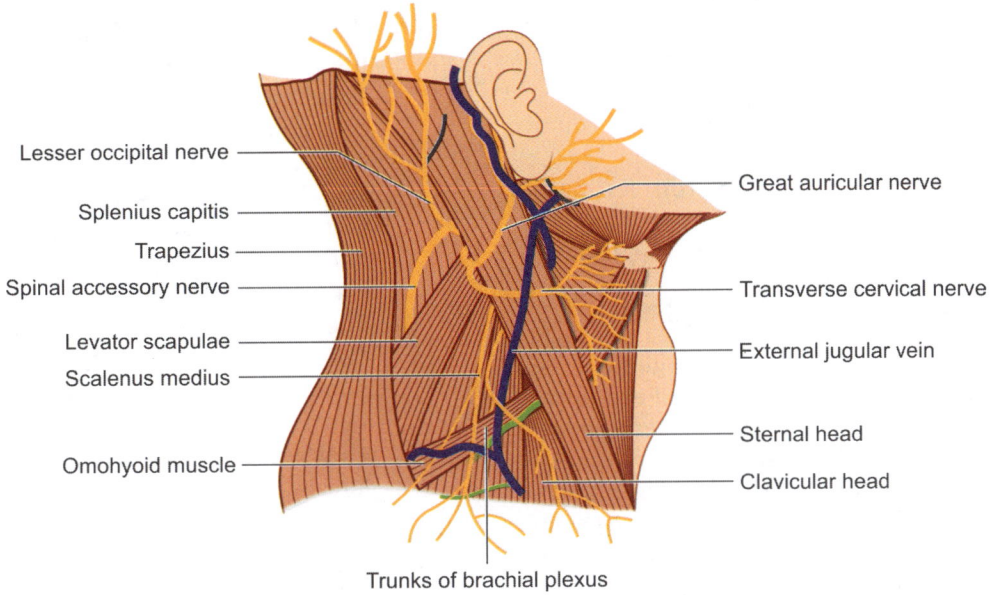

Fig. 26: Contents of posterior triangle.

- Injury to external jugular vein before it pierces the deep fascia results in air embolism
- Erb's palsy injury to Erb's point.

28. Extrinsic muscles of tongue.
Refer Short Notes 31 – 2005.

29. Brachiocephalic vein.

Formation: Brachiocephalic veins are formed by union of internal jugular vein and subclavian vein at the level of sternal end of clavicle. The left is longer than the right vein.

Termination: The right and left brachiocephalic veins unite to form superior vena cava at the level of 1st right costal cartilage

Relations
- **Right brachiocephalic vein:**
  – To its right side:
    - The right lung and pleura
    - The right phrenic nerve.
  – Posteromedially:
    - The brachiocephalic artery
    - The right vagus nerve.
  – Anteriorly:
    - The first costal cartilage
    - The sternal end of clavicle.
- **Left brachiocephalic vein:**
  – Anteriorly:
    - Manubrium sterni
    - Sternohyoid and sternothyroid muscles
    - Remnants of thymus.
  – Posteriorly:
    - Arteries arising from the arch of aorta, i.e. the brachiocephalic, left common carotid and left subclavian arteries
    - Trachea
    - Left vagus and left phrenic nerves.
- **Tributaries:**
  – Vertebral vein
  – First intercostal vein
  – Inferior thyroid vein
  – Superior intercostal vein (left brachiocephalic)
  – Internal thoracic vein (right brachiocephalic).

30. Development of atria.

- **Development of right atrium**
Refer Essay Q. No. 8 – 2009.

- **Development of left atrium**
  - It is developed from three sources
  - The posterior smooth part is by absorption of pulmonary veins
  - Anterior part is from left half of primitive atrium
  - A small ventral part from left half of atrioventricular canal.
- **Development of interatrial septum**
  Refer Short Notes 25 – 2006.

31. Histology of parotid gland.

- It is a serous type of salivary gland
- The secretory end pieces of the human parotid gland are mostly serous acini. Mucous acini are rare
- It is a compound tubuloalveolar gland
- The connective tissue forms the capsule and septae divide the gland into many lobes and lobules
- **Serous cells**
  - Pyramidal in shape
  - The spherical nucleus situated in the centre.
  - The cytoplasm above nucleus is filled by zymogen granules with amylase activity
  - Kallikrein, lactoferrin and lysozyme are secreted by serous cells.
- **Ducts:** The lining cells of **intercalated ducts** are lined with squamous cell or cuboidal cells
  - Striated ducts
    - Are lined by a low columnar epithelium
    - Basal striations are present in the cells and hence are called as striated cells
    - The infoldings of the basal cell membrane produce the striation
    - Between the folds mitochondria are situated
    - The nuclei are apically situated
    - The function of the cells are to carry potassium and bicarbonate into saliva
    - They reabsorb sodium and chloride ions in excess of water and produce a hypotonic saliva
    - Striated ducts modify electrolyte composition
    - Secrete IgA, lysozyme and kallikrein.
  - Collecting ducts
    - The lining epithelium of collecting ducts varies
    - It may be pseudostratified columnar, stratified cuboidal or columnar in the larger ducts
    - Near the termination, it becomes a stratified squamous epithelium.
  - **Myoepithelial cells** or basket cells are present between the basement membrane and the acinar cells which

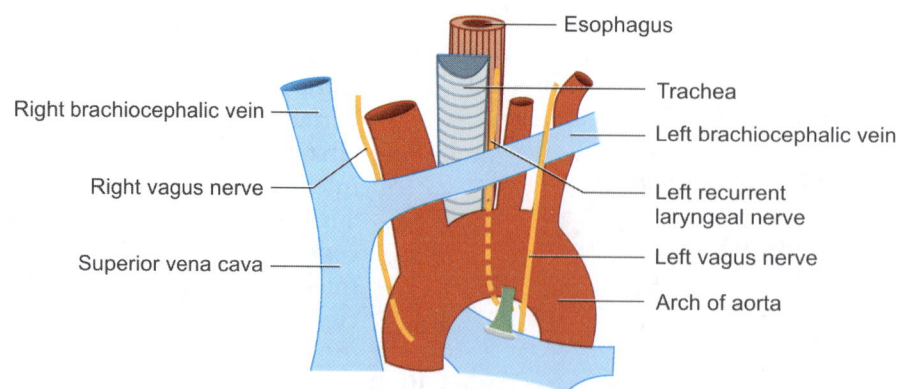

Fig. 27: Brachiocephalic vein.

help to empty the secretions from the acinus.

32. Histology of cornea.
Refer Short Notes 35 – 2009.

33. Development of lung.
- Around 4th week of intrauterine development a diverticulum grows from the ventral wall of the foregut in the region of pharynx, called tracheal diverticulum
- At first starts as a groove in the floor of the pharynx
- As the diverticulum grows caudally tracheo-esophageal ridges are formed
- These soon fuse and form tracheo-esophageal septum. This separates the trachea completely from esophagus
- Caudally the diverticulum bifurcates into two lung buds **(Fig. 29)**
- The two lung buds elongate and form the principal bronchi
- The right divides into three branches for the three lobes of the right lung
- The left divides into two branches for the two lobes of the left lung
- With successive divisions, the entire bronchial tree is formed. At least 17 generations of division take place before birth, 6 more divisions are formed after birth.

- Stages of lung development:
  - **Pseudoglandular stage** (6 – 16 weeks) **(Fig. 30A)**:
    - Repeated branching (14 times) to the level of terminal bronchioles
    - Lungs resemble an endocrine gland.
    - No respiratory bronchiole.
  - **Canalicular stage** (16 – 26 weeks) **(Fig. 30B)**
    - Lung tissue becomes highly vascular
    - Respiratory bronchioles develop
    - At the end of the phase some alveolar ducts are formed so that minimal gaseous exchange is possible
    - The lining epithelium also becomes thin simple squamous type I pneumocytes
    - Besides these alveolar surfactant type II pneumocytes are also formed in the alveoli.
  - **Terminal sac period** (26 weeks – birth)
    - Terminal sac formed
    - Capillaries establish close contact
    - Before birth the entire lung is filled with a fluid rich in chloride, surfactant and mucus secretions of bronchial glands
    - Only during 7th month of intrauterine life sufficient number pulmonary

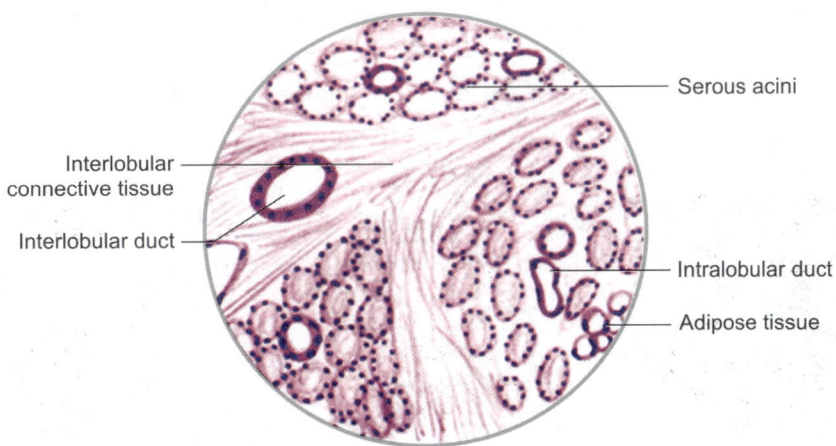

Fig. 28: Histology of parotid gland.

capillaries are present for adequate gaseous exchange.
- **Alveolar phase** (8th month – 8 years) **(Fig. 30C)**
  - Only one-sixth of the adult alveoli are present at birth
  - Epithelial endothelial contact is established
  - There is considerable increase in the alveoli after birth up to 8th year
  - The pulmonary circulation is established as early as 4th week
  - After birth, most of the fluid is absorbed by the capillaries
  - The surfactant forms a thin film lining the alveoli.

34. Internal capsule.
Refer Essay Q. No. 7 – 2005.

35. Typical intercostal nerve.
Refer Essay Q. No. 9 – 2006.

36. Cavernous sinus.
Refer Essay Q. No. 5 – 2008.

37. Connections of basal ganglia.
- Basal ganglion comprises the corpus striatum, the claustrum, the amygdaloid body
- Corpus striatum includes caudate nucleus, and lentiform nucleus
- Lentiform nucleus is divided into outer putamen and inner globus pallidus.
- Connections:

Afferent Fibers

- Corticostriate fibers—from entire neocortex to caudate nucleus, putamen
- Thalamostriate fibers from centromedian nucleus of thalamus to caudate nucleus and putamen
- Nigrostriate fibers from caudate and putamen to substantia nigra called **comb bundle**

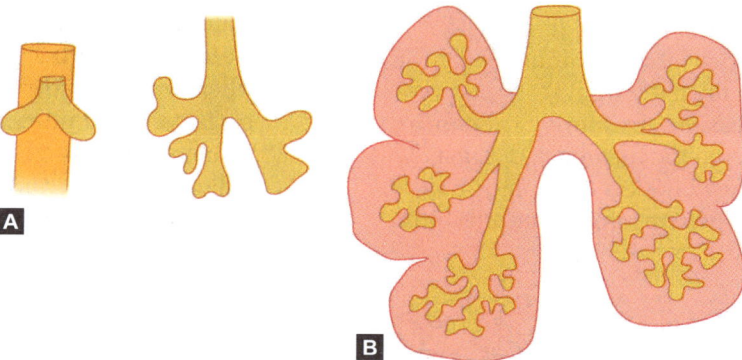

Figs. 29A and B: Divisions of diverticulum.

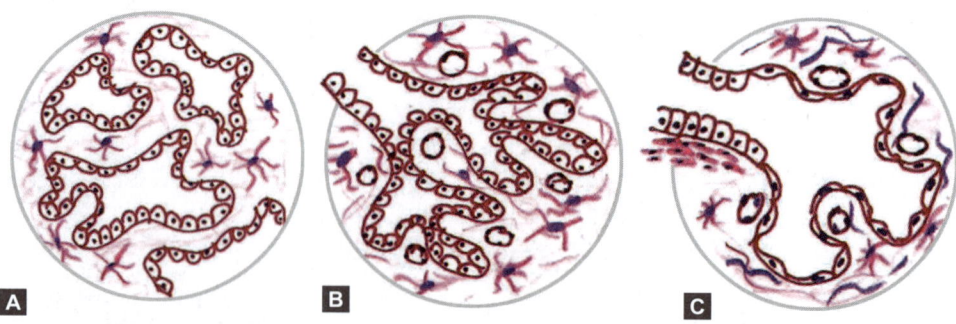

Figs. 30A to C: Development of lung: (A) Pseudoglandular stage; (B) Canalicular stage; (C) Alveolar phase.

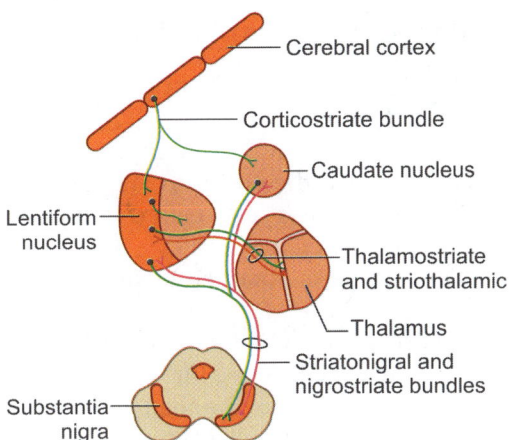

Fig. 31: Connections of basal ganglia.

- Pallidum receives fibers from striatum, substantia nigra.

Efferent Fibers

- Striatonigral fibers from striatum to substantia nigra
- Fasciculus lenticularis: Pallidum to sub thalamic nucleus
- Fasciculus subthalamicus—from globus pallidus to sub thalamic nucleus.

Applied Anatomy

Parkinsonism:

- It is due to deficiency of dopamine in corpus striatum
- The dopamine secreted by substantia nigra is carried to corpus striatum by the nigrostriate fibers. The disease is due to reduction of secretion of dopamine leads to degeneration of neurons of substantia nigra or nigrostriatal fibers
- It results in:
  – Increased muscle tone leading to rigidity, tremors, abnormal movements
  – Akinesia—slow movement
  – Cogwheel or lead pipe rigidity
  – Pill rolling movement
  – Mask like face
  – Shuffling gait
  – Stopped posture.

Huntington's chorea; reduction of GABA in striatonigral fibers.

38. Blood supply of thyroid gland.

Refer Short Notes 38 – 2008.

39. Lymphatic drainage of tongue.

Refer Essay Q. No. 6 – 2007.

40. Maxillary air sinus.

Refer Short Notes 25 – 2007.

III. SHORT ANSWER QUESTIONS

1. Buttonhole deformity.

A Buttonhole deformity is also called as **Boutonniere.**

- **Definition:** It is due to flexion deformity of the proximal interphalangeal joint
- **Reason for deformity:** The central slip of the extensor tendon, which is inserted into the base of the middle phalanx may be cut or lax
- **Effect of lesion:** The distal interphalangeal joint is hyperextended
- **Cause:** Trauma or rheumatoid arthritis may be the reason for the deformity.
- **Changes occurring:**
  – There is forward movement of the lateral bands of the extensor tendon
  – The head of the proximal phalanx to move posteriorly
  – In initial stage the deformity can be corrected. If prolonged, the soft tissues around the joint contract and results in a fixed deformity.

2. Brachioradialis muscle.

- It is one of the superficial muscle of the extensor compartment of forearm
- It forms lateral boundary for cubital fossa
- It is a fusiform muscle.
- **Origin:**
  – From proximal two third of the supracondylar ridge of humerus
  – Anterior surface of lateral intermuscular septa.
- **Insertion:**
  – Ends in a tendon in the middle of forearm
  – Distal end of lateral surface of radius just proximal to styloid process.

- **Nerve supply:** Radial nerve
- **Actions:**
  - Flexes forearm at the elbow joint
  - It is most powerful in mid-prone position of forearm
  - It is active in quick movements or flexion of forearm against resistance
  - Acts as a shunt muscle resisting subluxation of head of radius.

3. Muscle responsible for lateral rotation movement of shoulder joint.

- The rotation occurs in vertical axis.
- The humerus rotates about ¼ of a circle
- The range of movement is more when the arm hangs by the side
- In lateral rotation of shoulder the greater trochanter of humerus move under the coracoacromial arch
- **Muscles responsible:** Posterior fibers of deltoid, infraspinatus, teres minor.

4. Formation of superficial palmar arch.

- **Formation**
  - The superficial palmar arch is an anastomosis formed by the ulnar and radial artery
  - The ulnar artery enters the palm anterior to the flexor retinaculum.
- **Variations**
  - Usually the superficial palmar arch is formed by the ulnar artery alone
  - Sometimes completed by the superficial palmar branch of the radial artery
  - In some it is completed by the arteria radialis indicis.
- **Relations**
  - **Superficial:** Palmaris brevis and the palmar aponeurosis
  - **Deep:** Flexor digiti minimi, branches of the median nerve and the long flexor tendons and lumbricals.
- **Branches:** Four palmar digital branches: One passes to the medial side of little finger. The other three are common palmar digital branches. Each branch divides into two to supply adjacent sides of little, ring, middle and index fingers.

5. Histology of layers of aorta.

Refer Essay Q. No. 8 – 2010.

6. Palthi posture.

- Abduction and lateral rotator of thigh, and flexor of leg is the position of tailor
- This position is also called as palthi's posture
- This posture is obtained by the action of Sartorius
- Sartorius is attached to anterior superior iliac spine and inserted into the upper part of medial surface of the shaft of the tibia
- Femoral nerve supplies the muscle.

7. Gracilis muscles.

- It is one of the muscle of "guy ropes"
- It is situated in the medial side of thigh
- It belongs to adductor group
- **Origin:** From the lower half of body of the pubis along the medial margin, inferior ramus of the pubis, adjoining part of the ischial rami
- **Insertion:** Into the upper part of the medial surface of tibia in between sartorius (in front) and semitendinosus (behind)
- **Nerve supply:** Anterior division of obturator nerve
- **Actions:** Flexor and medial rotator of thigh, weak adductor of thigh.

8. Long saphenous vein.

Refer Short Notes 14 – 2005.

9. Allantois.

- The allantois or allantoenteric diverticulum arises around 16th day of development
- It is an **endodermal outgrowth** from the yolk sac into the mesenchyme of the connecting stalk
- It **divides the hindgut** into pre- and post allantoic parts
- With the development of the hindgut, the proximal part of the diverticulum unite with anterior abdominal wall. The distal part forms the allantoic duct
- The allantoic duct open into the terminal part of the hindgut anteriorly
- The allantois is a **site of development of blood vessels (angiogenesis)** gives rise

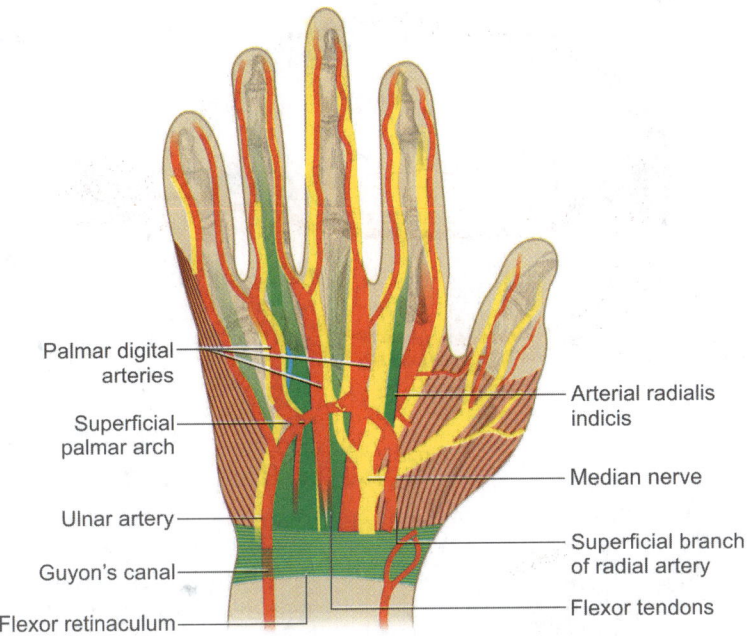

Fig. 32: Superficial palmar arch.

- to the umbilical vessels connecting to the placental circulation
- The connecting stalk if formed by the allantois and the extraembryonic mesenchyme around, which forms the **content** of the umbilical cord
- In the fetus, the allantoic duct, is present in the proximal end of the umbilical cord
- It persists as **median umbilical ligament/ urachus,** and continues into the **apex of the urinary bladder.**

10. Histology of cardiac muscle.

- It is striated and involuntary in function
- It is present in myocardium and large veins of heart
- **Shape**: It is cylindrical in shape.
- **Structure**
  - The muscle fiber branch at the ends and anastomose with each other
  - Each muscle fiber is made of a chain of cardiac myocytes each having their own nucleus
  - The nuclei one/two large in size, situated in the centre of each cell
  - The sarcolemma invaginates to form T tubules
  - Sarcoplasm contains abundant mitochondria and myofibrils
  - The cross-striations of cardiac muscle produced by A, I, Z, and H bands are less conspicuous than the skeletal muscle
  - Cells are joined together by inter-digitating junctional complexes, called the intercalated discs.
- **Intercalated disc**:
  - Intercalated discs are present only in cardiac muscle
  - In the ordinary microscope they are seen as irregular transverse lines, representing attachment point between the cardiac muscle fibers
  - The intercalated disc is seen opposite to the I-band
  - It allows the transmission of contractile and electrical force from one cell to the next by the firm attachment between the cells

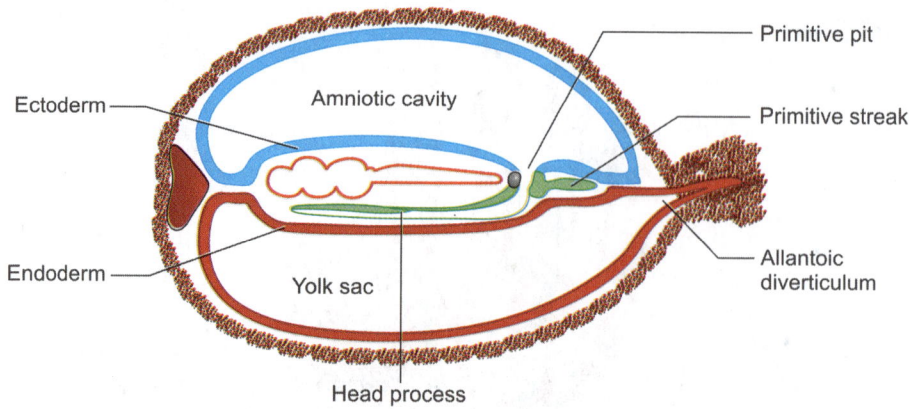

Fig. 33: Allantois.

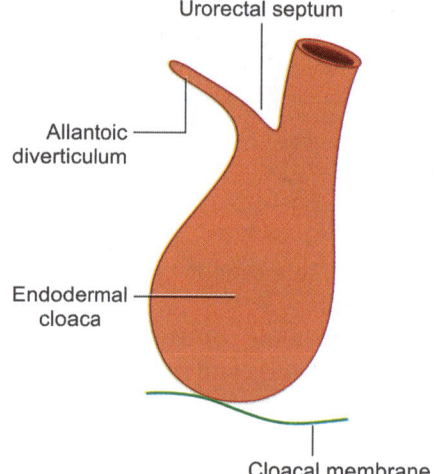

Fig. 34: Cloaca.

- In electron microscopy the intercalated disc is made of adherence of cell membrane
- The transverse portion formed by fascia adherens with desmosomes and lateral portion by the gap junctions, tight junctions
- Hence the intercalated disc appears to be broken steps.

11. Transpyloric plane.
Refer Short Answer 10 – 2008.

12. Branches of superior mesenteric artery.
- The superior mesenteric artery arises from abdominal aorta
- It arises at the level of L1, along the transpyloric plane
- It supplies the structures developed from midgut—from the second part of duodenum below major duodenal papilla to right two-third of transverse colon
- Branches:
  - Inferior pancreaticoduodenal artery
  - Ileal and jejunal branches
  - Ileocolic artery
  - Right colic artery
  - Middle colic artery.

13. Relations of inferior surface of liver.
- **Left lobe:** Impression for fundus of stomach and a part of lesser omentum
- **Quadrate lobe:**
  - It is adjacent to the left lobe
  - Structures related: Pylorus, first part of duodenum, lower part of lesser omentum, transverse colon (occasionally)
  - The quadrate lobe is between fossa for gallbladder and fissure for ligamentum teres.
- **Right lobe:**
  - Fissure for ligamentum teres close to midline and it contains the obliterated left umbilical vein
  - Fossa for gallbladder
  - To the right of gallbladder: Colic impression—right colic flexure
  - Renal impression—anterior surface of upper part of right kidney.

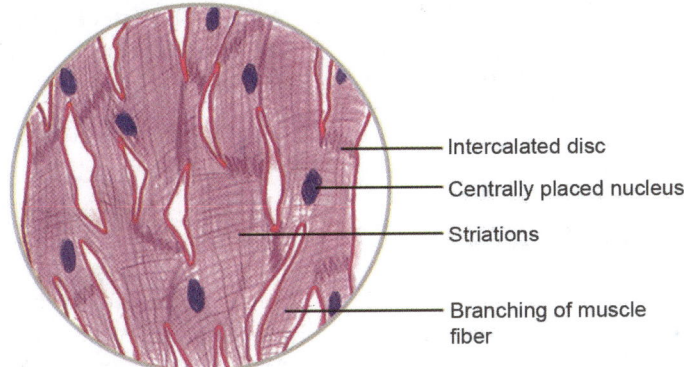

Fig. 35: Histology of cardiac muscle.

- Right suprarenal
- First part of duodenum.

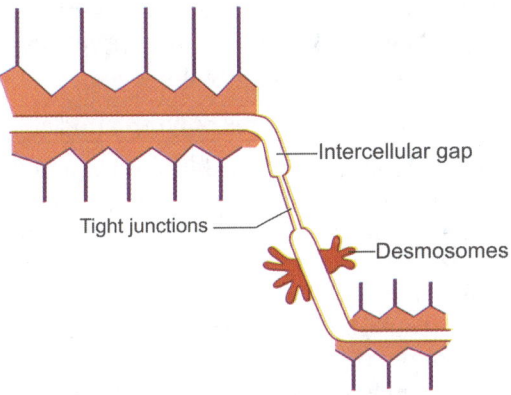

Fig. 36: Intercalated disc.

- **Porta hepatis**—hilum of liver
- **Caudate lobe:**
  - Lies posterior to porta hepatis
  - To the right of fissure for ligamentum venosum.

14. Perineal body.

Refer Short Notes 8 – 2004.

15. Anal fissure.

- Anal fissure is a painful condition of the anal canal because the area is supplied by sensory fibers inferior rectal nerve
- It is a tear in the mucosa of the anal canal at the level of anal valves
- It may extend into pecten
- It is usually found in the posterior wall in the midline

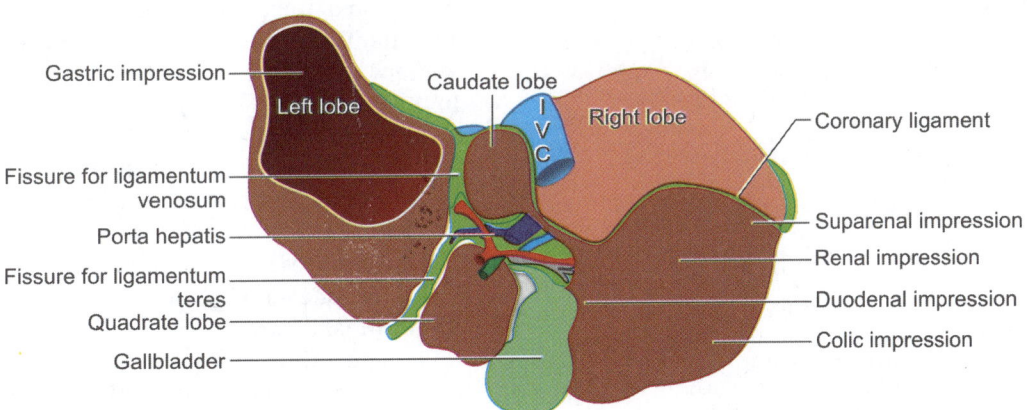

Fig. 37: Inferior surface of liver.

- The anal valves get torn due to the passage of hard feces
- A perianal abscess may follow an infection of anal fissure and result in ischioanal abscess
- It can spread to pelvis and form pelvirectal abscess.

16. Muscles attached to extensor expansion of hand.

Muscles forming are:
- The extensor digitorum forms the dorsal digital expansion
- The lumbrical is attached laterally to the expansion forming distal wing tendon
- The palmar and dorsal interossei attached either medially or laterally forming proximal wing tendon.

S. No.	Digit	Muscles forming	Muscles attached		
			Lumbricals	Palmar interossei	Dorsal interossei
1	Thumb	Extensor pollicis longus Abductor pollicis brevis Adductor pollicis	-------	1st interossei along ulnar side	------
2	Index finger	Extensor digitorum	1st lumbrical	2nd interossei along ulnar side	1st interossei along radial side
3	Middle finger	Extensor digitorum	2nd lumbrical	------	2nd and 3rd interossei along radial and ulnar side
4	Ring finger	Extensor digitorum	3rd lumbrical	3rd interossei along radial side	4th interossei along ulnar side
5	Little finger	Extensor digitorum Extensor digiti minimi	4th lumbrical	4th interossei along radial side	------

17. Name the structures piercing clavipectoral fascia.

Refer Short Answer 11 – 2009.

18. Remnants of notochord.

- Gastrulation begins with the formation of primitive streak on the surface of the epiblast
- Primitive streak appears by 15th day
- The primitive streak at the cephalic end extends between endoderm and the neuroectoderm called the **notochordal process or head process**
- Later forms solid **definitive notochord**
- It **induces differentiation** of neural tube from the medullary plate
- It also acts as **fore runner** in development of vertebral column
- **Remnants**: Notochord **persists** as **nucleus pulposus** in the center of intervertebral disc, and **apical ligament**.

19. Histological features of lymph node.

- Lymph node is divided into outer cortex and inner medulla. The cortex is absent at the hilum, where the medulla reaches the surface
- Afferent lymphatic vessels open into the **subcapsular sinus** on the periphery at different points
- From the subcapsular sinus numerous cortical sinuses pass to the medulla
- Larger medullary sinuses are formed by the union of the cortical sinuses
- The medullary sinus is continued as the efferent vessel from hilum.
- In the **cortex**:
  - Lymphocytes aggregate in the outer cortical area to form **lymphoid follicles** or nodules. The cells are densely packed
  - The follicle contains mainly B lymphocytes
  - Centre of each lymphoid follicle has a germinal centre
  - The germinal centre is paler stained made of larger antigen-stimulated B cells

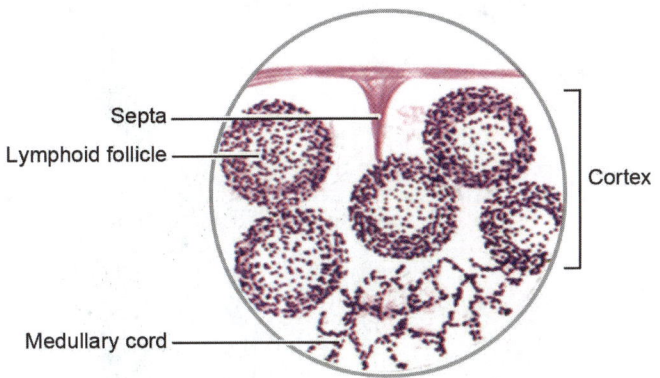

Fig. 38: Histology of lymph node.

- The cells in the germinal center divide rapidly than those at its periphery
- T cells are also present
- The mantle zone is seen surrounding the germinal center
- The cells in the mantle zone are mainly B cells, T cells, and macrophages
- The **deep cortex or Para cortex**
- Lies between the lymphoid follicles and the medulla.
- It is formed mainly by T cells
- They do not form follicles.
- In the **medulla:**
  - Lymphocytes are much less densely packed
  - The lymphocytes are arranged in irregular, branching pattern called **medullary cords**
  - It also contains macrophages, more in number in the medulla than in the cortex, plasma cells and a few granulocytes.

20. Contents of broad ligament.

- Uterine tube—the infundibulum, ampulla and isthmus parts are along the upper free margin of the broad ligament **(Fig. 39)**
- Proximal part of round ligament of uterus —below and in front of the uterine tube
- Ligament of ovary—below and behind the tube
- Ovarian vessels—runs through the suspensory ligament of the ovary. The artery is from abdominal aorta. The right vein drains to IVC, and the left to left renal vein
- Uterine vessels—enter through the base of the broad ligament. It arises from internal iliac artery. At the lateral cornu of the uterus it anastomoses with ovarian artery
- Tubules of epo-ophoron—the tubules are situated above the ovary. They are remnant of the proximal mesonephric tubules.
  - Duct of epo-ophoron (Gartner's duct)—the upper end of the tubules of epoophoron, unite to form the duct. It is remnant of proximal part of mesonephric duct
  - Tubules of paro-ophoron—situated between the ovary and the uterus. It is remnant of caudal part of mesonephric tubules
  - Lymphatics, nerves and smooth muscles of the uterus.

21. Lateral rotation of hip joint.

- Lateral rotation occurs around vertical axis passing through the center of head of femur
- Muscles producing are: Gluteus maximus, piriformis, obturator externus, obturator internus and two gemelli
- It is limited by the tension in medial rotators, iliofemoral ligament.

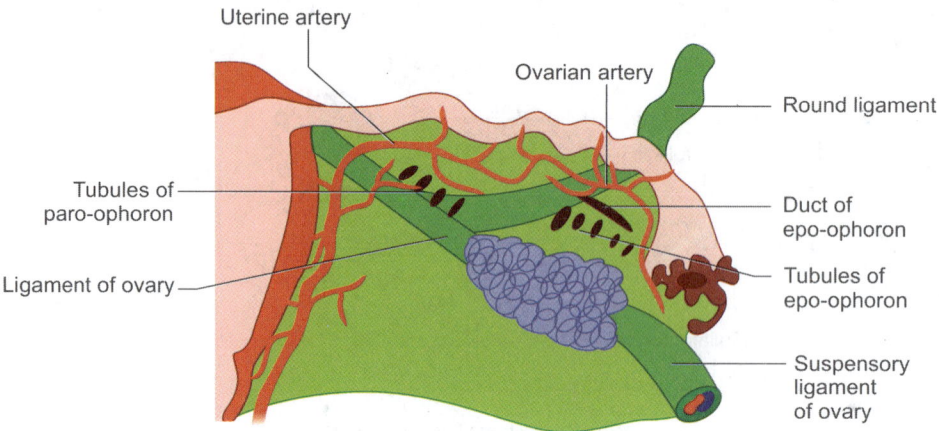

Fig. 39: Contents of broad ligament.

22. Name the PIN structures.

- P – Pudendal nerve
- I – Internal pudendal artery
- N – Nerve to obturator internus.

23. Name the ligaments related to spleen.

- Gastrosplenic ligament
- Lienorenal ligament
- Phrenicocolic ligament (sustentaculum lienis)
- Lienophrenic ligament (suspensory ligament).

24. Contents of pudendal canal.

- The pudendal canal is also known as **Alcock's canal**
- It is situated in the lateral wall of ischiorectal fossa
- It's about 3.75 cm in length
- It extends from lesser sciatic notch to deep perineal pouch
- It is formed by the splitting of obturator fascia.
- **Contents**
  - Internal pudendal vessels
  - Pudendal nerve(S2, 3, 4) situated lateral to the artery and divides into dorsal nerve of penis and perineal nerve within the canal.

25. Boundaries of auscultation triangle.

Triangular region at the back close to chest wall.

- **Boundaries**
  - Above—Trapezius
  - Below—Latissimus dorsi
  - Laterally—Medial border of scapula
  - Floor—parts of the sixth and seventh ribs and the interspace between them (overlying the apex of the lower pulmonary lobe) become subcutaneous.
- **Applied anatomy**
  - The apex of lower lobe of both lungs lie beneath this triangle
  - The cardiac orifice of stomach lies deep to this space on the left side. The splash of fluids swallowed can be heard in the esophageal obstruction.

26. Interventricular septum.

- It separates the right ventricle and left ventricle
- It is obliquely placed
- The anterior and posterior interventricular groove indicates the attachment of the interventricular septum
- It bulges towards the right ventricle and so the right ventricle is crescentic and left ventricle is circular in shape
- **Parts:** Its upper part is thinner called **membranous part** and the lower part is thicker called **muscular part**.

27. Costodiaphragmatic recess.

Refer Essay Q. No. 3 – 2003.

28. Tricuspid valve.

- Tricuspid valve guards the right atrio-ventricular orifice.
- It includes:
  - The atrioventricular orifice
  - The tricuspid annulus
  - Leaflets of tricuspid valve
  - Chordae tendineae
  - Papillary muscles.
- The **atrioventricular orifice** faces downwards forwards and to left. It is oval in shape. The circumference of the opening is about 10 – 12 cm
- **Tricuspid annulus** is a collagenous ring where the bases of the cusps are attached
- **3 cusps or leaflets**; anterior, posterior and septal are attached to the annulus
- **Chordae tendineae** are collagenous threads covered by endothelium connecting the various parts of cusps with the papillary muscles
- **Papillary muscles;** usually two in number—anterior and posterior.

29. Oblique fissure of lung.

- **Oblique fissure** separates the inferior lobe from middle and the upper lobes on right side and upper lobe from the lower lobe on left side
- In each lung the fissure begins from the mediastinal surface above and behind the hilum, passes upward and backward and cuts the posterior border of the lung about 2.5 cm lateral to the T4 spine
- Then it follows downward and forward along the costal surface coinciding with the 5th intercostal space in the mid-axillary line and cuts the inferior border of the lung at the 6th costochondral junction about 7.5 cm lateral to the mid line
- Finally, the fissure reaches the lower and anterior parts of the hilum
- Function: Acts as a plane of cleavage during inspiration.

30. Demilunes.

- Crescent-shaped serous demilunes are attached to the mucous acini

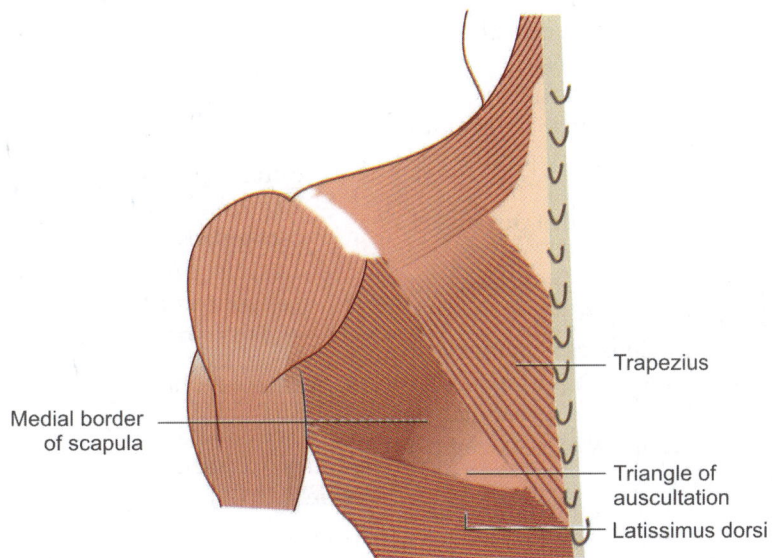

Fig. 40: Triangle of auscultation.

- The ducts of the demilunes open along with mucous acini
- The serous demilunes secrete an antibacterial enzyme.

31. Falx cerebelli.

- It is a sickle shaped fold of duramater
- Situated below tentorium cerebellai in the posterior cranial fossa
- Related to posterior cerebellar notch of cerebellum
- Parts: It has 2 borders, 2 surfaces
- Attachment: Convex margin is attached to internal occipital crest
- The concave margin is free
- The upper end is attached to inferior surface of tentorium cerebelli
- The lower end near foramen magnum divides into two, attached to margins of vermian fossa
- Sinus related: Occipital sinus.

32. Substantia nigra.

- It is a lamina of gray matter made of pigmented nerve cells situated in the midbrain
- The midbrain is divided into a ventral cerebral peduncle part and dorsal tectal by the cerebral aqueduct
- **Situation:** The cerebral peduncle of midbrain includes **crus cerebri**, **tegmental part** and **substantia nigra** which is between the two parts
- **Shape:** Crescent shaped band of gray matter
- **Parts:**
  - Dorsal part is called **pars compacta** and close to tegmentum
  - Ventral part is called **pars reticularis**. It is close to crus cerebri. It has a reticulated appearance due to the presence of intermingling of fibers of crus cerebri with the neurons
  - The nuclei contain melanin (dopamine) and iron.
- **Connections:**
  - Corpus striatum (caudate nucleus and putamen)
  - Red nucleus
  - Reticular formation.

- **Function:**
  - Synthesis of dopamine, and the dopamine reaches the corpus striatum
  - Concerned with muscle tone.
- **Applied anatomy:** In Parkinsonism the synthesis and transport of dopamine, from substantia nigra to striatum is defective.

33. List special somatic afferent nuclei.

- Vestibular nuclei—medial, lateral, superior and inferior vestibular nuclei
- Cochlear nuclei—ventral and dorsal nuclei.

34. Functional areas of superior temporal gyrus.

- **Area 41**
  - Situated in the transverse temporal (Heschl's) and superior temporal gyrus
  - It receives auditory radiation from medial geniculate body
  - It helps to identify the direction, intensity, and distance of the sound.
- **Area 42**
  - It is associated auditory area
  - It is situated in the superior temporal gyrus
  - It is essential for interpretation of sound impulses.
- **Area 22 (Wernicke's area)—sensory speech area**
  - It is called as Wernicke's area
  - Situated in the superior temporal gyrus
  - Comprehends spoken language, recognizes familiar sounds and words
  - Lesion produces **word deafness**/sensory aphasia, unable to interpret spoken words.

35. Waldeyer's ring.

It is a lymphoid ring around pharynx and belongs to **mucosa-associated lymphoid tissue** (MALT)

Situation: Surrounds the openings into the digestive and respiratory tracts

Function: Helps in the defensive mechanism of the respiratory and alimentary systems by destroying the entry of microorganisms from the external environment.

Formation of ring (Fig. 41):
- **Anteroinferiorly** by the **lingual tonsil:** Collection of lymphoid follicles deep to mucous membrane of posterior ⅓ of tongue
- **Laterally** by the:
  - **Palatine tonsil**
    - Situated in the lateral wall of oropharynx
    - By 5 – 6 years there is rapid increase in size, attaining maximum by puberty and
    - Involution of tonsil starts after puberty
    - The epithelial cells covering the tonsil has intimate relation with lymphocytes
    - Helps for direct transfer of antigen from external environment to tonsillar lymphoid tissue, resembling similar to M-fold (M cells) of gut.
  - **Tubal tonsils**: Collection of lymphoid mass near pharyngeal opening of auditory tube.
- Postero superior contains two parts:
  1. **Nasopharyngeal tonsil**
     - Collection of lymphoid follicles at the junction of roof and posterior wall of nasopharynx
     - The size of the tonsil is maximum by 5 years
     - The areas served by this tonsil are nasal cavity, nasopharynx, middle and internal ear, and auditory tube.
  2. **Aggregation of lymphoid tissue** in the intertonsillar intervals.

36. Middle cervical ganglion.
- It is the smallest of the three cervical sympathetic ganglions
- **Formation:** Formed by the fusion of ganglion of 5th 6th cervical ganglions
- **Situation**: In front of transverse process of C6 vertebra
- **Relations**:
  - Anteriorly—common carotid artery
  - Posteriorly—loop of the inferior thyroid artery.
- **Communications**: Connected to inferior cervical ganglion by two branches.
  1. One passes posteriorly and the nerve splits to enclose the vertebral artery
  2. Another passes anteriorly. It forms **ansa subclavia** which loops around the first part of the subclavian artery.
- **Branches**—lateral and medial
  - Lateral branches—gray rami communicants to the C5 and C6 spinal nerves
  - Medial branches—thyroid gland, trachea, esophagus, and cardiac branches join to form the deep cardiac plexus.

37. Parotid duct.
Refer Essay Q. No. 4 – 2004.

38. Fenestra vestibule.
- It is situated in the labyrinthine/medial wall of middle ear cavity
- It is also called as **oval window**
- The fenestra vestibuli is a kidney-shaped opening situated posterosuperior to the promontory
- Convex border faces upwards
- This opening connects the tympanic cavity with the vestibule of the inner ear
- The opening is closed by the base (the footplate) of the stapes
- Annular ligament attaches the margins of the footplate to the edges of the fenestra.

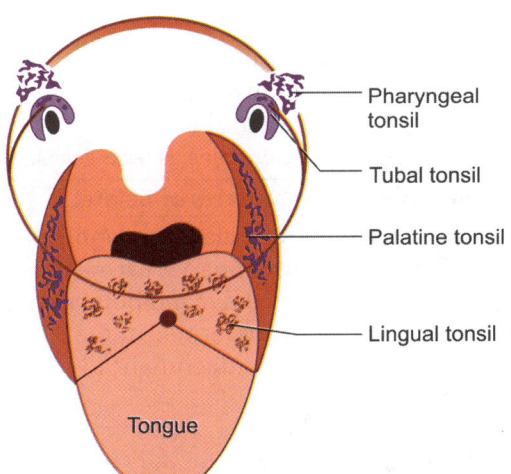

Fig. 41: Waldeyer's ring.

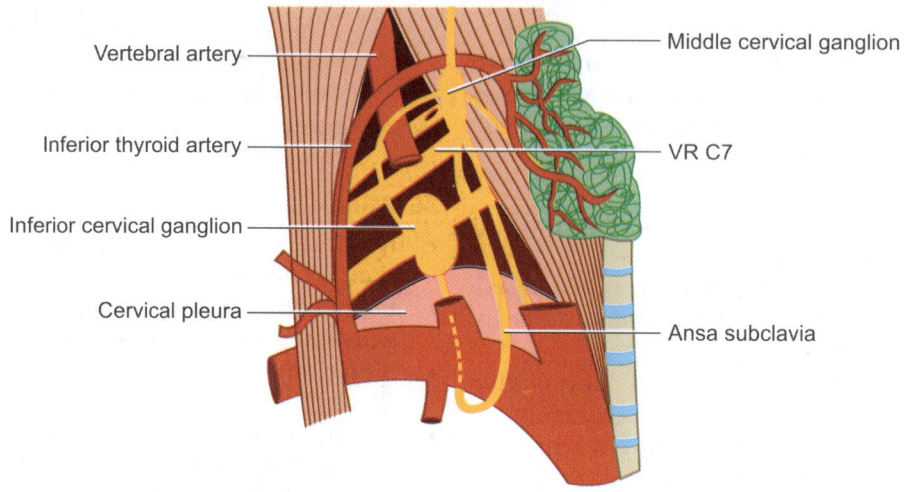

Fig. 42: Middle cervical ganglion.

39. Epicranial aponeurosis.

- It is the third layer of scalp
- It is also called as **galea aponeurotica**
- It is a sheet of fibrous tissue arranged longitudinally connecting occipital and frontal bellies
- Posteriorly, it extends between the two occipital bellies and is attached to the external occipital protuberance and highest nuchal lines
- Anteriorly, a narrow prolongation extends between the two frontal bellies and blends with the subcutaneous tissue at the root of the nose
- Laterally, it extends as a thin sheet superficial to the temporal fascia and is attached to the zygomatic arch
- This layer is attached to skin by fibrous septa and the first three layers form a single flap
- It is separated from pericranium by loose areolar tissue
- The **fibers are arranged** parallel to each other
- The **muscles attached** to the aponeurotica are auricularis posterior and superior, occipitofrontalis
- Galea is sensitive to pain
- The wounds of the scalp gape only when the galea is divided transversely
- **Applied anatomy**: The deep wound of the scalp gape, when it aponeurosis is cut horizontally due to pull of occipitofrontalis muscle.

40. Derivatives of third aortic arch.

- The aortic sac is divided by the spiral aorticopulmonary septum into pulmonary trunk and ascending aorta
- Initially six aortic arches appear
- Later the fifth one disappears
- The ascending aorta is connected to four arches and the pulmonary trunk to the sixth aortic arch.
- **Derivatives of third arch**
    - Common carotid artery
    - Part of internal carotid artery
    - External carotid arises as a new vessel.

41. Enumerate the muscles of palate.

- The muscles of the palate are supplied by the cranial accessory nerve, except tensor palate supplied by the mandibular nerve
- Palatine aponeurosis formed by the tensor palati muscle give attachment to all the muscles
- Levator veli palatini
- Tensor veli palatini
- Musculus uvulae
- Palatopharyngeus
- Palatoglossus.

42. Two features of nasopharynx.

Refer Essay Q. No. 8 – 2006.

43. Congenital anomalies of ventricles of heart.

- **Interventricular septal defects (VSD):**
  - Commonest congenital anomaly of the heart
  - The defect commonly involves the membranous part of the interventricular septum
  - It is due to failure of fusion of the endocardial cushions with the aortic pulmonary septum and muscular part of interventricular septum.
- **Cor triloculare**: Biatrial, monoventricular chamber
- **Fallot's tetralogy**: The components of Fallot's are:
  - Pulmonary stenosis.
  - Right ventricular hypertrophy
  - Ventricular septal defect
  - Overriding of aorta.

44. Derivatives of second pharyngeal arch.

Refer Short Notes 27 – 2005.

45. Arteries supplying the spinal cord.

Spinal cord is supplied by:
- **Branches of vertebral arteries**: Anterior and posterior spinal arteries
- **Segmental arteries**: Branches are received from vertebral, deep cervical, posterior intercostal, lumbar arteries
- **Radicular arteries**: The radicular arteries provide blood supply to the thoracic, lumbar, sacral, and coccygeal segments of the spinal cord. There are anterior and posterior radicular arteries.

46. Boundaries of submental triangle.

- It is one of the anterior triangle of neck
- Situated above the hyoid bone.

Boundaries:
- **Laterally**: Anterior bellies of digastric muscle
- **Base**: Body of hyoid bone
- **Apex**: Symphysis menti
- **Floor**: Mylohyoid muscle
- **Roof**: Skin, superficial fascia with platysma, investing layer of deep fascia.

47. Structures present at hilum of left lung.

Refer Essay Q. No. 3 – 2004.

48. Name the unpaired dural venous sinuses.

- **Classification of dural venous sinuses**: Paired and unpaired.
- **Unpaired**
  - Superior sagittal sinus
  - Inferior sagittal sinus
  - Straight sinus

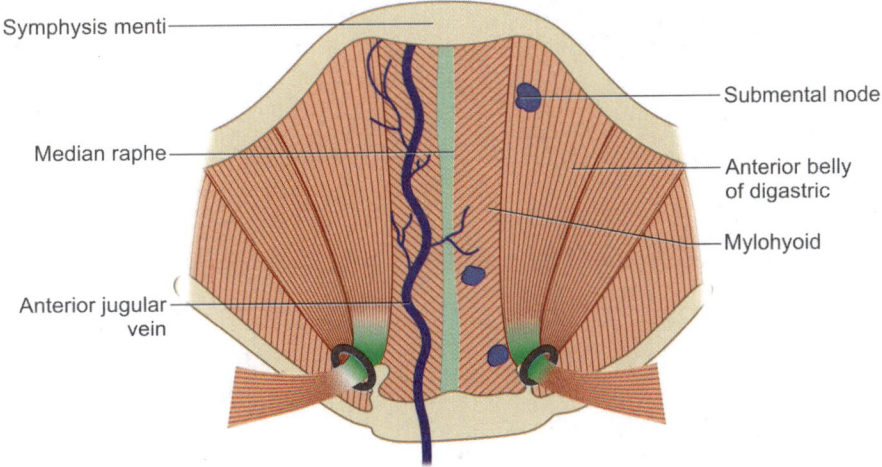

Fig. 43: Submental triangle.

- Occipital sinus
- Anterior intercavernous sinus
- Posterior intercavernous sinus
- Basilar plexus.

49. Intrinsic muscles of larynx.

- The intrinsic muscles of larynx are developed from sixth pharyngeal arch except the cricothyroid which is from 4th arch
- All the muscles are paired except transverse arytenoids
- All the muscles are supplied by recurrent laryngeal nerve except cricothyroid supplied by external laryngeal nerve
- The muscles are grouped into three according to their main actions:
  1. **Action on rima glottidis:** The posterior and lateral cricoarytenoid and oblique and transverse arytenoids
  2. **Action on vocal ligament:** The cricothyroid, posterior cricoarytenoid, thyroarytenoids and vocalis
  3. **Action on inlet of larynx:** The oblique arytenoids, aryepiglottic and thyroepiglottic muscles.

MBBS Examination 2012

ANSWER ALL QUESTIONS

I. Essay questions (15/10 Marks)

1. Describe anatomy of sciatic nerve under the following headings: (a) Root value and components, (b) Relations, (c) Arterial supply, (d) Branches and (e) Clinical importance.
2. Enumerate the parts of extrahepatic biliary apparatus. Describe gallbladder under the following headings: (a) Parts, (b) Peritoneal relations, (c) Arterial supply, (d) Development and (e) Applied anatomy.
3. Describe femoral triangle under the following headings: (a) Boundaries, (b) Contents, (c) Femoral sheath and (d) Applied aspect.
4. Describe stomach under the following headings: (a) Gross features, (b) Relations, (c) Blood supply and nerve supply and (d) Applied anatomy.
5. Classify the white matter of cerebrum and describe internal capsule under the following headings: (a) Parts and relations, (b) Constituent fibers, (c) Arterial supply and (d) Applied anatomy.
6. Define mediastinum. Name its subdivisions. Name the contents of posterior mediastinum and describe esophagus under the following headings: (a) Level of origin, (b) Parts and relations, (c) Level of constrictions, (d) Microscopic appearance and (e) Development.
7. Describe thyroid gland under following headings: (a) Gross features, (b) Relations, (c) Blood supply and (d) Applied anatomy.
8. Describe right lung under following headings: (a) Pleura, (b) Relations of medial surface, (c) Bronchopulmonary segments and (d) Applied anatomy.

II. Short notes (5/4 Marks)

1. Lymphatic drainage of mammary gland and its clinical importance.
2. Movements and muscles producing movements of shoulder joint.
3. Formation, termination and tributaries of portal vein.
4. Microscopic structure of kidney.
5. Superior radioulnar joint.
6. Erb's paralysis.
7. Formation, tributaries and termination of cephalic vein.
8. Descent of testes.
9. Supports of uterus.
10. Medial longitudinal arch of foot.
11. Deltoid muscle.
12. Flexor retinaculum.
13. Popliteal fossa.
14. Enumerate the ligaments and bursae around the knee joint.
15. Extrahepatic biliary apparatus.
16. Head of pancreas.
17. Prostatic part of urethra.
18. Blood supply of long bone.
19. Histology of kidney.
20. Descent of testis.
21. Lateral medullary syndrome.
22. Cavernous sinus.
23. Pterygopalatine ganglion.

24. Carotid triangle.
25. Interatrial septum.
26. Pathway of visual reflexes.
27. Circle of Willis.
28. Intrinsic muscles of larynx.
29. Median nasal septum.
30. External acoustic meatus.
31. Pterion.
32. Blood supply and nerve supply of scalp.
33. 2nd pharyngeal arch.
34. Histology of retina.
35. Fourth ventricle.
36. Name the muscles with nerve supply and action of tongue.
37. Digastric triangle.
38. Superior mediastinum.
39. Down syndrome.
40. Pericardial sinuses.

III. Short answe questions   (3/2 marks)

1. Name the muscles which produce inversion and eversion of foot.
2. Name the structures passing through the pudendal canal.
3. Give the root value of musculocutaneous nerve and name the muscles supplied by it.
4. Enumerate the intra-articular structures of knee joint.
5. Mention the boundaries and clinical importance of bare area of liver.
6. Name the contents of femoral sheath in order.
7. Enumerate the structures passing deep to the flexor retinaculum of hand.
8. Name the nerves which form the subsartorial plexus.
9. Name the parts of quadriceps femoris muscle.
10. Enumerate the short lateral rotators of thigh.
11. Contents of cubital fossa.
12. Nerve supply and action of lumbricals muscle of hand.
13. Name the branches of axillary artery.
14. Piriformis muscle.
15. Name the superficial vein of lower limb with one applied aspect.
16. Muscles attached with iliotibial tract.
17. Ligaments of spleen.
18. Blood supply of rectum.
19. Trigone of urinary bladder.
20. Histology of ureter.
21. Name the sesamoid bones.
22. Syndesmosis.
23. Layers of aorta with applied aspect.
24. Allantois.
25. Derivatives of midgut.
26. Formation and termination of external jugular vein.
27. Peculiarities of 1st intercostal nerve.
28. Lumbar puncture.
29. Structures lodged in the lateral sulcus of the cerebrum.
30. Dangerous area of face.
31. Formation and termination of left superior intercostal vein.
32. Suboccipital nerve.
33. Ligamentum denticulatum.
34. Structures pierced by parotid duct in order.
35. Origin and branches of middle meningeal artery.
36. Parts of corpus callosum.
37. Deep nuclei of cerebellum.
38. Tentorium cerebelli.
39. Name any four branches of external carotid artery.
40. Name the components of lacrimal apparatus.
41. Name the extraocular muscles of eyeball.
42. Development of pituitary gland (in brief).
43. Mention the boundaries of laryngeal inlet.
44. Right principal bronchus.
45. Pleural diaphragm.
46. Moderator band.
47. Triangle of Koch.
48. Simple squamous epithelium.
49. Mention the four features of Tetralogy of Fallot.
50. Mention the bones of middle ear cavity.

I. ESSAY QUESTIONS

1. **Describe anatomy of sciatic nerve under the following headings: a. Root value and components, b. Relations, c. Arterial supply, d. Branches and e. Clinical importance.**

Refer Essay Q. No. 5 – 2007.

2. **Enumerate the parts of extrahepatic biliary apparatus. Describe gall-bladder under the following headings: a. Parts, b. Peritoneal relations, c. Arterial supply, d. Development and e. Applied anatomy.**

Parts of extrahepatic biliary apparatus – Refer Essay Q. No. 2 – 2005.
Gallbladder – a, b and e—Refer Essay Q. No. 2 – 2005.

- **Arterial supply:**
  - Cystic artery branch from right hepatic branch
  - Reaches the neck of the gallbladder and divides into superficial and deep branch
  - Superficial branch ramifies on the inferior surface of body of gallbladder
  - The deep branch reaches superior surface
  - These arteries anastomose with each other around the body and neck
  - In addition, small **arterial branches from liver** supply the gallbladder.
- **Development (Fig. 1):**
  - Developed from endoderm of foregut
  - Development begins by middle of third week
  - A diverticulum called hepatic bud appears at the distal part of the ventral surface of foregut
  - The hepatic bud grows upwards in the ventral mesogastrium
  - Reaching the liver, it terminates by dividing into two. The upward growth forms the bile duct. Before termination an outgrowth appears from the upper part of the hepatic bud called cystic bud. It forms the gallbladder
  - The stalk of the outgrowth forms the cystic duct.

3. **Describe femoral triangle under the following headings: a. Boundaries, b. Contents, c. Femoral sheath and d. Applied aspect.**

It is an inverted triangular depressed intermuscular space.

Situation: In front of upper one-third of the thigh below the inguinal ligament.

Boundaries (Fig. 2)

- **Lateral**: By the medial border of the sartorius
- **Medial**: Medial border of the adductor longus
- **Base**: Inguinal ligament
- **Apex**: Point where the medial and lateral boundaries meet
- **Roof**: Skin, Superficial fascia with superficial inguinal nodes, femoral branch of genitofemoral nerve, branches of the ilioinguinal nerve, superficial branches of femoral artery with veins, upper part of great saphenous vein. Deep fascia with

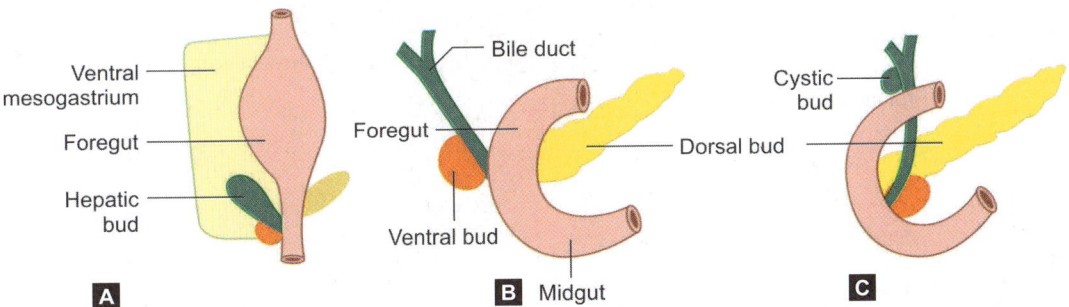

Figs.1A to C: Development of extrahepatic biliary apparatus.

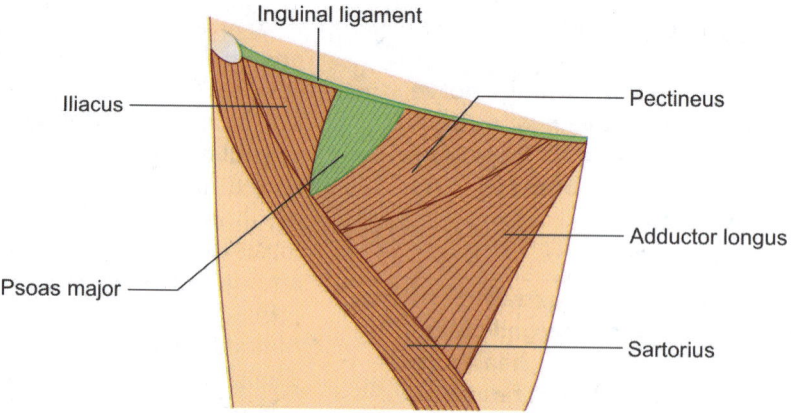

Fig. 2: Boundaries of femoral triangle.

saphenous opening and the cribriform fascia.
- **Floor**: It is formed from lateral to medial by:
  - Iliacus
  - Psoas major
  - Pectineus
  - Adductor longus.

Contents (Fig. 3)

- **Femoral artery** and its branches.
  - **Origin**: External iliac artery is continued as femoral artery behind the mid inguinal point
  - **Course**: It runs downwards in the femoral triangle and then in adductor canal. It is covered by femoral sheath for about 4 cm length
  - **Termination**: It leaves through the hiatus of adductor magnus and is continued as popliteal artery.
- **Relations**:
  - **In the triangle**:
    - **Anterior:** Skin, superficial fascia, fascia lata, anterior layer of femoral sheath, medial cutaneous nerve of thigh
    - **Posterior:** Posterior layer of femoral sheath, psoas, pectineus, adductor longus
    - **Medial**: Femoral vein
    - **Lateral**: Femoral nerve.

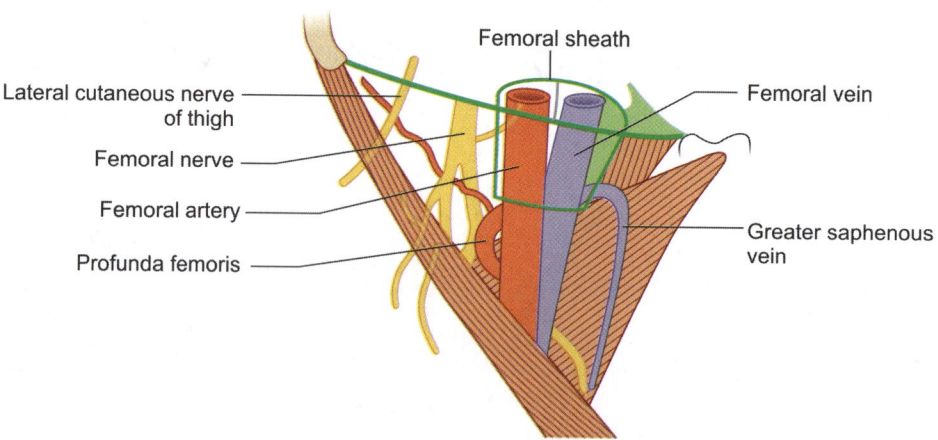

Fig. 3: Contents of femoral triangle.

- Branches:
  - Three superficial:
    1. Superficial epigastric artery
    2. Superficial circumflex iliac artery
    3. Superficial external pudendal artery
  - Three deep
    1. Deep external pudendal artery
    2. Muscular branches
    3. Profunda femoris artery
- **Femoral vein** and its tributaries:
  - **Formation**: Popliteal vein is continued as femoral vein from adductor opening
  - **Termination**: It is continued as external iliac vein
  - **At the base of triangle vein** is medial to the artery, but at its apex it is posteromedial to the artery.
  - **Tributaries**:
    - Great saphenous vein
    - Profunda femoris vein
    - Lateral and medial circumflex veins.
- **Femoral nerve and its branches:** It lies outside the femoral sheath lateral to the artery. The branches from femoral nerve are:
  - Nerve to pectineus and iliacus
  - Intermediate femoral cutaneous nerve
  - Medial femoral cutaneous nerve
  - Saphenous nerve.
- **Femoral branch of genitofemoral nerve**
- **Lateral cutaneous nerve of the thigh** medial to anterior superior iliac spine.
- **Inguinal lymph nodes**:
  - **Superficial group**: Horizontal group close to inguinal ligament and vertical group close termination of great saphenous vein
  - **Deep inguinal lymph nodes** medial to femoral vein.

Femoral Sheath

Refer Short Notes 4 – 2005.

Applied Anatomy

- Femoral pulse can be felt at mid inguinal point just below the inguinal ligament
- Femoral artery is superficial in position, it is used for various procedures namely angiography, for coronary angioplasty or catheterization
- Femoral hernia is common in female because of wider femoral canal. It is below and lateral to the pubic tubercle
- To control bleeding femoral artery can be compressed against the head of femur
- At the apex of femoral triangle, the femoral artery, femoral vein, profunda vein and profunda femoris artery are arranged one behind the other from superficial to deep. All the vessels will be involved in a stab injury at apex of triangle.

---

4. **Describe stomach under the following headings: a. Gross features, b. Relations, c. Blood supply and nerve supply and d. Applied anatomy.**

(a, b, c) (blood supply), (d) Refer Essay Q. No. 2 – 2007.

Nerve supply

- The stomach is supplied by sympathetic and parasympathetic nerves
- **Sympathetic**: They are vasomotor in function. They stimulate pyloric sphincter and inhibit the gastric musculature. The preganglionic motor fibers arise from T_6 to T_9 segments of spinal cord and reach through greater splanchnic nerves
- **Parasympathetic**: They stimulate gastric musculature and inhibit the pyloric sphincter. It is secretomotor to the glands. The parasympathetic fibers are derived from the vagus in the form of **anterior and posterior vagal trunks**. The anterior and posterior vagal trunks are formed by left and right vagus nerves respectively.
  - The **anterior vagal trunk (Fig. 4A)** gives rise to:
    - Hepatic branches—supplies liver, gallbladder and pylorus. The branch

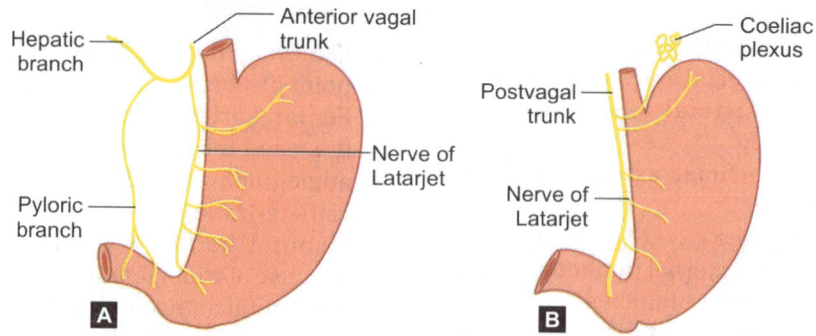

Figs. 4A and B: Nerve supply of stomach: (A) Anterior vagal trunk; (B) Posterior vagal trunk.

to pylorus is in the form of inverted 'y' and supplies the prepyloric part and pyloric sphincter
- Gastric branch—supplies the antero superiorsurface of the stomach and divides into 6 to 10 branches. The main gastric branch called the **nerve of Latarjet** runs close to lesser curvature within lesser omentum. Termination resembles crow's feet and supplies pyloric antrum.
- **Posterior vagal trunk (Fig. 4B):** It divides into
  - Celiac branches
  - Gastric branches: The main gastric branch called the **nerve of Latarjet** runs close to lesser curvature within lesser omentum and supplies the posteroinferior surface of the stomach
  - Sometimes the posterior vagal trunk gives off a branch to supply the fundus called the **nerve of Grassi (criminal nerve).**

Applied anatomy
- Vagotomy is performed to reduce the secretion of HCl in case of peptic ulcer.
- **Vagotomy** may be:
  - Truncal—section of both vagal trunks. As the stomach becomes atonic the patient has to undergo either pyloroplasty or gastrojejunostomy
  - Selective—section of nerve of Latarjet. It results in delayed emptying as the motility of pyloric antrum is reduced
  - Highly selective—only smaller branches from gastric nerves to prevent delayed gastric emptying.

5. **Classify the white matter of cerebrum and describe internal capsule under the following headings: a. Parts and relations, b. Constituent fibers, c. Arterial supply, d. Applied anatomy.**

Internal capsule—Refer Essay 7 – 2005.
Classification of white matter of cerebrum:
- The myelinated nerve fibers form the white matter of the cerebral hemispheres
- White matter is classified depending on the course and connections of the nerve fibers.
- Three types of fibers are present:
  1. **Association fibers**, are within the same cerebral hemisphere but connected to different cortical areas. It is of two types—short association and long association fibers. **Short association** are between adjacent gyri. **Long association** are from one gyrus to other gyrus at a distance, e.g. uncinate fasciculus, superior longitudinal fasciculus, cingulum, inferior longitudinal fasciculus
  2. **Commissural fibers**, crosses the midline and connect corresponding cortical areas in the two hemispheres, e.g. corpus callosum, commissure of fornix, posterior commissure, anterior commissure, Habenular commissure
  3. **Projection fibers**, which connect the cerebral cortex with the corpus

striatum, diencephalon, brainstem and spinal cord, e.g. internal capsule.

6. **Define mediastinum. Name its subdivisions. Name the contents of posterior mediastinum and describe esophagus under the following headings: a. Level of origin, b. Parts and relations, c. Level of constrictions, d. Microscopic appearance and e. Development.**

- **Definition:** The space in the thoracic cavity in between the right and left pleural sacs is called as mediastinum.
- **Boundaries (Fig. 5)**
    - Anteriorly: Sternum
    - Posteriorly: Thoracic vertebrae
    - Superiorly: Thoracic inlet
    - Inferiorly: Diaphragm
    - On each side: Mediastinal pleura.
- **Subdivisions (Fig. 5)**
    - Divided into superior mediastinum and inferior mediastinum by an **imaginary line** passing through the lower border of body of 4th thoracic vertebra behind and the sternal angle of Louis in front
    - The inferior is further subdivided into 3 by the pericardium:
        i. Anterior mediastinum—part in front of pericardium
        ii. Middle mediastinum—part enclosed within pericardium
        iii. Posterior mediastinum—part behind the pericardium.
- **Contents of posterior mediastinum:**
  Three veins:
  i. Azygos vein
  ii. Hemiazygos vein
  iii. Accessory azygos vein.
  Three nerves:
  i. Right and left sympathetic chain
  ii. Splanchnic nerves
  iii. Right and left vagi.
  Three tubes:
  i. Descending thoracic aorta
  ii. Esophagus
  iii. Thoracic duct.
  Posterior mediastinal lymph nodes
- **Esophagus**
  a, b, c Refer Short Notes 16 – 2003.
  d Refer Short Notes 31 – 2008.
- **Development**
  From post laryngeal part of foregut.

7. **Describe thyroid gland under following headings: a. Gross features, b. Relations, c. Blood supply and d. Applied anatomy.**

(a, b) Refer Short Notes 17 – 2004.
(c, d) Refer Short Notes 38 – 2008.

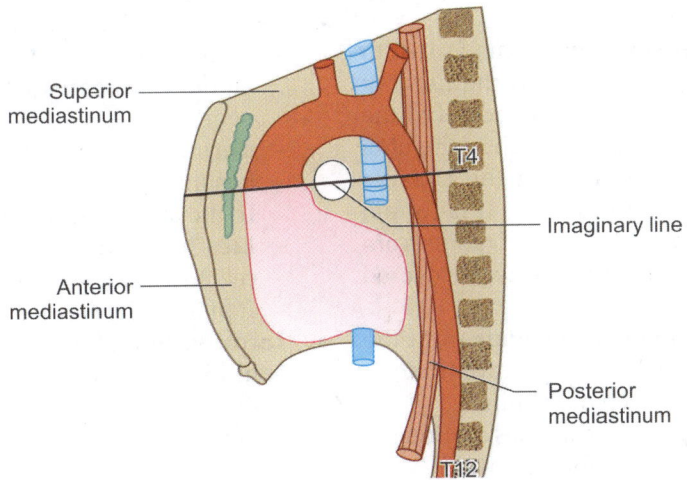

Fig. 5: Subdivisions of mediastinum.

8. **Describe right lung under following headings: a. Pleura, b. Relations of medial surface, c. Bronchopulmonary segments and d. Applied anatomy.**

(a) Refer Essay Q. No. 3 – 2003.
(b, c, d) Refer Essay Q. No. 3 – 2004.

II. SHORT NOTES

1. **Lymphatic drainage of mammary gland and its clinical importance.**

Refer Short Notes 19 – 2005.

2. **Movements and muscles producing movements of Shoulder Joint.**

Refer Essay 2 – 2006.

3. **Formation, termination and tributaries of portal vein.**

Refer Short Notes 6 – 2004.

4. **Microscopic structure of kidney.**

Refer Short Notes 3 – 2007.

5. **Superior radioulnar joint.**
   - **Type**: Synovial, uniaxial joint and pivot variety
   - **Articular surfaces:**
     – Circumference of head of radius
     – The radial notch of the ulna and the annular ligament form an osseofibrous ring.
   - **Ligaments (Fig. 6):**
     – **Annular ligament**: It forms four-fifth of the ring within which the head of the radius rotates. It is attached to the margins of the radial notch of the ulna and is continuous with the capsule of the elbow joint above. It is funnel shaped, to hold the head of radius from slipping down. Inner surface is covered with cartilage
     – **Quadrate ligament** extends from the neck of the radius to the lower margin of the radial notch of the ulna
     – **Blood supply:** Anastomosis around the lateral side of the elbow joint
     – **Nerve supply:** Musculocutaneous, median, and radial nerves
     – **Movements:** Supination and pronation.

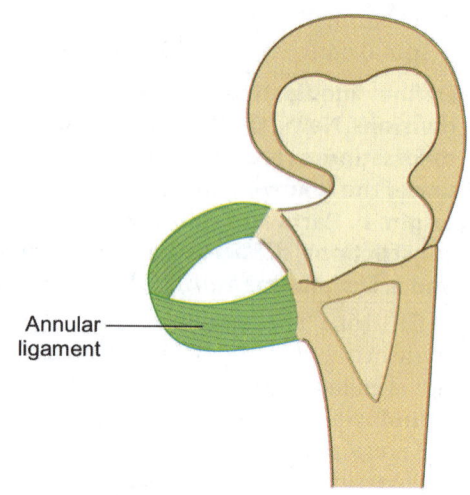

Fig. 6: Superior radioulnar joint.

6. **Erb's paralysis.**

Refer Essay Q. No. 3 – 2005.

7. **Formation, tributaries and termination of cephalic vein.**
   - **Formation:**
     – Starts over the anatomical snuff box
     – The lateral aspect of the dorsal venous arch is continued as cephalic vein.
   - **Course**:
     – The vein curves around the radial side of forearm and reaches the ventral surface. It receives veins from anterior and posterior sides in the forearm
     – Anterior to the elbow, the cephalic vein communicates with the median cubital vein
     – Through median cubital it joins the basilic vein
     – In the arm ascends lateral to biceps
     – Lies in the deltopectoral groove and reaches infraclavicular fossa
     – It pierces the clavipectoral fascia.
   - **Termination:** Drains to the axillary vein behind the clavicular head of pectoralis major.
   - **Tributaries:**
     – Veins of forearm
     – It may be connected to external jugular vein by a vein crossing superficial to clavicle.

8. Descent of testes.
Refer Short Notes 8 – 2007.

9. Supports of uterus.
Refer Essay Q. No. 2 – 2004.

10. Medial longitudinal arch of foot.
Refer Essay Q. No. 1 – 2003.

11. Deltoid muscle.

- Deltoid is a thick, triangular muscle
- The muscle surrounds the shoulder joint on all sides except inferomedially
- Rounded contour to the shoulder is produced by this muscle.
- **Origin (Fig. 7A):**
  - **Anterior fibers**—are oblique arises from the anterior border and superior surface of the lateral third of the clavicle
  - **Middle fibers**—are multipennate arises from the lateral margin and superior surface of the acromion process. It is arranged as four intramuscular septa from the acromion interdigitate with three septa ascending from the deltoid tubercle
  - **Posterior fibers**—are oblique arises the crest of the spine of scapula.
- **Insertion:** The fibers converge inferiorly to form a tendon which is attached to the deltoid tubercle on the lateral aspect of the middle of shaft of the humerus **(Fig. 7B).**
- **Nerve supply:** Axillary nerve
- **Actions:**
  - Anterior fibers draw the arm forwards and medially along with pectoralis major
  - The arm drawn backwards and laterally by the posterior fibers along with latissimus dorsi and teres major
  - The middle acromial fibers are multipennate and strong abductor. Along with supraspinatus it abducts the arm to 90°
  - The downward pull of arm with heavy load is resisted by the supraspinatus with the help of deltoid (action of paradox)
  - While walking **swinging of arm** is done by deltoid.
- **Relations: Structures deep to deltoid**
Refer Short Notes 4 – 2004.
- **Applied anatomy:** Injury to axillary nerve results in flat shoulder. The contour of shoulder is lost and loss abduction of arm.

12. Flexor retinaculum.

- It is a strong fibrous band bridging the anterior concavity of the carpal bones and converting it into a tunnel called the carpal tunnel
- It has in addition a superficial and a deep slip.
- **Attachments:**
  - **Medial:** Pisiform bone, hook of the hamate
  - **Lateral:** Tubercle of the scaphoid, crest of the trapezium
  - **Proximally:** It blends with the antebrachial fascia
  - **Distally:** It is continuous with palmar aponeurosis and gives attachment to thenar and hypothenar muscles

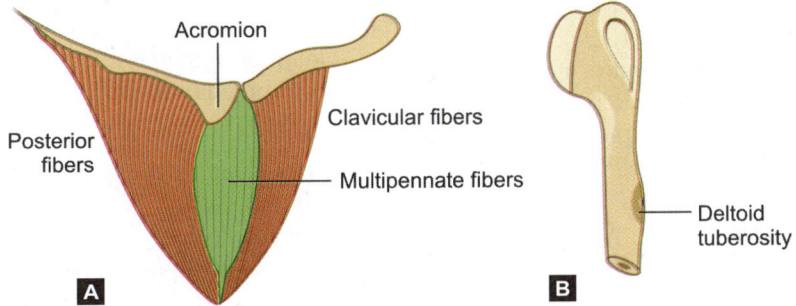

Figs. 7A and B: Deltoid muscle: (A) Origin; (B) Insertion.

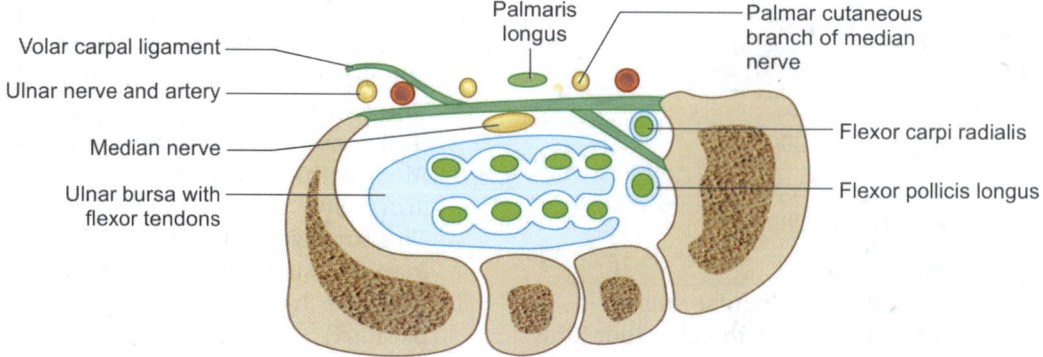

Fig. 8: Flexor retinaculum.

- The **deep slip** extends laterally and is attached to the lips of the groove of trapezium and lodges the tendon of flexor carpi radialis
- A **superficial slip** called **volar carpal ligament** extends medially to the pisiform enclosing a canal called **Guyon's canal**. The ulnar nerve and vessels pass through that.
- **Structures passing superficial** to the flexor retinaculum:
  - Superficial branch of radial artery
  - Palmar cutaneous branch of the median nerve
  - Tendon of palmaris longus
  - Palmar cutaneous branch of ulnar nerve
  - Ulnar vessels
  - Ulnar nerve.
- **Structures passing deep** to flexor retinaculum:
  - Median nerve
  - Tendons of flexor digitorum superficialis
  - Tendons of flexor digitorum profundus
  - Tendon of flexor pollicis longus
  - Tendon of flexor carpi radialis
  - Ulnar bursa
  - Radial bursa.
- **Applied anatomy**: **Carpal tunnel syndrome** Refer Short Notes 11 – 2010.

13. Popliteal fossa.
Refer Short Notes 8 – 2009.

14. Enumerate the ligaments and bursae around the knee joint.

Ligaments
- Fibrous capsule
- Ligamentum patellae
- Tibial collateral or medial collateral ligament
- Fibular collateral or lateral collateral ligament
- Oblique popliteal ligament
- Arcuate popliteal ligament
- Cruciate ligaments—anterior and posterior
- Meniscofemoral ligaments
- Coronary ligament
- Menisci—medial and lateral.

Bursae

Anterior
- Subcutaneous prepatellar bursa
- Subcutaneous infrapatellar bursa
- Deep infrapatellar bursa
- Suprapatellar bursa.

Lateral
- Bursa deep to the lateral head of gastrocnemius
- Bursa between the fibular collateral ligament and the biceps femoris

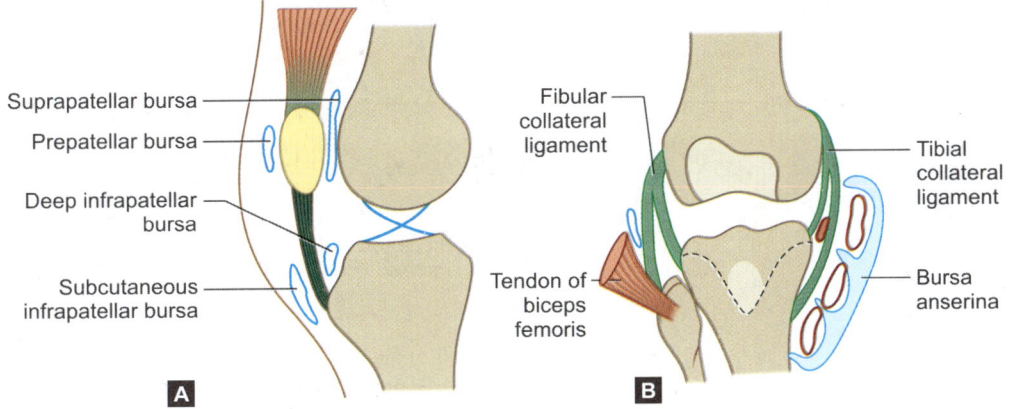

Figs. 9A and B: Ligaments and bursae of knee joint.

- Bursa between the fibular collateral ligament and the tendon of the popliteus
- Bursa between the tendon of the popliteus and the lateral condyle of the tibia.

Medial
- Bursa deep to the medial head of gastrocnemius
- Anserine bursa—separates the tendons of sartorius, gracilis and semitendinosus from one another, from the tibia and from the tibial collateral ligament
- Bursa deep to the tibial collateral ligament.
- Bursa deep to the semimembranosus.

15. Extrahepatic biliary apparatus.
Refer Essay Q. No. 2 – 2005.

16. Head of pancreas.
Refer Essay Q. No. 1 – 2006.

17. Prostatic part of urethra.
Refer Short Notes 2 – 2006.

18. Blood supply of long bone.
Refer Short Notes 2 – 2009.

19. Histology of kidney.
Refer Short Notes 3 – 2007.

20. Descent of testis.
Refer Short Notes 8 – 2007.

21. Lateral medullary syndrome.
Refer Short Notes 38 – 2009.

22. Cavernous sinus.
Refer Essay Q. No. 5 – 2008.

23. Pterygopalatine ganglion.
- It is the largest peripheral parasympathetic ganglion
- It is also called sphenopalatine/Hay fever ganglion
- It is concerned with supply of lacrimal gland, pharyngeal, nasal and palatine mucous glands
- It is anatomically connected to maxillary nerve, but functionally to facial nerve
- **Situation:** In the pterygopalatine fossa, near sphenopalatine foramen.
- **Roots (Fig. 10)**
  - **Parasympathetic root**
    Lacrimatory nucleus ------ facial nerve------ greater petrosal nerve + deep petrosal nerve ------- nerve of pterygoid canal.^Relays pterygopalatine ganglion ^Postganglionic fibers maxillary nerve ---------- zygomaticotemporal nerve ^Communicates lacrimal branch of ophthalmic nerve ---------- lacrimal gland
  - **Sympathetic root**
    Postganglionic fibers from superior cervical ganglion ------ deep petrosal nerve (plexus around internal carotid artery) ----- ganglion (do not relay). They are supply blood vessels and orbitalis muscle.
  - **Sensory root**
    General sensation is carried by branches of the maxillary division of

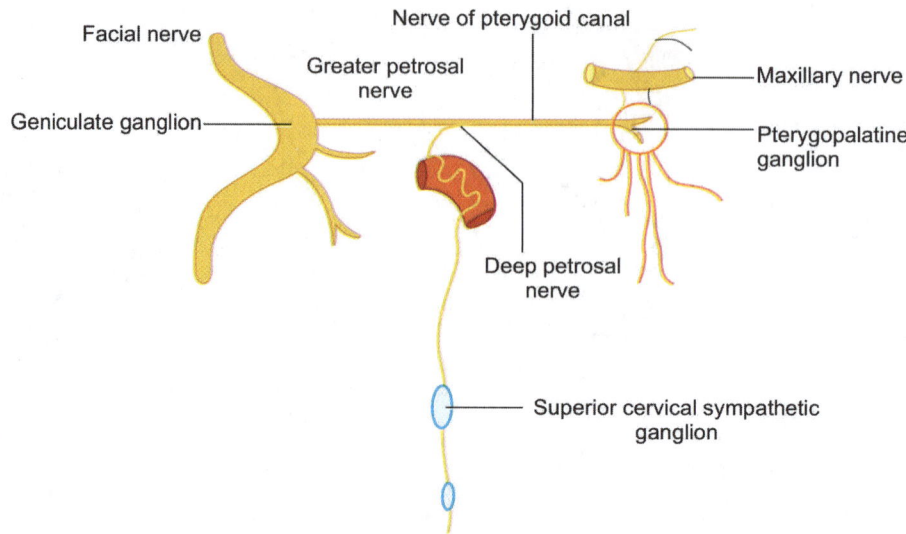

Fig. 10: Roots of pterygopalatine ganglion.

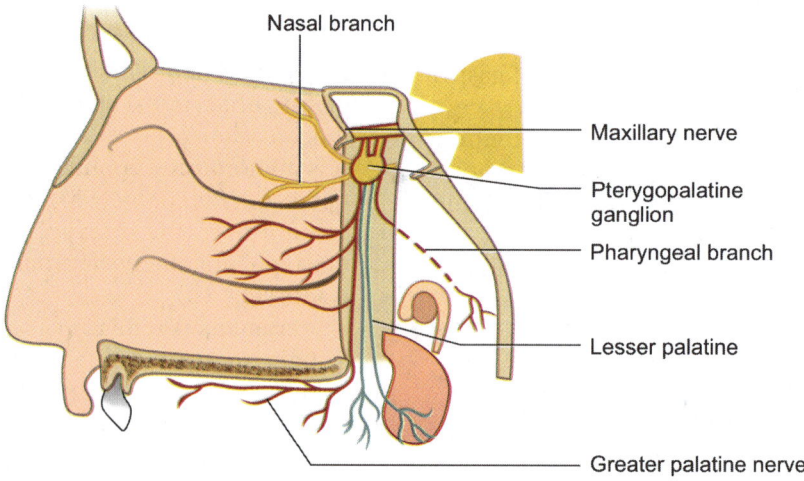

Fig. 11: Branches of pterygopalatine ganglion.

the trigeminal nerve pass through the ganglion without relaying.
- **Branches (Fig. 11)**
  - **Orbital branches**—supply periosteum of orbit. They pass through the inferior orbital fissure and enter the orbit. Some fibers by passing through posterior ethmoidal foramen supply the sphenoidal and ethmoidal sinuses
  - **Palatine branches**—are greater and lesser palatine branches.
- **Greater palatine nerve**
  - Runs down through the greater palatine canal, emerges through greater palatine foramen
  - On the inferior surface of the bony palate it runs forwards up to the incisor teeth
  - It supplies the gums, mucosa and glands of the hard palate
  - It gives off **posterior inferior lateral nasal branches** to supply

the mucous membrane of inferior nasal concha and the middle and inferior meatuses.
- **Lesser palatine branches** descend through the greater palatine canal.
  - Emerge through the lesser palatine foramina of the palatine bone
  - The structures supplied are, uvula, tonsil and soft palate
  - The taste sensation from palate is carried by the palatine branches.
- **Nasal branches**—are divided as medial and lateral branches.
  - **Posterior superior lateral nasal nerves** supply the mucous membrane of superior and middle conchae along its posterior part and the posterior ethmoidal sinuses
  - **Medial posterior superior nasal nerves** supply the mucosa of the posterior part of the roof and the nasal septum
    The nasopalatine nerve is a medial branch, supplies the inferior portion of the nasal septum and anterior part of the hard palate.
- **Pharyngeal branches**—enter the nasopharynx through palatovaginal canal and supply mucous membrane behind the tubal elevation.

24. Carotid triangle.
Boundaries—Refer Essay Q. No. 8 – 2011.
Contents—Refer Essay Q. No. 8 – 2011.

25. Interatrial septum.
Gross features—Refer Essay Q. No. 7 – 2006.
Development—Refer Short Notes 25 – 2006.

26. Pathway of visual reflexes.
- **Pupillary reflex**: The pupillary light reflex includes the direct and consensual responses
  - Direct light reflex: When light is thrown on one eye produces constriction of pupil in that eye. This is known as direct light reflex. The constriction of pupil is produced by the stimulation of Edinger Westphal nucleus
  - Consensual light reflex: The pupil of the other also constricts simultaneously with the direct light reflex.
- **Pathway:** From ganglionic cells of retina -------- optic nerve, optic chiasma, optic tract ---------- pretectal nucleus of midbrain -------- Edinger-Westphal nucleus --------- oculomotor nerve ---------- ciliary ganglion -------- short ciliary nerves ----------- sphincter papillae and ciliaris
- **Accommodation reflex (near triad) (CCC):** This is for looking near objects,

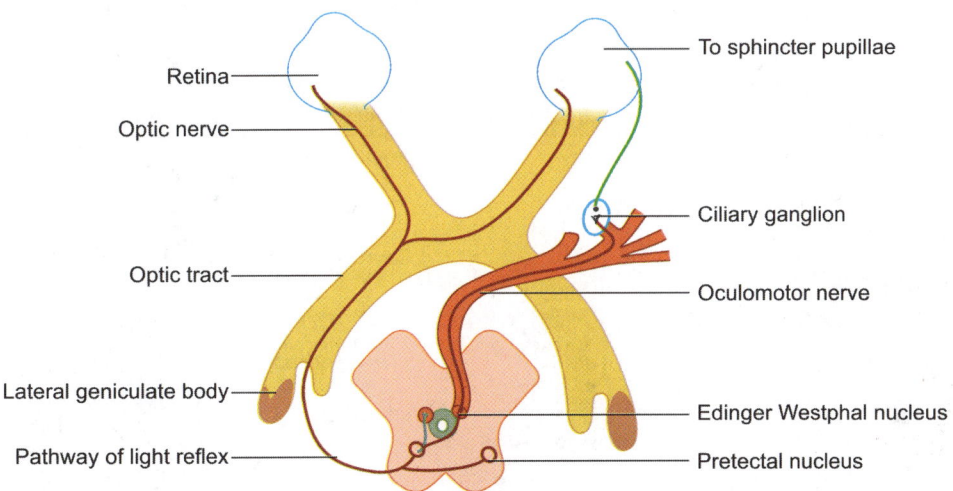

Fig. 12: Visual reflexes.

it includes ocular **c**onvergence, accommodation (**c**onvexity of lens), and **c**onstriction of pupil
  - **Ocular convergence**: Looking at a near object there is medial rotation of eye, helps to focus the light rays on the same points on both retina. The contraction of the medial rectus of both side produces this effect
  - **Accommodation:** Increase of the curvature of lens is called accommodation. This is done by contraction of ciliaris
  - **Constriction of pupil:** The pupil constricts with convergence and accommodation. This prevents the light rays entering and is responsible for sharpness of the image on the retina.
- **Pathway:** Optic nerve, tract ------- lateral geniculate body -------- optic radiation ----------- visual cortex (striate, para striate, peri striate areas) ----------- through long association fibers to frontal eye field. From cortex ------ oculomotor nucleus -------- Edinger-Westphal nucleus --------oculomotor nerve ----- ciliaris and sphincter papillae through ciliary ganglion for constriction of pupil and convexity of lens, to medial, superior and inferior recti, for convergence.

27. Circle of Willis.
Refer Short Notes 24 – 2005.

28. Intrinsic muscles of larynx.
- The intrinsic muscles of larynx are developed from sixth pharyngeal arch except the cricothyroid which is from 4th arch
- All the muscles are paired except transverse arytenoids
- All the muscles are supplied by recurrent laryngeal nerve except cricothyroid supplied by external laryngeal nerve
- The muscles are grouped into three according to their main actions:
  1. **Action on rima glottidis**: The posterior and lateral cricoarytenoid and oblique and transverse arytenoids
  2. **Action on vocal ligament**: The cricothyroid, posterior cricoarytenoid, thyroarytenoids and vocalis
  3. **Action on inlet of larynx**: The oblique arytenoids, aryepiglottic and thyro-epiglottic muscles.

S.No.	Name of the muscle	Origin	Insertion	Action
1	Posterior cricoarytenoid	From the posterior lamina of the cricoid cartilage. The upper fibers are horizontal, the middle fibers oblique and lower fibers are vertical.	Inserted into the muscular process of arytenoid cartilage	Abductor of vocal cord. Hence it is also known as safety muscle of larynx
2	Lateral cricoarytenoid	From upper border of arch of cricoid cartilage	To the muscular process of arytenoid cartilage	Adducts the vocal cord thereby closes the rima glottidis

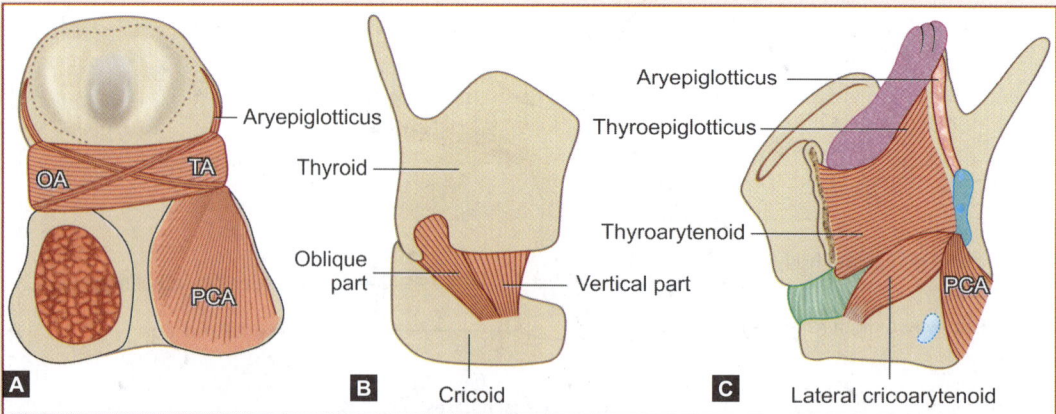

Figs. 13A to C: Intrinsic muscles of larynx.

Contd...

Contd...

S.No.	Name of the muscle	Origin	Insertion	Action
3	Transverse arytenoid	From lateral border and muscular process of arytenoid cartilage	To the corresponding parts of the other arytenoid cartilage	Adducts the arytenoid cartilage and closes the intercartilagenous part of rima glottidis
4	Oblique arytenoids	Muscular process of one arytenoid cartilage	To the apex of other arytenoid cartilage	Weak adductor of vocal cord
5	Cricothyroid	From external surface of anterior arch of cricoid cartilage. The anterior fibers ascend upwards called vertical part, and few fibers pass obliquely forming oblique part	Vertical part to inferior border of lamina of thyroid cartilage. Oblique part to inferior horn of thyroid cartilage	Tensor of vocal cord
6	Thyroarytenoids	From lower part of angle of thyroid cartilage	To anterolateral surface of arytenoids cartilage	Shortens and relaxes the vocal cord
7	Vocalis	Few deep fibers of thyroarytenoid muscle form a bundle lateral to vocal ligament. It extends from vocal process of arytenoids cartilage	To angle of thyroid cartilage	Shortens and relaxes the vocal cord
8	Aryepiglotticus	Few fibers of oblique arytenoids extend from apex of arytenoids cartilage	Pass along the aryepiglottic fold forming aryepiglotticus	closure of the inlet of larynx
9	Thyroepiglotticus	Some fibers of thyroarytenoid extend from angle of thyroid cartilage forming thyroepiglotticus muscle	To margins of epiglottis and aryepiglottic fold	Widens the inlet of larynx

29. Median nasal septum.

Refer Short Notes 17 – 2003.

30. External acoustic meatus.

- The external acoustic meatus **extends** from the concha to the tympanic membrane
- **Length** from the floor of the concha is about 2.5 cm and from the tragus 4 cm
- **Shape and division:** S-shaped and divided into pars externa, pars media and pars interna.
- **Direction**
  - Pars externa: Directed medially, anteriorly and slightly up
  - Pars media: Posteromedially and up
  - Pars interna: Anteromedially and slightly down.
- There are **two constrictions**, one in cartilaginous part near its medial end, the other is the isthmus junction between the two parts
- **Parts**: It has **two parts**—lateral third is **cartilaginous** and medial two-third is **osseous**.
  - **Cartilaginous part**
    - 8 mm long.
    - It is continuous with the cartilage of the external ear
    - Attached to osseous part by fibrous tissue
    - The cartilage is deficient posterosuperiorly completed by collagen fibers.
  - **Osseous part**
    - 16 mm long
    - Narrower than the cartilaginous part
    - The medial end is smaller than the lateral end
    - The lateral end is dilated and rough, gives attachment to the cartilaginous part
    - The tympanic plate of the temporal bone contributes for the anterior,

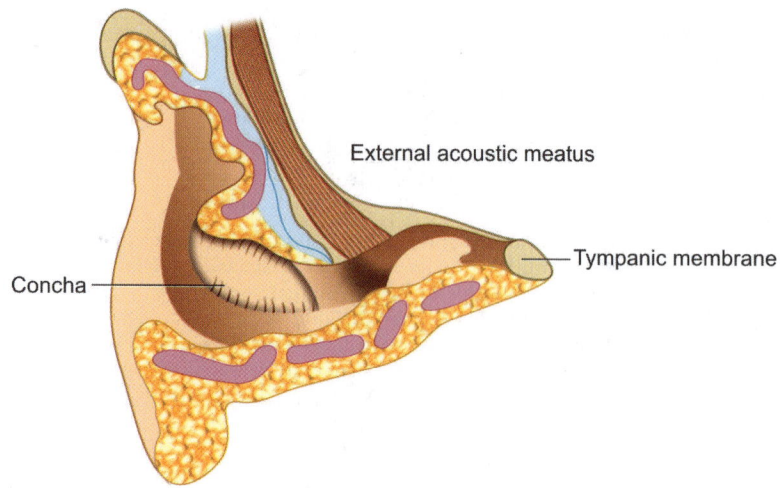

Fig. 14: External acoustic meatus.

inferior, posterior, parts of the osseous portion of the external acoustic meatus
- The squamous part of the temporal bone forms the posterosuperior part.
- **Blood supply**
  - Posterior auricular artery
  - Deep auricular branch of the maxillary artery
  - Auricular branches of the superficial temporal artery.
- **Venous drainage**—into the external jugular and maxillary veins and the pterygoid plexus
- **Nerve supply:** The sensory nerve supply—the auriculotemporal branch of the mandibular nerve, and the auricular branch of the vagus. The facial nerve through its communication with the auricular branch of vagus nerve.

31. Pterion.

- The pterion is seen in the floor of the temporal fossa
- It is an **H-shaped sutural junction**
- Four bones meet on one side
- **Formation:** Superiorly by the frontal and parietal bones and inferiorly by the greater wing of the sphenoid and squamous temporal.
- **Developmentally:** The anterolateral/sphenoidal fontanelle gets ossified by 3rd month of birth to form the pterion.
- **Structures related**:
  - The anterior branch of the middle meningeal artery
  - The lateral fissure of the cerebral hemisphere.
- **Surface marking**:
  - It usually lies 4 cm above the zygomatic arch and 3.5 cm behind the frontozygomatic suture
  - Its position can be marked about 3.5 cm above the centre of the zygomatic bone.
- **Sutural bone** seen between the antero-inferior angle of the parietal bone and the greater wing of the sphenoid called **pterion ossicles**.

32. Blood supply and nerve supply of scalp.
Refer Short Notes 23 – 2006.

33. 2nd pharyngeal arch.
Refer Short Notes 27 – 2005.

34. Histology of retina.
Refer Short Notes 24 – 2008.

35. Fourth ventricle.

- It is cavity of hindbrain
- **Situated** behind the pons and upper part of medulla, and in front of cerebellum

- **Communication:**
  - Above with third ventricle through cerebral aqueduct
  - Below with central canal of spinal cord
  - Laterally with cerebellomedullary cistern.
- **Boundaries:** It has two lateral walls, roof and floor
- The **roof** is formed above by superior medullary velum. Inferiorly by tela choroidea of fourth ventricle.
- **Lateral walls**
  - Superolaterally by superior cerebellar peduncles
  - Inferolaterally gracile tubercle, cuneate tubercle, and inferior cerebellar peduncle.
- **Floor** (Refer short notes on Q. No. 21 – 2008)
- **Openings:**
  - Lateral openings **(foramen Luschka)** – in the lateral recess
  - Median opening **(foramen Magendie)** – in the roof.

36. Name the muscles with nerve supply and action of tongue.

Refer Short Notes 31 – 2005.

37. Digastric triangle.

- It is one of the anterior triangle of the neck.

Boundaries (Fig. 15)

- **Base**—lower border of body of mandible and an imaginary line connecting angle of mandible and mastoid process
- **Apex**—intermediate tendon of digastrics muscle
- **Anteroinferiorly**—anterior belly of digastrics
- **Posteroinferiorly**—posterior belly of digastrics and stylohyoid muscle
- **Roof**—skin, superficial fascia with platysma, investing layer of deep fascia
- **Floor**—mylohyoid and hyoglossus.

Lesser's Triangle

The hypoglossal nerve crosses the triangle above the hyoid bone, and dips in-between the hyoglossus and the mylohyoid muscle. The hypoglossal nerve with diverging tendons of digastric form the Lesser's triangle. The lingual artery is the content of this triangle and lies deep to the hyoglossus.

Contents

- **Anterior part:**
  - Superficial part of submandibular gland
  - Facial artery and the glandular lie deep to the gland

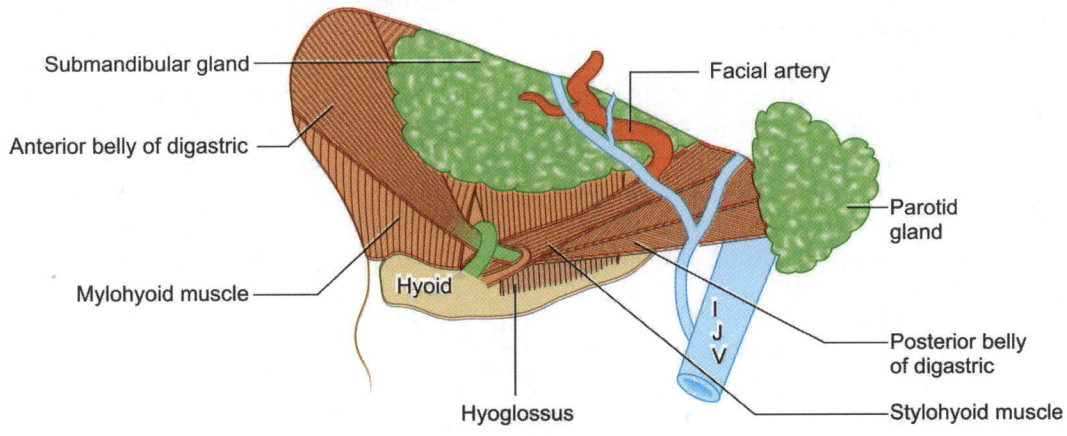

Fig. 15: Digastric triangle.

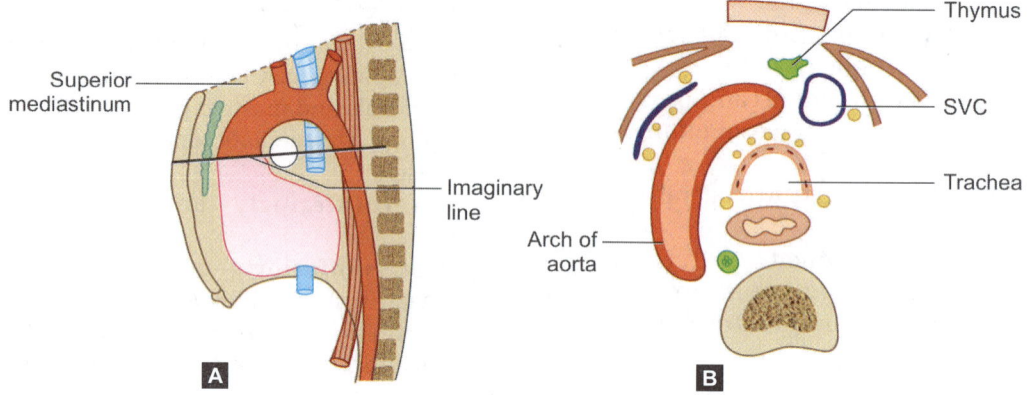

Figs. 16A and B: Superior mediastinum: (A) Boundaries; (B) Content.

- Facial vein superficial gland submental arteries and
- Nerve and artery to mylohyoid lie on mylohyoid muscle
- Hypoglossal nerve
- Submandibular nodes
- Posteriorly
  - Lower part of parotid gland
  - External carotid artery deep to stylohyoid
  - Carotid sheath with ICA, IJV, vagus
  - Glossopharyngeal nerve, styloglossus, stylopharyngeus lying between carotid sheath and ECA.

38. Superior mediastinum.

- **Boundaries (Fig. 16A)**
  - Anteriorly: Manubrium sterni
  - Posteriorly: Upper four thoracic vertebrae and intervertebral discs
  - Superiorly: Thoracic inlet
  - Inferiorly: Imaginary plane passing through sternal angle (front) and the lower border of the body of the fourth thoracic vertebra behind
  - On each side: Mediastinal pleura.
- **Contents (Figs 16B and 17)**
  4 arteries:
  1. Arch of aorta
  2. Brachiocephalic trunk
  3. Left common carotid artery
  4. Left subclavian artery.
- **4 veins:**
  1. Right brachiocephalic veins
  2. Left brachiocephalic veins
  3. Superior vena cava
  4. Left superior intercostal vein.
- **4 nerves:**
  1. Vagus
  2. Phrenic nerve
  3. Cardiac nerves
  4. Left recurrent laryngeal nerve.
- **3 muscles:** Origin of sternohyoid, sternothyroid, longus colli.
- **3 tubes:** Trachea, esophagus, thoracic duct
- **3 others:** Thymus, tracheobronchial lymph nodes, paratracheal lymph nodes
- **Applied Anatomy**
  - Neck infections between the pretracheal and prevertebral fasciae can spread into the superior mediastinum
  - Mediastinitis can result from infections in the neck.

39. Down syndrome.
Refer Short Notes 22 – 2005.

40. Pericardial sinuses.
Refer Short Notes 32 – 2007.

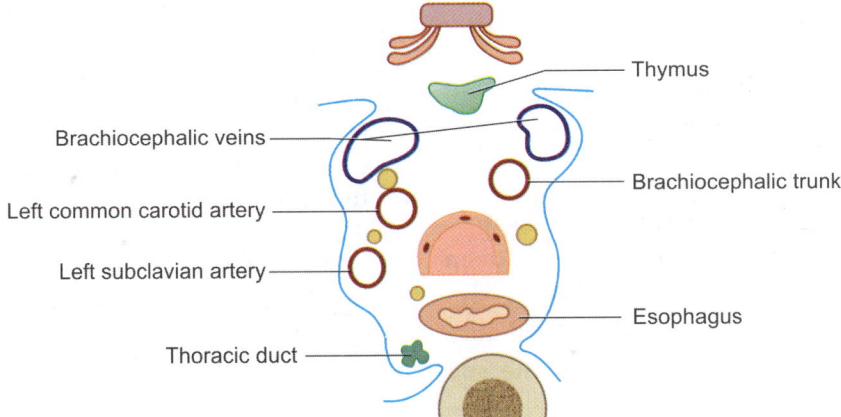

Fig. 17: Contents of superior mediastinum.

III. SHORT ANSWER QUESTIONS

1. Name the muscles which produce inversion and eversion of foot.

- **Inversion** takes place in subtalar joint.
  - In this movement the anterior part of foot is adducted and medial border of the foot is raised. The lateral border is depressed and sole is turned medially
  - **Muscles producing** inversion: Tibialis anterior and tibialis posterior
- **Eversion** is anterior part of foot is abducted and the lateral border is raised. The medial border is depressed and the sole faces lateral.
  - **Muscles producing** eversion: Peroneus longus and peroneus brevis.

2. Name the structures passing through the pudendal canal.

Refer Short Answer Questions 24 – 2011.

3. Give the root value of musculocutaneous nerve and name the muscles supplied by it.

- It is the nerve of anterior compartment of arm
- It arises from lateral cord of brachial plexus
- **Root value** is VR $C_5 - C_7$
- **Muscles supplied**—coracobrachialis, biceps brachii, brachialis.

4. Enumerate the intraarticular structures of knee joint.

Refer Short Answer Questions 6 – 2010.

5. Mention the boundaries and clinical importance of bare area of liver.

- Bare area is on the posterior surface of right lobe of liver.
- It is **bounded** by:
  - **Base**: Groove for inferior vena cava
  - **Above**: Superior layers of coronary ligament
  - **Below**: Inferior layers of coronary ligament
  - **Apex**: Right triangular ligament
- Structures related—right suprarenal gland, diaphragm
- **Clinical importance**: It is one of the sites of portocaval anastomosis.

6. Name the contents of femoral sheath in order.

- Femoral sheath is a flattened funnel shaped sleeve of fascia
- Encloses the upper 3 or 4 cm of the femoral vessels
- Sheath is divided into **3 compartments**
- **Contents**:
  - Lateral or arterial compartment— contains the femoral artery and the femoral branch of the genitofemoral nerve

- Intermediate or venous compartment contains femoral vein
- Medial or lymphatic compartment called **femoral canal.** The canal **contains** a lymph node called Cloquet's node or node of Rosenmuller which drains the glans penis/glans clitoris.

7. Enumerate the structures passing deep to the flexor retinaculum of hand.

Refer Short Answer Questions 13 – 2009.

8. Name the nerves which form the sub sartorial plexus.

- **Situation**: The plexus is deep to the fascia lata. It is in the roof of adductor canal, at the lower border of adductor longus and deep to the sartorius muscle.
- **Formation**:
  – Medial cutaneous nerve of the thigh
  – Branches of the saphenous nerve
  – Cutaneous branch from anterior division of obturator nerve
- **Structure supplied**: Skin of medial side of thigh.

9. Name the parts of quadriceps femoris muscle.

- Quadriceps is the anterior compartment muscle of thigh
- Four muscles end in a tendon and is inserted to the upper border of patella
- It is supplied by femoral nerve and extensor in function
- Made of four muscles which end in quadriceps tendon are:
  1. Rectus femoris
  2. Vastus medialis
  3. Vastus lateralis
  4. Vastus intermedius

10. Enumerate the short lateral rotators of thigh.

- Short lateral rotators are situated deep to gluteus maximus.
- The muscles are:
  – Piriformis
  – Obturator internus
  – Gamelli—superior and inferior
  – Quadratus femoris
  – Obturator externus.

11. Contents of cubital fossa.

From medial to lateral, the fossa contains **(MBBS)**
- **M**edian nerve
- **B**rachial artery—the terminal part
- **B**iceps the tendon
- **S**uperficial branch of radial nerve just under cover of brachioradialis.

12. Nerve supply and action of lumbricals muscle of hand.

Refer Short Answer Questions 4 and 12 – 2009.

13. Name the branches of axillary artery.

- Axillary artery is continuation of subclavian artery from the outer border of the 1st rib
- It terminates at the lower border of the teres major by continuing down as the brachial artery
- The pectoralis minor crosses the artery and divides it into 3 parts:
- **1st part** – Superior thoracic artery
- **2nd part**:
  – Thoracoacromial artery
  – Lateral thoracic artery.
- **3rd part**:
  – Subscapular artery
  – Anterior circumflex humeral artery
  – Posterior circumflex humeral artery.

14. Piriformis muscle.

- It is the key muscle of the gluteal region.
- It is triangular in outline.
- **Situation:** In the posterior wall of the pelvis and also in the gluteal region
- **Origin:** Middle three pieces of the sacrum along its pelvic surface
  – Upper margin of the greater sciatic notch
- **Course:** It comes out of pelvis through the greater sciatic foramen and reaches the gluteal region
- **Insertion:** Into the apex of the greater trochanter of femur
- **Nerve supply:** Ventral rami of S1, S2
- **Action:** Lateral rotator of thigh at the hip joint

- **Applied anatomy:** Piriform syndrome: pain is experienced in the gluteal region and along the course of the sciatic nerve as the nerve is compressed due to the hypertrophy of the muscle.

15. Name the superficial vein of lower limb with one applied aspect.

- Great and small saphenous veins and their tributaries.
- **Applied aspects:**
  - Great saphenous vein is used for by-passing the blocked coronary arteries
  - Varicose veins and ulcers: If the valves in the perforators or at the termination of superficial veins become incompetent, it may result in dilatation of the superficial veins and gradual degeneration of their walls producing varicose veins and varicose ulcers.

16. Muscles attached with iliotibial tract.

- Iliotibial tract is the thickening of lateral part of deep fascia (fascia lata) of thigh
- It stabilizes the knee in extension
- The muscles attached:
  - Gluteus maximus—three-fourth of it is inserted into iliotibial tract at its posterior border
  - Tensor fascia lata inserted into the iliotibial tract at its anterior border.

17. Ligaments of spleen.

Refer Short Answer Questions 23 – 2011.

18. Blood supply of rectum.

- **Arterial supply (Fig. 18A):**
  - Superior rectal artery—inferior mesenteric artery is continued as superior rectal. At the level of S3 it divides into anterior and posterior branches. It anastomose with inferior rectal artery. It is the main artery supplying the rectum supplies upper two-third of rectum
  - Middle rectal arteries—branch from the anterior division of internal iliac artery supplies middle third of rectum
  - Inferior rectal arteries—terminal branch of internal pudendal supply distal third of rectum
  - Median sacral artery branch of abdominal aorta supplies posterior wall of anorectal junction.
- **Venous drainage (Fig. 18B):**
  - Superior rectal vein starts from internal venous plexus and is continued as inferior mesenteric vein
  - The middle rectal drain to the anterior division of internal iliac vein.

19. Trigone of urinary bladder.

Refer Essay Q. No. 2 – 2003.

20. Histology of ureter.

It is made of three layers—from inner to outer are **(Fig. 19)**:

1. **Mucous layer:**
   - The mucous membrane is thrown into folds and the lumen appears stellate shape
   - It is made of epithelium and lamina propria
   - The **epithelium** is lined by transitional epithelium/urothelium
   - The lamina contains fibroelastic connective tissue, blood vessels and few lymphocytes.
2. **Muscular layer:** Made of inner longitudinal and outer circular bundles. In the middle part of the ureter, there is an additional outer longitudinal coat
3. **Adventitial layer:** Made of connective tissue and contains blood vessels.

21. Name the sesamoid bones.

Refer Short Notes 4 – 2007.

22. Syndesmosis.

- It is one type of fibrous joint
  - Restricted movements
  - The bones are connected by the interosseous membrane or a fibrous cord, or an aponeurotic membrane.
- **Example:**
  - Middle radioulnar joint—where radius and ulna are connected by the interosseous membrane; the movement between radius and ulna is supination and pronation
  - Posterior part of sacroiliac joint—connected by aponeurotic membrane

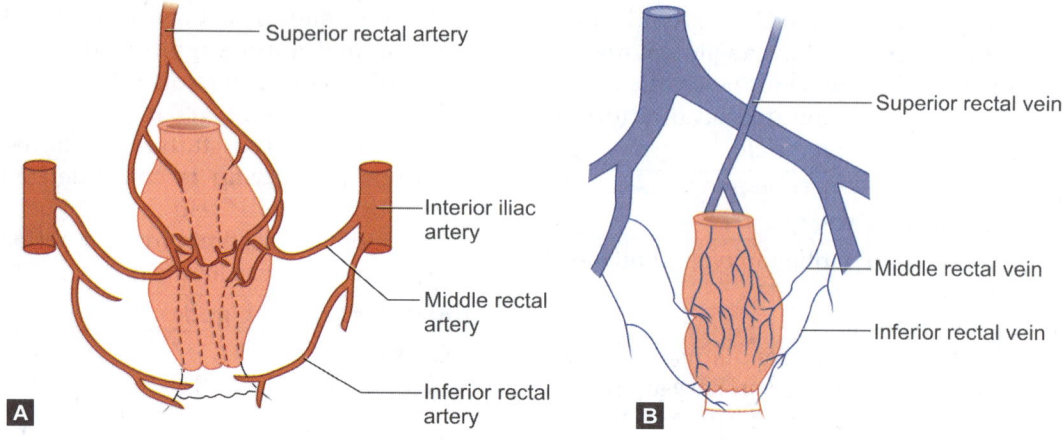

Figs. 18A and B: Blood supply of rectum: (A) Arterial supply; (B) Venous drainage.

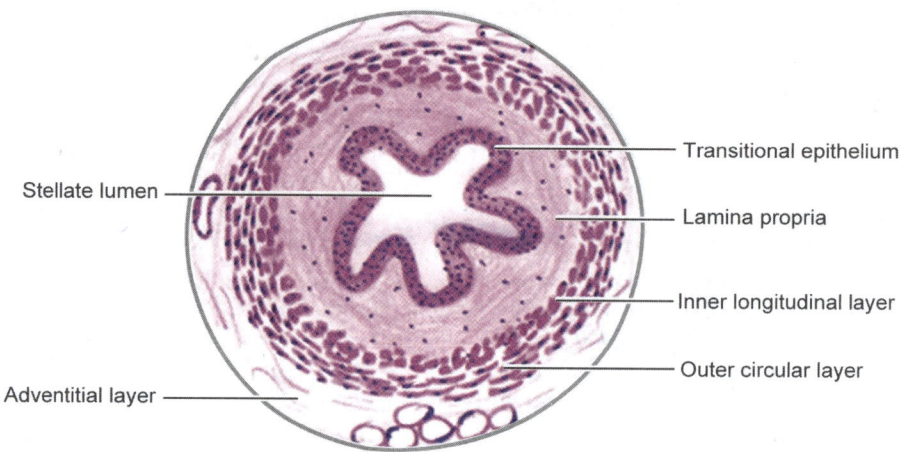

Fig. 19: Histology of ureter.

- Inferior tibiofibular joint—intervening interosseous ligament.

23. Layers of aorta with applied aspect.

- Aorta is also called as elastic artery
- Is made up of three layers from inner to outer are tunica intima, tunica media and tunica adventitia
- **Tunica intima** is made of endothelium lined by simple squamous epithelium, subendothelial layer (lamina propria), and inner elastic lamina is ill-defined.
- **Tunica media**
  - It contributes for more than half of the thickness of the wall of the artery
  - Mainly made of collagen and elastic fibers. The smooth muscle fibers are less.
- **Tunica adventitia** is formed of connective tissue, containing bundles of collagen fiber of varying thickness
- **Applied anatomy**
  - Aortic aneurysm (dilatation)
  - Dissecting aneurysm
  - Coarctation of aorta: Due to congenital stenosis or atresia of the arch of aorta distal to the origin of the left subclavian artery maybe preductal or postductal
  - Angiogram (diagnostic procedure to visualize the aorta and the coronary

arteries by injecting a radiopaque dye through the catheter into the aortic sinuses).

24. Allantois.
Refer Short Answer Questions 9 – 2011.

25. Derivatives of midgut.
- The midgut extends from anterior intestinal pore to posterior intestinal pore.
- The artery of the midgut is superior mesenteric artery
- **Structures derived** are:
  - Duodenum—second part distal to the major duodenal papilla, third and fourth parts
  - Jejunum
  - Ileum
  - Cecum and appendix
  - Ascending colon
  - Right two-thirds of transverse colon.

26 Formation and termination of external jugular vein.
- It is a superficial vein in the neck
- Formation: The posterior division of retromandibular vein joins with posterior auricular vein to form external jugular vein
- It descends down superficial to the investing layer of deep cervical fascia
- It crosses obliquely the sternocleidomastoid muscle and reaches posterior triangle
- About 5 cm above the clavicle the vein pierces the investing layer of deep fascia.
- Termination: Into subclavian vein
- Tributaries: Anterior jugular vein, transverse cervical vein, suprascapular vein.

27. Peculiarities of 1st intercostal nerve.
- The ventral ramus of first thoracic nerve divides unequally
- The larger branch crosses the neck of the first rib, to take part in the formation of the brachial plexus
- Formation: The **smaller branch of VR of first thoracic forms the first intercostal nerve**
- It runs in the first intercostal space
- Termination: Continued as the first anterior cutaneous nerve of the thorax
- The lateral cutaneous branch supplies the skin of axilla or sometimes may be absent
- It may communicate with the intercostobrachial nerve, and the medial cutaneous nerve of the arm
- Often it receives a communicating branch from 2nd intercostal nerve.

28. Lumbar puncture.
Refer Short Notes 34 – 2008.

29. Structures lodged in the lateral sulcus of the cerebrum.
- The lateral sulcus extends from anterior perforated substance of the inferior surface of cerebrum and passes between orbital and tentorial surfaces. It cuts the inferolateral border (sylvian point). Then it divides into three as anterior ramus, ascending ramus and posterior ramus. The portion from anterior perforated substance to sylvian point is known as stem
- The stem of the lateral sulcus lodges (related):
  - Free posterior margin of lesser wing of sphenoid
  - Sphenoparietal venous sinus
  - Middle cerebral artery
- The posterior ramus of lateral sulcus is related to:
  - Superficial middle cerebral vein
  - Branches of middle cerebral artery.

30. Dangerous area of face.
Refer Short Answer Questions 37 – 2009.

31. Formation and termination of left superior intercostal vein.
- Formation: Union of 2nd, 3rd, 4th, left posterior intercostal veins
- Termination: Ends into left brachiocephalic vein.

32. Suboccipital nerve.
- Suboccipital nerve is one of the content of suboccipital triangle
- It is dorsal rami of C1.

- It emerges between the posterior arch of atlas and third part of vertebral artery
- It divides immediately into branches
- Supplies rectus capitis posterior major and minor, obliquus capitis superior, obliquus capitis inferior and semispinalis capitis
- The branch to obliquus capitis inferior gives a communicating branch to greater occipital nerve
- It occasionally has a cutaneous branch to the scalp
- It may communicate with spinal accessory nerve.

33. Ligamentum denticulatum.

- They are extensions from spinal piamater
- They are tooth like lateral extensions
- Passes in-between the dorsal and ventral spinal roots
- They are attached laterally to the duramater
- There are 21 pairs of ligamentum denticulatum are present
- The first crosses posterior to the vertebral artery and is attached to margin of foramen magnum
- The spinal accessory nerve ascends behind the ligamentum denticulatum
- The last is between T_{12} and L_1 spinal nerves
- The form and position of the ligament changes during movement
- They help for anchorage of spinal cord
- Applied anatomy: During tractotomy surgeries this ligament is utilized as a guide by surgeons.

34. Structures pierced by parotid duct in order.

- The parotid duct emerges from the upper part of the gland, along the anterior border
- Runs horizontally, crosses masseter, turns at right angle medially. It pierces the structures mentioned below opposite the upper third molar tooth. Runs forwards between buccinator and the oral mucous membrane obliquely
- The oblique course of the duct acts as a valve preventing entry of air into the gland whenever there is raise in intraoral pressures.
- **Structures pierced are**:
  - Buccal pad of fat
  - Buccopharyngeal fascia
  - Buccinators muscle
  - Mucous membrane of the cheek.

35. Origin and branches of middle meningeal artery.

- **Origin:** It is a branch from the 1st part of maxillary artery
- **Termination:** Terminates as frontal and parietal branches
- **Branches:**
  - Ganglionic branch to supply trigeminal ganglion
  - Petrosal branch to supply facial nerve and geniculate ganglion
  - Superior tympanic to supply tensor tympani
  - Temporal branch anastomoses with deep temporal branch in the infratemporal fossa
  - Anastomotic branch anastomoses with recurrent meningeal branch of ophthalmic artery
  - Terminal branches: Frontal and parietal branches to supply meninges.

36. Parts of corpus callosum.

Refer Short Answer Questions 24 – 2009.

37. Deep nuclei of cerebellum.

Nuclei: From lateral to medial (Doctors **E**at **G**ood **F**ood**)**
- Dentate nucleus—neocerebellum
- Emboliformis nucleus—paleocerebellum
- Globosus nucleus—paleocerebellum
- Fastigii nucleus—archicerebellum.

38. Tentorium cerebelli.

- It is a fold of dura mater
- **Shape**—tent like fold of dura mater
- **Situation**—in the posterior cranial fossa
- It separates the occipital lobe of cerebrum from cerebellum
- It **divides** the cranial cavity into supra-tentorial- and infratentorial compartments

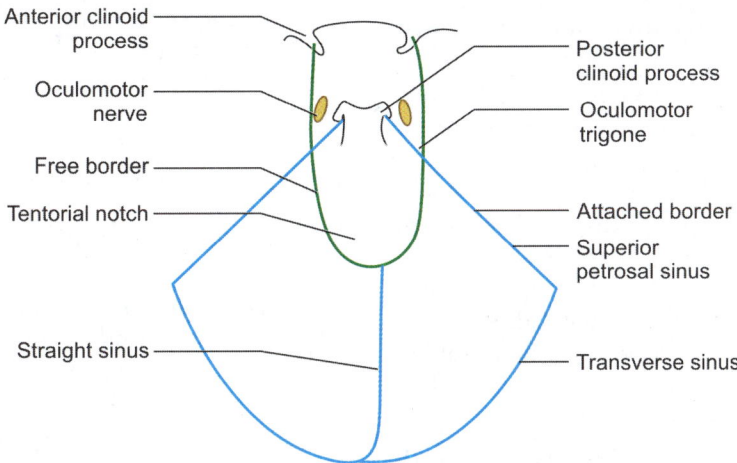

Fig. 20: Tentorium cerebelli.

- **Parts:** 2 borders attached and free 2 surfaces—superior and inferior
- **Attachment:**
  - **The attached posterior border** is convex
    - Posteriorly it is attached to the margins of transverse sinus
    - Laterally to the superior margin of petrous temporal
    - Anteriorly to posterior clinoid process.
  - **The free anterior border** is concave
    - It forms tentorial notch through which the brainstem passes
    - It is attached to the anterior clinoid process
    - The free and the attached borders cross to form a triangular part called **oculomotor trigone**
    - Near the apex of petrous bone, the inferior layer evaginates into middle cranial fossa covering the trigeminal ganglion called **cavum trigeminale.**
- **Sinuses related:**
  - Straight sinus
  - Transverse sinuses
  - Superior petrosal sinuses.
- **Nerve supply:** Tentorial nerve, a recurrent nerve from ophthalmic division
- **Applied anatomy:** When there is increase in intracranial pressure or a space occupying lesion, the brain herniates through tentorial notch and can compress the midbrain, arteries of inferior surface of cerebrum or oculomotor nerve.

39. Name any four branches of external carotid artery.

(**S**ister **L**ucy's **P**owdered **F**ace **O**ften **A**ttracts **M**edical **S**tudents)
- **S**uperior thyroid artery
- **L**ingual artery
- **P**osterior auricular artery
- **F**acial artery
- **O**ccipital artery
- **A**scending pharyngeal artery
- **M**axillary artery
- **S**uperficial temporal artery.

40. Name the components of lacrimal apparatus.

The structures concerned with secretion and drainage of the lacrimal fluid constitute the lacrimal apparatus
- Components of lacrimal apparatus are:
  - Lacrimal gland and its ducts
  - Conjunctival sac
  - Lacrimal puncta
  - Lacrimal canaliculi
  - Lacrimal sac
  - Nasolacrimal duct.

41. Name the extraocular muscles of eyeball.

- Extraocular muscles are seven in number
- They help in the movement of eyeball in all directions and elevation of the upper eyelid
- Four recti, two oblique muscles and levator palpabrae superioris
    - The **recti muscles** are strap muscles—superior, inferior, medial and lateral recti
    - The **oblique muscles** are superior and inferior oblique muscles
    - **Levator palpabrae superioris.**

42. Development of pituitary gland (in brief).

- Develops from **two** different sources
- Anterior lobe from ectoderm of stomodeum, posterior lobe from neuroectoderm
    1. **Anterior lobe** from ectodermal upward growth from the roof of stomodeum during 3rd week called **Rathke's pouch**.
        - It is situated in front of the cranial end of notochord
        - It extends up to the floor of forebrain vesicle
        - By 2nd month it is detached from the stomodeum
        - The cells of anterior wall form **pars anterior**
        - The cells of posterior wall form **pars intermedius**
        - The portion extending towards diencephalon persists as **pars tuberalis**
        - The cavity of the pouch persists as **cleft.**
    2. **Posterior lobe** from neuroectoderm.
        - It develops during 6th week as a diverticulum from the floor of the diencephalon
        - The lower end of the diverticulum differentiates to form **posterior lobe**
        - The narrow upper end of the diverticulum forms the **infundibulum**
        - It contains neuroglial cells
        - The nerve fibers from hypothalamus enter the posterior lobe.
- **Congenital anomaly**
    - Pharyngeal hypophysis: A small portion of Rathke's pouch persist in the roof of pharynx
    - Craniopharyngiomas arise from remnant of Rathke's pouch. It may be seen within or above sella turcica. It may cause hydrocephalus or pituitary dysfunction.

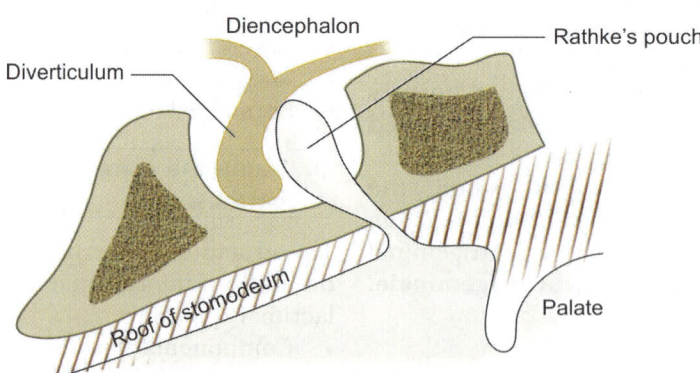

Fig. 21: Development of pituitary.

43. Mention the boundaries of laryngeal inlet.

- Situated at the level of C3
- The boundaries are:
  - Above and anteriorly—posterior surface of epiglottis
  - Laterally—aryepiglottic folds
  - Below and posteriorly—interarytenoid fold
- **Action on inlet of larynx**:
  - Aryepiglotticus, oblique arytenoids **closure/narrowing** of the inlet
  - Thyroepiglotticus **widens** the inlet.

44. Right principal bronchus.

- The principal bronchus is 2.5 cm in length
- It is wider, and shorter than the left bronchus
- It is more vertical and inclined at 25°
- The right principal bronchus gives of eparterial bronchi before entering the hilum of the right lung
- It enters the hilum of lung at T5 level
- The azygos arches over the bronchus
- The bronchus crosses posterior to pulmonary artery and enters the lung

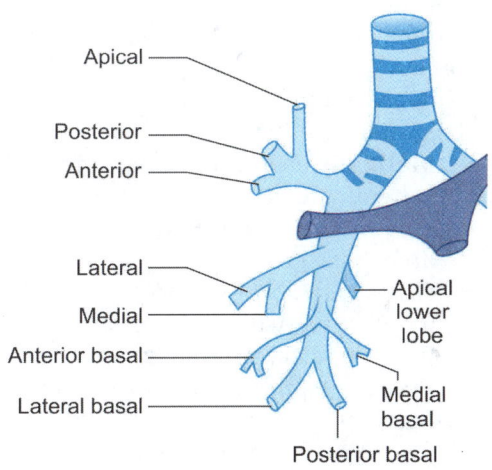

Fig. 22: Right principal bronchus.

- On entering the lung divides into two lobar bronchi, one for the middle lobe and the other for the lower lobe
- The eparterial bronchus enters the upper lobe and divides into **three**—apical, anterior and posterior tertiary or segmental bronchi.
- The middle lobar bronchus divides into **two**—medial and lateral segmental bronchi
- The lower lobar bronchus divides into **five**—apical of lower lobe, medial basal, lateral basal, anterior basal and posterior basal segmental bronchi
- **Applied anatomy**: As the right bronchus is vertical and wider the foreign body in the trachea is usually aspirated into the right lung.

45. Pleural diaphragm.

- The pleural diaphragm is the cervical pleura with suprapleural membrane
- **Cervical pleura** covers the apex of the lung
- Extends from inner border of 1st rib.
- The summit of the pleura is 3 to 4 cm above the 1st costal cartilage
- It is covered by **supra pleural membrane** called **Sibson's fascia**
- It extends from tip of 7th cervical vertebra to the inner border of 1st rib
- It contains few muscle fibers derived from scalenus medius muscle
- It is known as **scalenus minimus**
- It extends to the dome of pleura and produces tension.

46. Moderator band.

- Specialized bridge present in the right ventricle extending from the right side of interventricular septum to the base of the anterior papillary muscle
- This trabecula conveys the right branch of the atrioventricular bundle of His
- It is also called as septomarginal band

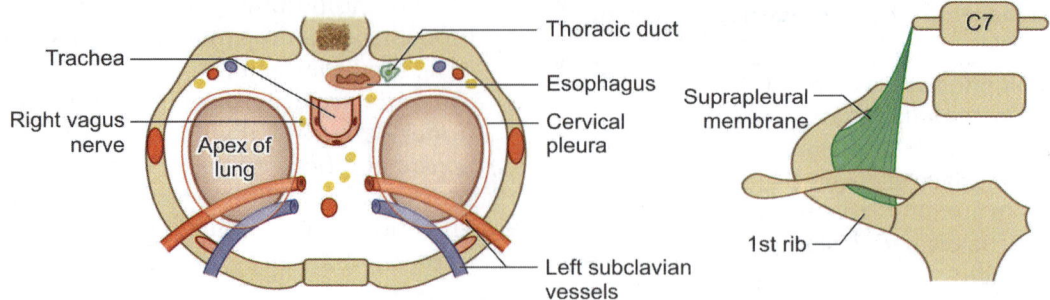

Fig. 23: Pleural diaphragm.

- According to some it prevents the over distension of the right ventricle and hence called as the moderator band.

47. Triangle of Koch.

Refer Short Answer Questions 27 – 2010.

48. Simple squamous epithelium.

- **Structure of squamous epithelium**
  - The cells are flat, polygonal, which are tightly apposed
  - They have irregular, interlocking borders
  - The nucleus usually bulges into the overlying space.
- **Functions**
  - Allows rapid diffusion of gases and water across its surface as it is thin
  - Materials pass through the cell because of the tight junctions between adjacent cells
  - Presence of numerous endocytic vesicles indicates that it helps in active transport
- **Situations**:
  - The alveoli of the lungs
  - Outer wall of renal corpuscles
  - Thin segments of renal tubules
  - Various parts of the inner ear
  - Blood vessels (endothelium)
  - Mesothelium.

49. Mention the four features of Tetralogy of Fallot.

The features of Fallot's are:
1. **Pulmonary infundibular stenosis:** Due to unequal division of conus resulting in a narrow right ventricular orifice
2. **Right ventricular hypertrophy:** Due to increase in pressure on right side
3. **Large ventricular septal defect:** Failure of fusion of bulbar septum
4. **Overriding of aorta:** Because of ventricular septal defect and orta arises directly above the defect.

50. Mention the bones of middle ear cavity.

- Three ear ossicles are inside the middle ear cavity
- They are the smallest bones in the body
- They are:
  - **Malleus** resembles a hammer, has a head, neck and three processes. Developed from 1st pharyngeal arch
  - **Incus** resembles premolar tooth with a body and two processes. Developed from 1st pharyngeal arch
  - **Stapes** resembles stirrup, presents a head, neck and two limbs. Developed from 2nd pharyngeal arch.

MBBS Examination 2013

ANSWER ALL QUESTIONS

I. Essay questions   (15/10 Marks)

1. Describe the arches of foot under following headings (a) Types of arches, (b) Constituents and support of each arch, (c) Functions and (d) Applied anatomy.
2. Describe the uterus under the following headings: (a) Normal position version and flexion, (b) Parts, (c) Peritoneal relations, (d) Supports and (e) Applied anatomy.
3. Describe the formation, prefixed and postfixed type, branches and applied anatomy of brachial plexus.
4. Describe the relations, blood supply, lymphatic drainage and applied anatomy of stomach.
5. Describe the Pancreas under the following headings: (a) Type of gland with ducts, (b) Gross features, (c) Relations, (d) Blood supply and (e) Applied aspect.
6. Describe the shoulder joint under the following headings: (a) Type with articulating bones, (b) Ligaments and Bursa, (c) Relations, (d) Movements with muscles involved and (e) Applied aspect.
7. Describe the temporomandibular joint under the following headings: (a) Type of joint, (b) Articular surfaces, (c) Articular disc, (d) Ligaments, (e) Movements and the muscles producing them and (f) Applied anatomy.
8. Describe the intercostal nerves under the following headings: (a) What are they branches of and what is their unique feature? (b) Classify them, (c) Communications, (d) Course, relation and branches of a typical intercostal nerve and (e) Applied anatomy.
9. Describe boundaries and contents of carotid triangle.
10. Describe origin, course, and branches of right coronary artery.
11. Describe the spinal cord under the following headings: (a) Extent with coverings, (b) External features and enlargements, (c) Cross section at mid thoracic level, (d) Blood supply and (e) Applied aspects.
12. Describe the Tongue under the following headings: (a) Gross features, (b) Papillae, (c) Muscles with action, (d) Nerve supply, (e) Lymphatic drainage and (f) Applied aspects.

II. Short notes   (5/4/3 Marks)

1. Sex linked inheritance.
2. Axillary nerve.
3. Portal vein.
4. Parts and blood supply of duodenum.
5. Levator ani muscle.
6. Inversion and eversion of foot.
7. Lymphatic drainage of mammary gland.
8. Lesser sac.
9. Gluteus medius muscle.
10. Erb's point.
11. Lumbricals of hand.
12. Histology of bone.
13. Development of suprarenal gland.
14. Lymphatic drainage of breast.
15. Pronation and supination.
16. Inguinal hernia.

17. Great saphenous vein.
18. Obturator nerve.
19. Popliteus muscle.
20. Ischiorectal fossa.
21. Biceps brachii muscle.
22. Applied aspects of hand.
23. Clavipectoral fascia.
24. Blood supply of long bone.
25. Structures under cover of gluteus maximus.
26. Urinary bladder (blood supply, nerve supply, trigone and applied aspects).
27. Draw a neat diagram of coronal section of kidney with its coverings.
28. Obturator nerve.
29. Popliteal fossa.
30. Enumerate the muscles of foot in each layer with nerve supply.
31. Blood supply of spinal cord.
32. Parts, deep nuclei, and arterial supply of cerebellum.
33. Ansa cervicalis.
34. Fourth ventricle.
35. Interior of right atrium.
36. Sternocleidomastoid.
37. Superior sagittal sinus.
38. Root of lung.
39. Arterial supply of heart.
40. Pleural recesses.
41. Parts of corpus callosum.
42. Name the extraocular muscles.
43. Facial artery in face.
44. Formation of superior vena cava.
45. Phrenic nerve.
46. Lateral pterygoid muscle.
47. Styloid process—structures attached.
48. Surfaces, borders of thyroid gland.
49. Muscles of tongue.
50. Posterior horn of lateral ventricle.
51. Thoracic duct.
52. Pericardium.
53. Mediastinal surface of left lung.
54. Venous drainage of heart.
55. Sagittal section of eyeball.
56. Paranasal air sinuses (name, functions, opening, area, applied aspects).
57. Part and constituent fibers of internal capsule.
58. Middle ear cavity.
59. Meninges with meningeal spaces.
60. Superolateral surface of cerebrum.

III. Short answer questions (3/2 Marks)

1. Name the quadrants of abdomen.
2. Name the peculiarities of popliteus muscle.
3. Name the muscles attached to the medial border of scapula.
4. Name the constituents of quadriceps femoris.
5. Name the cutaneous nerves that supply the anterior abdominal wall.
6. Name the rotator cuff muscles.
7. Name the nerves related to humerus.
8. Name the bones that form the floor of anatomical snuff box.
9. Bucket handle type of injury of semilunar cartilage of knee.
10. Boundaries of epiploic foramen.
11. Name the openings of diaphragm and their level.
12. Juxtaglomerular apparatus.
13. Contents of broad ligament.
14. Name the types of ossification with example.
15. Palmaris brevis muscle.
16. Root value and muscles supplied by axillary nerve.
17. Muscles attached to extensor expansion of hand.
18. Mention the areas drained by superficial inguinal lymph nodes.
19. Name the tributaries of portal vein.
20. Cruciate anastomosis.
21. Name the type of epiphysis of fibula at both ends.
22. Supracondylar fracture.
23. Superficial veins of upper limb with fate.
24. Foot drop.
25. Triceps surae.
26. Name the ligaments around hip joint.
27. Name the parts of vulva.
28. Hymenal membrane.
29. Perineal body (location in female with clinical importance).
30. Name any two sites of porta caval anastomosis.

31. Parts of the sensory nucleus of trigeminal nerve.
32. Dangerous area of scalp.
33. Surface marking of apex beat of heart.
34. Lobe of azygos.
35. Formation and termination of internal jugular vein.
36. Boundaries and applied anatomy of piriform recess.
37. Blood supply of internal capsule.
38. Parts of corpus callosum.
39. Root value of phrenic nerve and name the structures supplied by it.
40. Olive.
41. Terminal branches of external carotid artery.
42. Arterial supply to pituitary.
43. Dangerous area of face.
44. Opening of maxillary sinus.
45. Auditory tube openings.
46. Blood supply to tonsil.
47. Nerve supply and action of cricothyroid muscle.
48. Attachment of vocal cord.
49. Blood supply to lung.
50. Terminal branches of internal thoracic artery.
51. Suprasternal space of burns.
52. Dangerous area of face.
53. Structures passing through foreman ovale.
54. Boundaries of laryngeal inlet.
55. Branches of ascending and arch of aorta.
56. Lumbar puncture.
57. Pterion.
58. Apex beat.
59. Contents of posterior mediastinum.
60. Applied aspects of pleura.

I. ESSAY QUESTIONS

1. Describe the arches of foot under following headings: (a) Types of arches, (b) Constituents and support of each arch, (c) Functions and (d) Applied anatomy.

Refer Essay Q. No. 1 – 2003.

2. Describe the uterus under the following headings: (a) Normal position version and flexion, (b) Parts, (c) Peritoneal relations, (d) Supports, (e) Applied anatomy.

Refer Essay Q. No. 2 – 2004.

3. Describe the formation, pre fixed and post fixed type, branches and applied anatomy of brachial plexus.

Refer Essay on Q. No. 3 – 2005.

4. Describe the relations, blood supply, lymphatic drainage and applied anatomy of stomach.

Refer Essay on Q. No. 2 – 2007.
Lymphatic drainage Refer short notes on Q. No. 6 – 2007.

5. Describe the Pancreas under the following headings: (a) Type of gland with ducts, (b) Gross features, (c) Relations, (d) Blood supply and (e) Applied aspect.

Refer Essay Q. No. 1 – 2006.
Blood supply Refer Essay Q. No. 2 – 2008.

6. Describe the shoulder joint under the following headings: (a) Type with articulating bones, (b) Ligaments and Bursa, (c) Relations, (d) Movements with muscles involved, (e) Applied aspect.

Refer Essay Q. No. 2 – 2006.

7. Describe the temporomandibular joint under the following headings: (a) Type of joint, (b) Articular surfaces, (c) Articular disc, (d) Ligaments, (e) Movements and the muscles producing them and (f) Applied Anatomy.

Refer Essay Q. No. 4 – 2003.

8. Describe the intercostal nerves under the following headings: (a) What are they branches of and what is their unique feature? (b) Classify them, (c) Communications, (d) Course, relation and branches of a typical intercostal nerve and (e) Applied anatomy.

Refer Essay Q. No. 9 – 2006.

9. **Describe boundaries and contents of carotid triangle.**

Refer Essay Q. No. 8 – 2011.

10. **Describe origin, course, and branches of right coronary artery.**

Refer Essay Q. No. 5 – 2005.

11. **Describe the spinal cord under the following headings: (a) Extent with coverings, (b) External features and enlargements, (c) Cross section at mid thoracic level, (d) Blood supply and (e) Applied aspects.**

- **Extent (Fig. 1A):**
  - The spinal cord is continuation of medulla oblongata
  - **Upper end** is just below the level of foramen magnum
  - The **lower end** of spinal cord tapers called conus medullaris. In adult it is at the level of lower border of L1. In fetal life extends up to coccyx, and in newborn lies opposite to L3
  - The variation in the lower extent is due to disparity in the growth of vertebrae and spinal cord
  - The lower end of spinal cord below L1 vertebra resembles a horse tail and is known as **cauda equina** (Fig. 1A). The structures forming it are i) filum terminale, ii) coccygeal nerves, iii) S1 – S5 nerves, iv) L2 to L5 lumbar nerves.
- **Coverings (Figs. 1A and B):** The spinal cord is covered by dura mater, arachnoid mater, and pia mater
  - The **dura mater** is continuation of meningeal layer of cranial dura. The endosteal layer gets attached to the margins of foramen magnum.
    - The dura extends up to S_2 vertebra.
    - Below S_2, it unites with filum terminale and extends to the posterior surface of coccygeal vertebra and fuses with periosteum
  - The **arachnoid matter** and the subarachnoid space extends up to lower border of S_2 vertebra.
  - **The pia mater**
    - It invests the spinal cord completely
    - Below conus medullaris it is continued as **filum terminale**
    - Upper 15 cm of the filum terminale is covered by arachnoid and subarachnoid space, (L1 – S2) called **filum terminale interna**
    - The lower 5 cm named **filum terminale externa** is ensheathed by duramater and extends from S_2 to posterior surface of coccyx vertebra. It is also called as **coccygeal ligament**

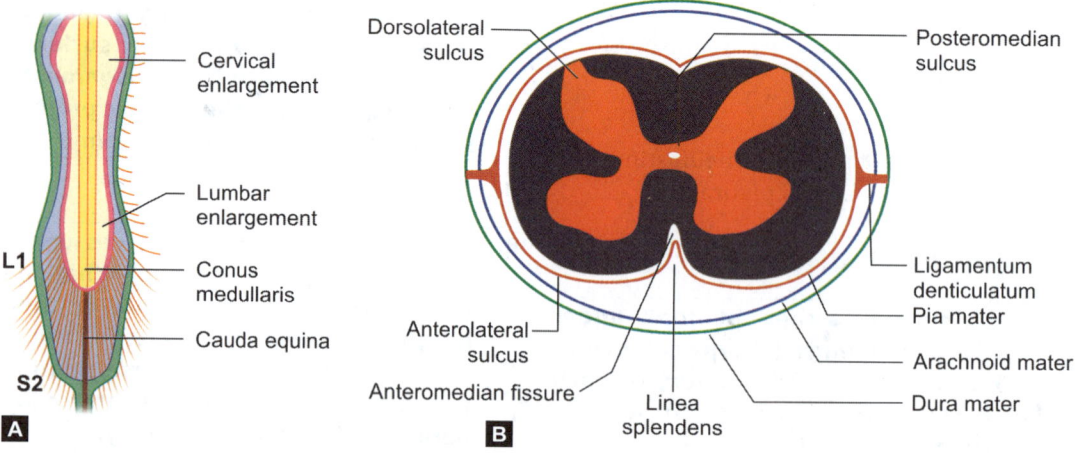

Figs. 1A and B: Extent and coverings of spinal cord.

- The other extensions of pia are ligamentum denticulatum, linea splendens.
- **External features**
  - Anteromedian fissure is a median cleft, and the linea splendens is lodged in it. The anterior spinal artery is related to it
  - The posteromedian sulcus along the posterior surface
  - The spinal cord is divided into two equal halves by these two grooves
  - The anterolateral sulcus is where the anterior roots emerge
  - The posterolateral sulcus the dorsal root fibers emerge
  - The spinal cord is divided into anterior, lateral and posterior funiculus or column
  - The portion from anteromedian fissure to anterolateral sulcus is anterior column
  - The portion in between the anterolateral and posterolateral sulcus as lateral column
  - The portion from posterolateral to posteromedian sulci is posterior column
  - The posterior column in turn is divided into fasciculus gracilis, and fasciculus cuneatus by posterointermedius sulcus.
- **Enlargements:** Two enlargements
  1. Cervical enlargement between C4 – T2 spinal segments to accommodate brachial plexus to supply upper limb
  2. Lumbar enlargement to supply muscles of lower limb. It extends from L2 – S3 spinal segments.
- **Cross section at mid thoracic level**
  - The gray matter is less in amount and white matter is more **(Fig. 2)**
  - The spinal cord at mid thoracic level is round in shape
  - It has inner gray matter and outer white matter
  - The **gray matter** is in H – shaped with a pair of ventral horns and a pair of dorsal horns connected by gray commissure.
    - The ventral horns and dorsal horns are slender
    - There is a lateral horn in addition to ventral and dorsal horn
    - The sympathetic fibers arise from the lateral horn
    - The gray commissure encloses the central canal
    - The gray horns consist of nerve cells, neuroglial cells and blood vessels.
  - The **white matter** consists of myelinated nerve fibers, neuroglia and blood vessels.

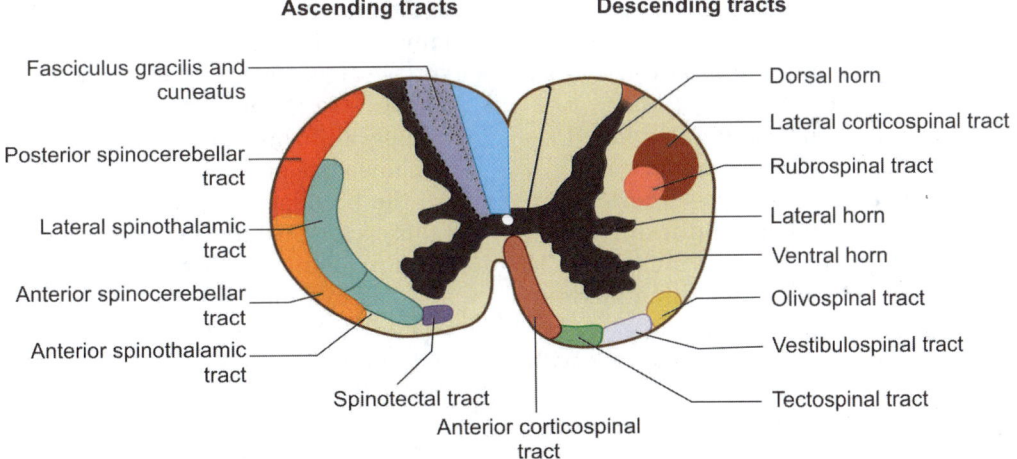

Fig. 2: Section at mid thoracic level.

- The white matter is arranged as three pairs of columns/funiculi
- The nerve fibers are arranged as tracts (ascending and descending tracts).
- **Ascending tracts**
  Posterior column:
  - Fasciculus gracilis in the posterior column carry sensation of proprioception, fine touch
  - Fasciculus cuneatus vibration and two-point discrimination.

  Lateral column:
  - Posterior spinocerebellar tract—is an uncrossed tract, and carries proprioceptive impulses from lower limb and caudal part of body. It reaches cerebellum through inferior cerebellar peduncle
  - Anterior spinocerebellar tract—crossed tract carrying proprioceptive and exterioceptive impulses from lower limb. It reaches the cerebellum through superior cerebellar peduncle
  - Lateral spinothalamic tract—is a crossed tract carrying pain and temperature sensation. Terminates in VPL nucleus of thalamus.

  Anterior column: Anterior spinothalamic tract – convey touch pressure, and itch sensation.
- **Descending tracts**
  - Lateral corticospinal tract—crossed 75 – 90% of pyramidal fibers from motor cortex
  - Anterior corticospinal tract—10 – 25% uncrossed pyramidal tract
  - Rubrospinal tract—fibers from red nucleus in midbrain, forms extrapyramidal system. It is responsible for regulating the tone in the flexor muscles
  - Tectospinal tract—concerned with spinovisual reflex
  - Vestibulospinal tract—concerned with maintenance of equilibrium of body
  - Olivospinal tract—from olivary nucleus in medulla.
- **Blood supply:** Refer Short Notes 27 – 2008.
- **Applied anatomy**
  - **Anterior spinal artery syndrome** – the anterior spinal artery may be occluded by thrombosis affecting the blood supply to the anterior two-third of spinal cord. This may lead to loss of motor functions as the nuclei in the anterior horn and corticospinal tract will be affected. There will be loss of pain and temperature on both sides due to involvement of spinothalamic tracts
  - Lesion of posterior column leads to loss of sense of position, vibration, stereognosis, and fine touch on the same side of lesion below the level of spinal cord lesion, e.g. tabes dorsalis.

12. Describe the tongue under the following headings: (a) Gross features, (b) Papillae, (c) Muscles with action, (d) Nerve supply, (e) Lymphatic drainage and (f) Applied aspects.

(a, b, e) Refer Essay Q. No. 6 – 2007.
(c) Refer Short Notes Q. No. 31 – 2005.

Papillae

- Papillae are projections of the mucosa covering the dorsal surface of the tongue
- They are present only in the presulcal part of the tongue
- Functions: It gives roughness, increase the surface area, and gustatory
- There are four types of papillae, namely filiform, fungiform, foliate and circumvallate papillae
- All the papillae are provided with taste buds except the filiform papillae.

1. **Circumvallate papillae (Fig. 3)**
   - 8 – 12 in number
   - Present in front and parallel to sulcus terminalis
   - It is surrounded by a deep circular sulcus
   - The papilla is narrow at the base and broad at apex

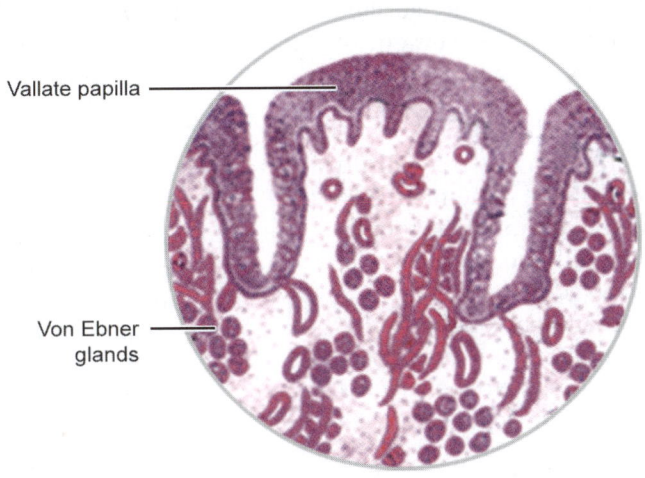

Fig. 3: Circumvallate papilla.

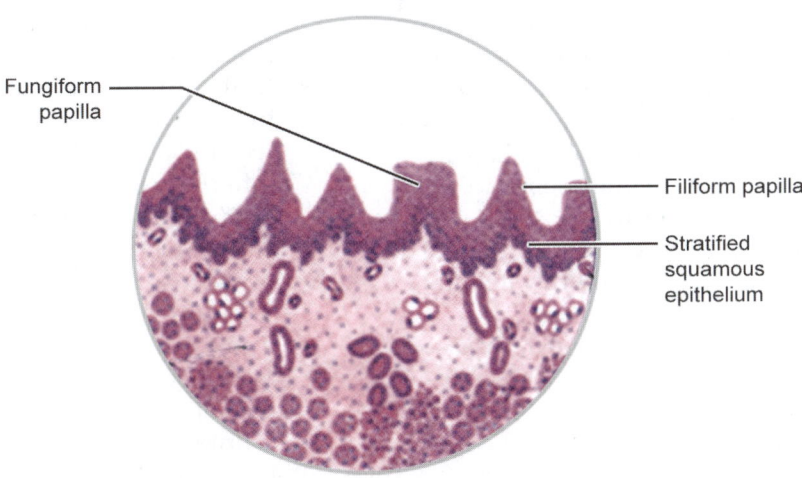

Fig. 4: Fungiform and filiform papillae.

- The mucous membrane covering the papilla is lined by non-keratinized stratified squamous epithelium
- Many taste buds are present in lateral walls of the sulcus
- Small serous (Von Ebner) glands are found in the floor of the sulcus.

2. **Fungiform papillae (Fig. 4)**
   - They are larger, rounded
   - Pink in color
   - Present along lateral margin with few scattered in the dorsum
   - Has few taste buds at the apex.

3. **Foliate papillae**
   - Present as linear leaf like mucosal ridges in front of sulcus terminalis
   - Lies along the lateral margin
   - Has numerous taste buds.

4. **Filiform papillae**
   - Small conical projections
   - More numerous covering most of anterior two-third of tongue
   - Lies in parallel to sulcus terminalis and towards tip horizontally placed
   - Surface is keratinized
   - Has no taste buds.

– Its function is to increase the surface area, and facilitate the movement of food particles.

Applied Anatomy

- Central regions of tongue may drain bilaterally, and should be remembered in removal of malignant tumor of the tongue that are nearer the midline. Both cervical nodes may be involved
- Glossitis—inflammation of tongue
- If genioglossus on one side is paralyzed, there is deviation of tongue to the affected side due to pull of the normal muscle medially.

II. SHORT NOTES

1. Sex linked inheritance.

- The inheritance patterns trace the transmission of genetically traits, diseases or conditions from parents to offspring
- In humans, there are hundreds of genes located on the X chromosome that have no counterpart on the Y chromosome.

Uses of inheritance pattern:
- For diagnosis of genetic disorders
- Suggest ways to prevent the genetic disorders
- To calculate the risk of the genetic disease appearing in offspring
- **Classification/Types:**
  – X-linked dominant inheritance
  – X-linked recessive inheritance
  – Y-linked inheritance.
- **Characteristic features**
  – **X-linked dominant inheritance**
    - If mother is carrier of the X-linked dominant disorder, 50% of the children born are normal. Only 50% are affected
    - If father is carrier of X-linked disorder, all the male children born are normal and all the female children are affected by the disorder
    - The sons who inherit the mutant gene will be hemizygotes and will manifest the trait.
  – **X-linked recessive inheritance**
    - If mother is a carrier of X-linked recessive disorder, chances of 50% of the children born are normal, 25% of female born is a carrier, and 25% male born is affected
    - The males are affected more than females
    - Daughter will be affected only if both parents are affected
    - Son of an affected mother will always be affected.
  – **Y-linked inheritance:** As the sons inherit Y chromosome from father, the affected father will have affected the son

  Example:
    - One of the most common of these diseases is **X-linked recessive** hemophilia
    - Color blindness, diabetes mellitus, Duchenne Muscular Dystrophy are X-linked recessive inheritance
    - An **X-linked dominant** form of the disease hypophosphatemia (a form of rickets)
    - **X-linked dominant** congenital hypertrichosis, Fragile-X syndrome, the most common form of inheritable mental retardation
    - **Y-linked diseases** has been linked to male infertility. Example: Sertoli-only cell syndrome, and hypertrichosis pinnae.

2. Axillary nerve.

- It is also known as **circumflex nerve**
- The nerve obeys the Hilton's law
- The nerve supplies the muscle, the joint on which the muscle acts and the skin covering the joint.
- **Formation:**
  – The axillary nerve arises from the posterior cord of brachial plexus
  – The root value is C5, 6.

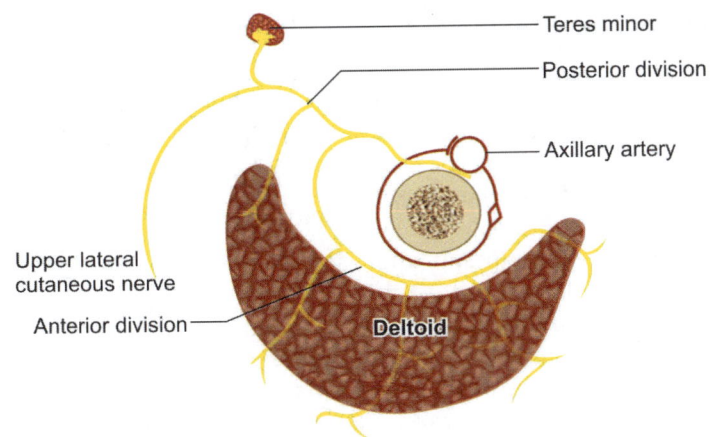

Fig. 5: Axillary nerve.

- **Course and Relation:**
  - In axilla: It is lateral to the radial nerve, behind the 3rd part of axillary artery and in front of subscapularis
  - Then passes through the quadrangular space accompanied by the posterior circumflex artery, inferior to capsule of shoulder joint
  - It divides as it passes through the space into anterior and posterior branches
  - The portion from origin to division is the trunk of axillary nerve.
- **Branches and distribution (Fig. 5):**
  - The **axillary trunk** supplies articular branch to the **shoulder joint**
  - **The anterior branch**—winds around the neck of the humerus, deep to deltoid accompanied by the posterior circumflex humeral vessels. It reaches the anterior border of the muscle and pierce deltoid. It terminates by dividing into many branches in the skin covering deltoid
  - Muscular branch—deltoid
  - Cutaneous branch—few small cutaneous branches which supplies the skin covering deltoid
  - **The posterior branch** runs medially and posteriorly, and is continued as upper lateral cutaneous nerve of arm
  - Muscular branch: Nerve to teres minor, posterior aspect of deltoid. The nerve to teres minor enters the inferior surface muscle and ends as pseudoganglion
  - Cutaneous branch: The posterior branch is continued as the upper lateral cutaneous nerve of the arm. The **upper lateral cutaneous nerve of the arm** pierces the deep fascia and supplies the skin over the lower part of deltoid and the upper part of the long head of triceps.
- **Applied anatomy:** Axillary nerve is injured when there is dislocation of shoulder or fracture surgical neck of humerus. It results in:
  - Loss of abduction of shoulder
  - Rounded contour of the shoulder is lost and appears flattened
  - Loss of sensation over lateral part of arm called regimental badge area.

3. **Portal vein.**

Refer Short Notes 6 – 2004.

4. **Parts and blood supply of duodenum.**

Refer Essay Q. No. 3 – 2007.

5. **Levator ani muscle.**

Refer Short Notes 18 – 2005.

6. Inversion and eversion of foot.

- **Definition**:
  - **Inversion**: Defined as the medial border is raised, the sole faces medially
  - **Eversion**: Defined the lateral border of foot is elevated and the sole turned laterally.
- **Joint**: The movement is at subtalar and talocalcaneonavicular joints
- **Axis of movement**: An oblique axis extending from posterior part of calcaneus through sinus tarsi, to the neck of talus
- **Associated movements**:
  - Inversion is accompanied by plantar flexion and adduction of the forefoot at mid tarsal joint, lateral rotation of foot at subtalar joint
  - Eversion is associated with dorsiflexion and abduction of the forefoot at mid tarsal joint and medial rotation at subtalar joint.
- **Range of movement**:
  - Inversion is more than eversion
  - The range is increased with plantar flexion.
- **Muscles producing**:
  - **Eversion**: Peroneus longus, peroneus brevis, assisted by long extensors of toe
  - **Inversion**: Tibialis posterior and tibialis anterior assisted by soleus and gastrocnemius through tendocalcaneus
- **Function**: Helps the foot to adjust while walking in uneven surfaces.

7. Lymphatic drainage of mammary gland.
Refer Short Notes 19 – 2005.

8. Lesser sac.
Refer Short Notes 10 – 2005.

9. Gluteus medius muscle

- It is fan shaped muscle and covers the lateral surface of the pelvis and hip
- **Origin:** Gluteal surface of ilium between the iliac crest and anterior gluteal line above and posterior gluteal lines below and the fascia covering it
- **Insertion:** Into the greater trochanter of femur on the oblique ridge on the lateral surface. The tendon is separated from bone by trochanteric bursa
- **Nerve supply:** Superior gluteal nerve (L4, L5, S1)
- **Actions:**
  - The gluteus medius and gluteus minimus are powerful abductors of the thigh. Their anterior fibers rotate the thigh medially
  - Acting from below both muscles, the unsupported side of the pelvis is prevented from sagging downward during walking. When a person stands on one foot and the foot of the other side is raised to take a step, the gluteus

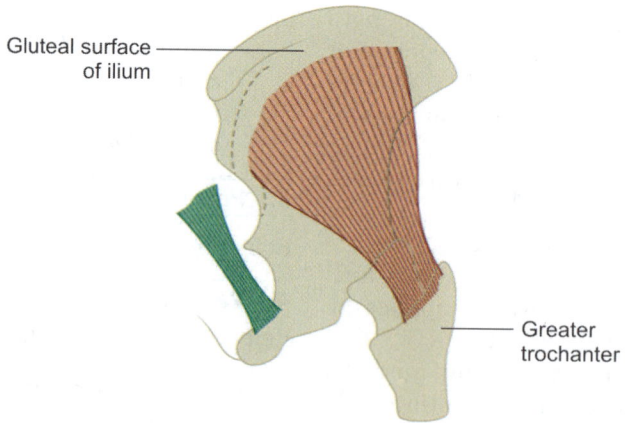

Fig. 6: Gluteus medius muscle.

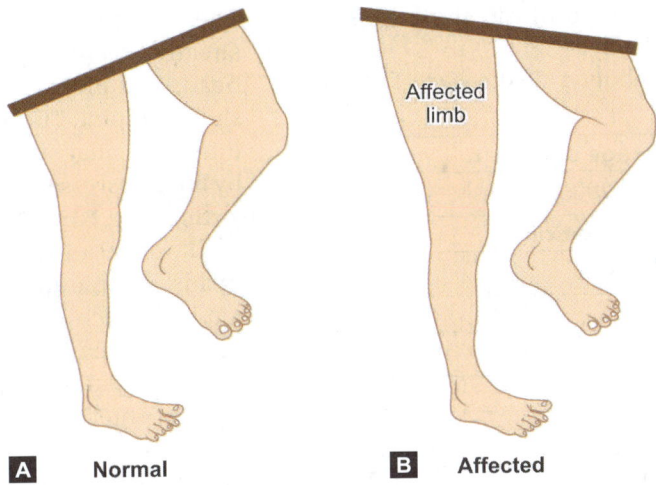

Figs. 7A and B: Trendelenburg's sign.

medius and minimus of the supported side contracts to raise the pelvis on the opposite side.

- **Relations:**
  - Superficial—gluteus maximus and fascia derived from deep fascia covering the muscle
  - Deep—gluteus minimus, branches of superior gluteal nerve and artery, hip joint.
- **Applied anatomy:**
  - When the gluteus medius and minimus are paralyzed, the patient cannot walk normally
  - Trendelenburg's sign: When paralyzed, if the patient stands on the affected limb (with paralyzed gluteus medius and minimus muscles), the pelvis sinks on the unsupported side.

10. Erb's point.
Refer Short Answer Q. No. 6 – 2009.

11. Lumbricals of hand.
Refer Short Notes Q. No. 15 – 2008.

12. Histology of bone.
Refer Short Notes on Q. No. 1 – 2003.

13. Development of suprarenal gland.
The suprarenal gland is developed from two sources.

- Mesoderm forms the cortex and ectoderm forms the medulla
- The **cortex is from mesoderm**
  - The mesothelial cells situated between the dorsal mesentry of gut and mesonephric ridge form the suprarenal ridge by fifth week
  - This cells of the ridge proliferate and penetrate into mesenchyme to form the large acidophilic cells filled **primitive cortex**
  - Second time the mesothelial cells of the ridge proliferate and enter the mesenchyme. It surrounds the acidophilic cells and form **definitive cortex**
  - Numerous capillaries grow and communicate with venous sinuses.
- The **medulla** is developed from the ventral sympatho chromaffin masses of **neural crest cells**
- A **fibrous capsule** is developed around the ridge
- **Fetal cortex:** The cells of the cortex secrete a pre-hormone, dehydroepiandrosterone
- It reaches the placenta and is converted to androgen or estrogen, thereby a feto-placental unit is formed
- At birth the gland is large and ⅓ the size of the kidney

- Within two weeks after birth the cortex regresses completely
- At puberty it is about 1/30 the size of the kidney.

14. Lymphatic drainage of breast.
Refer Short Notes 19 – 2005.

15. Pronation and supination.
Refer Short Notes 7 – 2005.

16. Inguinal hernia.
Refer Short Notes 20 – 2008.

17. Great saphenous vein.
Refer Short Notes 14 – 2005.

18. Obturator nerve.
Refer Short Notes 17 – 2010.

19. Popliteus muscle.
Refer Short Notes 19 – 2009.

20. Ischiorectal fossa.
Refer Short Notes 8 – 2003.

21. Biceps brachii muscle.
- It is called biceps as it has two heads—long and short
- It is also known as **supinator longus**
- **Attachments (Fig. 9)**
  Origin:
  - The **short head** arises by a thick flattened tendon from the apex of coracoid process, together with coracobrachialis
  - The **long head** origin is intracapsular. Arises as a long narrow tendon, from the supraglenoid tubercle of the scapula. The tendon is enclosed by synovial sheath. It arches over the humeral head, and pierces the capsule of the shoulder joint. Then it descends in the intertubercular sulcus, where it is held by the transverse humeral ligament.

  Insertion (Fig. 8):
  - At the level of elbow joint both the heads unite and end in a flattened tendon, which is attached to the rough posterior area of the radial tuberosity. A bursa separates the tendon from the smooth anterior area of the tuberosity. The tendon spirals near radius, its anterior surface becoming lateral
  - The tendon has **the bicipital aponeurosis,** a medial expansion, which crosses the brachial artery and merges with deep fascia of the forearm.
- **Nerve supply:** Musculocutaneous nerve
- **Action:**
  - Flexor of elbow
  - Powerful supinator
  - Keeps the head of humerus in position during abduction of shoulder joint
- **Relation:** In the cubital fossa the brachial artery pulsation can be felt medial to the tendon of biceps
- **Applied anatomy:** When the tendon of long head of biceps ruptures as in case of weight lifters the detached part of the muscle appears as a ball in the lower part of the arm called **Popeye's deformity.**

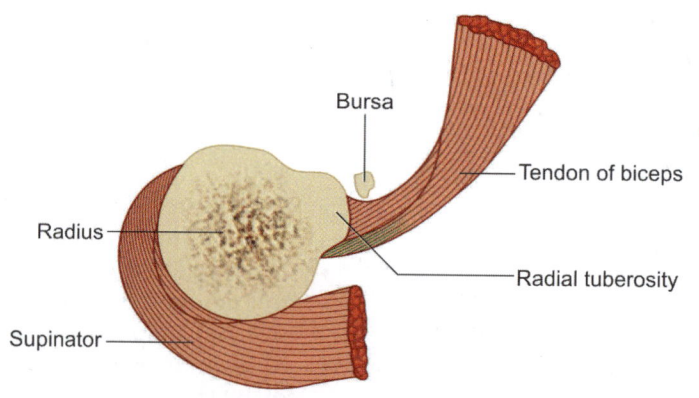

Fig. 8: Insertion of biceps brachii.

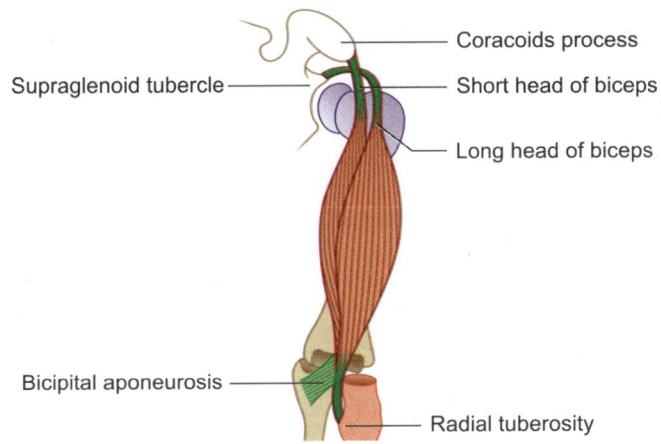

Fig. 9: Attachment of biceps brachii muscle.

22. Applied aspects of hand.

Applied Functional Aspects of Hand

- The hand is the chief sensory organ of touch and is uniquely adapted for grasping
- The radial side of the hand performs a **pinch grip** between the fingers and thumb
- The ulnar side performs a **power grip** between the fingers and palm
- The flexible, elongated digits which extend from palm has the ability to grip, manipulate, or perform complex tasks involving multiple and individual motions (e.g. when typing or playing a piano)
- The **bones of the hand** can be **divided into**
- **Central, fixed unit** for stability formed by eight carpal bones and
- **Three mobile units** for skill and power. They are:
  1. The thumb—the first carpometacarpal joint permits extension, flexion, abduction, and adduction for powerful **pinch and grasp** and fine manipulations
  2. The index finger, with independent extrinsic extensors and flexors and powerful intrinsic muscles—for **precise movements** alone or with the thumb
  3. The middle, ring, and little fingers—for **power grip**.

Applied Clinical Aspects of Hand

- Nerve injuries
  - **Ulnar nerve injury**—
    - Manifests in the form of Claw partial **claw hand** of the medial two fingers
    - This results in flexion of interphalangeal joints and extension of metacarpophalangeal joints of the little and ring fingers of the hand. This occurs due to paralysis of interossei and medial two lumbricals
    - The patient is unable to spread the fingers due to paralysis of dorsal interossei
    - Loss of adduction of thumb. Usually tested by Froments sign
    - Sensory loss on the dorsal and palmar aspect of medial 1½ fingers.
  - **Radial nerve injury**—
    - Presents as **finger drop and thumb drop**
    - Loss of extension at metacarpophalangeal joints of fingers and thumb due to paralysis of extensor digitorum and extensor pollicis longus and brevis
    - Sensory loss on the dorsum at the base of the thumb

- **Median nerve injury**
  - **Benediction deformity**: Paralysis of the FDS and FDP tendons of the middle and index fingers gives this position. Lateral two lumbricals are paralyzed
  - Injury to median nerve in forearm results in:
    * **Ape thumb deformity** paralysis of thenar eminence
    * Sensory loss to the palmar aspect of the lateral three and a half fingers
    * Injury of **median nerve is at mid forearm** affects only the tendon of flexor digitorum superficialis to index finger and results in **pointing index finger**.
- **Tendon sheaths injuries**:
  - **Dequevervain's tenosynovitis:** It is tenovaginitis of the common extensor sheath of APL and EPB resulting in painful limitation of the thumb movement
  - **Trigger finger:** It is tenovaginitis of the fibrous flexor sheath of the fingers and thumb. The sheath thickens and the tendon distal to it bulges to form a nodule. When an attempt is made to flex the finger the nodule passes through the constricted sheath and the finger snaps
  - **Button hole finger:** Boutonniere deformity rupture of the central slip of dorsal digital expansion results in flexion at PIP and hyperextension of DIP joints
  - **Swan neck finger:** This is due to degeneration of the tendon of flexor digitorum superficialis and insertion of dorsal digital expansion, resulting in hyperextension of proximal interphalangeal and flexion at distal interphalangeal joints
  - **Mallet finger/baseball finger:** Due to injury of insertion of extensor expansion at distal phalanx, so the distal phalanx remains flexed.

- **Palmar aponeurosis injury: Dupuytrens contracture**—occurs due to shortening of the medial half of the palmar aponeurosis causing flexion deformity of the ring and little fingers.
- **Spaces infection**: **Felon/whitlow**—an infection of the pulp space of the finger. Presents with throbbing pain and may be complicated with avascular necrosis of the distal 4/5 of the distal phalanx.

23. Clavipectoral fascia.
Refer Short Notes 5 – 2006.

24. Blood supply of long bone.
Refer Short Notes 2 – 2009.

25. Structures under cover of gluteus maximus.

- The sacrotuberous ligament converts the sciatic notch into foramen
- This foramen is subdivided into an upper greater sciatic and a lower lesser sciatic foramen by the sacrospinous ligament.
  - Greater sciatic foramen is above ischial spine and directs from pelvis to gluteal region
  - The lesser sciatic foramen situated below the ischial spine and leads from gluteal to perineum
  - The nerves, arteries and a muscle enters the gluteal region from pelvis
  - The corresponding veins enter the pelvis from gluteal region.
- **Nerves and vessels** which enter the gluteal region may be of three groups:
  1. Remain in the gluteal region—superior and inferior gluteal nerve and vessels
  2. Structures descend from gluteal to thigh—sciatic nerve, posterior cutaneous nerve of thigh, branches from inferior gluteal vessels
  3. Turn towards lesser sciatic foramen into the perineum—the internal pudendal nerve, pudendal artery, nerve to obturator internus.

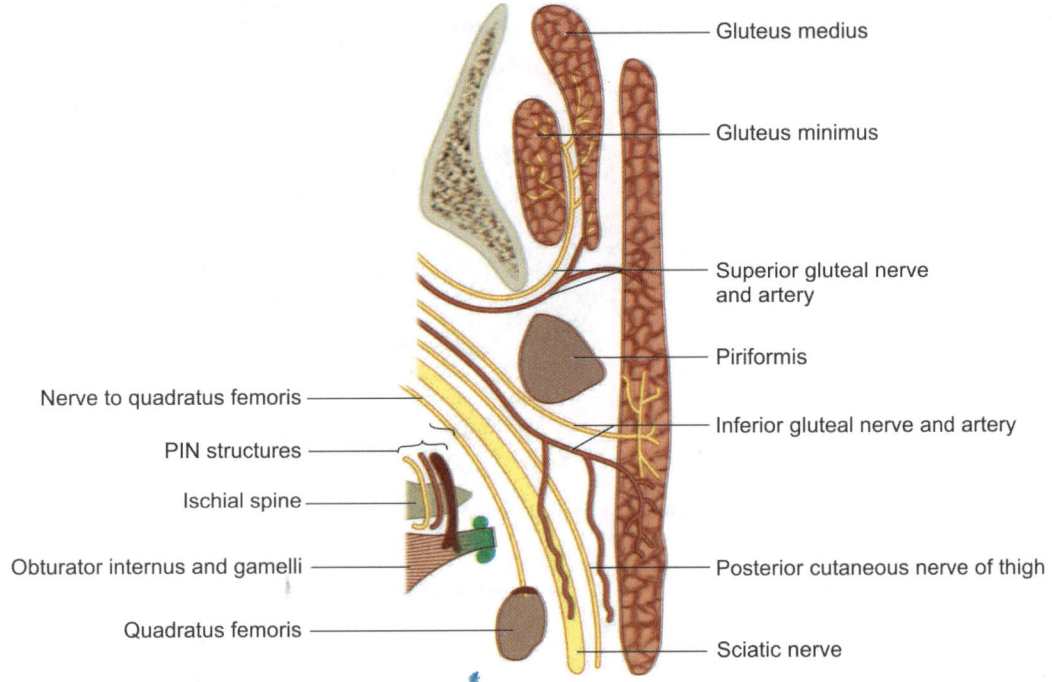

Fig. 10: Structures deep to gluteus maximus.

- **Muscles:**
  - Piriformis enter through greater sciatic foramen
  - Obturator internus enter through lesser sciatic foramen
  - Gluteus medius
  - Gamelli—superior and inferior
  - Quadratus femoris
  - Origin of hamstring muscles.
- **Ligaments:**
  - Sacrotuberous ligament—vestigial part of long head of biceps femoris
  - Sacrospinous ligament—vestigial part of ischiococcygeus muscle.
- **Bones:**
  - Sacrum
  - Coccyx
  - Ischial tuberosity
  - Ischial spine
  - Greater trochanter of femur
  - Ilium of hip bone.
- **Bursae:**
  - Trochanteric bursa over greater trochanter
  - Gluteofemoral bursa between gluteus maximus and vastus laterals
  - Ischiofemoral over gluteal tuberosity.
- **Applied anatomy**
  - **Weaver's bottom:** The lower and medial part of ischial tuberosity is covered by the ischial bursa. While sitting this part of bone supports the body. The bursa gets inflamed due to constant irritation and the condition is known as weaver's bottom.

26. Urinary bladder (blood supply, nerve supply, trigone and applied aspects).

Blood supply Refer Essay 3 – 2010.
Nerve supply, trigone, applied aspect Refer Essay Q. No. 2 – 2003.

27. Draw a neat diagram of coronal section of kidney with its coverings.

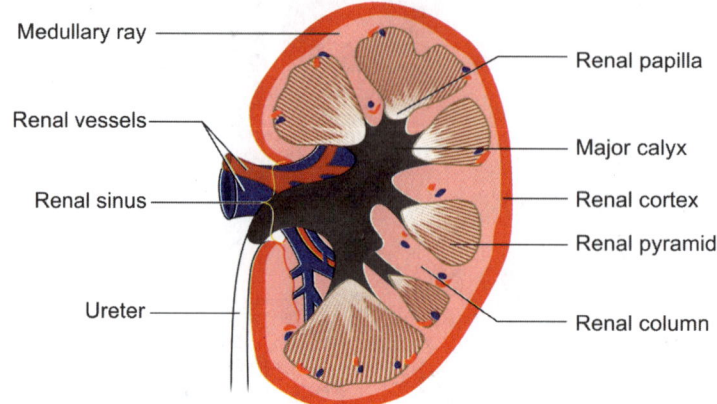

Fig. 11: Coronal section of kidney.

28. Obturator nerve.
Refer Short Notes 17 – 2010.

29. Popliteal fossa.
Refer Short Notes 8 – 2009.

30. Enumerate the muscles of foot in each layer with nerve supply.

S. No.	Layers	Tendons	Muscles	Nerve supply
1	First	-------	Abductor hallucis	Medial plantar
			Abductor digiti minimi	Lateral plantar
			Flexor digitorum brevis	Medial plantar
2	Second	Tendon of flexor hallucis longus Tendon of flexor digitorum longus	Flexor accessorius	Lateral plantar
			Lumbricals—four in number	1st - Medial plantar 2nd, 3rd, 4th Lateral plantar
3	Third	-------	Flexor hallucis brevis	Medial plantar
			Flexor digiti minimi brevis	Lateral plantar
			Adductor hallucis	Lateral plantar
4	Fourth	Tendon of tibialis posterior Tendon of peroneus longus	Dorsal interossei (four)	Lateral plantar
			Plantar interossei (three)	Lateral plantar

31. Blood supply of spinal cord.
Refer Short Notes 27 – 2008.

32. Parts, deep nuclei, and arterial supply of cerebellum.
Refer Essay Q. No. 7 – 2011.

33. Ansa cervicalis.
Refer Short Notes 26 – 2008.

34. Fourth ventricle.
Refer Short Notes 35 – 2012.

35. Interior of right atrium.
Refer Essay Q. No. 7 – 2006.

36. Sternocleidomastoid.
Refer Short Notes 31 – 2006.

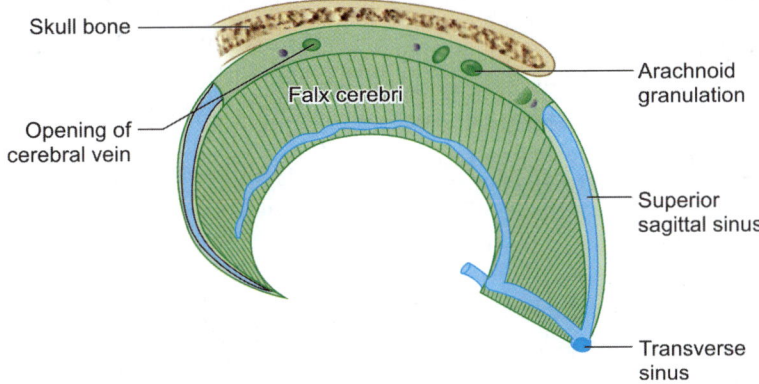

Fig. 12: Superior sagittal sinus.

37. Superior sagittal sinus.
- It is an unpaired sinus
- **Situation:** Along the superior convex border of the falx cerebri
- **Relation:** Related to the groove for sagittal sinus along inner surface of frontal, parietal, squamous part of occipital bones
- **Formation:** Formed by union of frontal lobe veins and ascending frontal vein. It is narrow anteriorly and broader posteriorly
- **Termination:** It is continued as right transverse sinus, from the level of confluence of sinuses
- **Tributaries:** Superior cerebral veins, emissary vein through foramen caecum, parietal emissary vein, meningeal and diploic veins drain into it
- There are three lacunae present along the sinus namely frontal, parietal, and occipital. Into these lacunae the arachnoid granulations project and drain cerebrospinal fluid
- **Applied anatomy:** Thrombosis of the sinus can result in accumulation of cerebrospinal fluid and lead to hydrocephalus.

38. Root of lung.
- The pulmonary root connects the medial surface of the lung to the heart and trachea
- The group of structures related to the hilum form the root covered by a tubular sheath of pleura
- The pleura extends inferiorly as a fold called pulmonary ligament
- **Contents:**
  - The principal bronchus/divisions of bronchus
  - Pulmonary artery
  - Two pulmonary veins
  - Bronchial artery – one/two
  - Bronchial veins
  - Anterior and posterior pulmonary autonomic plexus
  - Lymphatic of lung
  - Bronchopulmonary lymph nodes and
  - Loose connective tissue.
- **Level:** The pulmonary roots, is situated opposite the bodies of the fifth to seventh thoracic vertebrae.
- **Relations: Both hila**
Refer Essay Q. No. 3 – 2004.

39. Arterial supply of heart.
Refer Essay 5 – 2005.

40. Pleural recesses.
Refer Essay 3 – 2003.

41. Parts of corpus callosum.
Refer Short Notes 25 – 2011.

42. Name the extraocular muscles.
Refer Short Notes 25 – 2009.

43. Facial artery in face.
Refer Short Notes 26 – 2007.

44. Formation of superior vena cava.

Superior vena cava is a large vein which **collects** blood from the upper half of the body and drains into the right atrium. Valve is absent.

- **Situation**:
  - Extrapericardial part: In superior mediastinum
  - Intrapericardial part: In middle mediastinum.
- **Formation:** The right and the left brachiocephalic veins unite to form SVC, behind the lower border of the first right costal cartilage close to the sternum.
- **Course**:
  - Begins behind the lower border of sternal end of the first right costal cartilage
  - Opposite the second right costal cartilage pierces the pericardium.
- **Termination:** Opens into the upper part of sinus venarum part of right atrium behind the third right costal cartilage.
- **Development**:
  - Intrapericardial part from right common cardinal vein (duct of Cuvier)
  - Extrapericardial part from right anterior cardinal vein below oblique anastomoses.
- **Applied Anatomy**
  - Superior venacava may be obstructed above or below the termination of the azygos vein
  - If obstructed above, collateral circulation may be established through the tributaries of internal thoracic vein and lateral thoracic vein
  - When obstructed below, collateral circulation follows the azygos vein, superior and inferior epigastric veins, lateral thoracic and thoracoepigastric veins, hence to inferior vena cava and finally into the right atrium
  - Important channel through which blood from lower half of the body drains in obstruction of inferior vena cava through the azygos vein.

45. Phrenic nerve.

- The phrenic nerve is a mixed nerve—the motor fibers to the diaphragm and carries sensation from pericardium, pleura, and diaphragm
- It is formed by the ventral rami of C3, C4, C5
- Terminates by supplying the diaphragm
- The pericardiacophrenic vessels accompany the nerve
- In the thorax, each phrenic nerve supplies branches to the mediastinal pleura, fibrous pericardium and parietal layer of serous pericardium and carries sensation from the structures
- The relations of right and left phrenic nerves differ in their **intrathoracic course.**

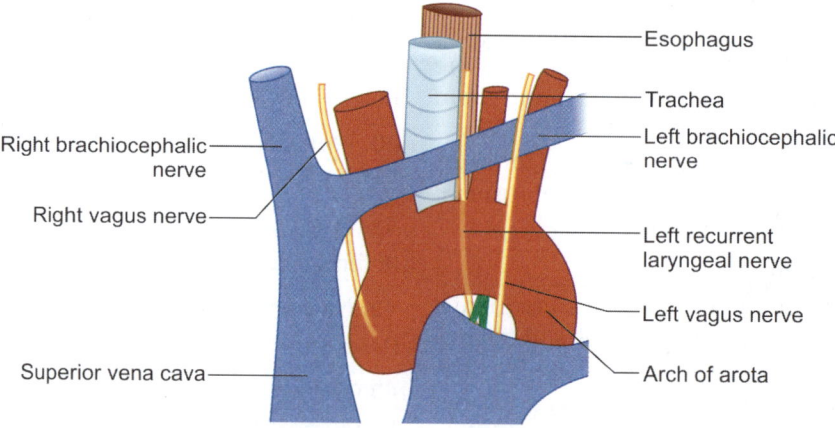

Fig. 13: Superior vena cava.

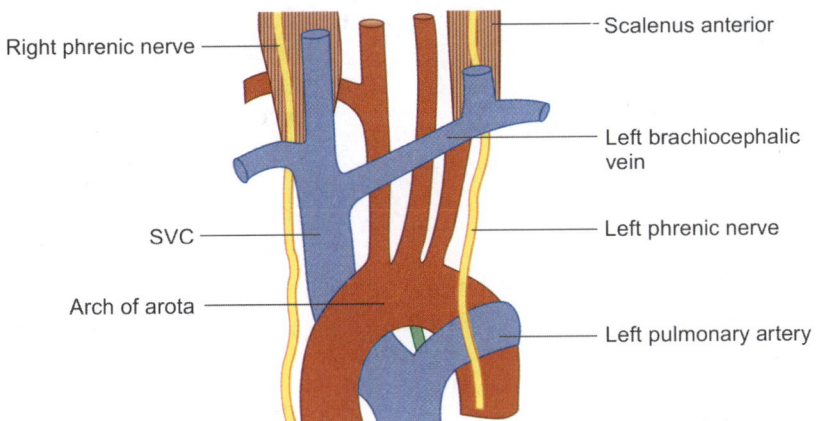

Fig. 14: Phrenic nerves.

- **Right phrenic nerve**
  - At the root of the neck the right phrenic nerve is anterior to scalenus anterior which separates it from the second part of the right subclavian artery
  - It is situated lateral to the right brachiocephalic vein, the superior vena cava, the right surface of the right atrium with fibrous pericardium and inferior vena cava
  - Leaves the thorax through the IVC orifice
  - Terminates by supplying the diaphragm.
- **Left phrenic nerve**
  - At the root of the neck, the left phrenic nerve leaves the medial edge of scalenus anterior
  - It passes anterior to the first part of the left subclavian artery and behind the thoracic duct
  - Then the nerve crosses anterior to the left internal thoracic artery
  - Descends to medial side of the apex of the left lung and pleura
  - Then it runs in the groove between the left common carotid and left subclavian arteries
  - It descends anteromedially, superficial to the left vagus nerve and behind the left brachiocephalic vein
  - The nerve is superficial to the aortic arch and the left superior intercostal vein
  - Lies anterior to the hilum of left lung, and is situated between the left ventricle with pericardium and the mediastinal pleura
  - Leaves the thorax by piercing the left dome of diaphragm
  - Terminates by supplying the diaphragm.
- **Applied anatomy**
  - Avulsion of the phrenic nerve in the neck results in complete paralyses the corresponding half of the diaphragm
  - If an accessory phrenic nerve is present, injury of the main nerve as it lies on scalenus anterior will not result in complete paralysis
  - Referred diaphragmatic pain is frequently felt at the tip of the shoulder. It is usually due to inflammation/irritation of the diaphragmatic pleura e.g. in basal pneumonia, pleural effusions or malignant disease.

46. Lateral pterygoid muscle.
Refer Short Notes 30 – 2005.

47. Styloid process-structures attached.
Refer Short Notes 38 – 2005.

48. Surfaces, borders of thyroid gland.
Refer Short Notes 17 – 2004.

49. Muscles of tongue.
Refer Short Notes 31 – 2005.

50. Posterior horn of lateral ventricle.
Refer Short Notes 26 – 2011.

51. Thoracic duct.

- Is the largest lymph duct
- **Length:** 38 – 45 cm
- **Extends** from the second lumbar vertebra to the base of the neck
- **Course (Fig. 16):**
  - Starts from the **upper end of the cisterna chyli**
  - At the level of lower border of the twelfth thoracic vertebra, passes through the **aortic orifice** of the diaphragm
  - Passes upwards in the **posterior mediastinum**, on the right of the midline
  - The duct crosses from right to left at the level of the body of the fifth thoracic vertebra
  - Reaches the **superior mediastinum**
  - Then runs upwards to the **thoracic inlet** along the left border of the esophagus
  - In the **neck**, at the level of the transverse process of the C_7 vertebra it arches laterally about 3 – 4 cm above the clavicle.
- **Termination:** By opening into the junction of the left subclavian and internal jugular veins

- **Relations**
  - **Aortic orifice (Fig. 17):** Anteriorly—diaphragm and is related to the aorta, azygos and hemiazygos veins
  - **In the posterior mediastinum (Fig. 18):**
    - On its left—the descending thoracic aorta
    - On its right—the azygos vein
    - Posterior—the vertebral column, the right posterior intercostal arteries and terminal part of the hemiazygos and accessory hemiazygos veins
    - Anterior—The diaphragm and esophagus.
  - **In the superior mediastinum (Fig. 19)**
    - Anteriorly—the aortic arch and the left subclavian artery.

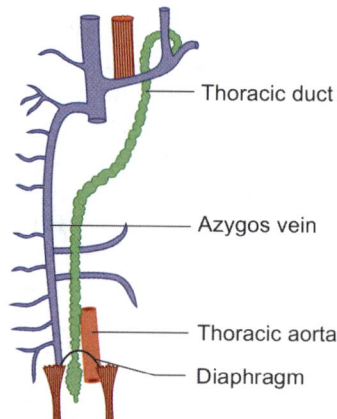

Fig. 16: Course of thoracic duct.

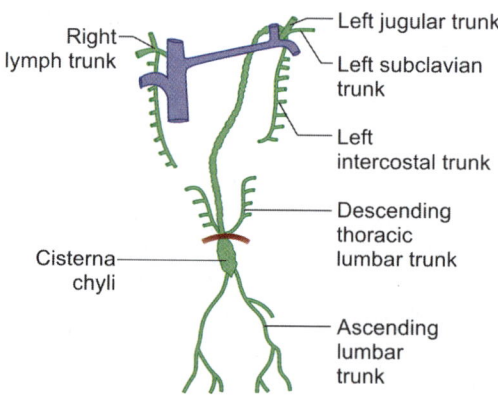

Fig. 15: Tributaries of thoracic duct.

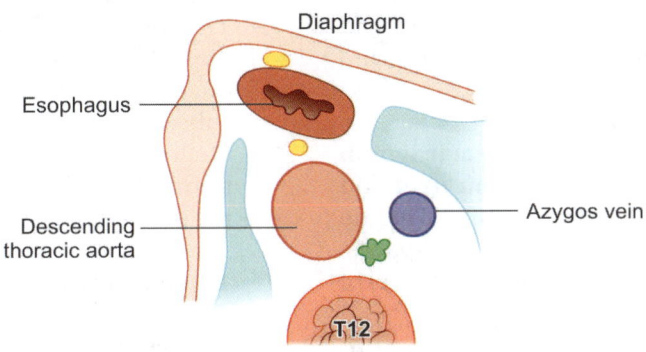

Fig. 17: Relation at aortic orifice of diaphragm.

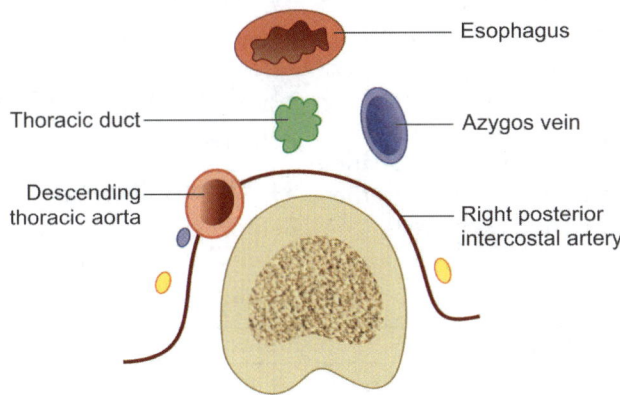

Fig. 18: Relation in posterior mediastinum.

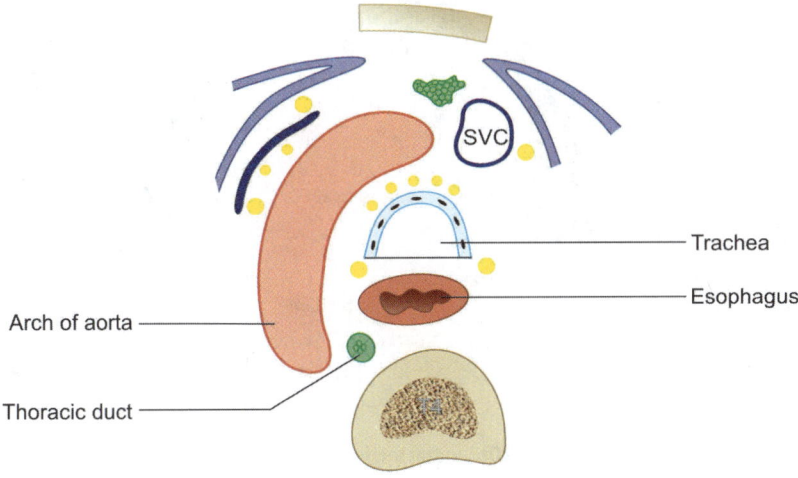

Fig. 19: Relations in superior mediastinum.

- **In the neck**:
  - Posterior—the vertebral artery and vein, the left sympathetic trunk, the thyrocervical trunk or its branches, the left phrenic nerve and the medial border of scalenus anterior, first part of the left subclavian artery.

- Anterior—the left common carotid artery, vagus nerve and internal jugular vein.
- **Tributaries**
  - **Bilateral descending thoracic lymph trunks** collects lymph from right and left intercostal lymph nodes of the lower six or seven intercostal spaces. Ends in the thoracic duct at the level of formation in the abdomen
  - **Bilateral ascending lumbar lymph trunks** receiving the upper lateral aortic nodes, ascend to drain into the thoracic duct within the thorax
  - The **left upper intercostal trunk** drain the intercostal nodes in the left upper five or six left intercostal spaces
  - The **mediastinal trunks** drain the groups of nodes from the diaphragmatic surface of the liver, the diaphragm, the pericardium, heart and esophagus
  - The **left subclavian trunk** drain the left upper limb and opens into the thoracic duct, but may open directly into the left subclavian vein
  - The **left jugular trunk** receives lymph from left side head and neck and joins the thoracic duct, but may open directly into the left internal jugular vein
  - The **left bronchomediastinal trunk** drains the left lung and left half of mediastinum occasionally joins the thoracic duct.

52. Pericardium.

Refer Short Notes 32 – 2007.

53. Mediastinal surface of left lung.

Refer Essay Q. No. 3 – 2004.

54. Venous drainage of heart.

Refer Essay Q. No. 5 – 2005.

55. Sagittal section of eyeball

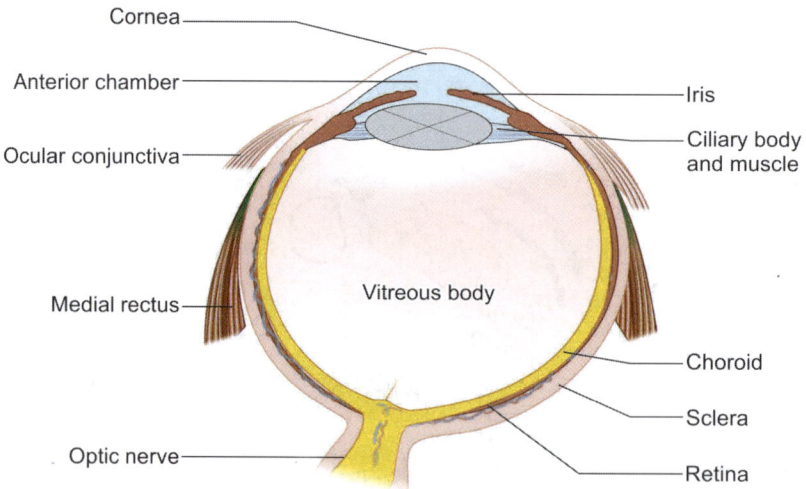

Fig. 20: Sagittal section of eyeball.

56. Paranasal air sinuses (name, functions, opening, area, applied aspects).

Refer Short Notes 37 – 2008.

57. Part and constituent fibers of internal capsule.

Refer Essay Q. No. 7 – 2005.

58. Middle ear cavity.

Refer Short Notes 37 – 2005.

59. Meninges with meningeal spaces.

- The cranial meninges are arranged as three layers—dura mater, arachnoid mater, and pia mater
- The **dura mater** is called pachymeninges
  It is the outer layer.
  It is made of two layers. Outer endosteal layer and inner meningeal layer
  The **endosteal layer** covers the skull bones and form periosteum
  Inner **meningeal layer** forms dural folds and dural venous sinuses are present
- The middle layer is **arachnoid mater.**
  It does not dip into the sulci or grooves of the brain
  This layer is made of mesothelial cells with connective tissue fibers
  Protrusion from arachnoidmater called arachnoid granulations. It protrudes into dural venous sinuses and helps in drainage of CSF.
- The **pia mater** is the inner layer
  It is a thin vascular layer
  It invests into all contours of brain
  It consists of two layers, outer epi pia and inner pia glial.
- **Spaces:**
  – The **extradural space** is absent in the cranium
  – **The subdural space** contains a capillary layer of fluid
  – The **subarachnoid space** contains cerebrospinal fluid. The space is large in base of brain forming subarachnoid cisterns
  – The arachnoid and pia maters form a prolongation along with subarachnoid space for the blood vessels penetrating the brain. The space is called **Virchow Robin perivascular space.**
- **Applied anatomy**
  – Subarachnoid bleeding is usually from arterial and due to rupture of small aneurysms
  – Extradural hemorrhage is due to rupture of meningeal vessels
  – Subdural bleeding is usually venous as a result of head injury.

60. Superolateral surface of cerebrum.

Refer Essay Q. No. 7 – 2007.

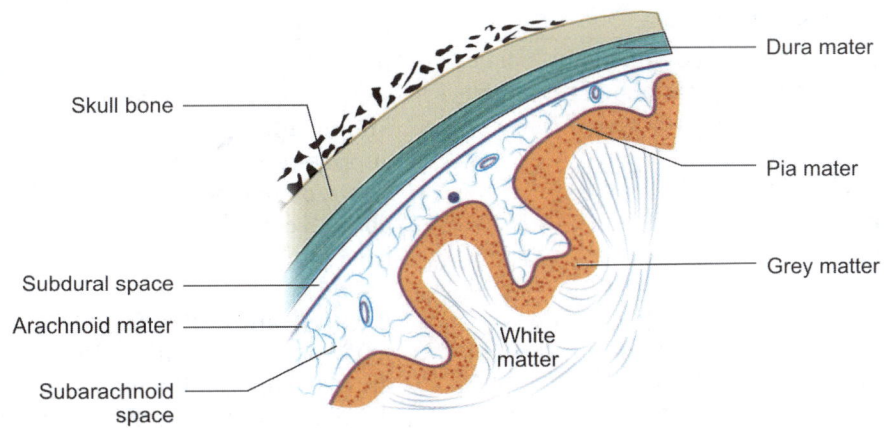

Fig. 21: Meninges and meningeal spaces.

III. SHORT ANSWER QUESTIONS

1. Name the quadrants of abdomen.

- The abdomen is divided into nine quadrants by two horizontal and two vertical planes
- The vertical planes are right and left mid clavicular/mid inguinal planes
- The horizontal planes are transpyloric plane at the level of L1 and transtubercular plane at the level of upper border of body of L5
- The **nine quadrants** formed are:
  - **Upper three quadrants**
    - Epigastrium, right and left hypochondrium.
  - **Middle three quadrants**
    - Central umbilical, right and left lumbar.
  - **Lower three quadrants**
    - Hypogastrium, right and left iliac fossae.

2. Name the peculiarities of popliteus muscle.

- The origin of popliteus is intracapsular
- Origin is extra synovial
- Origin is tendinous in nature
- Insertion is fleshy
- The nerve to the muscle winds around the lower border of the muscle to supply the anterior surface.

3. Name the muscles attached to the medial border of scapula.

- The medial border has dorsal and costal surfaces. The muscles attached to medial border of the scapula are:
  - Serratus anterior
  - Levator scapulae
  - Rhomboidus minor
  - Romboidus major.
- **Mode of attachment along costal surface—serratus anterior.**
  - Superior angle: First digitation of serratus to a triangular area of both surfaces of the angle
  - Entire medial border: The next two or three digitations form a triangular sheet along medial border.
  - Inferior angle: The musculotendinous fibers of the lower four or five digitations converge to be attached by to a triangular impression on the costal surface of the inferior angle.
- **Mode of attachment along dorsal surface**
  - Superior angle to the root of the spine: **Levator scapulae** is attached
  - Opposite the root of the spine: **Rhomboid minor** is attached
  - Remainder of the border: **Rhomboid major** is attached.

4. Name the constituents of quadriceps femoris.

Refer Short Answer Q. No. 9 – 2012.

5. Name the cutaneous nerves that supply the anterior abdominal wall.

- The **ventral rami of seventh to the 12th lower thoracic and ventral rami of L1 supply the anterior abdominal wall**
- The **seventh and eighth** nerves supplying the upper portion of the anterior abdominal wall muscles, pierce the anterior rectus sheath and supply the skin of the epigastrium
- The ninth to 11th intercostal nerves emerges from their intercostal spaces between digitations of the diaphragm and transversus abdominis. The ninth nerve courses forward horizontally. The tenth and 11th pass inferomedially
- The **ninth nerve** supplies skin above the umbilicus, the **tenth** supplies skin, including the umbilicus, and the **11th** supplies skin below the umbilicus
- **Subcostal nerve the 12th** thoracic nerve supplies above hypogastric area
- **Iliohypogastric nerve** (VR L1) emerges about 3 cm above the superficial inguinal ring, and supplies the skin of suprapubic region
- **Applied anatomy:** The iliohypogastric nerve is occasionally injured above the anterior superior iliac spine, in an oblique surgical approach to the appendix. It can result in weakness of the posterior wall of the inguinal canal and can influence a direct hernia.

- Referred pain in appendicitis is to umbilicus supplied by T10.

6. Name the rotator cuff muscles.

- The shoulder joint is covered by articular capsule and is strengthened by tendons of muscles around the joint
- The muscles fuse with the lateral part of articular capsule of the shoulder joint are called as **musculo tendinous cuff/rotator cuff of Codman**
- When the humerus is abducted, flexed and internally rotated, the cuff usually impinges against the coracoacromial arch. This position is known as the impingement position
- **Components of rotator cuff:**
  - Anteriorly: Subscapularis
  - Superiorly: Supraspinatus
  - Posteriorly: Infraspinatus
  - Teres minor.

7. Name the nerves related to humerus.

Refer Short Answer Q. No. 9 – 2008.

8. Name the bones that form the floor of anatomical snuff box.

- Anatomical snuff box is a triangular depression seen when the thumb is fully extended
  - Situated on the lateral side of the wrist between the tendons of abductor pollicis longus, extensor pollicis brevis anteriorly and tendon of extensor pollicis longus posteriorly
  - **Floor** is formed by scaphoid and trapezium
  - **Applied anatomy:** Fracture of scaphoid is common in a fall with outstretched hand. It may result in avascular necrosis, and there will be tenderness in this region.

9. Bucket handle type of injury of semilunar cartilage of knee.

- The bucket handle type of injury of semilunar cartilage of knee commonly affects the **medial meniscus**
- **Reason:**
  - The menisci may be torn/injured due to twisting strain applied to the flexed knee
  - It is common in football players
  - The medial meniscus is more affected because of its attachment to the tibial collateral ligament and the rotatory movement is more than the lateral.
- **Cause of lesion:** The medial rotation of thigh in semiflexed position of knee, induces forced abduction of tibia on the femur
- **Effect of lesion:** The detached portion may get displaced to the centre of the joint, restricting all the movements.

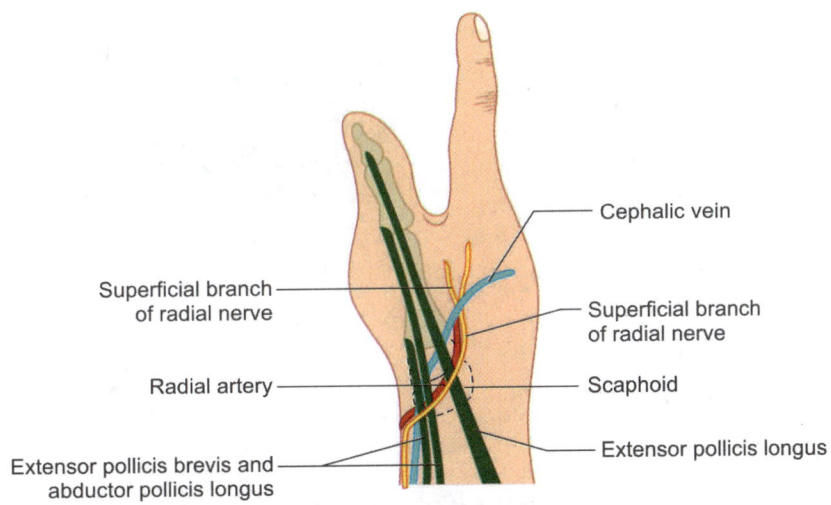

Fig. 22: Anatomical snuff box.

10. Boundaries of epiploic foramen.
Refer Short Answer Q. No. 14 – 2009.

11. Name the openings of diaphragm and their level.
Refer Essay on Q. No. 8 – 2005.

12. Juxtaglomerular apparatus.
- The juxtaglomerular apparatus consists of macula densa, polkissen cells and juxtaglomerular cells.
    - **Macula densa**:
        - Cells of distal convoluted tubule in close contact with the afferent glomerular arterioles
        - The cells become columnar and closely packed, with apical nucleus and basal golgi complexes
        - It is a sensory structure concerned with regulation of renal blood flow and thus filtration rate.
    - **Polkissen/Lacis cells**:
        - Cells lying between the vascular pole of nephrons and the distal convoluted tubules
        - They are supportive in function.
    - **Juxtaglomerular cells**:
        - Are epitheloid cells in the tunica media of the afferent glomerular arterioles.
        - The smooth muscle fibers are modified
        - Also transmit signals from macula densa to glomerulus.
- **Functions:**
    - Autoregulation of glomerular filtration rate
    - JG cell releases renin which helps for conversion of angiotensinogen into angiotensin I.

13. Contents of broad ligament.
Refer Short Answer Q. No. 20 – 2011.

14. Name the types of ossification with example.
- Ossification is the process of formation of new bone including proliferation of collagen and ground substance and deposition of calcium salts by cells called osteoblasts.
- **Two types** of ossification:
    1. **Endochondral ossification**:
        - Most bones are formed by a process of endochondral ossification
        - The mesenchyme condenses and differentiates into cartilage
        - The cartilage cells proliferate and form cartilage models
        - Calcium salts are deposited by cartilage cells.

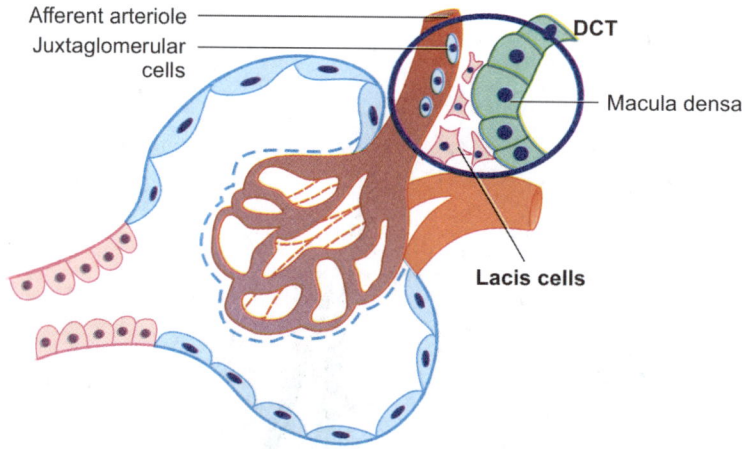

Fig. 23: Juxtaglomerular apparatus.

- The surrounding vascular layer is converted to perichondrium and becomes periosteum with formation of osteoblasts
- Example—long bones of limbs.
2. **Intramembranous ossification:**
    - Intramembranous ossification is the direct formation of bone within highly vascular membranes of condensed primitive mesenchyme
    - The mesenchymal cells differentiate into osteoblast which in turn proliferate to produce collagen fibers and hyaline matrix
    - Example—the cranial vault.

15. Palmaris brevis muscle

- Palmaris brevis is a thin, quadrilateral subcutaneous muscle, on the medial/ulnar side of the palm
- **Origin:** From the flexor retinaculum and the medial border of the central part of the palmar aponeurosis
- **Insertion:** To the dermis on the medial border of the hand
- **Nerve supply:** The superficial branch of the ulnar nerve
- **Action:** Wrinkles the skin on the ulnar side of the palm of the hand
    - Deepens the hollow of the palm by increasing the hypothenar eminence.
    - It helps in the palmar grip.

16. Root value and muscles supplied by axillary nerve.

- Axillary nerve is also known as **circumflex nerve**
- The axillary nerve arises from the posterior cord of brachial plexus
- The **root value** is C5, 6
- **Muscles supplied**
- The nerve divides into anterior and posterior divisions
- Anterior division supplies deltoid
- Posterior division—deltoid and teres minor.

17. Muscles attached to extensor expansion of hand

Refer Short Answers Q. No. 16 – 2011.

18. Mention the areas drained by superficial inguinal lymph nodes.

- The superficial inguinal nodes are **arranged** in the form of letter 'T'
- They are **grouped** as a vertical group and an upper horizontal group.
- **The upper horizontal group**
    - The lymph nodes lie parallel to and below the inguinal ligament
    - It is **subdivided** into the **upper lateral** and **upper medial** groups.
    - **Area of drainage:**
        - **Upper lateral group** drains lymph from infra umbilical part of anterior abdominal wall and gluteal region
        - **Upper medial group** drains lymph from anterior abdominal wall below umbilicus, external genital the terminal part of the urethra, lower part of anal canal, and in female the lower part of vagina, and cornua of uterus.
- **Vertical group:** The nodes are situated along the terminal part of great saphenous vein
- **Area of drainage:** It drains lymph from most of the lower limb except areas drained by popliteal nodes.

19. Name the tributaries of portal vein.

Refer Short Notes 6 – 2004.

20. Cruciate anastomosis.

- Cruciate anastomosis is seen in the lower limb
- It establishes connection between internal iliac and femoral arteries
- **Situated** in the upper part of back of thigh, undercover of gluteus maximus and between the upper border of adductor magnus and lower border of quadratus femoris.
- **Formation:**
    - From above: Descending branch of inferior gluteal artery branch of internal iliac artery
    - From below: Ascending branch of first perforator of profunda femoris

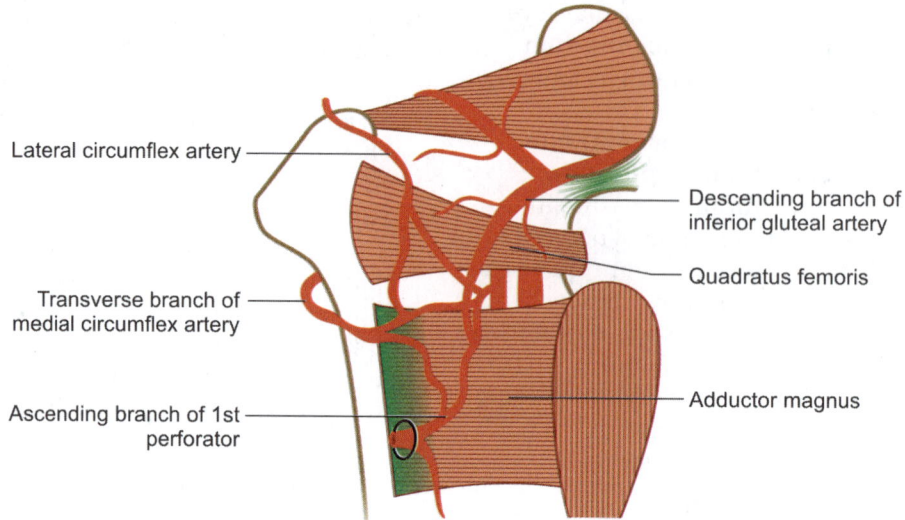

Fig. 24: Cruciate anastomosis.

- **Medially:** Transverse branch of medial circumflex artery branch of femoral artery
- **Laterally:** Transverse branch of lateral circumflex artery branch of femoral artery
- **Applied anatomy**
  - Collateral circulation will take place if femoral artery is ligated above the origin of profunda femoris
  - Medial and lateral circumflex femoral arteries with first perforator of profunda femoris and inferior gluteal artery
  - Inferior gluteal branch of internal iliac with perforating branches of profunda femoris artery.

21. Name the type of epiphysis of fibula at both ends

- Upper end—traction epiphysis
- Lower end—pressure epiphysis
- **The law for appearance of epiphysis** is, the pressure epiphysis appears before the traction epiphysis
- As per the above mentioned law the center for ossification for the lower end of fibula appears first
- The law **of ossification** is the center which appears first unites with shaft later, than the other epiphysis
- The fibula disobeys the law of ossification.
- The lower end, the pressure epiphysis appears early and fuses first with the shaft
- The upper end, the traction epiphysis appears later and fuses later and forms the growing end.

22. Supracondylar fracture.

- A **supracondylar fracture** is a fracture, of the distal end of humerus just above the epicondyles
- It is rare in adults but very common in children and is often associated with serious complications
- The history of the case is, that the child fell down with an outstretched hand followed by pain, swelling and inability to move the affected elbow
- On examination, the lower end of humerus is displaced posteriorly, there will be unusual prominence of olecranon process
- **Complications**
  - Tear or entrapment or compression of the brachial artery
  - Compression of median nerve.

- **Effects of lesion**
  - Ischemia due to compression of brachial artery
  - Lack of blood supply to flexor group of muscles of forearm known as **Volkmann's ischemic contracture.**

23. Superficial veins of upper limb with fate.

- The main superficial veins of the upper limb, the cephalic and basilic veins, formed in the subcutaneous tissue on the dorsum of the hand from the dorsal venous arch. Perforating veins form communications between the superficial and deep veins.
- The **cephalic vein**
  - Formed in the subcutaneous tissue from the lateral end of the dorsal venous arch
  - Anterior to the elbow, the cephalic vein communicates with the median cubital vein, and joins the basilic vein
  - Ascends lateral to biceps
  - Reaching infraclavicular fossa it pierces the clavipectoral fascia
  - It terminates by joining the axillary vein behind the clavicular head of pectoralis major
  - It may be connected to external jugular vein.
- The **basilic vein** is formed in the subcutaneous tissue from the medial end of the dorsal venous network. It pierces the brachial fascia and reaches axilla, where it joins with the venae comitantes of the axillary artery to form the axillary vein
- The **median cubital vein** begins at the base of the dorsum of the thumb, curves around the wrist laterally, and runs in the middle of the anterior aspect of the forearm between the cephalic and the basilic veins.

24. Foot drop

- It is a clinical condition due to injury to common peroneal nerve or its branches
- Level of lesion: Usually at the neck of fibula
- Cause of lesion:
  - Superficial as it winds around the neck of fibula
  - The nerve may be trapped by origin of peroneus longus
  - Compression by application of plaster casts
  - Traction of nerve in dislocation of knee.
- It is a painless lesion
- Deep peroneal supplies tibialis anterior, extensor hallucis longus, extensor digitorum longus, peroneus tertius and are dorsiflexors of the ankle
- Superficial peroneal supplies peroneus longus, peroneus brevis, and the action is eversion of foot
- The ankle is fully plantar flexed and foot is inverted and adducted
- Ankle jerk is normal.

25. Triceps surae.

- It is formed by two heads of gastrocnemius and soleus
- Soleus is superficial to gastrocnemius
- The muscles belong to superficial group of muscles in the posterior compartment of leg
- Near the middle of the calf the muscles end in a tendon called calcanean/achilles tendon
- The tendon is about 15 cm in length
- The tendon spirals laterally through 90°, so that the fibers of gastrocnemius are lateral towards insertion

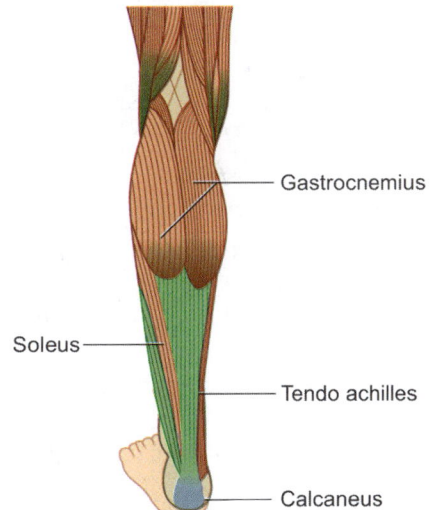

Fig. 25: Tendo Achilles.

- The muscles are inserted through the tendon to the middle of posterior surface of calcaneus
- The muscles are supplied by tibial nerve
- Action: Plantar flexion of foot
- Gastrocnemius is for propulsion in walking, running and leaping with force
- Soleus, is made of slow, fatigue—resistant type of muscle fibers and hence, helps to steady the leg on the foot in standing
- **Applied anatomy:**
  - **Calcaneal tendinitis**: Inflammation of the calcanean tendon due to injury to the collagen fibers in the tendon, which causes pain while walking
  - **Calcaneal tendon rupture**: In complete rupture of the tendon, the person cannot plantar flex, and there will be excessive dorsiflexion.

26. Name the ligaments around hip joint
- Fibrous capsule
- Iliofemoral ligament
- Pubofemoral ligament
- Ischiofemoral ligament
- Acetabular labrum
- Transverse acetabular ligament
- Ligament of head of femur.

27. Name the parts of vulva
- Female external genitalia is also known as vulva.
- It includes
  - Mons pubis
  - Labia majora
  - Labia minora
  - Clitoris
  - Bulbs of the vestibule
  - Greater vestibular glands.

28. Hymenal membrane
- The hymen is an incomplete mucous fold
- Situated within the external orifice of vagina
- It is of various shapes—annular, crescentic or cribriform
- Sometimes, the hymen is congenitally absent or may be imperforate
- The first sexual intercourse causes rupture of hymnal ring, but can rupture earlier during nonsexual physical activity
- Small round carunculae hymenales are the remnants after it has been ruptured.

29. Perineal body (location in female with clinical importance).
Refer Short Notes 8 – 2004.

30. Name any two sites of porta caval anastomosis.
Refer Short Notes 6 – 2004.

31. Parts of the sensory nucleus of trigeminal nerve.
- The sensation carried by the trigeminal nerve is sensation from face, scalp, upper and lower jaw teeth, eye, nasal cavity, paranasal air sinuses, general sensation from anterior ⅔ of tongue, floor of mouth, external ear and proprioceptive impulses from muscles of mastication, temporomandibular joint
- The sensory nuclei concerned are—spinal nucleus, chief sensory nucleus, and mesencephalic nucleus
- The **spinal nucleus** of trigeminal is situated in the medulla and extends above to pons and below to spinal cord upper cervical segment. it receives pain and temperature sensation from ipsilateral half of face, general sensory fibers of glossopharyngeal, vagus, and facial nerves
- The **chief sensory nucleus** situated in the pons receives tactile impulses
- **Mesencephalic nucleus** in the midbrain receives proprioceptive impulses.

32. Dangerous area of scalp.
- Fourth layer of scalp is known as danger area of scalp
- It contains loose areolar layer tissue and forms a potential space deep to aponeurosis
- This space contains emissary veins blood vessels and nerves
- Emissary veins are devoid of valves and connects extracranial veins with intracranial venous sinus
- Hence it is known as **danger area of scalp.**
- **Applied anatomy:** Infection from scalp can spread into venous sinuses resulting in thrombosis.

33. Surface marking of apex beat of heart.

- The left ventricle forms the apex of the heart
- It is covered by the left lung and pleura
- The apex beat is felt in the 5th left intercostal space a little medial to midclavicular plane.

34. Lobe of azygos.

Refer Essay Q. No. 6 – 2008.

35. Formation and termination of internal jugular vein.

- Internal jugular vein is **formed** by the continuation of the sigmoid sinus
- The sigmoid sinus passes through the jugular foramen and is continued as superior bulb of internal jugular vein
- It descends downwards lateral to the carotids, within the carotid sheath
- At the lower end forms inferior bulb which is a content of lesser supraclavicular triangle
- **Termination**: At the level of medial end of clavicle it unites with the subclavian vein to form brachiocephalic vein.

36. Boundaries and applied anatomy of Piriform recess.

Refer Short Answer 32 – 2009.

37. Blood supply of internal capsule.

Refer Essay Q. No. 7 – 2005.

38. Parts of corpus callosum.

Refer Short Answer Q. No. 24 – 2009.

39. Root value of phrenic nerve and name the structures supplied by it.

- Root value—ventral rami of C 3, 4, 5.
- VR C3, C4 from cervical plexus and C5 contribution is from brachial plexus
- Structure supplied –
  - **Motor**—diaphragm
  - **Sensory**—pericardium, pleura, diaphragm.

40. Olive.

- It is an elevation seen in the medulla oblongata
- It is situated lateral to pyramid
- Between pyramid and olive is the anterolateral sulcus
- The hypoglossal nerve rootlets emerge
- The posterolateral sulcus is lateral to olive
- The glossopharyngeal, vagus and cranial part of accessory nerves emerge through posterolateral sulcus
- Between the lower border of pons and olive the facial nerve emerges
- The olive is produced by the inferior olivary nucleus
- The olivary nucleus is large and hollow with crenate edges. The hilum faces dorsomedially
- Afferent: Cerebello-olivary fibers from cerebellum to olivary nuclei
- Efferent: The fibers arising from the nuclei are olivocerebellar, olivospinal fibers.

41. Terminal branches of external carotid artery.

The external carotid artery ascends up and at the level of the neck of mandible terminates as superficial temporal and maxillary arteries.

42. Arterial supply to pituitary

Arterial Supply

- One inferior and several superior hypophysial arteries on each side supply the gland.
- **The inferior hypophyseal**
  - The artery is branch from cavernous part of internal carotid artery
  - The inferior hypophysial artery divides into medial and lateral branches
  - An arterial ring is formed around infundibulum by the anastomosis of the branches
  - Neurohypophysis is supplied by the branches from the anastomosis.
- **The superior hypophyseal**
  - It is from supraclinoid part of internal carotid artery and from the anterior cerebral and posterior cerebral arteries
  - These arteries supply the median eminence, upper infundibulum
  - The lower infundibulum is supplied through trabecular arteries

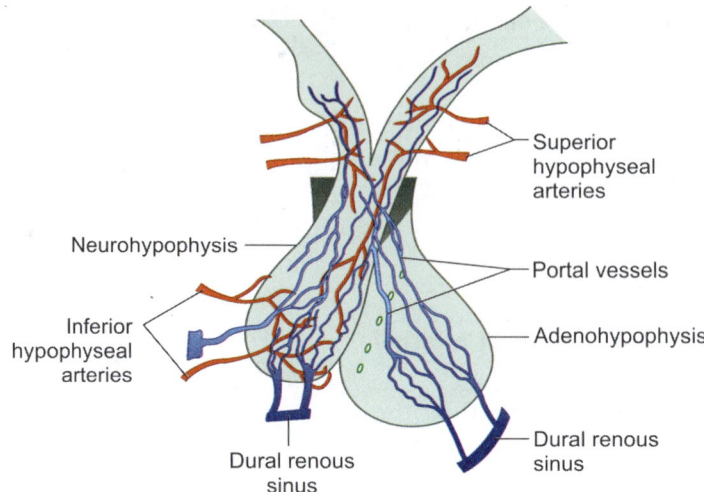

Fig. 26: Blood supply of pituitary.

- External and an internal plexus are formed by the arteries in the median eminence
- These plexuses are continuous with plexus in the infundibulum
- Long portal vessels drain the external and internal plexus, and enter the pars anterior
- Short portal vessels drain the lower infundibulum and reach the pars anterior.
- In the adenohypophysis long and short portal vessel open into vascular sinusoids
- Adenohypophysis does not have direct arterial supply
- Hormone-releasing factors are carried by the portal system
- **Pars intermedius** is avascular.

43. Dangerous area of face.

Refer Short Answer Q. No. 37 – 2009.

44. Opening of maxillary sinus.

- Maxillary sinus opening is usually seen as two openings
- Opens into the hiatus semilunaris of middle meatus
- The opening of the sinus is at a higher level than the floor of the sinus
- The opening is made small in living by articulation with lacrimal bone anteriorly, inferior concha inferiorly, uncinate process of ethmoid superiorly, and perpendicular plate of palatine bone posteriorly
- **Applied anatomy:** Drainage of the sinus is difficult. In case of collection of fluid inside the sinus, should be drained by postural drainage.

45. Auditory tube openings

- Bony part of the auditory tube opens laterally into anterior/carotid wall of middle ear cavity
- The opening of the auditory tube is situated in the nasopharynx about 1.2 cm behind and below the posterior end of inferior concha of nasal cavity
- Above and behind the opening is the **tubal elevation,** produced by the cartilaginous part of tube
- Sometimes there is collection of lymphoid tissue near the pharyngeal orifice called the **tubal tonsil**
- At birth the pharyngeal orifice is seen as narrow slit, level with the palate and tubal elevation is absent.

46. Blood supply to tonsil

Refer Short Notes Q. No. 32 – 2008.

47. Nerve supply and action of cricothyroid muscle

- Cricothyroid is one of the intrinsic muscle of the larynx
- Nerve supply—external laryngeal nerve
- Action—tensor of vocal cord. Rotation occurs at cricothyroid joint and posterior part of the muscle pulls the thyroid cartilage forwards. Thus the vocal cord is stretched.

48. Attachment of vocal cord

- **True vocal cord**:
  - Upper margin of cricovocal membrane (conus elasticus) is thickened to form the vocal ligament
  - **Vocal fold/cord** is formed by vocal ligament, vocalis muscle, lamina propria and mucous membrane
  - It extends between the angle of thyroid cartilage to tip of vocal process of arytenoid cartilage
  - The lining epithelium of vocal cord is stratified squamous epithelium
  - The ligament is attached to the underlying lamina, hence appears pearly white in color.
- **False vocal cord**:
  - The lower end of the quadrangular membrane is thickened to form the vestibular ligament
  - The mucous membrane together with the ligament forms the vestibular fold/false vocal cord
  - Extends from angle of thyroid cartilage to the anterolateral surface of arytenoid cartilage.

49. Blood supply to lung

- Each lung has a pulmonary artery supplying blood to it and two pulmonary veins draining blood from it
- The right and left **pulmonary arteries** arise from the pulmonary trunk at the level of the sternal angle
- Two **pulmonary veins**, a superior and an inferior pulmonary vein on each side, carry "oxygenated" blood from corresponding lobes of each lung to the left atrium of the heart. The middle lobe vein of right lung drains to the right superior pulmonary vein

- **Bronchial arteries** supply blood for the structures of the root of the lungs, the supporting tissues of the lungs, and the visceral pleura
- On the left side two bronchial arteries, usually arise from the thoracic aorta. The single right bronchial artery usually from the right 3rd posterior intercostal artery.

50. Terminal branches of internal thoracic artery.

The artery descends vertically downwards at sixth intercostal space terminates by dividing into two terminal branches:
- Musculophrenic artery and
- Superior epigastric artery.

51. Suprasternal space of burns.

- Above manubrium the investing layer of deep cervical fascia splits into two as superficial and deep layers
- The superficial layer is attached to the anterior border of manubrium and posterior layer to posterior border of manubrium and interclavicular ligament
- It encloses a space called suprasternal space of burns
- Contents
  - Sternal head of sternocleidomastoid muscle
  - Interclavicular ligaments
  - Areolar tissue
  - Anterior cervical lymph node
  - Lower part of anterior jugular vein and jugular venous arch.

52. Dangerous area of face.

Refer Short Answer 37 – 2009.

53. Structures passing through foreman ovale.

Refer Short Answer 27 – 2009.

54. Boundaries of laryngeal inlet.

Refer Short Answer 43 – 2012.

55. Branches of ascending and arch of aorta.

- Branches of ascending aorta:
  - Right coronary artery from anterior aortic sinus
  - Left coronary artery from left posterior aortic sinus.

- Branches from arch of aorta:
  - Brachiocephalic trunk
  - Left common carotid artery
  - Left subclavian artery
  - Occasional branches—thyroidea ima, vertebral artery, right subclavian.

56. Lumbar puncture.
Refer Short Notes 34 – 2008.

57. Pterion.
Refer Short Notes 31 – 2012.

58. Apex beat.
Refer Short Answer Q. No. 33 – 2013.

59. Contents of posterior mediastinum.
Refer Essay Q. No. 6 – 2012.

60. Applied aspects of pleura.
- Inflammation of the pleura is called as **pleurisy**
- Presence of air in the pleural cavity is called **pneumothorax**
- Presence of serous fluid is referred to as **pleural effusion**
- Presence of blood in the pleural cavity is called **hemothorax**
- Presence of pus is called **empyema**
- If the thoracic cavity is injured, lymph may enter the pleural cavity and is called as **chylothorax**
- Paracentesis thoracis: Tapping fluid from the pleural cavity by inserting a needle through the intercostal space.

MBBS Examination 2014

ANSWER ALL QUESTIONS

I. Essay questions   **(15/10 Marks)**

1. Describe type, ligaments, relations, movements muscles producing the movements and applied anatomy of shoulder joint.
2. Describe boundaries, contents and applied anatomy of femoral triangle.
3. Describe great saphenous vein under the following headings: (a) Formation and termination, (b) Course and relations, (c) Tributaries and perforators and (d) Applied anatomy.
4. Describe the anal canal under the following headings: (a) Interior, (b) Blood supply, (c) Development including congenital anomalies and (d) Applied anatomy.
5. Classify the white matter of cerebrum with examples and describe the internal capsule in detail. Add a note on its applied anatomy.
6. Describe the interior of right atrium in detail and add a note about its development and clinical anatomy.
7. Describe sulci, gyri, and functional areas in the superolateral surface of brain with neat labeled diagrams.
8. Describe extraocular muscles in detail.

II. Short notes   **(5/4 Marks)**

1. Inguinal canal.
2. Femoral artery.
3. Portal vein.
4. Elbow joint.
5. Mid palmar space.
6. Musculocutaneous nerve.
7. Extensor expansion of middle finger.
8. Ischiorectal fossa.
9. Vascular segments of liver.
10. Ligaments of knee joint.
11. Flexor retinaculum.
12. Classify the joints of the body giving suitable examples and describe a typical synovial joint.
13. Short lateral rotators of the thigh.
14. Ligaments of uterus.
15. Eustachian tube.
16. Typical intercostal nerve.
17. Lateral wall of nose.
18. Midbrain at superior colliculus level.
19. Ansa cervicalis.
20. Ciliary ganglion.
21. Parts, arterial supply of interventricular septum.
22. Cardiac plexus.
23. Middle ear.
24. Origin, termination, applied anatomy of internal mammary artery.
25. Digastric triangle.
26. Third ventricle.
27. Medulla oblongata at mid-olivary level.
28. Superior mediastinum.

III. Short answer questions   **(3/2 Marks)**

1. Mesentery.
2. Cartilage.
3. Somites.
4. Wrist drop.
5. Histology of ovary.
6. Stomach bed.
7. Axillary vein.
8. Developmental anomalies of kidney.

9. Adductor canal.
10. Boundaries and contents of popliteal fossa.
11. Clavipectoral fascia.
12. Blood supply of gonads.
13. Quadrangular space.
14. Cryptorchism.
15. Histology of duodenum.
16. Perineal body.
17. Gluteus medius.
18. Results of fertilization.
19. Skin.
20. Sciatic nerve.
21. Name the thenar muscles.
22. Name the branches given off by the radial nerve in the spiral groove.
23. Meckel's diverticulum.
24. Name the structures crossed by the root of mesentery in order.
25. Parts of fallopian tube.
26. Name the bones that form the first carpometacarpal joint.
27. Boundaries of epiploic foramen.
28. Constituents of quadriceps femoris.
29. Root value, branches and applied anatomy of pudendal nerve.
30. Name the boundaries of femoral ring.
31. Inferior constrictor of pharynx.
32. Blood supply of spinal cord.
33. Carotid sheath.
34. Left brachiocephalic vein.
35. Histology of thyroid gland.
36. Parkinsonism.
37. Pterygopalatine ganglion.
38. Structures present at T4 level.
39. Hilum of right lung.
40. Development of pituitary gland.
41. Orbicularis oculi muscle.
42. Blood supply of thyroid gland.
43. Azygos vein.
44. Pleural recesses.
45. Histology of thymus.
46. Boundaries and contents of sub-occipital triangle.
47. Pineal gland.
48. Lateral medullary syndrome.
49. Lumbar puncture.
50. Development of tongue.
51. Formation of basal vein.
52. Surface marking of apex beat of heart.
53. Blood supply of internal capsule.
54. Parts of caudate nucleus.
55. Dangerous area of scalp.
56. Patent ductus arteriosus.
57. Formation and distribution of spinal part of the accessory nerve.
58. Name any four branches of external carotid artery.
59. Define typical intercostals nerve with example.
60. Tributaries of cavernous sinus.

I. ESSAY QUESTIONS

1. **Describe type, ligaments, relations, movements, muscles producing the movements and applied anatomy of shoulder joint.**

Refer Essay Q. No. 2 – 2006.

2. **Describe the boundaries, contents and applied anatomy of femoral triangle.**

Refer Essay Q. No. 3 – 2012.

3. **Describe the great saphenous vein under the following headings: (a) Formation and termination, (b) Course and relations, (c) Tributaries and perforators and (d) Applied anatomy.**

Refer Short Notes on Q. No. 14 – 2005.

4. **Describe the anal canal under the following headings: (a) Interior, (b) blood supply, (c) Development including Congenital anomalies and (d) Applied anatomy.**

(a, b, d) Refer Essay Q. No. 4 – 2005.

(c) **Development and congenital anomalies**

- The anal canal is developed from two sources
- Up to pectinate line is **endodermal** in origin developed from **primitive rectum**. Below the line it is **ectodermal** in origin developed from **proctodeum**
- **Up to pectinate line**
  - The **post-allantoic part** of the hindgut dilates to form endodermal cloaca
  - It extends up to cloacal membrane.

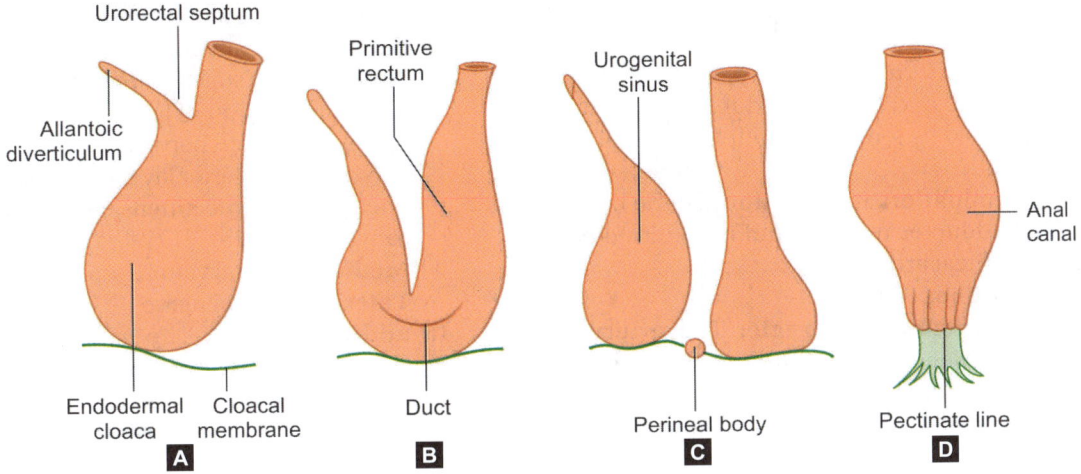

Figs. 1A to D: Development of anal canal.

- The endodermal cloaca is divided into a ventral primitive urogenital sinus and dorsal part called primitive rectum by the urorectal septum
- By 7th week the septum fuses with the cloacal membrane, and divides the cloaca into two
- The cloacal membrane is divided into anal membrane and urogenital membrane
- Primitive rectum gives rise to upper part of anal canal up to pectinate line.
- **Below pectinate line:**
  - Developed from anal membrane
  - A depression is formed in the anal membrane called anal pit or proctodeum.
- Both the parts **fuse** and the membrane **ruptures** and communication is established to the exterior.
- **Congenital anomaly:**
  - Imperforate anus—is due to failure of perforation of anal membrane and it persists
  - Ectopic anus—the anal pit lies close to vagina in female and root of scrotum in male
  - Rectovesical/rectourethral fistula—failure of closure of cloacal duct and a communication is seen between the structures.

5. **Classify the white matter of cerebrum with examples and describe the internal capsule in detail. Add a note on its applied anatomy.**

Classification—Refer Essay Q. No. 5 – 2012.
Internal capsule—Refer Essay Q. No. 7 – 2005.

6. **Describe the interior of right atrium in detail and add a note about its development and clinical anatomy.**

Interior—Refer Essay Q. No. 7 – 2006.
Development—Refer Essay Q. No. 8 – 2009.

7. **Describe the sulci, gyri, and functional areas in the superolateral surface of brain with neat labelled diagrams.**

Refer Essay Q. No. 7 – 2007.

8. **Describe the extraocular muscles in detail.**

Refer Essay Q. No. 6 – 2005.

II. SHORT NOTES

1. **Inguinal canal**

Refer Short Notes 20 – 2008.

2. **Femoral artery**
- It is the main artery of lower limb
- **Origin**
  - External iliac artery is continued behind the mid inguinal point which

is midpoint between anterior superior iliac spine to pubic symphysis.
- **Course:** It runs downwards in the femoral triangle and then in adductor canal. It is covered by femoral sheath for about 4 cm length
- **Termination:** It leaves through the hiatus of adductor magnus and is continued as popliteal artery.
- **Relations (Fig. 2)**
  - **In femoral triangle:** The artery is crossed anteriorly by the medial cutaneous nerve of thigh from lateral to medial, and the femoral vein crosses from medial to posterior.
    - **Anterior:** Skin, superficial fascia, fascia lata, anterior layer of femoral sheath, medial cutaneous nerve of thigh
    - **Posterior:** Posterior layer of femoral sheath, psoas, pectineus, adductor longus
    - **Medial:** Femoral vein
    - **Lateral:** Femoral nerve
  - **In adductor canal:** The saphenous nerve crosses the artery from lateral to medial **(Fig. 3)**.

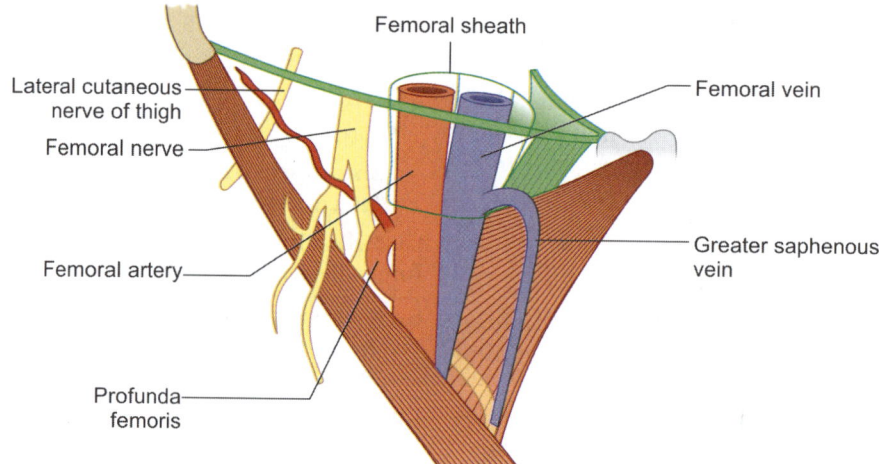

Fig. 2: Relations in femoral triangle.

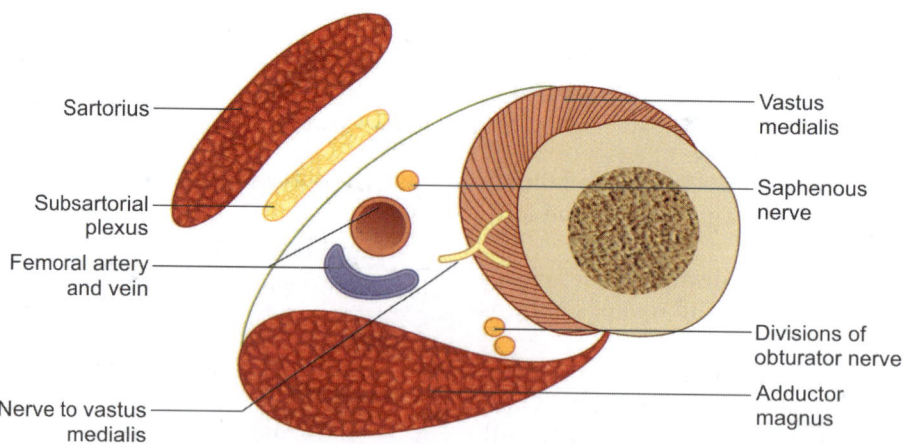

Fig. 3: Femoral artery in adductor canal.

- **Anterior:** Sartorius, saphenous nerve
- **Posterior:** Adductor longus and magnus, femoral vein
- **Medial:** Saphenous nerve (in the lower part)
- **Lateral:** Nerve to vastus medialis, saphenous nerve in the upper part.

- **Branches (Fig. 4)**
  In the femoral triangle:
  – Superficial branches:
    - Superficial epigastric
    - Superficial external pudendal
    - Superficial circumflex iliac.
  – Deep branches:
    - Deep external pudendal
    - Profunda femoris
    - Muscular branches.
  In the adductor canal:
    - Descending genicular
    - Muscular branches
  – Superficial epigastric artery—arises 1 cm below the inguinal ligament. Runs in the fascia of abdomen up to umbilicus. Supplies inguinal nodes and skin
  – Superficial external pudendal artery—runs medially deep to great saphenous vein and supply the skin of external genitalia
  – Superficial circumflex iliac artery—passes towards anterior superior iliac spine. Supply the skin and inguinal nodes.
  – **Profunda femoris:**
    - Arises laterally about 3.5 cm below the inguinal ligament
    - It is continued as fourth perforator
    - It is the main artery of adductor, flexor and extensor compartment muscles
    - It also anastomose above with internal and external iliac arteries and popliteal artery below
    - The branches from it are medial circumflex, lateral circumflex and perforators arteries.
  – Deep external pudendal artery—passes medially and supply skin of perineum and scrotum or labia majora
  – Descending genicular artery—is the branch given in adductor canal. It gives of a saphenous branch, which takes part in anastomosis around knee joint.
- **Anastomosis formed by femoral artery**
  – Cruciate anastomosis—medial and lateral circumflex arteries (from femoral), first perforator and superior and inferior gluteal arteries (from internal iliac)
  – Trochanteric anastomosis—superior and inferior gluteal arteries with medial and circumflex arteries

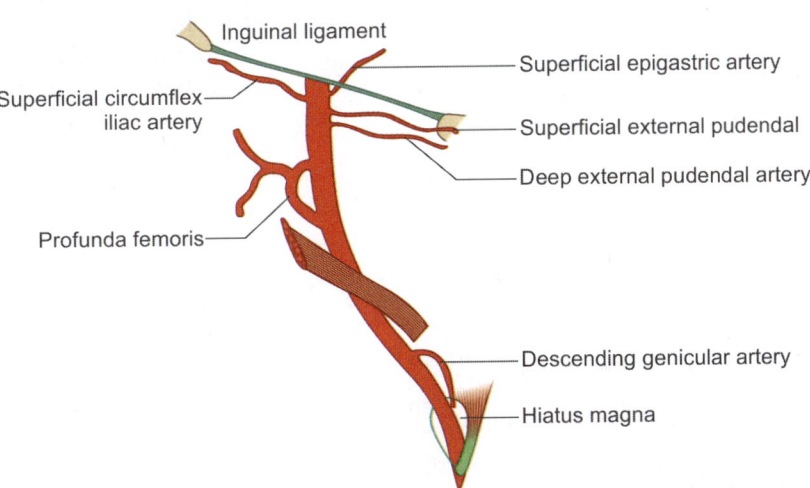

Fig. 4: Branches of femoral artery.

- Spinous anastomosis—deep (from external iliac), superficial and medial and lateral circumflex iliac arteries with superior gluteal artery
- Genicular anastomosis—descending genicular artery, fourth perforator and popliteal artery
- Anastomosis on the back of thigh—longitudinal anastomosis by the perforators branch of profunda
- In perineum—internal pudendal (from internal iliac) with superficial and deep external pudendal arteries (from femoral artery).
- **Applied anatomy**
  - At the apex of femoral triangle, the arrangement of vessels one behind the other from superficial to deep are the femoral artery, femoral vein, profunda vein and profunda femoris artery. All the vessels will be involved in a stab injury at apex of triangle
  - Femoral artery pulsation felt at mid inguinal point
  - The femoral artery is used for cannulation as it is superficial
  - If the femoral artery is ligated collateral circulation is established between the femoral, internal external iliac arteries through the anastomosis mentioned above.

3. Portal vein.
Refer Short Notes 6 – 2004.

4. Elbow joint.
Type: Synovial, uniaxial, hinge variety.

Bones Taking Part
- It is divided into humeroulnar and humeroradial joints
- The humeroulnar is between trochlea of humerus and trochlear notch of ulna
- The humeroradial is capitulum of humerus and radial head.

Articular Surfaces (Fig. 5)

Humeroulnar joint
- The trochlea of humerus—shape of a pulley, with medial edge projecting 6 mm lower than the lateral. The trochlear articular surface is larger posteriorly than anterior
- The coronoid fossa is a depression just above the anterior aspect of the trochlea. The coronoid process of the ulna fits into it when the elbow is flexed
- The olecranon fossa lies just above the posterior aspect of the trochlea. The olecranon process of the ulna is accommodated in the fossa when the elbow is extended
- Trochlear notch of ulna: The coronoid and olecranon articular surfaces of the notch are separated by a nonarticular part of bone.

Humeroradial joint
- Capitulum of humerus like a ball and articular surfaces are in front and below
- The radial fossa is a depression present just above the capitulum. It accommodates the head of the radius in flexion of the elbow
- The head of radius—superior surface is disc like.

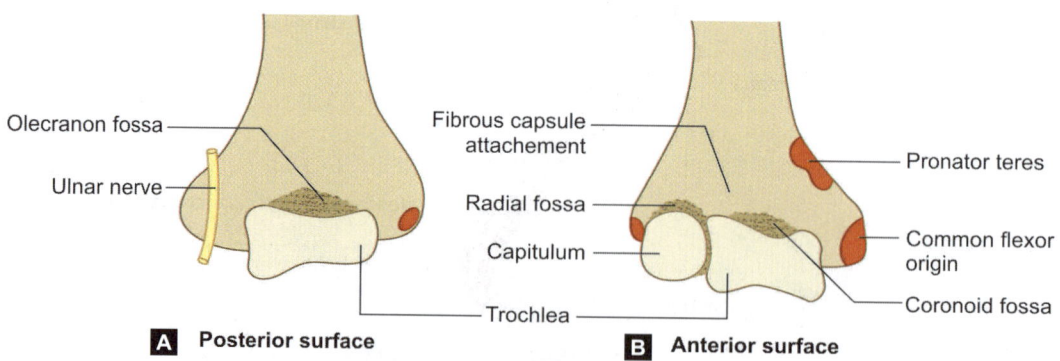

Figs. 5A and B: Articular surfaces.

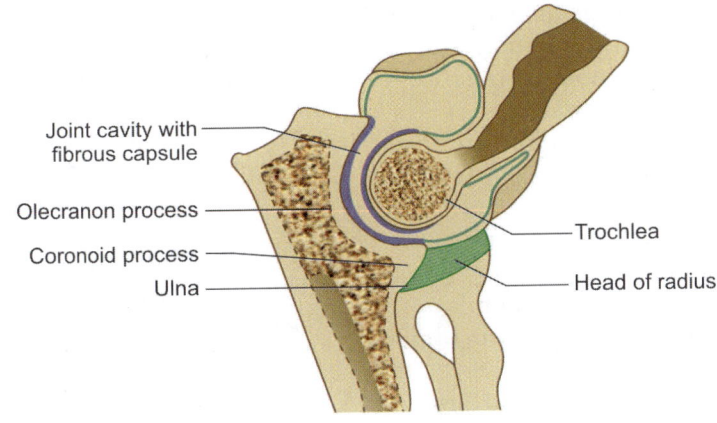

Fig. 6: Fibrous capsule.

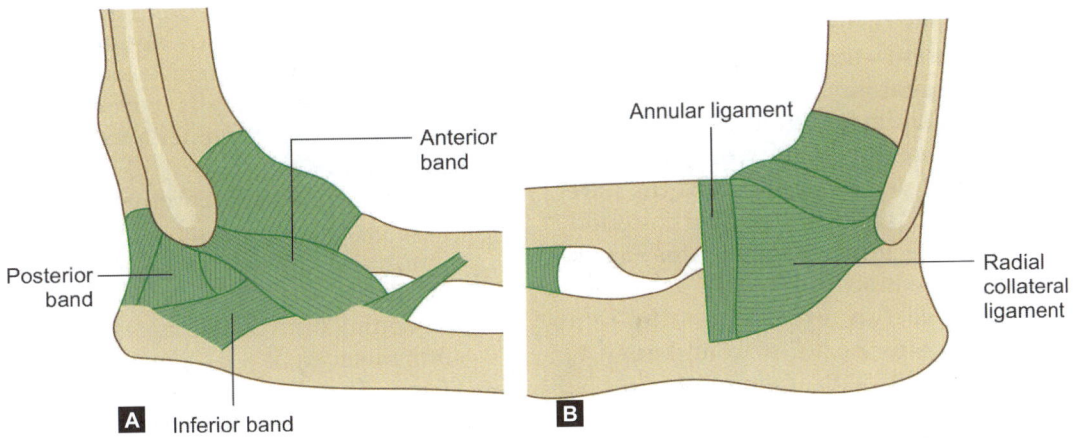

Figs. 7A and B: Ligaments of elbow joint: (A) Ulnar collateral ligament; (B) Radial collateral ligament.

Ligaments

- **Fibrous capsule (Fig. 6):**
  - Capsule is complete
  - It is thin anteriorly
  - It is attached **above** to the humerus to the margins of the three fossae. The epicondyles are extracapsular
  - **Below** to margins of trochlear notch and blends with annular ligament of superior radio ulnar joint
  - The synovial membrane lines the inner surface of the capsule.
- **Ulnar collateral ligament (Fig. 7A)**
  - Is triangular in shape
  - The ligament is thickened to form three bands—anterior, inferior, and posterior
  - The anterior band is from the front of medial epicondyle to the tubercle on the medial margin of the coronoid process
  - The posterior band is from back of medial condyle to the medial margin of olecranon process
  - The inferior band extends between olecranon and coronoid process.
- **Radial collateral ligament**—from lateral epicondyle to the annular ligament **(Fig. 7B)**
- **Relations**
  - Anteriorly—brachialis, tendon of biceps, median nerve, brachial artery
  - Posteriorly—triceps, anconeus
  - Medially—common origin of flexors of forearm, ulnar nerve

- Laterally—common origin of superficial extensors of forearm, supinator, radial nerve and its terminal branches—superficial and deep branches
- Blood supply: From anastomosis around elbow
- Nerve supply: Musculocutaneous nerve, radial nerve, ulnar nerve.
- **Movements:**
  - Flexion—the range of flexion is 150° and the flexor surface of forearm comes in contact with the arm
  - Extension—when the arm and forearm are in straight line.
- **Muscles producing the movements**
  - Flexion—brachialis, biceps brachii, brachioradialis
  - Extension—triceps, anconeus.
- **Applied anatomy:**
  - **Supracondylar fracture of humerus**—usually fall on outstretched hand. More common in children. The lower fractured segment is pushed posteriorly and the upper segment may cause injury to brachial artery
  - **Dislocation of elbow**—the joint dislocates posteriorly and may be associated with fracture of coronoid process
  - **Tennis elbow**—while playing tennis sudden pronation may produce sprain or tear of the radial collateral ligament causing pain and tenderness over lateral epicondyle
  - **Student's elbow/Dart thrower's elbow/Minor's elbow**—when the olecranon bursa gets injured during fall and become inflamed resulting in subcutaneous olecranon bursitis.

5. **Midpalmar space.**

- The palmar spaces are called as fascial spaces of palm
- It is divided by a midpalmar septum into thenar and mid palmar space
- Midpalmar space communicates with 3rd and 4th lumbrical canals which open to web spaces
- **Boundaries (Fig. 8):**
  - **Anteriorly**—palmar aponeurosis, superficial palmar arch, flexor tendons of medial three digits, covered with synovial sheath the ulnar bursa medial three lumbricals
  - **Posteriorly**—fascia covering the third and fourth interossei muscles and fourth and fifth metacarpal bones
  - **Medially**—the medial palmar septum extending from palmar aponeurosis to fifth metacarpal
  - **Laterally**—the midpalmar septum extending from palmar aponeurosis to third metacarpal
  - **Proximally**—up to flexor retinaculum
  - **Distally**—up to distal palmar crease

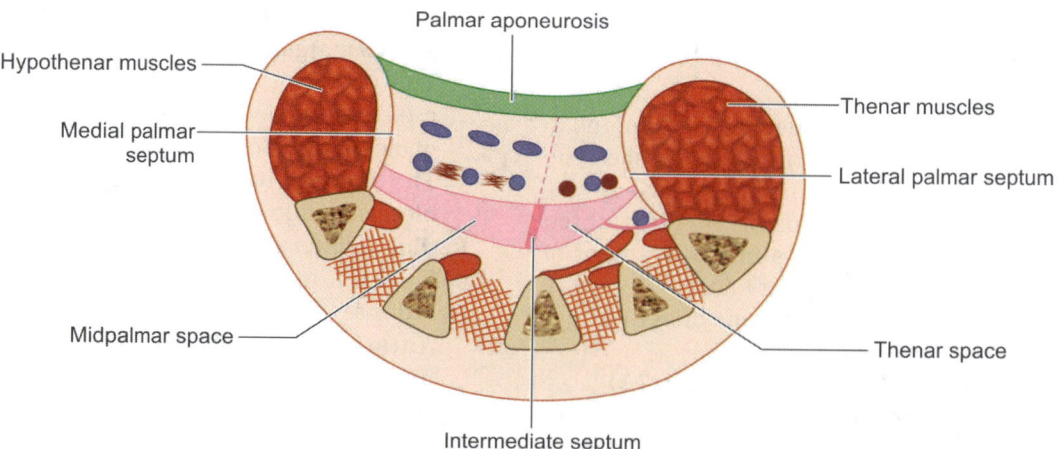

Fig. 8: Palmar spaces.

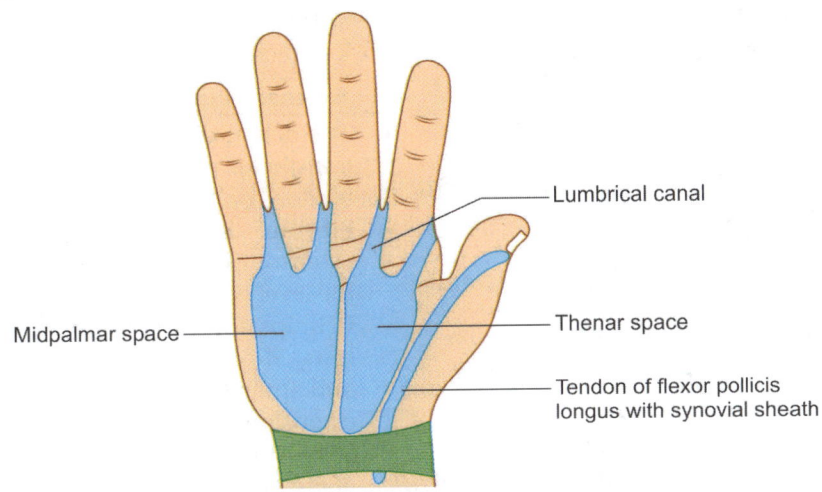

Fig. 9: Communication of midpalmar space.

- **Communication (Fig. 9):** Distally the space communicates with third and fourth lumbrical canals
- **Applied anatomy:** Infection of midpalmar space, the pus can be let out through web space as the midpalmar space communicates with web space via lumbrical canal.

6. **Musculocutaneous nerve.**

- It is the nerve of anterior compartment of arm
- It arises from lateral cord of brachial plexus
- Root value is VR $C_5 - C_7$
- **Course and relation:**
  - In the axilla: It is situated lateral to third part of axillary artery

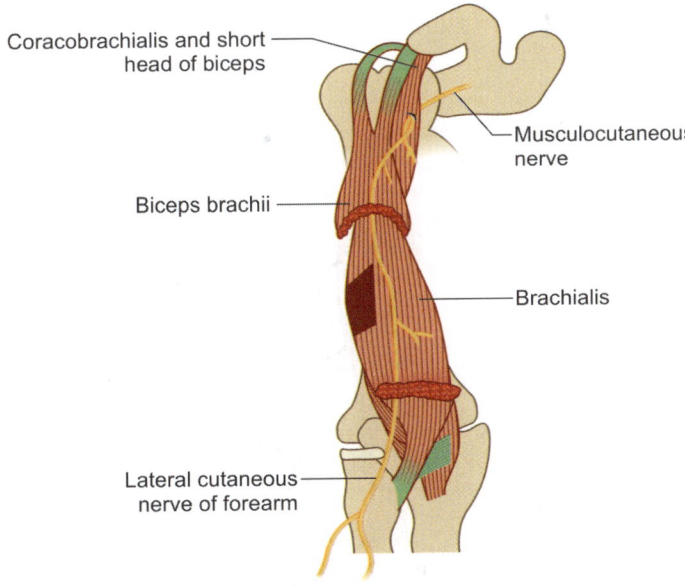

Fig. 10: Musculocutaneous nerve.

- In the arm: It descends downwards and passes between the two heads of the coracobrachialis
- Then it lies between biceps and brachialis muscles
- Below the elbow: It pierces the deep fascia and lies lateral to the tendon of biceps.
- **Termination:** It is continued as lateral cutaneous nerve of forearm
- **Branches**
  - Muscular branches—coracobrachialis, biceps brachii, brachialis
  - Articular branch—shoulder joint
  - Cutaneous—lateral region of anterior surface of forearm
  - Variations:
    - Musculocutaneous nerve may replace superficial branch of radial nerve
    - Median nerve may send a branch to musculocutaneous nerve.
- **Applied anatomy:**
  - Injury to musculocutaneous nerve is rare. If injured there is weakness of flexion of elbow as biceps and brachialis muscles are affected
  - In Erb's palsy the nerve roots injured are VR C5, 6. Hence the muscles supplied by the musculocutaneous nerve are affected.

7. **Extensor expansion of middle finger.**
- The dorsal digital expansion is a fibrous hood like expansion of the extensor tendons on the dorsal surface of hands
- Fibrous extensor expansion hold the extensor digitorum tendon in position at the level of metacarpophalangeal joint
- It helps for the coordinated action of long flexors, extensors, lumbricals, and interossei so that the flexion and extensions are carried out smoothly
- **Extent:** The expansion covers the dorsum of the proximal phalanx of each digit
- **Formation:** The expansion is formed by extensor tendon and joined by lumbricals, interossei muscles. The attachment of these tendons are named as wing tendons
- **Level of attachment of wing tendons:**
  - The interossei at the proximal portion of proximal phalanx
  - Lumbrical at mid portion of proximal phalanx.
- **Shape:**
  - The expansion is triangular in shape
  - Transverse fibers (sagittal bands) are present connecting the expansion to transverse metacarpal ligament

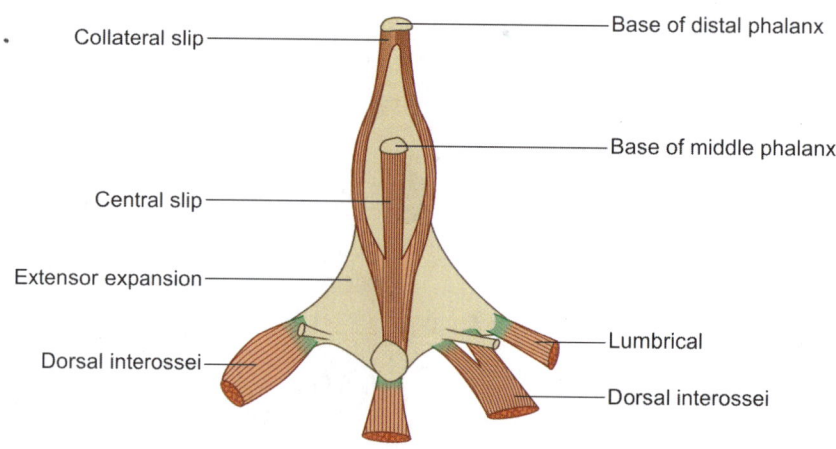

Fig. 11: Extensor expansion.

- **Components of the extensor expansion of middle finger:**
  - Extensor digitorum tendon of middle finger
  - 2nd lumbricals on the lateral side
  - 2nd dorsal interossei on lateral side
  - 3rd dorsal interossei on the medial side
  - There is no contribution from palmar interossei for the middle finger.
- **Mode of attachment:**
  - The expansion divides into three slips—central and two lateral.
  - The central slip contains extensor tendon and also fibers from lumbricals and interossei
  - The central slip is inserted to the dorsum of base of middle phalanx
  - The lateral slips fuse and inserted to the base of the distal phalanx.
- **Functions:**
  - It moves during flexion and extension of metacarpophalangeal joint
  - A bursa separates the expansion from the joint.
- **Applied anatomy:**
  - Injuries to transverse fibers results in subluxation of extensor tendon
  - **Trigger finger**—due to anterior dislocation of extensor tendon following a direct injury detaching the extensor tendon from the hood
  - **Mallet finger**—due to the tear of the terminal portion of hood, over distal interphalangeal joint. The terminal phalanx remains flexed. It is also known as baseball finger.
- **Buttonhole deformity**—rupture of insertion of extensor expansion into the base of middle phalanx. An attempt to extend the terminal interphalangeal joint will produce flexion in the middle phalanx.

8. **Ischiorectal fossa.**

Refer Short Notes 8 – 2003.

9. **Vascular segments of liver.**

- Vascular segments are considered as functional segments
- Couinaud divided the liver into segments, based on the number of branches of portal vein and position of hepatic vein
- According to the main branches of portal veins there are four portal sectors—right lateral, right medial, left lateral and left medial
- Three main hepatic veins lie in-between these sectors, called intersectorial veins
- Each sector is divided into two depending upon the tertiary division of biliary sheath
- So there are eight segments
- Each segment is supplied by a branch of hepatic artery, portal vein, hepatic duct
- Segment I—is caudate lobe
- Segments II, III, IV are confined to left lobe
- Segments V, VI, VII, VIII involves the right lobe

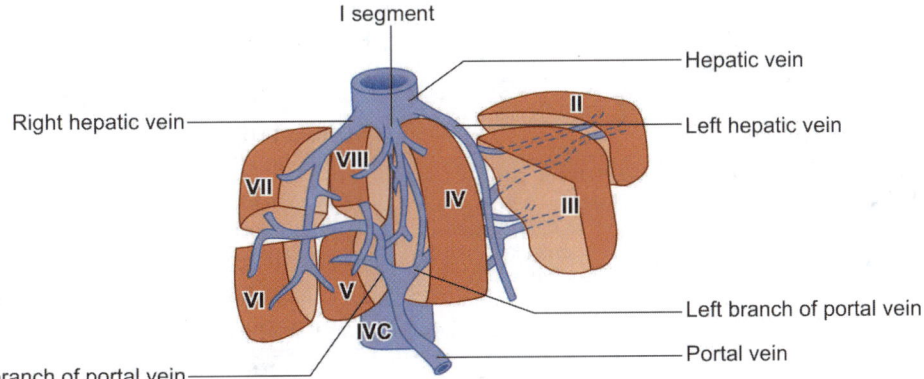

Fig. 12: Vascular segments of liver.

- **Clinical importance** – in CT and MRI segment I lies behind and to the right of IVC
  - Segments VII, VIII, IV, II are above the portal vein
  - Segments VI, V, IV, III are below portal vein.
- **Applied anatomy**: The **hepatic segmentectomies** are possible to perform. The laser surgery procedure makes it possible to remove the segment which is injured or affected by tumor. The right, intermediate and left hepatic veins serve as guide to the planes between the hepatic divisions.

10. Ligaments of knee joint.

- **Fibrous capsule**
  - **Attachments:**
    - Proximal:
      * Posteriorly: Margins of intercondylar notch, 1cm above and parallel to medial and lateral condyles of femur
      * Anterior: It is deficient above patella.
    - Distal:
      * Posteriorly: Adjoining margins of medial, lateral condyles and intercondylar area of tibia
      * Anteriorly: Sides of triangular surface and tibial tuberosity, attached to margins of patella and blends with ligamentum patella.
- **Tibial collateral ligament**: Refer Short Notes 5 – 2003.
- **Fibular collateral ligament:**
  - **Attachment:** Lateral epicondyle of femur to head of fibula
  - **Morphology:** Degenerated part of peroneus longus
  - **Function:** Stability in extension and strengthens the lateral part of capsule
- **Ligamentum patella:**
  - **Attachment:** Apex of patella to tibial tuberosity
  - **Morphology:** Degenerated part of quadriceps femoris
- **Oblique popliteal ligament:**
  - **Attachment:** Forms floor of popliteal fossa. Medial condyle of tibia to lateral part of intercondylar line
  - **Morphology:** Expansion of semi-membranous
  - **Function:** Strengthens the posterior part of joint
- **Arcuate ligament:**
  - **Attachment:** Styloid process of head of fibula to lateral condyle of tibia (posterior band) and lateral condyle of femur (anterior band)
  - **Cruciate ligaments:** Refer short note Q. No. 2 – 2007.
- **Meniscofemoral ligament:**
  - Two in number, one anterior (ligament of Humphry), and other posterior (ligament of Wrisberg), related to the posterior cruciate ligament correspondingly.
  - **Attachment:** Extends from posterior end of lateral meniscus to the lateral surface of medial condyle of femur.
- **Menisci of knee joint**: Refer Short Notes Q. No. 20 – 2010.
- **Transverse ligament:**
  - **Attachment:** Anterior margin of lateral meniscus to anterior horn of medial meniscus
  - **Function:** Helps to decrease tension.

11. Flexor retinaculum.

Refer Short Notes 12 – 2012.

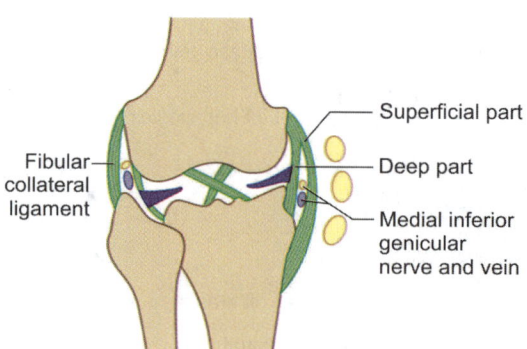

Fig. 13: Ligaments of knee joint.

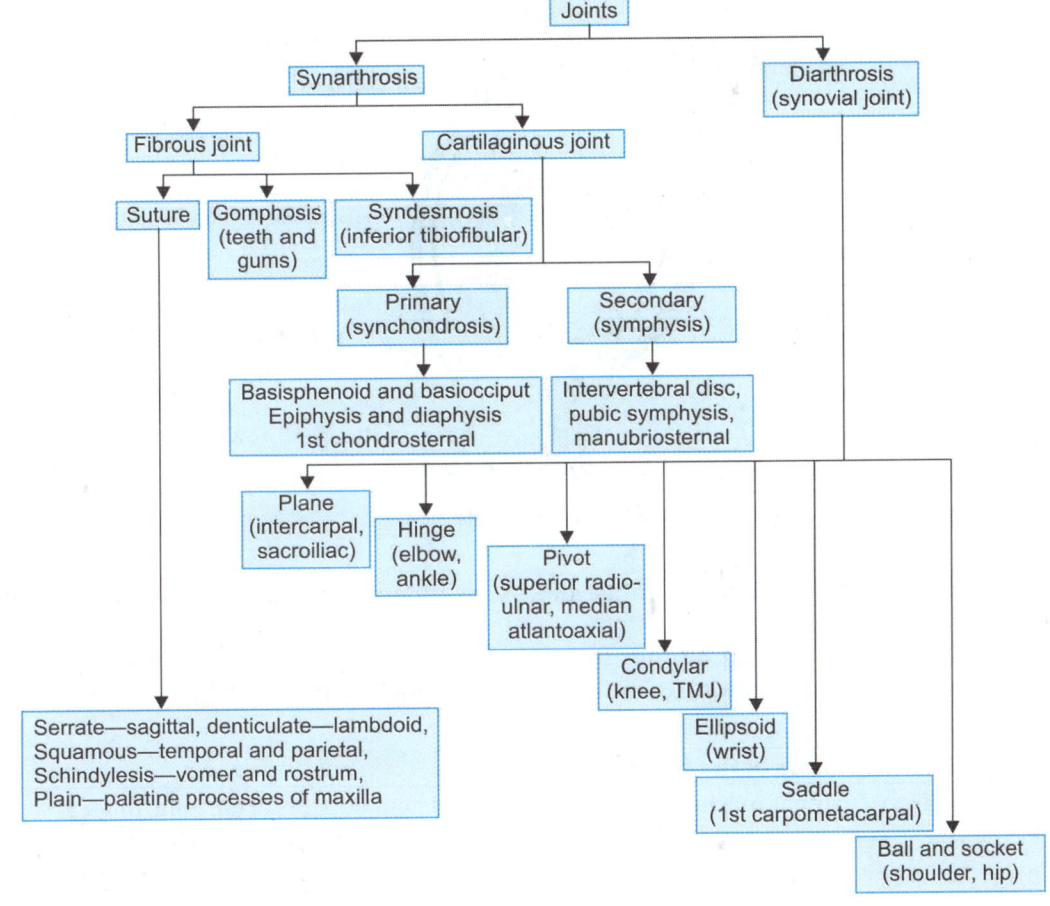

Fig. 14: Classification of joints.

12. Classify the joints of the body giving suitable examples and describe a typical synovial joint.

- Joints of the body are classified depending on structure and function.
- **Depending on structure intervening between the bones**
  - Fibrous
  - Cartilaginous
  - Synovial
- **Depending on movements**
  - Immovable (synarthrosis)
  - Movable (diarthrosis)
  - Synarthrosis is divided into fibrous and cartilaginous joints
  - Diarthrosis include the synovial joint
- **Depending on axis of movement**
  - Uniaxial joint
  - Biaxial joint
  - Multiaxial joint
- **Features of typical synovial joints (Fig. 15)**
  - Articular capsule covers the joint and supports it.
  - Articular cartilages made of hyaline cartilage are present covering the articular surfaces of the bones which reduces the friction during movements.
  - Joint cavity is present and is lined by synovial membrane.
  - Joint cavity is filled with synovial fluid secreted by the synovial membrane. Synovial fluid lubricates the articular surfaces and provides nutrition to the articular cartilages.

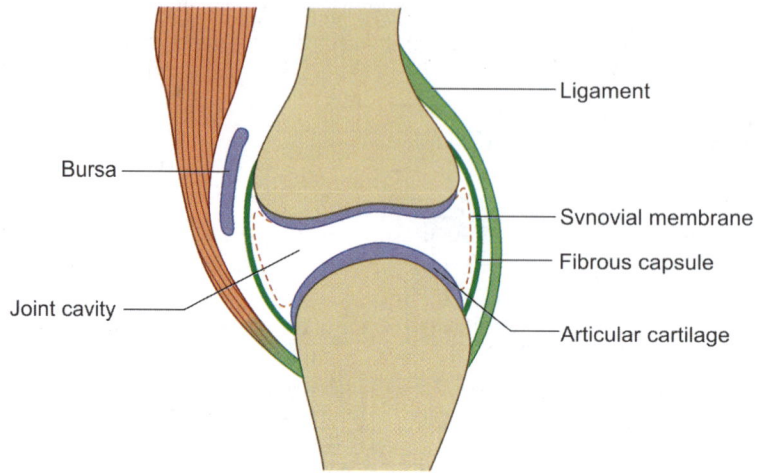

Fig. 15: Typical synovial joint.

- As there is joint cavity the range of movement is more.
- Joint receives arterial supply from periarticular arterial plexuses and are innervated by articular branches of the nerves
- A lymphatic plexus drains along blood vessels to the regional deep lymph nodes.

13. Short lateral rotators of the thigh

- Situated deep to gluteus maximus. All the muscles are lateral rotators of hip joint/thigh

S.No	Name of muscle	Origin	Insertion	Nerve supply
1	Piriformis	Front of sacrum, margin of greater sciatic notch, sacrotuberous ligament	Depression on the superior border of greater trochanter of femur	Branches from L5, S1 and 2
2	Obturator internus	Ramus of ischium and pubis, obturator membrane and fascia, pelvic surface of ilium	The impression which is anterosuperior to the trochanteric fossa, and lies on the greater trochanter along its medial surface	Nerve to obturator internus, L5 and S1
3	Gamelli	Superior: Posterior surface of ischial spine
Inferior: Upper part of the lateral surface of the tuberosity of ischium	Joins with the upper border of obturator internus tendon, and is inserted into the medial surface of the greater trochanter
Joins with the lower border of obturator internus tendon, and is inserted into the medial surface of the greater trochanter.	Nerve to obturator internus, L5, S1 and S2. Nerve to quadratus femoris, L4, L5 and S1
4	Quadratus femoris	Upper part of the external aspect of the ischial tuberosity	Tubercle above the middle of the trochanteric crest of the femur	Nerve to quadratus femoris, L4, L5 and S1
5	Obturator externus	External surface of the obturator membrane, pubic and ischial rami	Trochanteric fossa of the femur	Branch from posterior division of obturator nerve

- **Applied anatomy:** Piriformis syndrome: Due to the hypertrophy of the muscle piriformis, the sciatic nerve is compressed, resulting in pain along the course of the sciatic nerve in the gluteal region.

14. Ligaments of uterus.

Refer Essay on Q. No. 2 – 2004.

15. Eustachian tube.

It is also called as **pharyngotympanic tube** or **auditory tube**.
- **Function:** Provides communications between nasopharynx and the middle ear; and equalizes the pressure on either side of the tympanic membrane.
- **Length:** 36 mm
- **Direction:** Directed downwards forwards and medially and inclined at 45°
- **Ends**
  - Lateral end opens in the anterior wall of middle ear
  - Medial end opens on the lateral wall of nasopharynx, situated about 1.25 cm below and behind the inferior concha
- **Parts:** It has two parts:
1. **Outer bony part**
   - 12 mm in length.
   - It is related to the anterior wall of middle ear cavity.
   - Extends up to the junction of the squamous and petrous parts of the temporal bone.
   - The margins are irregular to give attachment to cartilaginous part
2. **Inner cartilaginous part:**
   - 24 mm in length.
   - It is triangular.
   - The apex attached to bony part and base opens into the lateral wall of nasopharynx.
   - It is related to base of skull and is lodged in the groove present between the petrous part of the temporal bone and the greater wing of the sphenoid.
   - It enters the nasopharynx by passing through sinus of Morgagni.
   - The opening is about 1.25 cm behind and just below the posterior end of inferior nasal concha.
   - It produces an elevation in the mucous membrane of nasopharynx called **tubal elevation** (torus tubarius/Eustachian cushion).
   - It is hook like in section, deficient below and laterally, and the gap is bridged by fibrous tissue.
   - The junction of bony and cartilaginous part is the narrowest part called **isthmus**, and greatest at cartilaginous opening.
- **Lining epithelium:** The mucous membrane of the tube is lined by ciliated columnar epithelium. Mucous glands are present in the cartilaginous part. Sometimes collection of lymphoid mass called the **tubal tonsil** present at tubal elevation.
- **In children:** The auditory tube is half the length of adult in newborn and is more

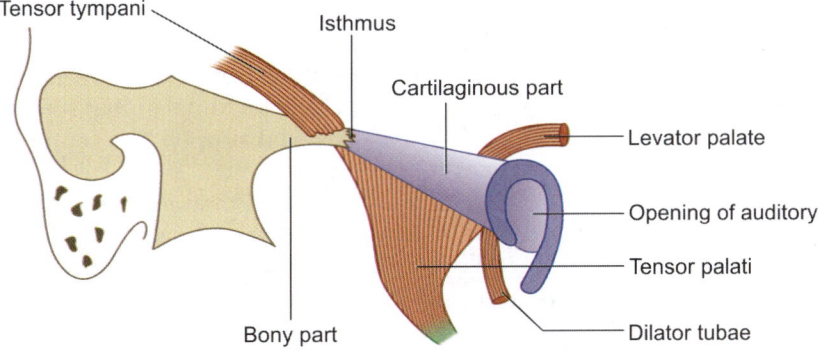

Fig. 16: Auditory tube.

horizontal. The pharyngeal opening is a slit, at the level of palate. Tubal elevation is not produced.
- **Relations:**
  - Anterolaterally—tensor veli palatine, mandibular nerve, chorda tympani, middle meningeal artery and otic ganglion
  - Posteromedially—levator veli palatine
- **Muscles attached**
  - Laterally some fibers of tensor palati arises from the tube called **dilator tubae**
  - Inferiorly salpingopharyngeus
  - Medially levator palati
- **Blood supply:** Ascending pharyngeal, middle meningeal and artery of pterygoid canal
- **Nerve supply:** Glossopharyngeal nerve through tympanic plexus and pharyngeal branch of pterygopalatine ganglion
- **Development:** From tubotympanic recess of first pharyngeal pouch
- **Applied anatomy:**
  - Auditory tube block for a longer period results in chronic otitis media.
  - Middle ear infections are common in children as the auditory tube is short and horizontal.

16. Typical intercostal nerve.
Refer Essay Q. No. 9 – 2006.

17. Lateral wall of nose.
Refer Short Notes 16 – 2004.

18. Midbrain at superior colliculus level.
Refer Short Notes 40 – 2009.

19. Ansa cervicalis.
Refer Short Notes 26 – 2008.

20. Ciliary ganglion.
Refer Short Notes 31 – 2009.

21. Parts, arterial supply of interventricular septum.

- It separates the right ventricle and left ventricle.
- It is obliquely placed
- The anterior and posterior interventricular groove indicates the attachment of the interventricular septum
- It bulges towards the right ventricle and so the right ventricle is crescentic and left ventricle is circular in shape.
- **Parts:** Its upper part is thinner called **membranous part** and the lower part is thicker called **muscular part**.
- **Membranous part:**
  - Extends from right aortic semilunar valve to the anterior cusp of bicuspid valve.
  - It connects the muscular part with fibrous rings surrounding the atrioventricular and aortic orifices.
  - The posterior part of the membranous septum is **atrioventricular septum** extending between right wall of aortic orifice to muscular wall of right atrium under the septal cusp of tricuspid valve
  - It is developed from right edge of septum intermedium
- **Muscular part:**
  - Thick extends from floor of the ventricle.
  - The development of the membranous part is different from muscular part and it may be deficient leaving an interventricular foramen inferior to aortic orifice
  - On the right surface of the septum, the **septomarginal band** passes from septum to anterior papillary muscle which carries the right crus of atrioventricular bundle (bundle of His).
  - Left surface carries left bundle branch of AV bundle
  - It is developed from ventricular septum and proximal bulbar septum.
- **Arterial supply:** The septum is **supplied** by:
  - Septal branches of anterior interventricular artery
  - Septal branches of posterior interventricular artery
  - The anterior two-third of interventricular septum is supplied by anterior

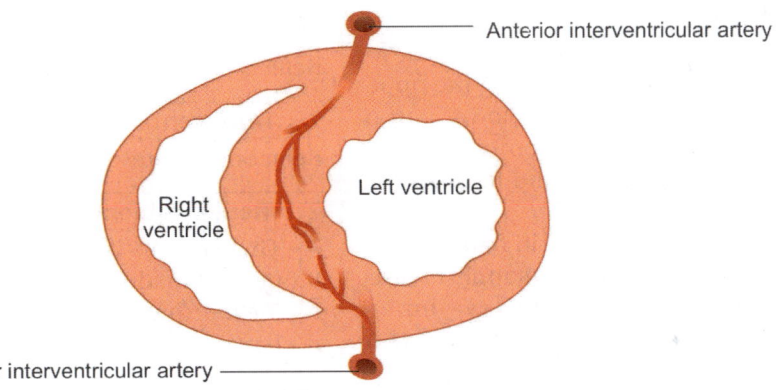

Fig. 17: Blood supply of interventricular septum.

interventricular branch of left coronary artery
- Posterior one-third by the posterior interventricular artery branch of right coronary artery.
- **Variation in blood supply:** In left coronary artery dominance the posterior interventricular artery arises from its circumflex branch. Hence in left dominance the entire septum is supplied by left coronary artery.
- **Applied anatomy:**
  - Ventricular septal defect (VSD):
    - Commonest congenital anomaly of the heart.
    - The defect commonly involves the membranous part of the interventricular septum.
    - It is due defect in partition of conotruncal region.
    - Interventricular septal defect in the muscular part is rare.

22. Cardiac plexus.
Refer Short Notes 17 – 2007.

23. Middle ear.
Refer Short Notes 37 – 2005.

24. Origin, termination, applied anatomy of internal mammary artery.

- **Origin:** Arises from inferior aspect of first part of subclavian artery about 2 cm above the sternal end of clavicle.
- **Course:**
  - Runs vertically downwards
  - 1 cm from lateral border of sternum
  - Terminates at sixth intercostal space
  - The venae comitantes accompany the artery.
- **Termination:** Divides into two terminal branches:
  1. Musculophrenic artery and
  2. Superior epigastric artery
- **Branches:**
  - Pericardiophrenic artery—accompanies phrenic nerve and supplies pericardium and diaphragm

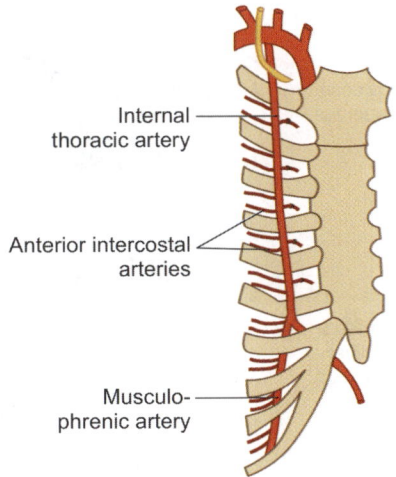

Fig. 18: Internal thoracic artery.

- Mediastinal arteries
- Two anterior intercostal arteries for upper six spaces. One along the upper part and other along the lower part of each space. They anastomose with the posterior intercostal and its collateral branch
- Perforating branches—in female 2nd – 4th branches enlarge to supply breast
- Superior epigastric artery—enters rectus sheath and anastomose with inferior epigastric artery
- Musculophrenic artery—provides anterior intercostal arteries for 7th – 9th spaces.

- **Applied Anatomy:**
  - In cardiac surgery, sometimes the internal thoracic artery is anastomosed with a coronary artery distal to the site of obstruction, in an attempt to improve coronary circulation
  - In coronary artery bypass surgery, the internal thoracic artery is used as a graft (LIMA Graft). Because, this artery has more elastic fibers in its wall and less prone to atherosclerosis.

25. Digastric triangle.
Refer Short Notes 37 – 2012.

26. Third ventricle.
Refer Short Notes 12 – 2003.

27. Medulla oblongata at mid olivary level.
- This section is in the upper part (open part) of medulla, which forms the floor of the fourth ventricle
- It passes through the olive.

Features
- **White matter:**
  - Deep to pyramid elevation, the corticospinal tract is seen as a bundle
  - Medial lemniscus (crossed sensory fibers of posterior column of spinal cord) dorsal to corticospinal tract
  - The section of inferior cerebellar peduncle, more laterally
  - Medial longitudinal bundle and tectospinal tract ventral to hypoglossal nucleus
  - Reticular formation situated lateral to medial lemniscus

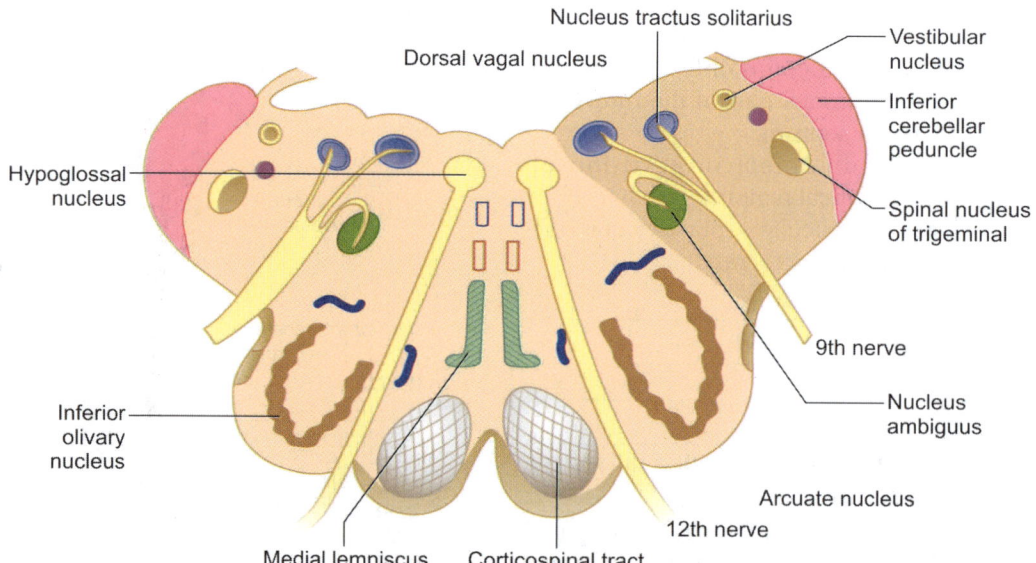

Fig. 19: Section of medulla oblongata at mid olive level.

- **Gray matter**
  - Ventral to pyramid is the arcuate nucleus, from which the external arcuate fibers arise
  - Deep to olive the inferior olivary nucleus is situated. The nucleus edges are crenate; the hilum faces medially. The nucleus is surrounded by a myelinated fibre called amiculum
  - The olivocerebellar tract starts from olivary nucleus, crosses to reach the cerebellum through inferior cerebellar peduncle
  - The medial and dorsal accessory olivary nuclei are situated close to inferior olivary nucleus
  - Deep to tuberculum cinerium the spinal nucleus and tract of trigeminal nerve
  - In the floor of fourth ventricle, the hypoglossal nucleus present deep to hypoglossal triangle
  - The hypoglossal nerve emerges between olive and pyramid in the anterolateral sulcus
  - Lateral to it the dorsal vagal nucleus deep to vagal triangle
  - Nucleus solitarius and tractus solitarius lateral to vagal nucleus
  - The vestibular nuclei deep to vestibular area
  - In the deep part of reticular formation nucleus ambiguus is present
  - The ambiguus nucleus is branchio-motor gives rise to 9th, 10th, and 11th cranial nerve fibers. These nerves emerge along the posterolateral sulcus, lateral to olive.
- **Applied anatomy:** Injury to medulla due to hard blow on the head may be fatal as the vital centers—the respiratory and cardiovascular are present in medulla
- **Lateral medullary syndrome:** Refer Short Notes on 38 – 2009.
- **Medial medullary syndrome.**
  - Also, called **anterior medullary syndrome/hypoglossal hemiplegia alternans**.
  - Vascular lesion due to anterior spinal artery
  - The hypoglossal nerve rootlets and corticospinal tract are affected
  - Lesion—contralateral hemiplegia with ipsilateral paralysis of tongue.

28. Superior mediastinum.

Refer Short Notes 38 – 2012.

III. SHORT ANSWER QUESTIONS

1. Mesentery.

Refer Short Notes 13 – 2008.

2. Cartilage.

- It is a modified connective tissue
- It forms skeletal framework for some parts of the body
- **Features:**
  - It is firm but not rigid like bone
  - It is **avascular**, limited ability to regenerate.

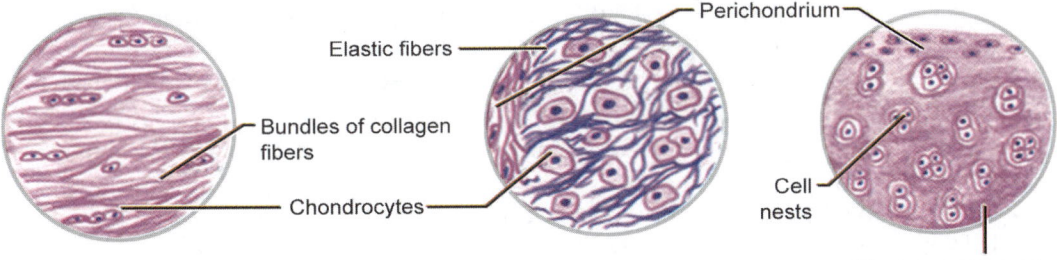

A Fibro cartilage **B** Elastic cartilage **C** Hyaline cartilage

Figs. 20A to C: Types of cartilage.

- The cells receive their nutrition by diffusion
- It has no nerves and is **insensitive**.
- **Microstructure:**
  - It is **made of** cells and matrix
  - The cells are called **chondrocytes**. They are surrounded by a space known as lacunae. The cells are provided with nucleus, mitochondria, golgi complex, and endoplasmic reticulum
  - The matrix is made of ground substance and fibers
  - The ground substance is made of molecules containing proteins and carbohydrates (proteoglycans), water and dissolved salts
  - The fibers are type II collagen. But in fibrous cartilage type I collagen is seen
  - The cartilage is surrounded by a fibrous membrane the **perichondrium**
- **Types of cartilage**: Hyaline, fibroelastic, elastic cartilages.
- **Differences:**

Features	Hyaline cartilage (Fig. 20C)	Elastic cartilage (Fig. 20B)	Fibrous cartilage (Fig. 20A)
Perichondrium	Present	Present	Absent
Matrix	Homogenous matrix, refractive index same as ground substance	Heterogeneous	Heterogeneous
Fibers	Collagen type II fibers	Elastic fibers	Collagen Type I fibers
Cells	Arranged in groups—cell nest	Singly	Rows of chondrocytes Cells are rounded
Ossification	Gets ossified	Does not ossify	Does not ossify

- **Distribution:**
  - **Hyaline cartilage** is present in costal cartilage, articular cartilage, thyroid, cricoid part of arytenoid cartilages of larynx, trachea, large bronchi, epiphyseal cartilage, septum of nose.
  - **Elastic cartilage** is seen in auricle, auditory tube, epiglottis, and part of arytenoid, cuneiform, cornuculate cartilages of larynx
  - **Fibrous cartilage** is present in secondary cartilaginous joints (symphysis), articular discs glenoidal labrum and acetabular labrum.
- **Applied anatomy:** Enchondroma, chondroblastoma are benign tumor.

3. Somites.

The intraembryonic mesoderm extends over whole of the embryonic area except in midline, prochordal plate and caudal to primitive streak.

- The mesoderm is divided by longitudinal groove into three parts **(Fig. 21)**.
  1. Paraxial mesoderm—on each side of notochord and developing neural tube
  2. Intermediate mesoderm—floor of longitudinal groove
  3. Lateral plate mesoderm—extends up to periphery.
- **Paraxial mesoderm:**
  - It extends from prochordal plate to primitive streak
  - It passes on either side of hindbrain, close to otic vesicle
  - The post otic part of paraxial mesoderm forms bilateral solid cords on either side of notochord
  - The paraxial mesoderm undergoes segmentation to form **somites or somitomere**
  - The process of segmentation extends craniocaudally
  - Somites appear between 20th to 30th days
  - Three pairs of somite appear each day.

Days	No. of somites
20 – 21	1 – 4
22 – 23	5 – 12
24 – 25	13 – 20
26 – 27	21 – 29
28 – 30	30 – 35

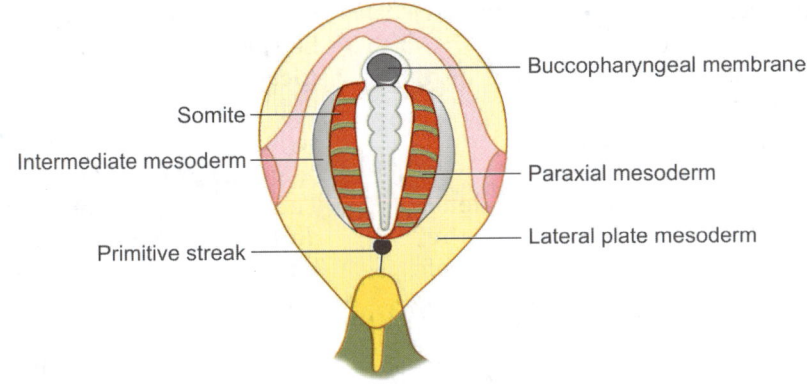

Fig. 21: Intraembryonic mesoderm.

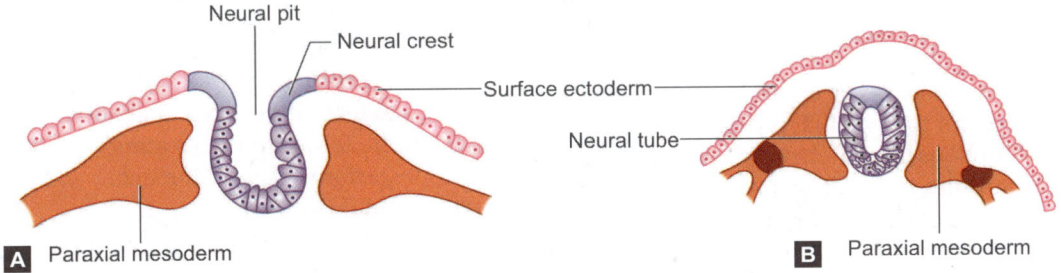

Figs. 22A and B: Divisions of intraembryonic mesoderm.

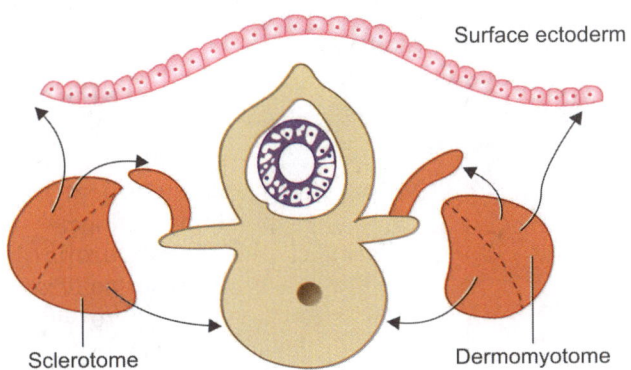

Fig. 23: Differentiation of somites.

- By end of 5th week there will be 44 pairs of somites.
- 44 pairs of somites are seen.
  - 4 occipital somites
  - 8 cervical
  - 12 thoracic
  - 5 lumbar
  - 5 sacral
  - 8 – 10 coccygeal
- The first occipital and 5 – 7 coccygeal somites disappear.
- **Differentiation of somites:**
  - Each somite divides into a ventromedial **sclerotome** and dorsolateral **dermomyotome.**
  - **Sclerotome** cells become polymorphous and migrate ventromedially around the notochord and neural

tube to form primitive vertebrae and ribs
- The **dermomyotome** is divided into **dermatome** and **myotome**
- The cells of dermal plate forms dermis of skin and subcutaneous tissue
- The myotome gives rise to skeletal muscle. The myotome forms the striated muscles of trunk, and most of the muscles of limbs
- The muscle is innervated by a spinal nerve and does not lose it even if the muscle migrates.

4. Wrist drop.

- It is a clinical condition due to lesion of the radial nerve, a nerve of posterior compartment of the arm and forearm
- The radial nerve arises from the posterior cord of the brachial plexus
- Supplies the extensors of arm and forearm muscles
- The root value is $C_5 - C_8, T_1$
- **Course:**
  - It runs along posterior wall of the axilla lies posterior to third part of axillary artery
  - It enters the posterior compartment of arm along with the profunda brachii vessels by passing through the lower triangular space

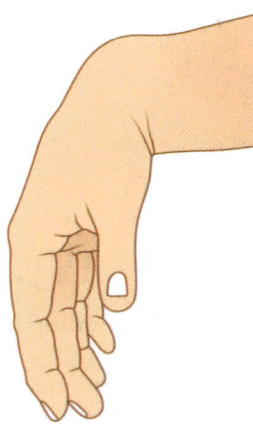

Fig. 24: Wrist drop.

- Enters the spiral groove of humerus between the lateral and medial head of triceps
- It pierces the lateral intermuscular septum and reaches the front of lateral epicondyle of humerus
- The nerve terminates into superficial and deep (posterior interosseous) branches
- **The deep branch** called posterior interosseous nerve passes through two heads of the supinator and supplies the extensors of forearm.

- **Level and cause of injury**
  - In the arm:
    - Fracture of humerus (nerve in spiral groove)
    - Fracture shaft of humerus proximal to termination of radial nerve.
  - In the forearm: Penetrating wounds of posterior surface of forearm
- **Effect of lesion:**
  - The person affected by this, assumes a flexed position of wrist
  - The wrist and hand drop
- **Reasoning the effect of lesion:**
  - Wrist drops due to paralysis of extensor carpi radialis longus and brevis and extensor carpi ulnaris
  - Hand drops due to paralysis of extensor digitorum and so there is loss of extension at metacarpophalangeal joints of fingers
  - Thumb drops due to paralysis of extensor pollicis longus and brevis
  - When there is injury in the spiral groove the triceps will not be completely paralysed, only weakness of muscle. Because medial head of triceps alone will be affected.

5. Histology of ovary.

Refer Short Notes 11 – 2007.

6. Stomach bed.

- The relations of posteroinferiorly surface of stomach is known as stomach bed
- It is covered with peritoneum of lesser sac

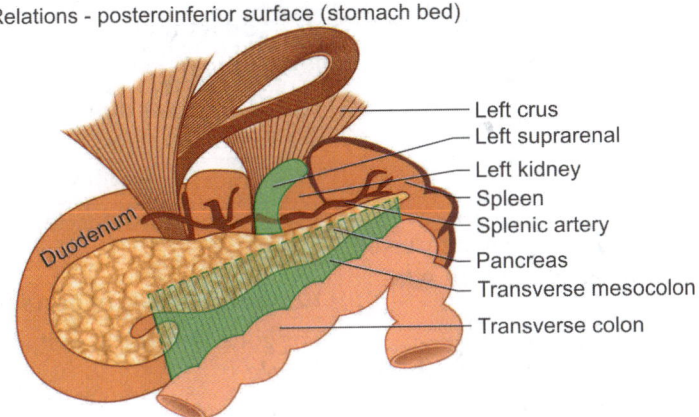

Fig. 25: Stomach bed.

- The **lesser sac separates** the stomach from stomach bed structures
- **Function:** Allows the stomach to slide whenever there is distension
- The **bed is formed** by:
  - Left crus and dome of diaphragm
  - Left suprarenal gland
  - Anterior surface of left kidney
  - Splenic artery
  - Anterior surface of pancreas
  - Anterior layer of transverse mesocolon
  - Gastric area of spleen
  - Inferior phrenic vessels

- **Applied anatomy:**
  - Perforation of posterior wall of stomach can result in accumulation of fluid in the omental bursa
  - Inflamed or injured pancreas can result in pseudopancreatic cyst which is due to collection of pancreatic fluids in the lesser sac.

7. Axillary vein.

- Axillary vein lies outside the axillary sheath.

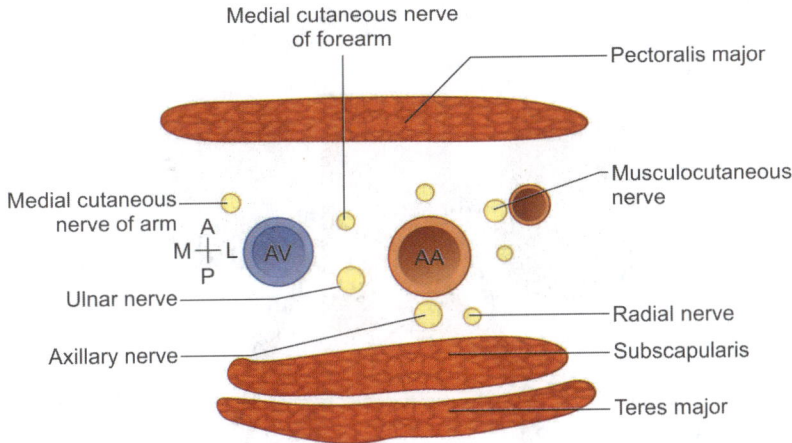

Fig. 26: Relations of axillary vein.

- **Formation:** Continuation of basilic vein from the level of lower border of teres major
- **Termination:** Continued as subclavian vein from outer border of 1st rib. A valve present near termination
- **Relations:**
  - Medially—medial cutaneous nerve of arm, lateral group of axillary lymph nodes
  - Laterally—axillary artery
  - Between artery and vein—medial cord of brachial plexus, medial cutaneous nerve of forearm, ulnar nerve, medial pectoral nerve.
- **Tributaries:** Brachial vein, cephalic vein, veins accompanying branches of axillary artery
- **Applied anatomy:**
  - Axillary arch—a muscular band extending from latissimus dorsi near its insertion across the axillary vein to the pectoralis major compresses the vein leading to thrombosis of the axillary vein
  - Thrombosis of axillary vein at the apex of the axilla may occur due to traction, as seen in people who keep the arm hyperabducted for a prolonged period.

8. Developmental anomalies of kidney.

Refer Short Notes 10 – 2006.

9. Adductor canal.

Refer Short Notes 3 – 2006.

10. Boundaries and contents of popliteal fossa.

Refer Short Notes 8 – 2009.

11. Clavipectoral fascia.

Refer Short Notes 5 – 2006.

12. Blood supply of gonads.

The gonads are testis in male, and ovary in the female.

Testis

Arterial supply:
- Main artery is testicular artery from abdominal aorta
- In addition, it is also supplied by artery to vas branch from superior vesical artery.

Venous drainage: Pampiniform plexus of veins helps for countercurrent heat exchange. At superficial inguinal ring join to form four veins. In turn it forms two veins at deep inguinal ring. In the posterior abdominal wall, a testicular vein is formed. The right vein drains to IVC and left to left renal vein.

Ovary

Arterial supply:
- Ovarian artery branch from abdominal aorta

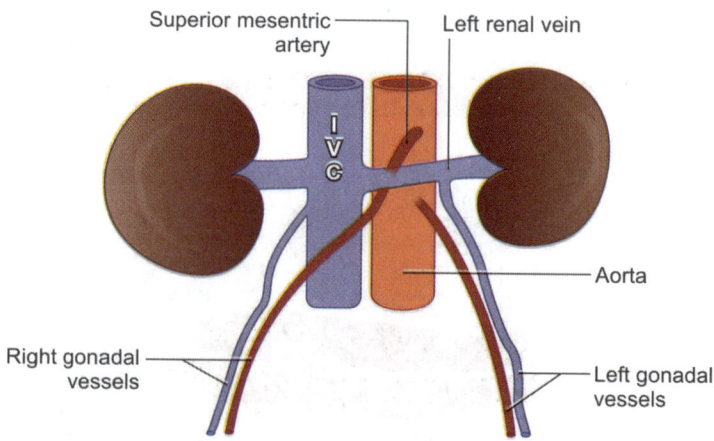

Fig. 27: Blood supply of gonads.

- In addition, partly supplied by uterine artery of internal iliac artery
- **Venous drainage:** The venous plexus joins to form single vein in the suspensory ligament of ovary. Right vein joins IVC and left drains to left renal vein.

Applied Anatomy

- Varicocele of left testicular vein is more common than the right side.
- The reasons are
  - Left vein is longer than right
  - The vein ends at right angles to left renal vein
  - The compression effect of the left renal vein between aorta and superior mesenteric artery – nutcracker/left renal vein entrapment syndrome
  - Pressure effect by loaded sigmoid colon.

13. Quadrangular space.
Refer Short Notes 13 – 2007.

14. Cryptorchism.
Refer Short Notes 8 – 2007.

15. Histology of duodenum.
Refer Short Notes 9 – 2004.

16. Perineal body.
Refer Short Notes 8 – 2004.

17. Gluteus medius.
Refer Short Notes 9 – 2013.

18. Results of fertilization.

- Fertilization is a process of fusion of mature male and female gametes
- Diploid zygote is formed
- It occurs in the ampulla of the uterine tube
- Before fusion the spermatozoa undergo capacitation and acrosomal reaction to acquire the capacity to fuse

The **effects of fertilization** are:
- Restoration of diploid number of chromosomes: Half of chromosome from father and half from mother and the number is 44 + sex chromosome (XY/XX)
- Completion of second meiotic division of ova: Meiosis II is initiated but arrested at metaphase 3 hours before ovulation. So completion of second meiotic division is only after fertilization.

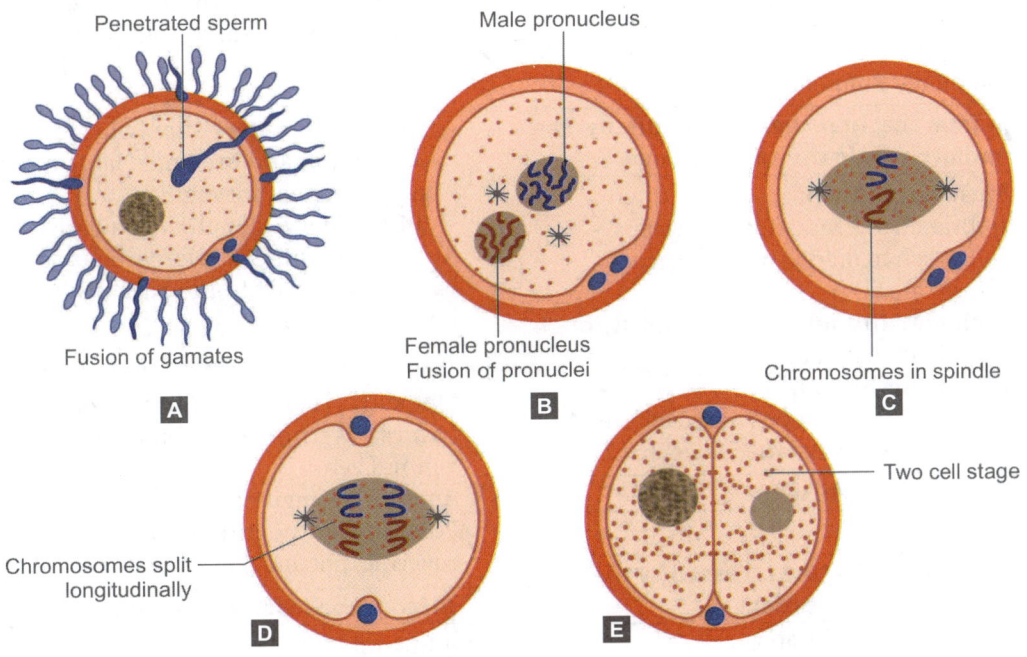

Figs. 28A to E: Changes after fertilization.

- Initiation of cleavage: If there is no fertilization the oocyte degenerates 24 hours after ovulation. The zygote when it reaches two cell stage then undergoes series of mitotic divisions
- Sex determination: Chromosomal sex determination is depending on sperm. The sperm with Y chromosome results in male child and X chromosome female child
- It prevents polyspermy by producing the vitelline block
- The line of entry of spermatozoa decides the plane of cleavage division, polarity and cephalocaudal axis.

19. Skin.
Refer Short Notes 20 – 2011.

20. Sciatic nerve.
Refer Essay Q. No. 5 – 2007.

21. Name the thenar muscles.
- The muscles which act on the thumb are grouped as **thenar muscles**
- Flexor pollicis brevis
- Abductor pollicis brevis
- Opponens pollicis
- Adductor pollicis
- The adductor pollicis does not take part in the thenar eminence.

22. Name the branches given off by the radial nerve in the spiral groove.
- **Muscular branches:**
  - Branch to lateral head of triceps
  - Branch to medial head of triceps
  - Anconeus.
- **Articular branch:** Elbow joint through branch to anconeus
- **Cutaneous branch**
  - Posterior cutaneous nerve of forearm
  - Lower lateral cutaneous nerve of arm.

23. Meckel's diverticulum.
Refer Short Notes 12 – 2005.

24. Name the structures crossed by the root of mesentery in order.
Refer Short Notes 13 – 2008.

25. Parts of fallopian tube.
Refer Short Answer Questions 17 – 2010.

26. Name the bones that form the first carpometacarpal joint.
Distal surface of trapezium and base of first metacarpal bone.

27. Boundaries of epiploic foramen.
Refer Short Answer Questions 14 – 2009.

28. Constituents of quadriceps femoris.
Refer Short Answer Questions 9 – 2012.

29. Root value, branches and applied anatomy of pudendal nerve.
- **Root value**—from sacral plexus—ventral division of ventral rami of S2, S3, S4
- **Branches:**
  - **Muscular branches** supplies the superficial transverse perineii, bulbospongiosus, ischiocavernosus, deep transverse perineii, sphincter urethrae and the anterior parts of the external anal sphincter and levator ani
  - In males, the corpus spongiosum penis and the urethral mucosa are supplied by **nerve to the bulb of the urethra**
  - **Inferior rectal nerve**—supplies external sphincter, lower part of anal canal, perianal skin
  - **Perineal branch**—supply in male skin of scrotum and in female labia majora and lower part of vagina
  - **Dorsal nerve of penis/clitoris.**
- **Applied anatomy:** The nerve block is done by infiltration with a local anesthetic to numb the perineal and anal skin.

30. Name the boundaries of femoral ring.
- Medially—lacunar/Gimbernat's ligament
- Laterally—the septa separating the femoral vein
- Anteriorly—inguinal ligament
- Posteriorly—pectineus and the fascia covering, pectineal ligament.

31. Inferior constrictor of pharynx.
Refer Essay 8 – 2006.

32. Blood supply of spinal cord.
Refer Short Answer Questions 45 – 2011.

33. Carotid sheath.
Refer Short Notes 40 – 2010.

34. Left brachiocephalic vein.
Refer Short Notes 29 – 2011.

35. Histology of thyroid gland.
Refer Essay Q. No. 8 – 2007.

36. Parkinsonism.

- It is a clinical condition due to lesion in corpus striatum
- It is also called as paralysis agitans
- It is due to deficiency of dopamine in corpus striatum
- Corpus striatum includes caudate nucleus, and lentiform nucleus
- Lentiform nucleus is divided into outer putamen and inner globus pallidus
- **Mechanism of action:**
  - The dopamine secreted acts in pathways
  - The pathway is: Dopamine—acts on GABA – SP neurons in putamen which in turn acts on pallidum thereby reducing the inhibition of thalamocortical neurons. This leads to facilitation of movements.
- **Connections:**
  - **Afferent fibers:**
    - Corticostriate fibers—from entire neocortex to caudate nucleus, putamen
    - Thalamostriate fibers from centromedian nucleus of thalamus to caudate nucleus and putamen
    - Nigrostriate fibers from caudate and putamen to substantia nigra called comb bundle
    - Pallidum receives fibers from striatum, substantia nigra.
  - **Efferent fibers:**
    - Striatonigral fibers from striatum to substantia nigra
    - Fasciculus lenticularis—pallidum to subthalamic nucleus
    - Fasciculus subthalamicus—from globus pallidus to subthalamic nucleus.
- Dopamine secreted by substantia nigra is carried to corpus striatum by the nigrostriate fibers
- **Reason:** The disease is due to reduction of secretion of dopamine leads to degeneration of neurons of substantia nigra or nigrostriate fibers.

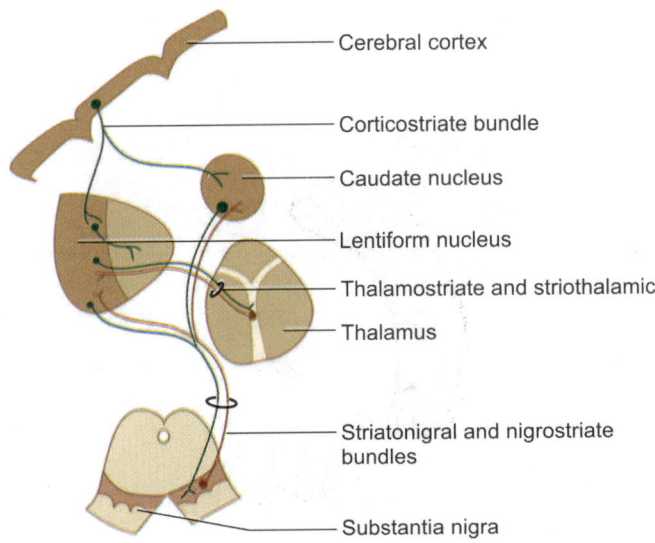

Fig. 29: Connections of corpus striatum.

- **Effect of lesion**:
  - Increased muscle tone leading to rigidity, tremors, abnormal movements. This occurs due to increased activity in globus pallidus which causes increased inhibition of thalamocortical neurons
  - Akinesia—slow movement
  - Cogwheel or lead pipe rigidity
  - Pill rolling movement
  - Mask like face
  - Shuffling gait
  - Stopped posture.

37. Pterygopalatine ganglion.
Refer Short Notes 23 – 2012.

38. Structures present at T4 level.
- T4 corresponds to sternal angle
- It lies at the junction of manubrium and body of sternum
- **Events occurring at this level are:**
  - The plane that divides the superior and inferior mediastinum passes through T4
  - 2nd costal cartilages are attached to the sternum at this level and hence useful in counting the ribs
  - Azygos vein arches over the root of the lung and drains into the superior vena cava
  - Ascending aorta ends at this level
  - Arch of aorta begins and ends at this level
  - Descending aorta begins at this level
  - Trachea bifurcates into two principal bronchi at this level
  - Pulmonary trunk bifurcates below this level
  - The discontinuous dermatomes, C4 segment above and T2 segment below at this level
  - Superior vena cava pierces the fibrous pericardium
  - Anterior margins of both the lungs and pleurae approximate at this level.

39. Hilum of right lung.
Refer Essay Q. No. 3 – 2004.

40. Development of pituitary gland.
Refer Short Answer Questions 42 – 2012.

41. Orbicularis oculi muscle.
- It is one of the muscle of facial expression, **developed** from 2nd branchial arch
- It is a muscle which surrounds the circumference of the orbit and eyelids and extends to anterior temporal, infraorbital cheek and superciliary regions.
- **Parts:**
  - Orbital part
  - Palpebral part
  - Lacrimal part.

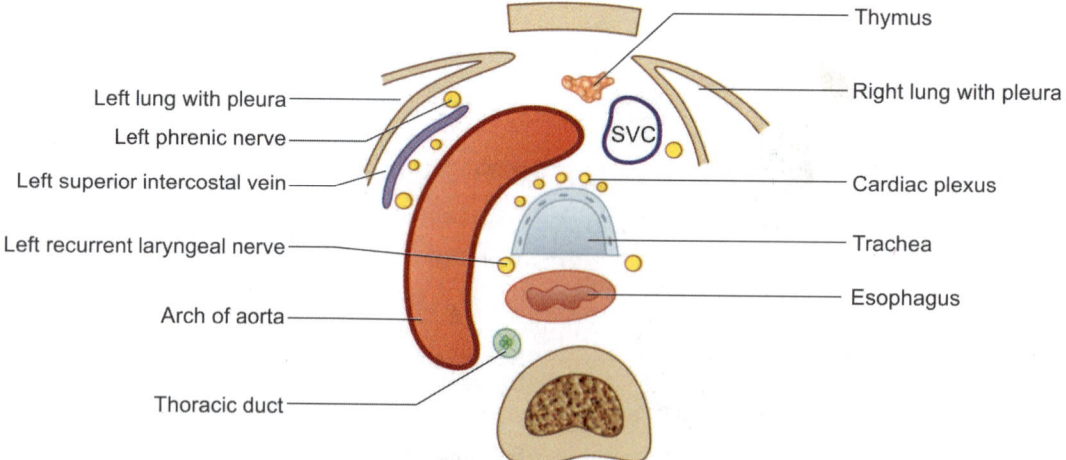

Fig. 30: Section at the level of T4.

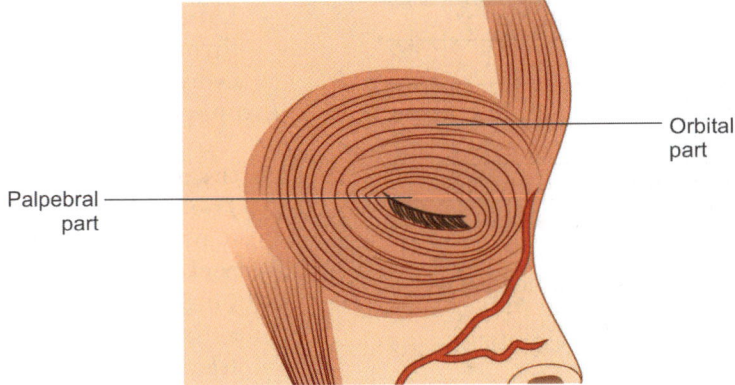

Fig. 31: Parts of orbicularis oculi.

- **Attachments:**
  - **Orbital part:**
    - *Origin:* Nasal process of the frontal bone, the frontal process of the maxilla and from the medial palpebral ligament
    - *Insertion:* Winds around the orbital margin to forms a complete circle and are inserted into the skin and subcutaneous tissue of the eyebrow.
  - **Palpebral part:**
    - *Origin:* From the medial palpebral ligament, and from the adjacent bone above and below the ligament
    - *Insertion:* The fibres pass across the eyelids, decussate at the lateral angle of eye to form the lateral palpebral raphe.
  - **Lacrimal part:**
    - It is also known as **Horner's muscle**.
    - *Origin:* Arises from the superior part of the lacrimal crest, and the lateral surface of the lacrimal bone
    - *Insertion:* Passes laterally and divides into two as upper and lower slips posterior to the nasolacrimal sac and are inserted into the tarsi of the corresponding eyelids.
- **Nerve supply:** Temporal and zygomatic branches of the facial nerve

- **Actions:**
  - Orbital fibers helps in narrowing of the palpebral fissure, thereby the amount of light entering the eye is reduced
  - Upper orbital fibres contract to produce vertical folds above the bridge of the nose
  - The palpebral portion gentle closure of the eyelids as in sleep, or reflexly as in blinking
  - The lacrimal part of the muscle pulls the eyelids and the lacrimal papillae medially, and so the lacrimal sac is dilated and helps in drainage of tears
  - When the entire orbicularis oculi muscle contracts, produces folds in the skin which extend from the lateral angle of the eyelids ('crow's feet').
- **Applied anatomy:**
  - Paralysis of orbital part produces inability to close the eyelid leading to dryness of cornea and exposure keratitis
  - Paralysis of lacrimal part produces loss of dilation of lacimal sac. Hence tear fluid accumulates in conjunctival sac and dripples through palpebral fissure called epiphora
  - The lower eyelid falls away from eyeball (ectropion).

42. Blood supply of thyroid gland.

Refer Short Notes 38 – 2008.

43. Azygos vein.
Refer Short Notes 21 – 2011.

44. Pleural recesses.
Refer Essay Q. No. 3 – 2003.

45. Histology of thymus.
- It is a lymphoid organ situated in superior mediastinum
- It is covered by a fibrous connective tissue capsule
- The thymus is divided into lobules by the septae from capsule
- Each lobule is made up of outer **cortex** and inner **medulla**
- The lobules are incomplete and the medulla is continuous with adjacent lobule
- The cells present in the thymus are epitheliocytes, lymphocytes, non-lymphocytic cells
    - **Epitheliocytes**:
        - The supportive framework is formed by reticular epitheliocytes derived from pharyngeal endoderm
        - The epitheliocytes form a continuous sheet on which the cells are arranged
        - Epitheliocytes vary in size and shape depending on the position within the thymus
        - Large epitheliocytes are called thymic **nurse cells** as many thymocytes are attached to it.
    - **Lymphocytes**:
        - The lymphocytes are called as **thymocytes**
        - The cortex is made of mainly T lymphocytes which are densely packed
        - The medulla contains loosely arranged lymphocytes
        - **Hassall's corpuscles** are seen in the medulla, start appearing before birth and increase in number throughout life
        - The corpuscles contain cellular debris, degenerating thymocytes forming a homogenous eosinophilic mass encircled by concentrically arranged epitheliocytes.
    - The other **nonlymphocytic cells** present are: i) mature macrophages, monocytes, present more in cortex, ii) fibroblasts present in perivascular space, capsule and medulla, and iii) myoid cells in medulla.

46. Boundaries and contents of suboccipital triangle.
- It is a triangle situated back of neck, below the occipital bone

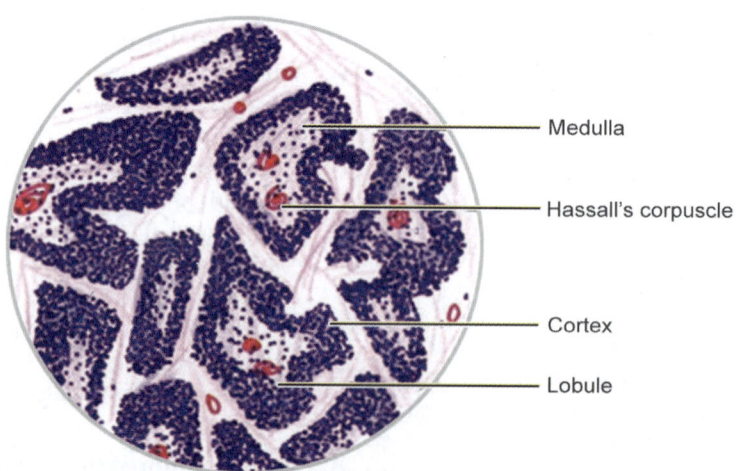

Fig. 32: Histology of thymus.

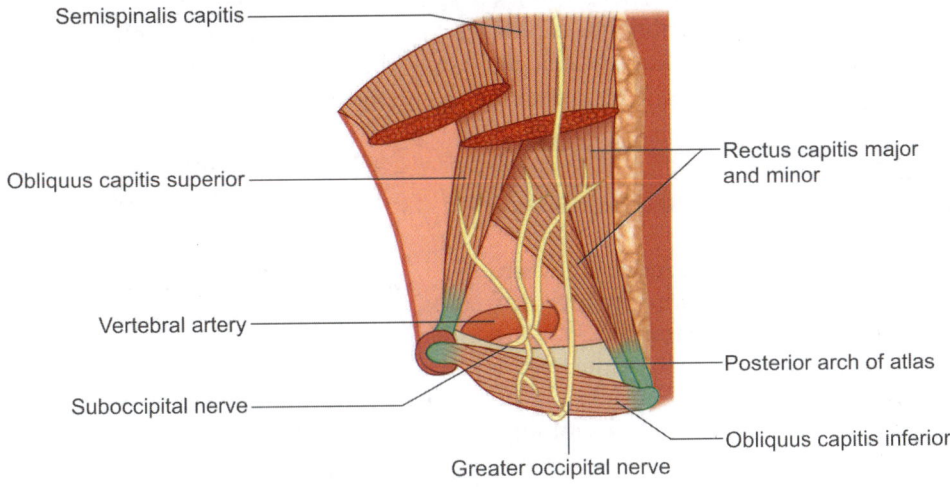

Fig. 33: Suboccipital triangle.

- **Boundaries:**
  - *Medially:* Rectus capitis posterior minor, and major
  - *Superolaterally:* Obliquus capitis superior
  - *Inferolaterally:* Obliquus capitis inferior
  - *Floor:* Posterior-atlanto-occipital membrane, and posterior arch of atlas
  - *Roof:* Dense connective tissue, semispinalis capitis.

- **Contents:**
  - **3rd part of vertebral artery**—passes from foramen transversarium of atlas to the foramen magnum. It is separated from the posterior arch of atlas by the suboccipital nerve
  - **Suboccipital nerve:** Refer Short Answer Questions 32 – 2012
  - **Suboccipital plexus of veins**—draining the posterior part of scalp

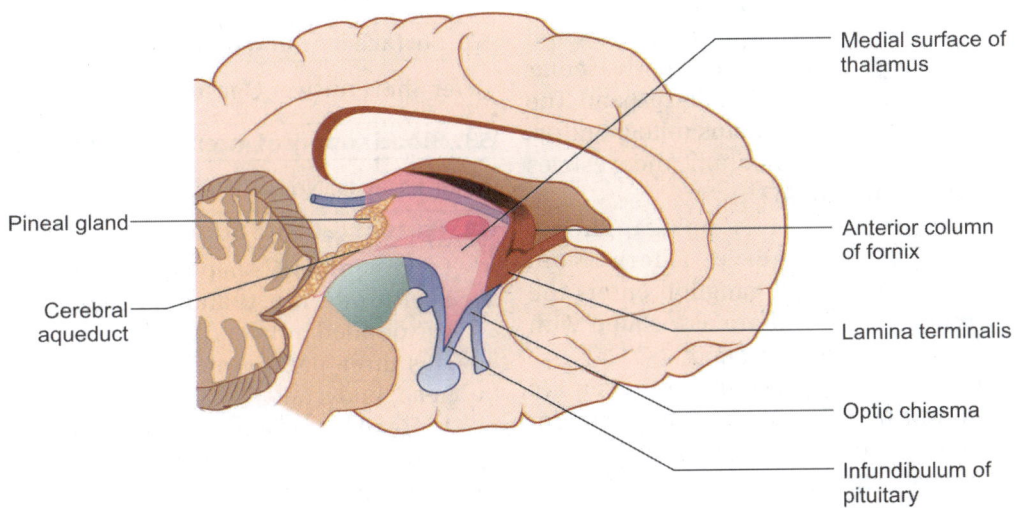

Fig. 34: Pineal gland and its relations.

- **Greater occipital nerve** (DR C2) hooks around lower border of obliquus capitis inferior, receives a communicating twig from suboccipital nerve. It ascends up to supply the scalp.

47. Pineal gland.

- It is also known as **epiphysis cerebri**
- It is **part** of epithalamus
- It is situated in the pineal recess between the superior colliculi and below the splenium of corpus callosum
- It is attached by a stalk which is attached to the posterior wall of third ventricle
- The stalk divides into two—superior and inferior laminae
- The two laminae are separated by the pineal recess
- The laminae contain posterior and Habenular commissure
- The gland is **supplied** by posterior choroidal branches from posterior cerebral artery
- It is covered by pia mater
- **Microscopic structure**:
  - From pia septae extend inside and divides the gland into lobules
  - It contains pinealocytes arranged as cords, and neuroglial cells
  - The pinealocytes are highly modified neurons
  - The processes of the pinealocytes extend from cell body towards perivascular spaces and the terminal part expand. The expanded part contains mitochondria, endoplasmic reticulum and vesicles storing melatonin
  - **Nervus conarii** is postganglionic sympathetic nerve fibers from superior cervical ganglion enters the pineal gland and are associated with parenchyma of the gland
  - Brain sand or **corpora arenacea** are found in old age which are calcium deposits in extracellular matrix of the pineal gland.
- **Functions:**
  - It is an endocrine gland
  - Secretes serotonin and melatonin
  - It controls the pituitary, endocrine part of pancreas, parathyroid, adrenal and gonads and is inhibitory in action
  - The melatonin is associated with circadian rhythm and is influenced by light.
- **Applied anatomy:** Pinealomas—causes delayed puberty, depression of gonadal functions.

48. Lateral medullary syndrome.

Refer Short Notes 38 – 2009.

49. Lumbar puncture.

Refer Short Notes 34 – 2008.

50. Development of tongue.

Refer Short Notes 20 – 2003.

51. Formation of basal vein.

- Basal vein is one of the external cerebral vein: It is formed by
  - Deep middle cerebral vein which drains the insula
  - The anterior cerebral vein drains medial surface of cerebrum
  - Striate veins
- **Level of formation:** Formed in the region of anterior perforated substance.

52. Surface marking of apex beat of heart.

Refer Short Answer Questions 33 – 2013.

53. Blood supply of internal capsule.

Refer Essay Q. No. 6 – 2006.

54. Parts of caudate nucleus.

- Large comma/C-shaped gray matter
- Surrounds the thalamus and itself is surrounded by lateral ventricle
- Has three parts: Anterior to posterior—head, body, tail
  1. **Head:** Large and rounded. Forms floor of antetrior horn of lateral ventricle. It is connected to lentiform nucleus

2. **Body:** Forms floor of central part of lateral ventricle
3. **Tail:** Forms roof of the inferior horn of lateral ventricle. It ends in amygdaloid body.

55. Dangerous area of scalp.

Refer Short Answer 32 – 2013.

56. Patent ductus arteriosus.

- Ductus arteriosus is formed from dorsal part of left 6th aortic arch
- It connects in fetal life the left pulmonary artery and arch of aorta distal to origin of left subclavian artery
- The duct is closed functionally soon after birth by contraction of muscular wall of the artery
- Anatomical closure occurs 3 months after birth by proliferation of tunica intima
- It forms about 10% of cardiac defects
- Patent ductus arteriosus is due to failure of obliteration of ductus arteriosus
- If there is failure of closure, a shunt is established between the arch of aorta and left pulmonary artery
- It is more common in females and in population living in high altitude.

57. Formation and distribution of spinal part of the accessory nerve.

- Formed by the ventral rami of $C_1 - C_5$
- It enters the cranial cavity through the foramen magnum
- It joins with the cranial part of accessory nerve
- It emerges out from cranial cavity through jugular foramen
- It separates from the cranial part as it passes through the jugular foramen
- It supplies the sternocleidomastoid and trapezius muscles.

58. Name any four branches of external carotid artery.

Refer Short Answer Questions 39 – 2012.

59. Define typical intercostals nerve with example.

Refer Essay Q. No. 9 – 2006.

60. Tributaries of cavernous sinus.

Refer Essay Q. No. 5 – 2008.

MBBS Examination 2015

ANSWER ALL QUESTIONS

I. Essay questions   (15/10 Marks)

1. Describe the root value, course, relations branches and distribution and applied anatomy of sciatic nerve.
2. Describe the type, ligaments, relations, movements and muscles producing the movements and applied anatomy of hip joint.
3. Describe the position, peritoneal and visceral relations, supports, microstructure and applied anatomy of uterus.
4. Describe the origin, course, relations, branches, and clinical anatomy of abducent nerve.
5. Classify dural venous sinuses. Describe the cavernous sinus in detail. Add a note on its applied anatomy.
6. Describe the blood supply of heart. Add a note on its clinical significance.

II. Short notes   (5/4 Marks)

1. Radioulnar joint.
2. Vermiform appendix.
3. Superior mesenteric artery.
4. Formation and branches of brachial plexus.
5. Axillary artery.
6. Ligaments of knee joint.
7. Draw a labeled diagram of blood supply of thyroid gland with its development.
8. Left coronary artery.
9. Nucleus, course, distribution and applied anatomy of hypoglossal nerve.
10. Blood supply of brain.
11. Lacrimal apparatus.
12. Sulci, gyri, and functional areas of Superolateral surface of cerebrum.

III. Short answer questions   (3/2 Marks)

1. Histology of cardiac muscle.
2. Blood supply of pancreas.
3. Spermatogenesis.
4. Rotator cuff.
5. Histology of suprarenal gland.
6. Supports of uterus.
7. Flexor retinaculum of hand.
8. Cloaca and its derivatives.
9. Popliteus muscle.
10. Cruciate anastomosis.
11. Ossification.
12. Spermatic cord.
13. Carpal tunnel syndrome.
14. Histology of kidney.
15. Notochord.
16. Rectouterine pouch.
17. Biceps brachii muscle.
18. Annular pancreas.
19. Peripheral heart.
20. Great saphenous vein.
21. Median nerve in hand.
22. Rectus sheath.
23. Hamstring muscles.
24. Microscopic anatomy of lymph node.
25. Pronation and supination.
26. Second part of duodenum.
27. Synovial joints.
28. Deep peroneal nerve.
29. Development of kidney.
30. Winging of scapula.
31. Histological layers of cornea.
32. Cricoid cartilage characteristic features.
33. Branches of descending thoracic aorta.
34. Pleural recesses.

35. Waldeyer's ring.
36. Buccinator muscle.
37. Subclavian vein formation course and termination.
38. Derivatives of neural tube.
39. Area of epistaxis.
40. Thoracic duct area of drainage.
41. Nasal septum.
42. Floor of fourth ventricle.
43. Histology of the palatine tonsil.
44. Otic ganglion.
45. Cross sectional diagram of typical intercostal space.
46. Fallot's tetralogy.
47. Corpus callosum.
48. Interior of right atrium.
49. Boundaries and content of posterior mediastinum.
50. Muscles of tongue.
51. Falx cerebri.
52. Superior laryngeal nerve.
53. Histology of cerebellum.
54. Muscles of mastication.
55. Development of interatrial septum.
56. Maxillary sinus.
57. Basilar artery.
58. Vocal cord.
59. Bell's palsy.
60. Bronchopulmonary segments.

I. ESSAY QUESTIONS

1. **Describe the root value, course, relations branches and distribution and applied anatomy of sciatic nerve.**

Refer Essay Q. No. 5 – 2007.

2. **Describe the type, ligaments, relations, movements and muscles producing the movements and applied anatomy of hip joint.**

Refer essay Q. No. 1 – 2004.
Relations Refer Essay Q. No. 3 – 2008.

3. **Describe the position, peritoneal and visceral relations, supports, microstructure and applied anatomy of uterus.**

Refer Essay Q. No. 2 – 2004.
Microstructure Refer Essay Q. No. 3 – 2006.

4. **Describe the origin, course, relations, branches, and clinical anatomy of abducent nerve.**

- Abducent nerve is the sixth cranial nerve.
- It is motor in nature
- **Supplies the** lateral rectus of the extraocular muscle which is **developed** from 5th somitomere
- It has a long subarachnoid course.

Functional Component

Somatic efferent—supplies lateral rectus
- **Origin:**
  – Arises from abducent nucleus situated in lower pons deep to facial colliculus in the floor of fourth ventricle
  – The nucleus is surrounded by the loop of facial nerve.

Course and Relations

- Intrapontine part **(Fig. 1):** From the nucleus, the nerve fibers pass through pons, ventrally through the corticospinal fibers and emerges along the pontomedullary junction just above the pyramid of the medulla
- The course of the nerve after it emerges from pons is **divided** into four segments:
  1. **Cisternal segment (Fig. 2)**
     - It enters the pontine cistern, and is called **cisternal segment**
     - After emerging from the brainstem it runs upwards, forwards, and laterally and is dorsal to anterior inferior cerebellar artery
     - The two abducent nerves are separated by the basilar artery.
  2. **Petroclival segment (intracranial course)**
     - It pierces the dura mater lateral to dorsum sellae of sphenoid bone
     - Then makes a bend to ascend up and cross the superior border of petrous temporal bone close to apex, deep to petrosphenoid ligament (Gruber's ligament)
     - Sometimes the ligament gets ossified results in a foramen called

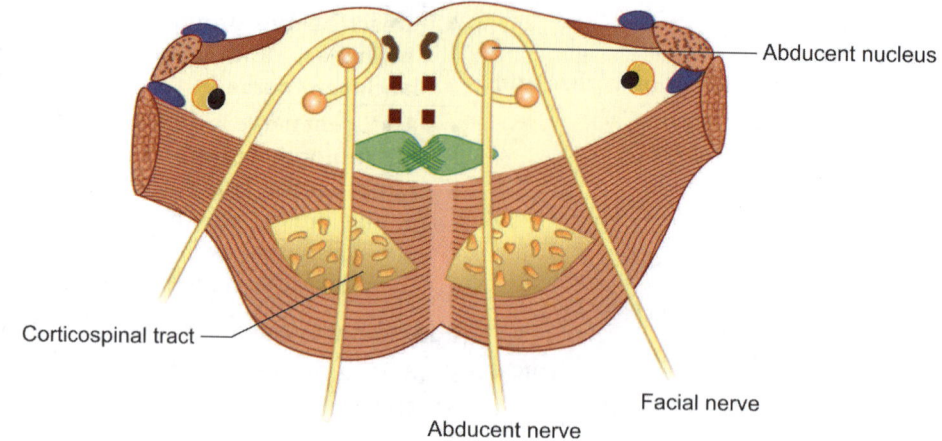

Fig. 1: Intrapontine course.

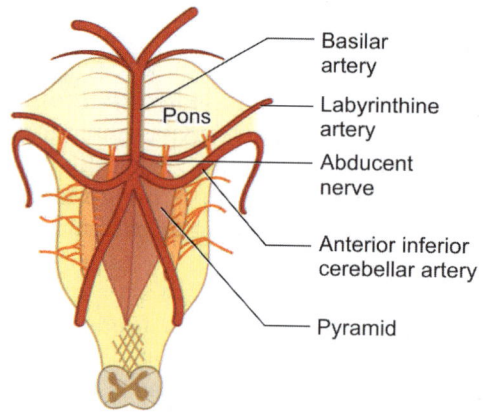

Fig. 2: Cisternal segment.

Dorello's canal, and if the foramen is present the abducent nerve passes through it.
3. **Cavernous segment (Fig. 3)**
   - The part related to cavernous sinus is called **cavernous segment**
   - It enters the cavernous sinus, and becomes a content of it, along with internal carotid artery
   - Here it is lateral initially and then inferolateral to the artery.
4. **Orbital segment (Fig. 4):** Enters the orbit, through the middle compartment of superior orbital fissure accompanied by oculomotor and nasociliary nerves.
- **In the orbit (Fig. 5):** It terminates by supplying the ocular surface of the lateral rectus.
- **Branches**
  - **Communicating branches:** With sympathetic plexus around ICA in the cavernous sinus
  - **Distributing branch:** To lateral rectus.
- **Connections**
  - Connected to precentral gyrus through corticobulbar fibers
  - Through medial longitudinal bundle (MLB) to the 3rd, 4th, and 8th cranial nerve for coordination.
- **Applied anatomy:**
  - Injury to abducent nerve sometimes is due to fracture of the base of skull. If injured, results in paralysis of lateral rectus leading to medial (convergent) squint and diplopia
  - **Raymond's syndrome:** It is a vascular lesion resulting in involvement of abducent nerve and corticospinal tract. It results in ipsilateral 6th nerve palsy and contralateral hemiplegia
  - **Foville's syndrome:** It affects the dorsal and medial part of inferior pons. In this lesion the abducent, facial nerve nuclei

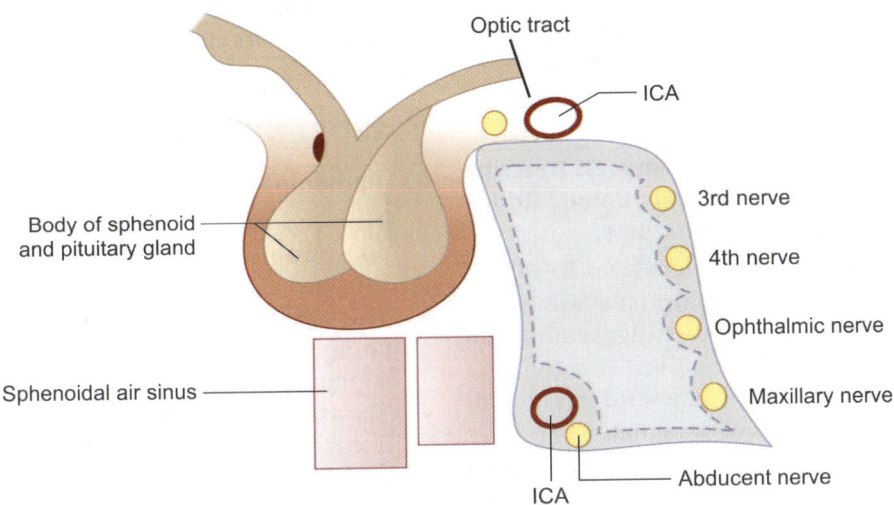

Fig. 3: Cavernous segment.

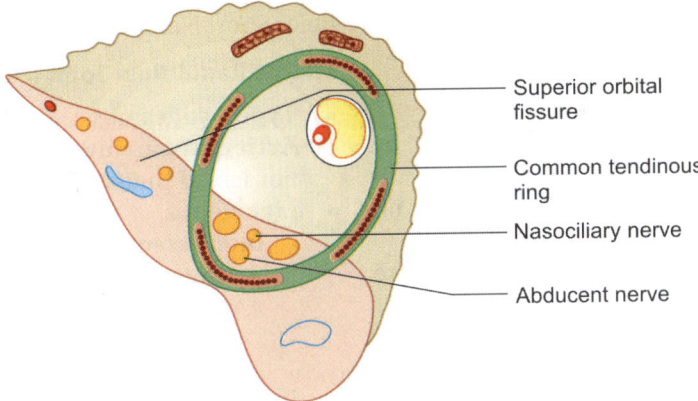

Fig. 4: Orbital segment.

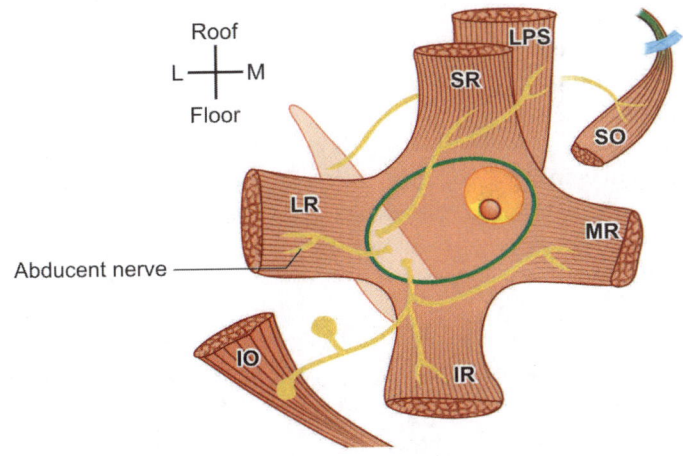

Fig. 5: In the orbit.

and corticospinal tract are affected. The effect is paralysis of lateral rectus leading to medial squint, paralysis of facial muscles on same side, and hemiparesis.

5. Classify dural venous sinuses. Describe the cavernous sinus in detail. Add a note on its applied anatomy.

Cavernous sinus Refer Essay Q. No. 5 – 2008.
- The dural venous sinuses are veins draining the brain, meninges, and skull bones
- Situated between the endosteal and meningeal layers of dura mater
- CSF is drained into the venous system through arachnoid villi and granulations which open into the sinuses.

Features

- Lined by endothelium
- No valves
- No muscular tissue in their walls
- Connected to extracranial veins by emissary veins
- Not seen as a tube like veins and so no lumen
- The cerebrospinal fluid drains into these sinuses.

Classification

Paired and unpaired
- **Paired**
  - Cavernous sinus
  - Sphenoparietal sinus
  - Superior petrosal sinus
  - Inferior petrosal sinus
  - Transverse sinus
  - Sigmoid sinus
  - Middle meningeal veins.
- **Unpaired**
  - Superior sagittal sinus
  - Inferior sagittal sinus
  - Straight sinus
  - Occipital sinus
  - Anterior intercavernous sinus
  - Posterior intercavernous sinus
  - Basilar plexus.

6. Describe the blood supply of heart. Add a note on its clinical significance.

Refer Essay Q. No. 5 – 2005.

II. SHORT NOTES

1. Radioulnar joint.

- The radioulnar joint has got three components—**superior, middle and inferior**
- The movement produced by the three components together is pronation and supination
- The **axis of the movement** passes obliquely from the center of the head of the radius to the ulnar attachment of the articular disc below.

Superior Radioulnar Joint

Refer Short Notes 5 – 2012.

Middle Radioulnar Joint (Figs. 6A and B)

- **Type**: Syndesmosis
- **Articular surfaces**: The interosseous borders of shafts of radius and ulna
- **Ligaments**:
  - **Interosseous membrane**
    - **Nature:** Fibrous sheath
    - **Direction:** Directed downwards and medially from radius to ulna
    - **Attachment:** Interosseous borders of radius and ulna
    - **Deficiencies:** About 2 – 3 cm below the radial tuberosity along upper border for the passage of posterior interosseous artery.
      * An oval opening in the lower part of membrane through which the anterior interosseous artery passes.
    - **Functions:** Connects the two bones together.
      * Gives attachment to the muscles of forearm
      * Transmits force from radius to ulna.
    - **Changes during movements:**
      * It is relaxed in complete pronation and supination

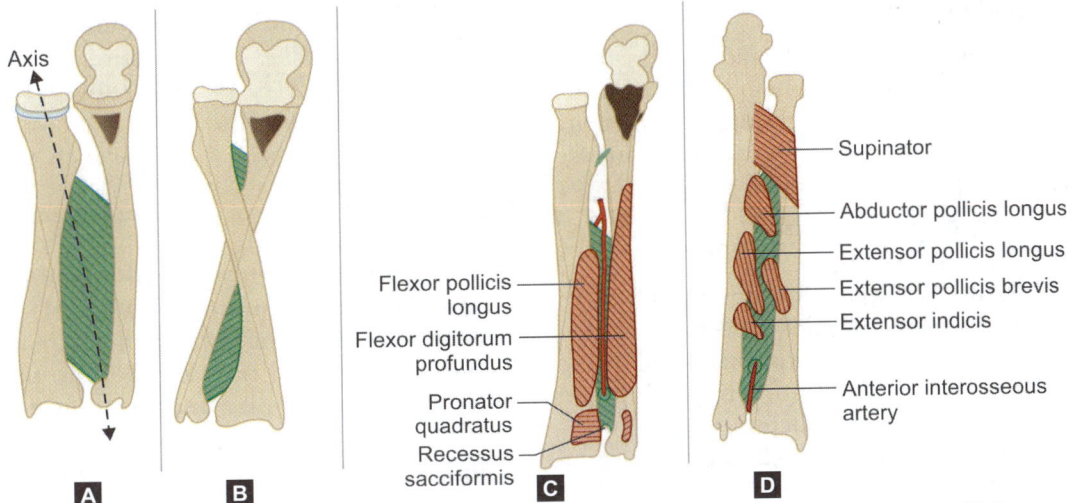

Figs. 6A to D: Middle radioulnar joint movements and relations: (A) Supination; (B) Pronation; (C) Anterior; (D) Posterior.

* Tensed during mid prone position
* It is spiralized in pronation and despiralized in supination
- **Relation:**
- Anteriorly—flexor pollicis longus, flexor digitorum profundus, anterior interosseous nerve and vessel, pronator quadratus, recessus sacciformis (Figs. 6C and D)
    * Posteriorly—supinator, extensor indicis, extensor pollicis longus and brevis, abductor pollicis longus, posterior interosseous nerve and vessels
- **Oblique cord:** It is a fibrous band extending from ulnar tuberosity to radius below radial tuberosity at right angles to interosseous membrane. **Morphologically:** It is vestigial part of flexor pollicis longus.

Distal Radioulnar Joint (Fig. 7)

- **Type:** Synovial, uniaxial joint, and pivot type
- **Articular surfaces**
    - Head of ulna
    - Ulnar notch of radius.
- **Ligaments**
    - **Fibrous capsule:** Attached around the joint loosely attached. It is thicker anteriorly. The synovial membrane projects upwards as recess in front of interosseous membrane called recessus sacciformis
    - **Articular disc:** It is triangular in shape. Made of fibrous cartilage it is attached to the depression between the styloid process and head of ulna to the ridge between ulnar notch and carpal articular surface of radius. It undergoes degeneration as age advances.
- **Nerve supply:** Interosseous nerves
- **Movement:** Pronation, supination
- **Muscles producing the movements**
    - **Supination:** Biceps brachii, supinator and brachioradialis
    - **Pronation:** Pronator teres and pronator quadratus.

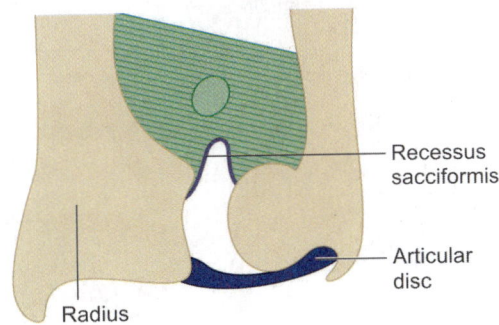

Fig. 7: Distal radioulnar joint.

Applied Anatomy

Pulled elbow: The head of radius slips out of the annular ligament due to traction on the wrist. It is common in children below 6 yrs as the size of the head and neck of radius are same.

2. Vermiform appendix.

- It is a vestigial organ
- Worm like diverticulum attached to posteromedial surface of cecum
- It is also called **abdominal tonsil** due to the presence of numerous lymphoid follicles in the submucosa
- **Length**: It ranges from 2 – 20 cm, average being 9 cm
- **Situation** in the right iliac fossa
- **Parts**: It has a base, tip and body
- **Base** is attached to the posteromedial surface of cecum and identified by convergence of teniae coli
- The **body** is narrow and tubular
- The **tip** is the least vascular part and is directed in various positions
- The **position** of the appendix depends on the direction of its tip **(Figs. 8A and B).**
    - Retrocecal/retrocolic (12° clock)—commonest position. Behind the cecum
    - Splenic (2° clock)—directed upwards and to left. It is of two types:
        1. Preileal in front of ileum (most dangerous position)
        2. Postileal behind ileum
    - Promontoric (3° clock) towards sacral promontory
    - Pelvic (4° clock) second commonest position towards pelvis
    - Inguinal/iliac (6° clock) lies below cecum
    - Paracolic/subcecal (11° clock) directed upwards and to right.
- **The peritoneum** covering the appendix is called **mesoappendix (Fig. 9)**. It is attached to the posterior layer of mesentry. It does not extend up to the tip of the appendix, hence the artery is directly in contact with the walls of appendix. The gangrenous perforation seen in appendicitis is due to this reason.

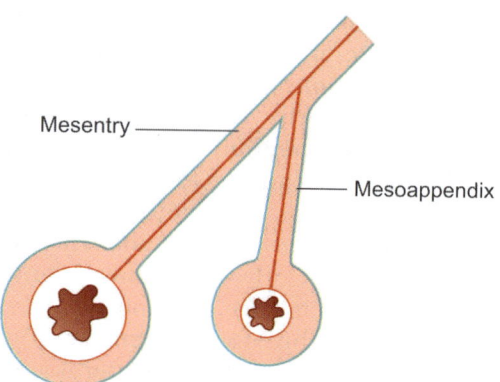

Fig. 9: Mesoappendix.

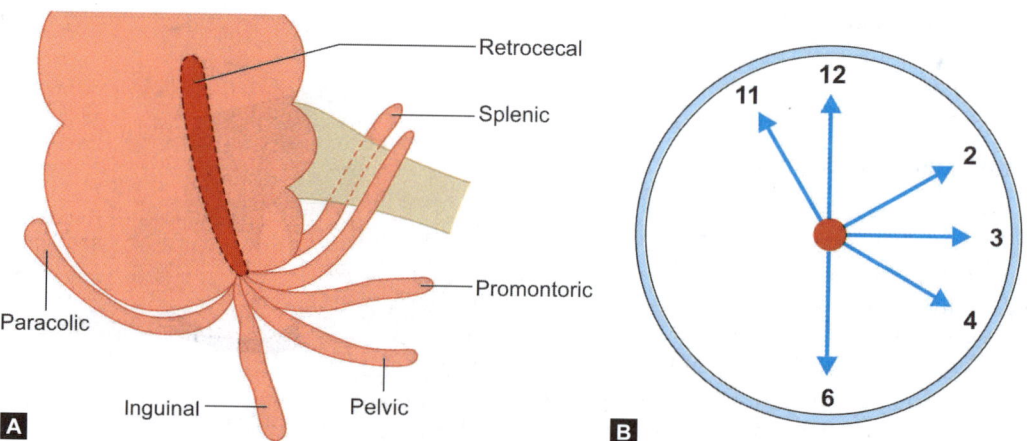

Figs. 8A and B: Positions of appendix.

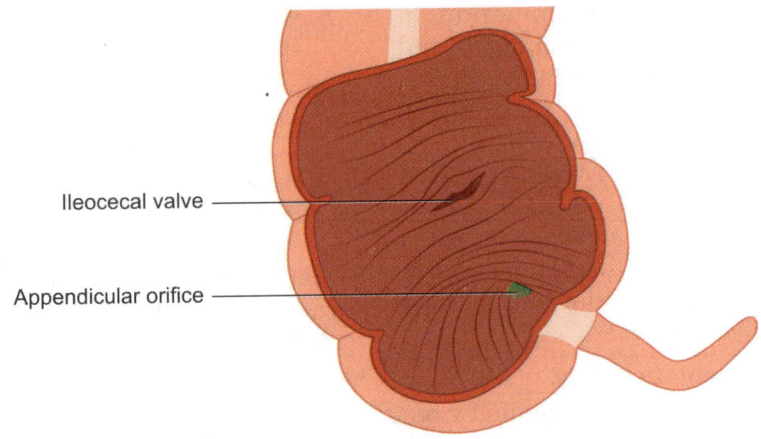

Fig. 10: Opening of appendix.

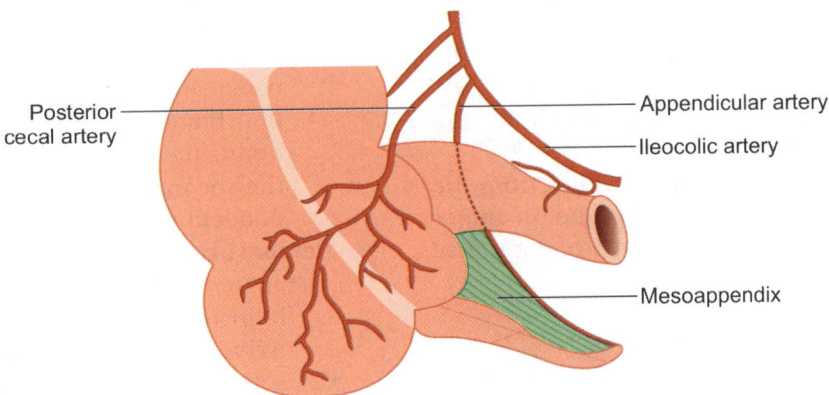

Fig. 11: Arterial supply.

- The orifice of appendix (base opens into) is situated 2 cm below the ileocecal orifice along the posteromedial surface of cecum. The opening is guarded by a valve called valve of Gerlach **(Fig. 10)**.
- **Blood supply**:
  - **Arterial supply (Fig. 11)**
    - The appendicular artery branch from ileocolic branch of superior mesenteric artery. It is an end artery
    - Accessory appendicular artery (of Seshachalam) from posterior cecal artery is common.
  - **Venous drainage**: Superior mesenteric vein—portal system
- **Nerve supply**: Sympathetic T_{10} segment: Parasympathetic—vagus
- **Surface marking**:
  - 2 cm below the intersection of transtubercular and right lateral plane
  - McBurney's point is at the junction of lateral ⅓ and medial ⅔ of a line drawn from umbilicus to anterior superior iliac spine, where maximum tenderness is felt in case of appendicitis
- **Microscopic structure** Refer Short Notes 11 – 2005.
- **Development** from postarterial part of midgut, as a diverticulum from the cecal bud

- **Applied anatomy:** Inflammation of appendix is known as appendicitis and removal of appendix is appendicectomy
- In appendicitis there is referred pain to umbilicus, as the dermatome is T10
- Care should be taken to avoid injury, when incision (gridiron) is made for appendicectomy, to the cutaneous branches of iliohypogastric and ilioinguinal nerves as they pass between the internal and external oblique muscles.

3. **Superior mesenteric artery.**

It supplies the structures developed from midgut.
- **Origin:**
  - From abdominal aorta
  - It is one of the ventral branch
- **Level:**
  - Arises at the level of L1.
  - The level of origin is along the transpyloric plane.
- **Structures supplied:** Supplies from the second part of duodenum below major duodenal papilla to right ⅔ of transverse colon
- **Course and relations:**
  - The artery runs inferiorly
  - Anterior to the uncinate process of the pancreas and the third part of the duodenum **(Fig. 12)**
  - Posterior to the splenic vein and the body of the pancreas
  - The left renal vein lies behind it and separates it from the aorta
  - The artery enters the root of the mesentery
  - Crosses anterior to the inferior vena cava, right ureter and right psoas major.
- **Termination:** Terminates by anastomosing with its branch the ileocolic artery in the right iliac fossa.
- **Branches (Fig. 13)**
  - **Inferior pancreaticoduodenal artery**
    - Divides into anterior and posterior branches
    - The anterior and posterior branches anastomose with the anterior and posterior branches of superior pancreaticoduodenal artery
    - Both branches supply the pancreatic head, its uncinate process and the second and third parts of the duodenum.
  - **Jejunal branches**
    - There are usually five to ten jejunal branches
    - Arise from the left side of the superior mesenteric artery
    - They are distributed to the jejunum as short arcades

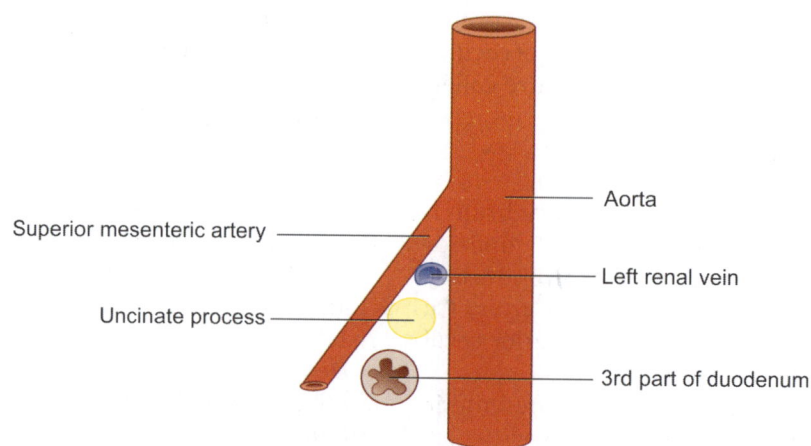

Fig. 12: Superior mesenteric artery course.

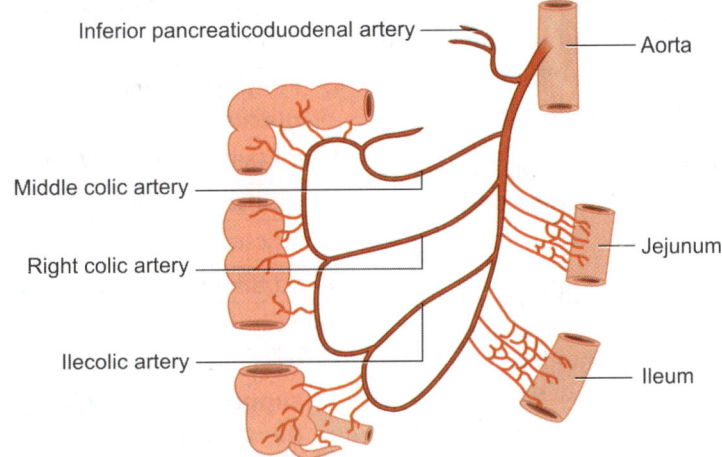

Fig. 13: Branches of superior mesenteric artery.

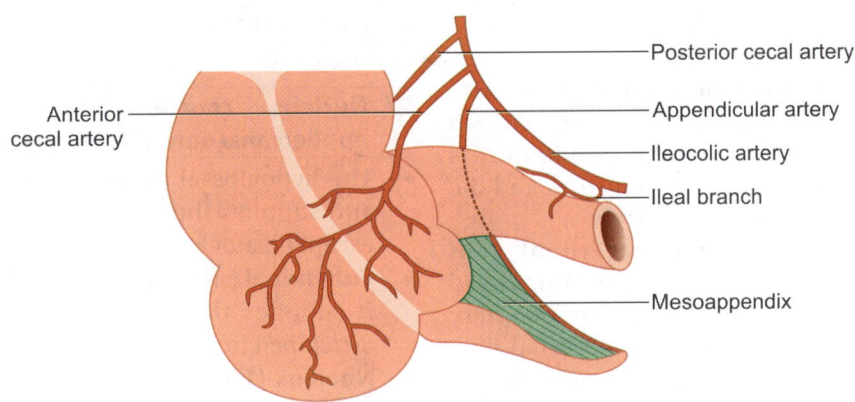

Fig. 14: Ileocolic artery.

- Arcades give rise to multiple long vasa recta.
- **Ileal branches**
    - Ileal branches are more numerous
    - Smaller in caliber than the jejuna branches
    - They arise from the left of the superior mesenteric artery
    - The length of the branches is greater in the ileum
    - Form three, four arcs within the mesentery
    - From the arcade multiple vasa recta are given which are short
    - The ileal branches run parallel and are distributed to alternate aspects of the ileum.
- **Ileocolic artery (Fig. 14)**
    - The ileocolic artery arises from the right side of the superior mesenteric artery
    - It descends to the right towards the caecum
    - Crosses anterior to the right ureter, gonadal vessels and psoas major to reach the right iliac fossa
    - It anastomoses with the right colic artery and terminal part of superior mesenteric artery
    - It gives rise to the following branches: ascending colic, anterior caecal, posterior caecal, appendicular artery and ileal branch.

- **Right colic artery**
  - Branch from the right side of the superior mesenteric artery
  - Near the colon it divides into a descending branch
  - Anastomoses with the ileocolic artery, and the right branch of the middle colic artery
- **Middle colic artery**
  - Arises just inferior to the uncinate process of the pancreas and anterior to the third part of the duodenum
  - It runs within the root of the transverse mesocolon, divides into a right and left branch
  - The right branch anastomoses with the right colic artery, and the left branch anastomoses with the left colic artery.
- **Applied anatomy**
  - **Superior mesenteric artery syndrome:** It is a gastrovascular disorder, in which the third part of the duodenum is compressed in-between aorta and the superior mesenteric artery
  - **Nutcracker syndrome/renal vein entrapment syndrome:** Downward traction of superior mesenteric artery may compress on the left renal vein resulting in renal vein entrapment syndrome. It is also called as nutcracker syndrome by the appearance of vein in the acute arterial angle.

4. **Formation and branches of brachial plexus.**
Refer Essay Q. No. 3 – 2005.

5. **Axillary artery.**
Refer Essay Q. No. 4 – 2007.

6. **Ligaments of knee joint.**
Refer Short Notes 10 – 2014.

7. **Draw a labeled diagram of blood supply of thyroid gland with its development.**
Blood supply Refer Short Notes 38 – 2008.
Development Refer Essay 8 – 2007.

8. **Left coronary artery.**
Refer Essay Q. No. 5 – 2005.

9. **Nucleus, course, distribution and applied anatomy of hypoglossal nerve.**
- The hypoglossal nerve is a motor nerve and supplies the muscles of the tongue except palatoglossus
- **Functional component:** Somatic efferent: It supplies the muscles of the tongue developed from occipital myotomes
- **Nucleus (Fig. 15):** Hypoglossal nucleus situated in the medulla in the floor of

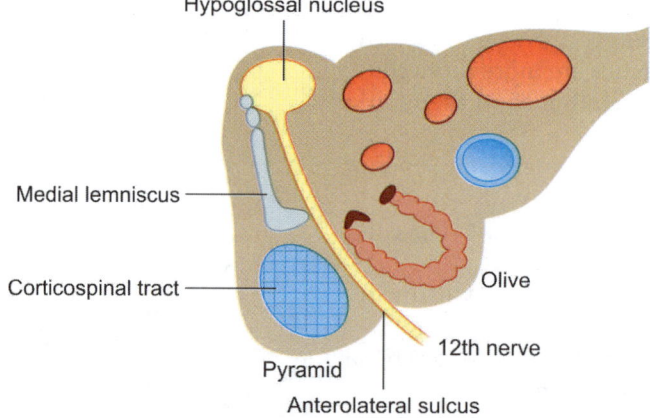

Fig. 15: Section of medulla oblongata.

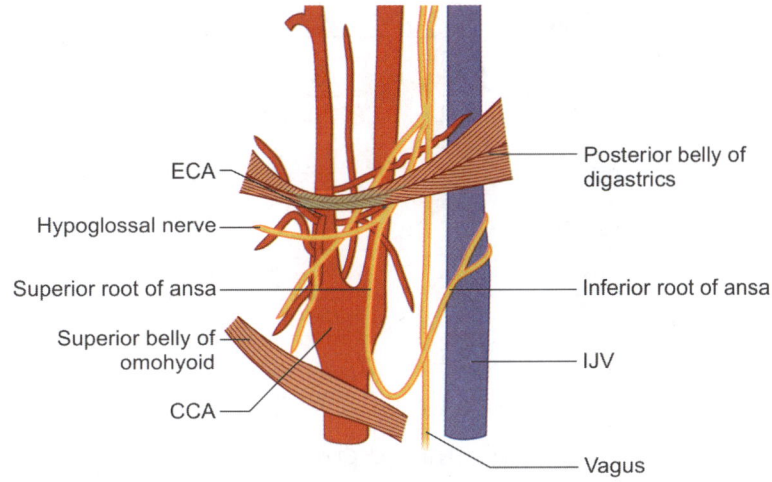

Fig. 16: Extracranial course.

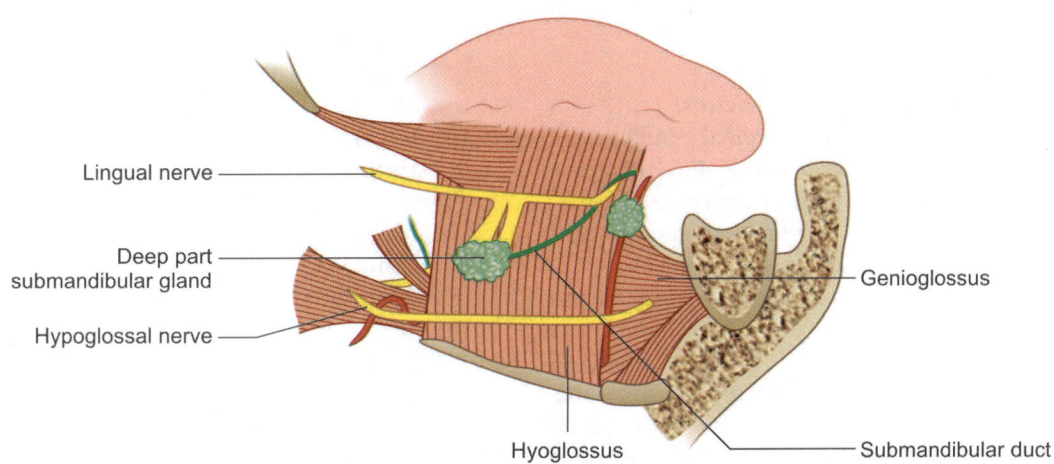

Fig. 17: Hyoglossus.

the fourth ventricle, deep to hypoglossal triangle.
- **Course:**
  - **Intracranial (Fig. 15)**
    - From hypoglossal nucleus the nerve passes through medulla
    - Emerges between pyramid and olive along the anterolateral sulcus of medulla oblongata
    - It leaves the cranial cavity through hypoglossal canal.
  - **Extracranial (Fig. 16)**
    - As soon it emerges out of cranial cavity, it is medial to IJV, ICA, and 9th, 10th, 11th cranial nerves
    - Then it descends downwards and laterally to reaches in between ICA and IJV
    - It turns forward winding around the inferior sternomastoid branch of occipital artery
    - It crosses the ICA and ECA and the loop of lingual artery in the carotid triangle
    - Lies on hyoglossus muscle
    - On hyoglossus it is related above to deep part of submandibular gland and duct, submandibular ganglion and lingual nerve (Fig. 17)

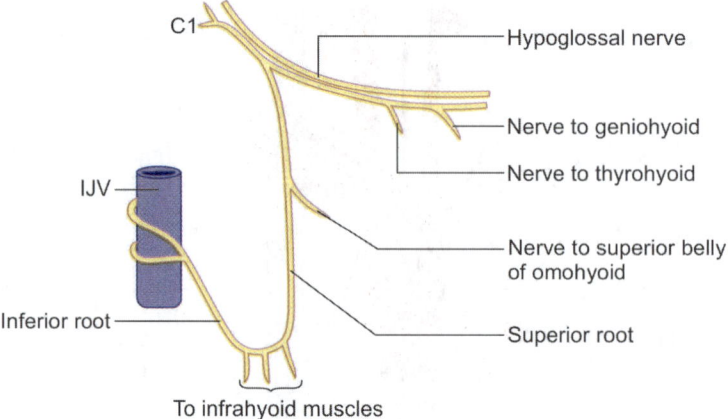

Fig. 18: Branches through C1 communication.

- It then dips into genioglossus, and continues forward up to the tip of the tongue.
- **Branches (Fig. 18):**
  - **Communicating branches:**
    - With superior cervical ganglion
    - With ventral rami of C_1 fibers—through this communication it supplies the strap muscles and geniohyoid muscle
    - With vagus—receives a branch from pharyngeal plexus called ramus lingualis vagi
    - With lingual nerve—by this communication the proprioceptive impulses from the tongue muscles are transmitted to the lingual nerve.
  - **Distributing branches:**
    - Meningeal branch—containg C_1 fibers to meninges of the posterior cranial fossa
    - Descendens hypoglossai or superior root of ansa—containing C_1 fibers. It is given as it loops the occipital artery. It lies on the anterior surface of carotid sheath. It supplies superior belly of omohyoid and then joins with the inferior root at the level of cricoid cartilage to form ansa cervicalis. The ansa cervicalis ($C_{1,2,3}$) supplies the infrahyoid muscles namely sternothyroid, sternohyoid, inferior belly of omohyoid
    - Nerve to thyrohyoid (C_1 fibers)
    - Nerve to geniohyoid (C_1 fibers)
    - Terminal branch to extrinsic and intrinsic muscles of tongue except palatoglossus.
- **Applied anatomy**
  - Complete hypoglossal nerve injury causes unilateral lingual paralysis and atrophy of muscles on the side of the lesion. When the patient protrudes the tongue it deviates to the paralyzed side
  - Due to paralysis of the infrahyoid muscles on the side of lesion, the larynx may deviate towards the normal side in swallowing.

10. Blood supply of brain.

Refer Essay Q. No. 5 – 2011.

11. Lacrimal apparatus.

Refer Short Notes Q. No. 27 – 2006.

12. Sulci, gyri, and functional areas of superolateral surface of cerebrum.

Refer Essay Q. No. 7 – 2007.

III. SHORT ANSWER QUESTIONS

1. Histology of cardiac muscle.

Refer Short Answer 10 – 2011.

2. Blood supply of pancreas.

Refer Essay Q. No. 2 – 2008.

3. **Spermatogenesis.**

Refer Short Notes 12 – 2007.

4. **Rotator cuff.**

Refer Short Notes 4 – 2003.

5. **Histology of suprarenal gland.**

Refer Short Notes 3 – 2010.

6. **Supports of uterus.**

Refer Essay Q. No. 2 – 2004.

7. **Flexor retinaculum of hand.**

Refer Short Notes 12 – 2012.

8. **Cloaca and its derivatives.**

- The hindgut is divided by allantoic diverticulum into a pre and postallantoic parts
- The **postallantoic part** of the hind gut dilates to form endodermal cloaca
- It extends up to cloacal membrane
- The endodermal cloaca is divided into a ventral part called primitive urogenital sinus and a dorsal part the primitive rectum by urorectal septum **(Fig. 19A)**
- Initially a gap is seen between the septum and cloacal membrane is called **cloacal duct.** Through this gap the primitive rectum and urogenital sinus communicate
- By 7th week the septum fuses with the cloacal membrane, and divides the cloaca into two **(Figs. 19B and C)**
- The cloacal membrane is divided into anal membrane and urogenital membrane

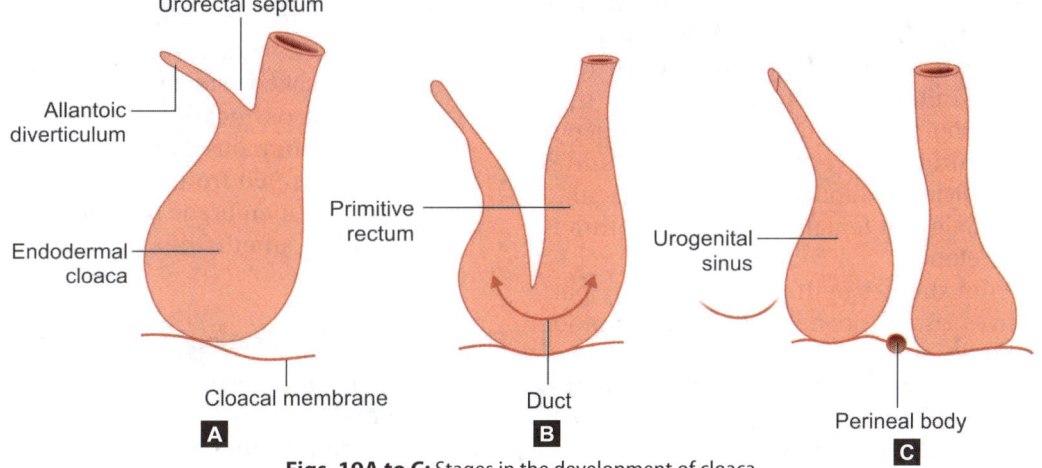

Figs. 19A to C: Stages in the development of cloaca.

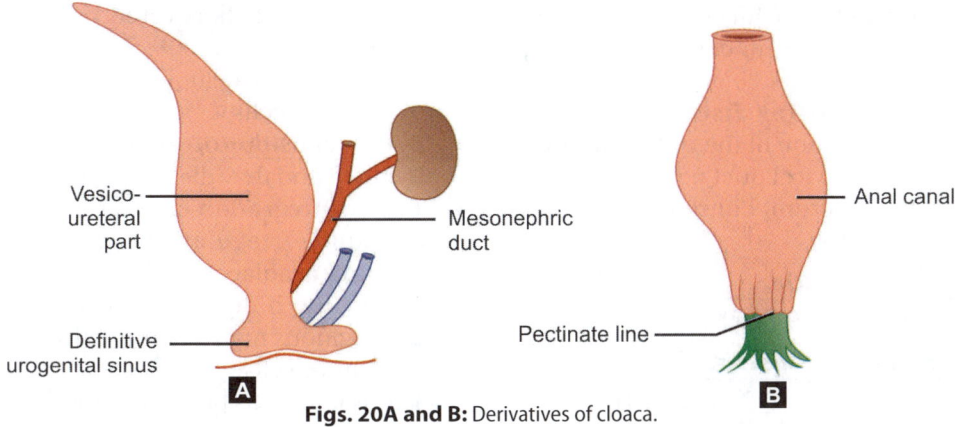

Figs. 20A and B: Derivatives of cloaca.

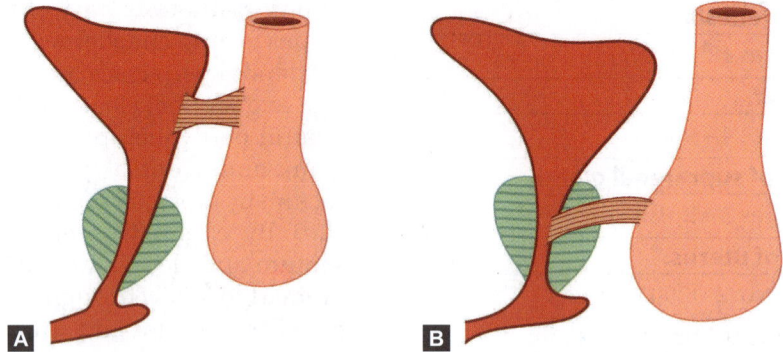

Figs. 21A and B: Congenital anomalies of cloaca: (A) Rectovesical fistula; (B) Rectourethral fistula.

- Primitive rectum gives rise to rectum below Houston's valve and upper part of anal canal up to pectinate line
- Primitive urogenital sinus is divided by the opening of mesonephric ducts into a **vesicourethral** part and **definitive urogenital sinus (Fig. 20A)**
- Vesicourethral canal gives rise to mucous membrane of entire urinary bladder except trigone and part of prostatic urethra in males. In female the entire urethra is developed
- From the urogenital sinus—pelvic part gives rise to prostatic and membranous part of urethra in male. Phallic part of spongy urethra (up to the glans penis) is developed.
- **Congenital anomaly (Fig. 21)**
  - **Rectovesical fistula**: Failure of approximation of the urorectal septum and the cloacal duct persists at a higher level. The rectum communicates with urinary bladder
  - **Rectourethral fistula**: Failure of approximation of the urorectal septum and the cloacal duct persists at a lower level. Rectum communicates with urethra.

9. Popliteus muscle.
Refer Short Notes 19 – 2009.

10. Cruciate anastomosis.
Refer Short Answers Q. No. 20 – 2013.

11. Ossification.
- It is the process of formation of new bone
- It also includes the proliferation of collagen and ground substance
- It is completed by deposition of calcium salts by cells called osteoblasts
- Two types of ossification—enchondral and intramembranous ossification
- The bones ossified from membrane are called dermal/membrane bones
- The bones ossified from cartilage are cartilage bones.

Endochondral Ossification

- Most bones are formed by a process of endochondral ossification
- The mesenchyme condenses and differentiates into cartilage
- The cartilage cells proliferate and form **cartilage models** covered by perichondrium
- Deposition of calcium salts are enhanced by cartilage cells
- By the **deposition of calcium,** the nutrition is cut off and they die and degenerate
- The **disintegration** of cartilage cell leads to empty irregular spaces known as **primary areolae**
- Later the blood vessels invade the cartilaginous matrix along with the osteoprogenitor cells
- This is known as periosteal bud

- The primary areolae fuse to form **secondary areolae**
- The osteoprogenitor cells are converted to osteoblasts
- The osteoblast produces collagen fibers and bone matrix
- Osteoid is calcified to form lamellae. In-between the lamellae the osteoblast are converted to osteocyte
- The periosteum deposits bones to the sides
- After birth the ends of long bones are formed similarly to form epiphysis
- The epiphyseal cartilage multiply and form 4 zones—zone of resting cartilage, zone of proliferating cartilage, zone of maturing cartilage, zone of calcified cartilage **(Fig. 22)**
- Example—long bones of limbs.

Intramembranous Ossification

- Intramembranous ossification is the direct formation of bone within highly vascular membranes of condensed primitive mesenchyme
- The mesenchymal cells differentiate into osteoblast
- In turn osteoblasts proliferate to produce collagen fibers and hyaline matrix
- Example—the cranial vault

- **Ossification centers** appear during bone growth
- The center appears before birth (in embryonic life) is called the **primary center of ossification**
- The primary center appears for shaft of all long bones, talus, calcaneus, cuboid and lower end of femur
- The center appears after birth (in the postnatal growing period) is known as **secondary center of ossification**
- Ends of long bones except lower end of femur, are cartilaginous at birth, and converted into bone from secondary centers.
- **Laws of ossification**
  - The secondary center which appears first will unite with diaphysis last. The fibula disobeys the law
  - The direction of nutrient foramen is away from growing end of bone
  - The growing end fuses later than the other end.

Applied Anatomy

- Defect in enchondral ossification causes a condition called **achondroplasia**, in which the limbs are short and trunk normal resulting in dwarfism
  - Defect in membranous ossification results in a syndrome called **cleidocranial**

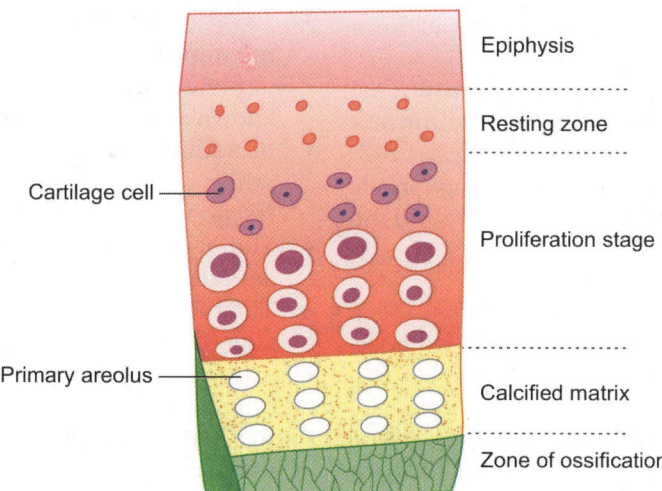

Fig. 22: Four zones of epiphyseal cartilage.

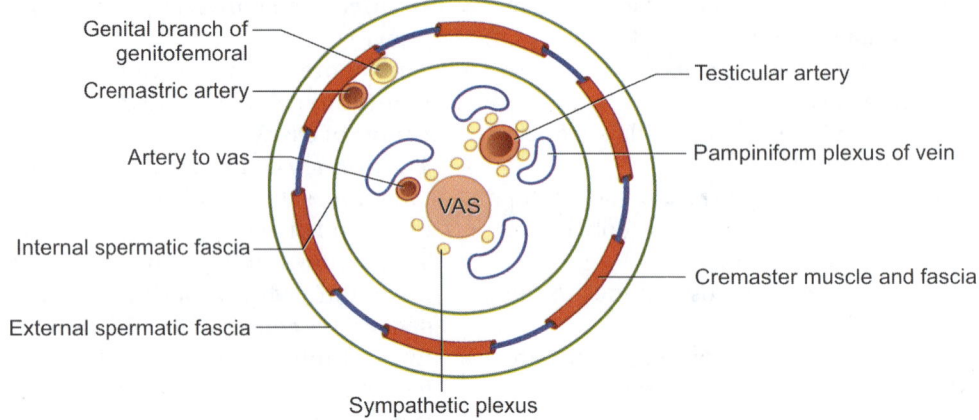

Fig. 23: Contents of spermatic cord.

dysostosis. The features are aplasia of clavicle, unossified fontanelle, and transverse diameter of cranium is more.

12. Spermatic cord.
- It is a tubular sheath containing vas deferens, vessels, nerves of testis and epididymis
- Extent—from deep inguinal ring to posterior aspect of the testis
- Length—7.5 cm. The left cord is longer than the right.

Contents: Refer Short Answers Q. No. 1 – 2009.

Coverings of spermatic cord (Fig. 23)
- External spermatic fascia derived from external oblique aponeurosis
- Cremaster muscle and fascia from internal oblique and transverses abdominis muscle
- Internal spermatic fascia from transversalis fascia forms a thin loose layer around the cord.

Applied Anatomy
- Vasectomy—ligation of both side vas deferens is a method used for contraception
- Encysted hydrocele—the processus vaginalis persists in the middle between deep inguinal ring and testis and undergo cystic changes.

13. Carpal tunnel syndrome.
Refer Short Notes 11 – 2010.

14. Histology of kidney.
Refer Short Notes 3 – 2007.

15. Notochord.
Refer Short Notes 15 – 2005.

16. Rectouterine pouch.
Refer Short Answer Q. No. 15 – 2009.

17. Biceps brachii muscle.
Refer Short Notes Q. No. 21 – 2013.

18. Annular pancreas.
Refer Short Answer Q. No. 16 – 2009.

19. Peripheral heart.
- In standing position the lower limb depends on the muscular contraction known as **muscle pump**
- In addition the efficiency of the muscle pump is increased by tight sleeve of deep fascia
- The perforators connect deep veins with superficial veins
- The blood flow in the lower limb is from superficial veins to deep veins
- The valves are so arranged, they prevent blood flow from deep to superficial veins
- At rest the pressure is equal to the pressure in heart
- When the muscle contract the blood is pumped in the deep veins

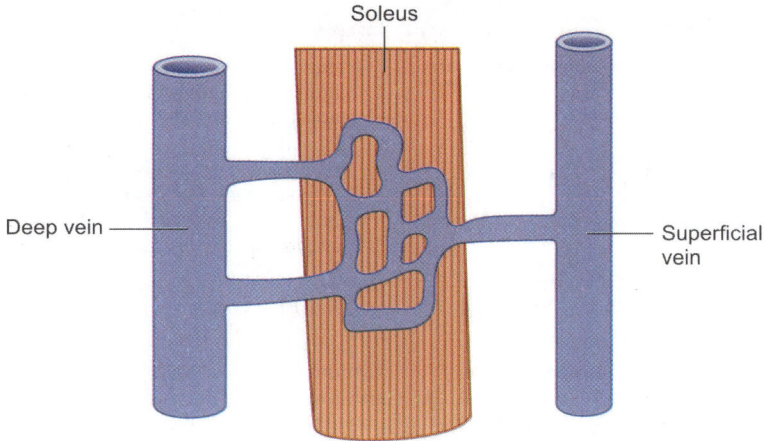

Fig. 24: Venous plexus connecting superficial and deep veins.

- During relaxation of the muscle, the blood from superficial veins flow into the deep veins
- Soleus and lateral pterygoid muscles are known as peripheral heart
- **Soleus** muscle is known as peripheral heart as it helps in venous return from the lower limb.
  - It contains large venous sinuses which are provided with valves
  - The contraction of the muscle pumps the blood out of venous plexus
  - At rest the venous blood gets collected in the sinuses.
  - The muscle is multipennate and situated deep to gastrocnemius
  - Origin is from upper ⅓ of posterior surface of fibula, soleal line and medial border of tibia
  - Forms tendocalcaneus along with gastrocnemius and is inserted to middle of posterior surface of calcaneus
  - Nerve supply is by tibial nerve
  - Action is plantar flexion and steadies the leg on foot.
- **Lateral pterygoid** muscle is a muscle of mastication, situated in the infratemporal fossa and is intimately related to the pterygoid venous plexus. When the muscle contracts help in propulsion of blood in the pterygoid venous plexus into the maxillary vein
- **Applied anatomy**: Incompetence of the valves in the perforating veins, will lead to leakage of blood from deep veins during muscular contraction and results in dilatation and varicosity of superficial veins.

20. Great saphenous vein.
Refer Short Notes 14 – 2005.

21. Median nerve in hand.
Refer Short Notes 5 – 2007.

22. Rectus sheath.
Refer Short Notes 6 – 2003.

23. Hamstring muscles.
- The muscles of the back of thigh are known as hamstring
- The **features** of it are:
  - **Origin** is from ischial tuberosity
  - **Inserted** to any bone of leg
  - **Nerve supply** is by tibial component of sciatic nerve
  - **Action** is flexors of knee and extensors of hip.
- The hamstring muscles are semitendinosus, semimembranosus, long head of biceps, hamstring part of adductor magnus.

Name of muscle	Origin	Insertion
Semimembranosus	Superolateral impression on the ischial tuberosity	The tendon divides at the level of the knee into five slips. 1. Is attached to a tubercle on the posterior aspect of the medial tibial condyle. 2. To the medial margin of the tibia; 3. To the fascia over popliteus; 4. Tendon to the lower lip and adjacent part of the groove on the back of the medial condyle of tibia. 5. Oblique popliteal ligament of the knee joint.
Semitendinosus	Inferomedial impression on the upper area of the ischial tuberosity	Upper part of the medial surface of the tibia behind the attachment of sartorius
Long head of biceps	Inferomedial impression on the upper area of the ischial tuberosity	Tendon splits to enclose the fibular collateral ligament and is attached to the head of the fibula. The vestigial part of the muscle is sacrotuberous ligament.
Hamstring part of adductor magnus	From the inferolateral aspect of the ischial tuberosity.	To the adductor tubercle on the medial condyle of the femur and expansion to the medial supracondylar line. Tibial collateral ligament is degenerated part of adductor magnus

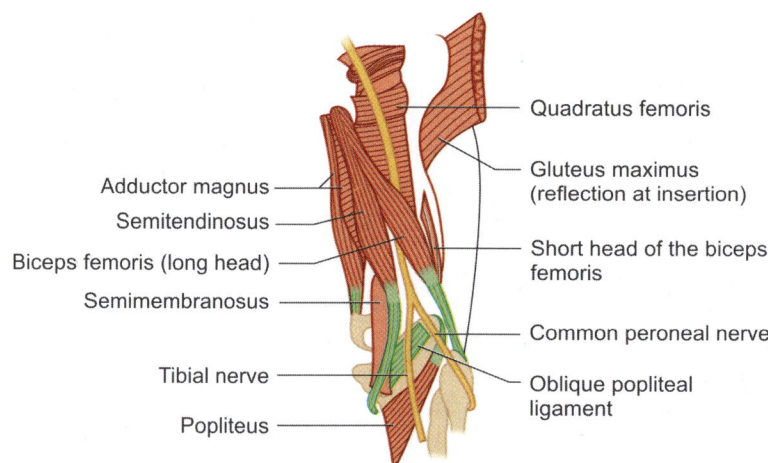

Fig. 25: Hamstring muscles.

24. Microscopic anatomy of lymph node.
Refer Short Answer Q. No. 19 – 2011.

25. Pronation and supination.
Refer Short Notes 7 – 2005.

26. Second part of duodenum.
Refer Short Notes 13 – 2006.

27. Synovial joints.
Features of synovial joint: Refer Short Notes 12 – 2014.

Classification of Synovial Joins
- **Uniaxial joint:**
  - **Hinge joints:** The articular surfaces resemble hinges. Movements are permitted only in one plane, e.g. elbow joint, interphalangeal joints
  - **Pivot joints:** The pivot (Part of bone) rotates within an osseo-ligamentous ring, e.g. superior radioulnar joint, median atlantoaxial joint

- **Condylar joints:** The convex condylar articular surface of one bone fits into concave or flat articular surface of another bone, e.g. right and left temporomandibular joints, knee joint.
- **Biaxial joint:**
  - **Ellipsoidal joints:** The oval convex surface of one bone articulates with the oval concave surface of another bone, e.g. radiocarpal joint, atlanto-occipital joint
  - **Saddle or sellar joints:** The articular surfaces are reciprocally saddle shaped, i.e. concavo-convex, e.g first carpometacarpal joint, sternoclavicular joint.
- **Multiaxial joint: Ball and socket or spheroidal joints:** Rounded convex surface of one bone fits into the cup-like socket of another bone, e.g hip joint, shoulder joint
- **Plane joint:** The articular surfaces are nearly flat, permits gliding movements in various directions, e.g. intercarpal joints, intertarsal joints, intermetatarsal, intermetacarpal, joints between the articular processes of adjacent vertebrae.

28. Deep peroneal nerve.
Refer Short Notes 6 – 2006.

29. Development of kidney.
Refer Short Notes 10 – 2004.

30. Winging of scapula.
- This condition is mainly due to injury to long thoracic nerve of bell
- The long thoracic nerve arises from root stage of brachial plexus
- Root value—C_5 C_6 C_7
- The nerve supplies serratus anterior muscle
- **Causes for winging:**
  - Blunt trauma
  - Contusion of shoulder
  - Sport's or pressure injury
  - Osteochondroma
  - Weakness of scapular stabilizers—the fascioscapulohumeral dystrophy
  - Loss of scapular suspensory mechanism – dislocation of acromioclavicular joint or fracture of lateral third of clavicle with rupture of coracoclavicular ligament
  - Neuralgic amyotrophy—usually affects the long thoracic nerve
  - Brachial plexus injury or brachial neuritis.
- **Attachment of the muscle (Fig. 26):**
  - The serratus anterior origin is from upper eight ribs as eight digitations, and is inserted to the medial border of scapula along the costal surface
  - The mode of insertion is first digitation to superior scapular angle, 2nd and 3rd digitation to complete medial border,

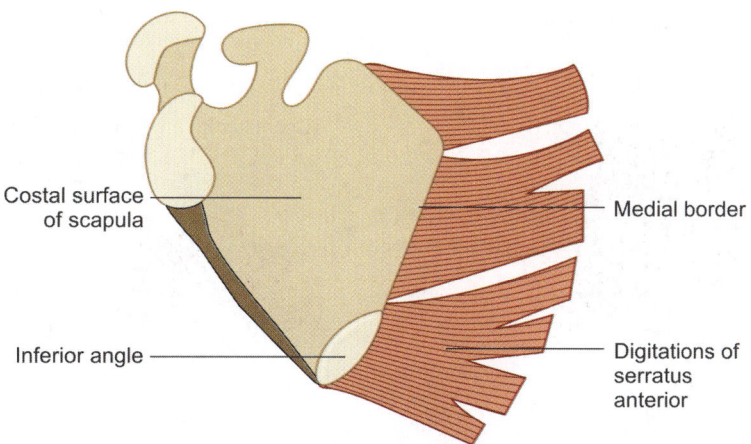

Fig. 26: Attachment of serratus anterior muscle.

the lower four or five slips to the inferior angle.

- **Actions:**
  - The muscle protracts the scapula in pushing and punching movements
  - The bulk insertion to the lower part pulls the inferior angle of scapula forwards around thorax
  - The action of serratus anterior is antagonized by retraction of scapula by the rhomboids and middle fibers of trapezius.
- **Effect of lesion:**
  - Patient may complain of pain, weakness, restricted elevation of shoulder
  - Inferior angle rotates towards midline.
  - Prominence of the medial border of scapula **(Fig. 27)**
  - Because of the unopposed action of paralyzed serratus anterior muscle, the medial border of the scapula is elevated by the actions of rhomboids and middle fibers of trapezius
  - When the patient makes an attempt to push, the protrusion of medial border becomes more prominent.

31. Histological layers of cornea.
Refer Short Notes 35 – 2009.

32. Cricoid cartilage characteristic features.
- It is an unpaired cartilage of larynx
- It is the only cartilage which is complete
- Situated at the **level** of C_6
- **Developed** from mesoderm of 6th pharyngeal arch
- **Type of cartilage**: Hyaline cartilage
- **Shape**: Signet ring
- **Parts**: A narrow anterior arch and broader posterior lamina
- **Lamina**: A ridge is present in the center of lamina and gives attachment to the tendon of esophagus **(Fig. 28A)**
- On either side of ridge the posterior cricoarytenoid muscle is attached
  - The **arch (28B)** has a sloping superior border, straight inferior border internal and external surfaces
  - Superior border gives attachment for lateral cricoarytenoid muscle, cricothyroid ligament
  - Inferior border to cricotracheal ligament.

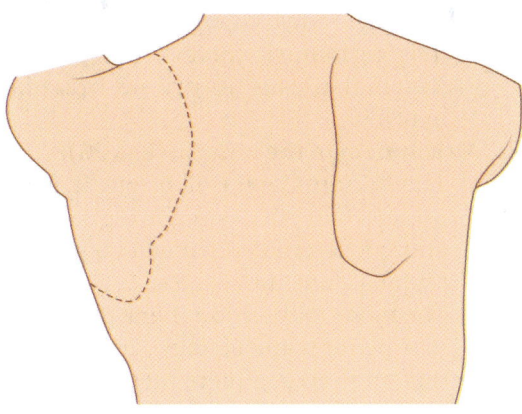

Fig. 27: Winging of scapula.

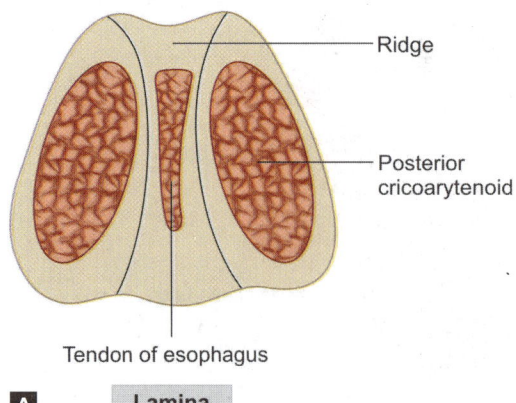

A Lamina

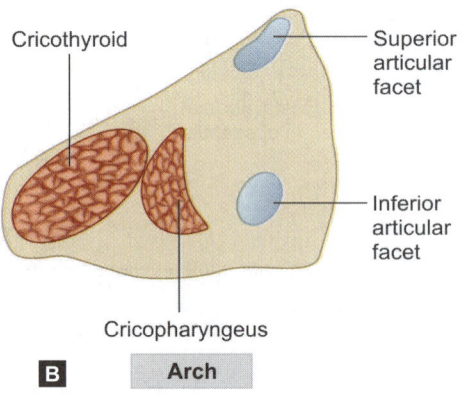

B Arch

Figs. 28A and B: Cricoid cartilage.

- The internal surface is covered with mucous membrane
- To the external surface the cricothyroid muscle and cricopharyngeal part of inferior constrictor are attached
- Between arch and lamina two articular facets are seen
- The base of arytenoids cartilage articulates with upper facet and inferior horn of thyroid cartilage articulates with the lower facet, forming cricothyroid and cricoarytenoid synovial joints respectively.
- **Applied anatomy**
  - During tracheostomy the cricoid cartilage should be taken care to avoid injury, as it is the only cartilage which is complete to support the laryngeal framework
  - Subglottis stenosis—may be congenital or acquired. Congenital stenosis results in respiratory obstruction. Acquired may be due to trauma and scaring after prolonged endotracheal intubation in case of premature babies.

33. Branches of descending thoracic aorta

- Thoracic aorta is the continuation of arch of aorta
- It is a content of posterior mediastinum
- It extends from T_4 to T_{12}
- It is continued as abdominal aorta through aortic orifice
- It provides branches to pericardium, lung, bronchi, esophagus, and thoracic wall
- Branches:
  - **Pericardial** branches
  - **Bronchial** arteries
    - One on right side and two on left side
    - The **right** branch sometimes arises from right 3rd posterior intercostals artery and is posterior to right bronchus
    - One of the **left** bronchial branch is given at T5 vertebral level and the other below left bronchus.
  - **Mediastinal** branches to supply lymph nodes and areolar tissue
  - **Superior phrenic** artery to supply diaphragm
  - **Posterior intercostals** arteries.
    - One in each intercostal space
    - Lower nine from thoracic aorta
    - The right branches are longer than left
    - Runs in the costal groove.
- Anastomose with upper anterior intercostals artery.
  - **Subcostal artery**: Last pair of arteries, is accompanied by the subcostal nerve, runs along the lower border of 12th rib,

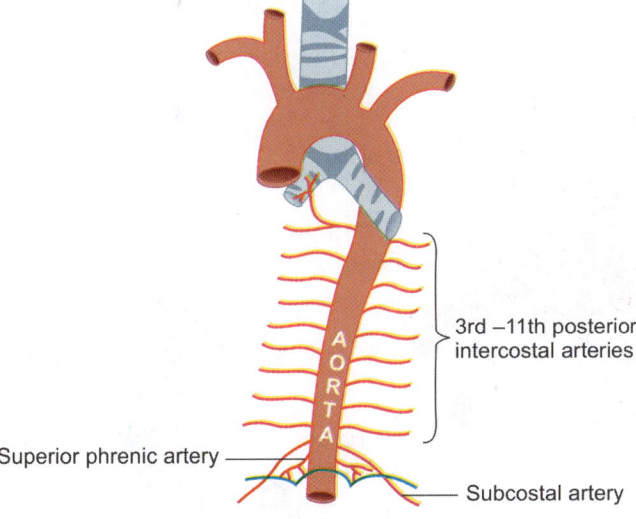

Fig. 29: Descending thoracic aorta.

and passes deep to the lateral arcuate ligament
- **Aberrant artery**: Sometimes given near right bronchial artery. It is developmentally remnant of right dorsal aorta. When it is enlarged it replaces the 1st part of right subclavian artery sometimes.
- **Applied anatomy**: Aortic rupture in case of accidents results in blunt injury, where there is horizontal tear in intima extending to media. It can lead on to formation of false aneurysm.

34. Pleural recesses.
Refer Essay Q. No. 3 – 2003.

35. Waldeyer's ring.
Refer Short Answer 35 – 2011.

36. Buccinator muscle.
Refer Short Notes 18 – 2007.

37. Subclavian vein formation course and termination.
- **Formation**: The axillary vein is continued from the level of outer border of 1st rib as subclavian vein **(Fig. 30A)**.
- **Extent**: From outer border of 1st rib to medial border of scalenus anterior
- **Course**
  - It arches upwards but the artery is posterosuperior to vein separated by scalenus anterior
  - It lies behind the clavicle and is related to the groove on the upper surface of first rib
- **Termination**: Joins with internal jugular vein to form brachiocephalic vein **(Fig. 30B)**.

38. Derivatives of neural tube.
- The neuroectodermal cells become thickened to form medullary/neural plate
- The neural plate form neural pit, groove and gradually the groove fuses to form neural tube
- The fusion starts from cervical region extending caudally with appearance of two pores
- The anterior pore closes by middle of 4th week and the posterior pore by end of 4th week
- The cephalic part of tube enlarges to form 3 vesicles – fore, mid and hindbrain vesicles.
  1. **Fore brain** vesicle gives rise to—telen and diencephalon
  2. **Midbrain**—mesencephalon
  3. **Hind brain**—myelin and metencephalon.
- The rest of the tube forms the **spinal cord**.

39. Area of epistaxis.
- The anteroinferior part of nasal septum is called as the area of epistaxis
- It is also known as Little's area (Kisselbach's plexus)

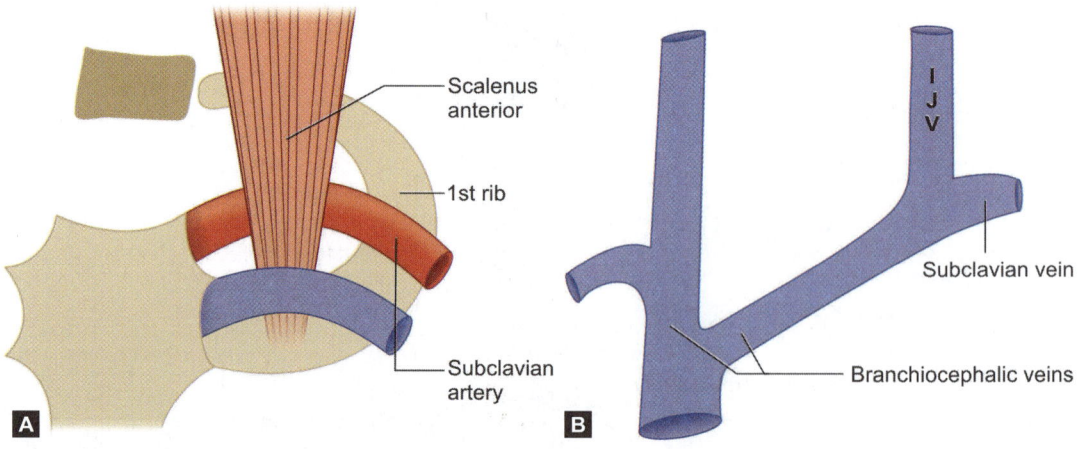

Figs. 30A and B: Subclavian vein.

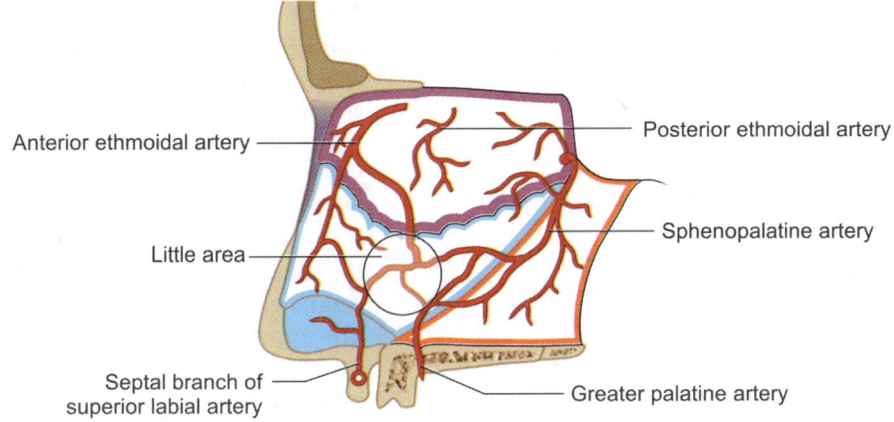

Fig. 31: Area of epistaxis.

- It is highly vascular
- Common site for bleeding from nose
- The septal branch of superior labial, anterior ethmoidal, greater palatine, and branches of sphenopalatine arteries anastomose in the anteroinferior part of nasal septum
- There is arteriovenous anastomosis between these arteries in the anteroinferior part of septum
- This area is called **Little's area (Kisselbach's plexus) (Fig. 31)** which is the commonest site of epistaxis (bleeding from nose)
- Even a small ulcer produces profuse bleeding
- Causes for bleeding—high blood pressure, nose picking, trauma.

40. Thoracic duct area of drainage.

Refer Short Notes 51 – 2013.

41. Nasal septum.

Refer Short Notes 17 – 2003.

42. Floor of fourth ventricle.

Refer Short Notes 21 – 2008.

43. Histology of the palatine tonsil.

Refer Short Notes 34 – 2005.

44. Otic ganglion.

Refer Short Notes Q. No. 22 – 2009.

45. Cross sectional diagram of typical intercostal space.

Refer Essay Q. No. 9 – 2006.

46. Fallot's tetralogy.

Refer Essay Q. No. 6 – 2010.

47. Corpus callosum.

Refer Short Notes 25 – 2011.

48. Interior of right atrium.

Refer Essay Q. No. 7 – 2006.

49. Boundaries and content of posterior mediastinum.

- **Boundaries of posterior mediastinum (Fig. 32):**
    - Anteriorly—bifurcation of trachea, pulmonary vessels, pericardium, diaphragm

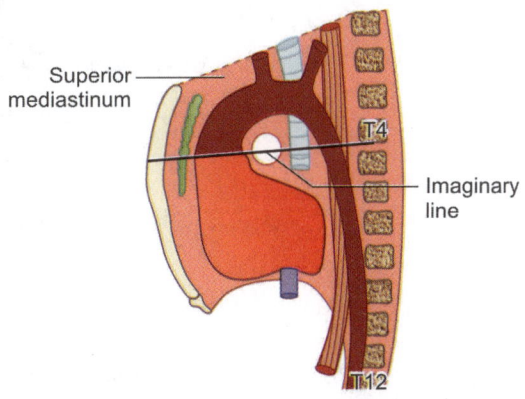

Fig. 32: Posterior mediastinum boundaries.

- Posteriorly—lower 8 thoracic vertebrae and the intervertebral disc and ligament
- Laterally—mediastinal pleura
- Above—sternal angle passing through lower border of body of T4 vertebra
- Below—diaphragm.
• **Contents of posterior mediastinum**: Refer Essay Q. No. 6 – 2012.

50. Muscles of tongue.
Refer Short Notes Q. No. 31 – 2005.

51. Falx cerebri.
Refer Short Notes Q. No. 29 – 2007.

52. Superior laryngeal nerve.

Origin
- It is a branch from middle of inferior ganglion of vagus given in the neck
- It is a mixed nerve.

Course
- It descends downwards initially posterior and then medial to internal carotid artery
- Descends along the pharynx.

Termination
- It terminates by dividing into internal and external laryngeal nerve about 1.5 cm below the inferior ganglion of vagus.

Branches
- The **internal laryngeal nerve**
  - It is the larger terminal branch of superior laryngeal nerve
  - It is above the superior thyroid artery
  - Pierces the thyrohyoid membrane along with superior laryngeal vessels
  - It lies in the floor of piriform fossa
  - It divides into upper, middle and lower branches
  - The upper branches supply the mucous membrane of vallecula of the epiglottis, aryepiglottic fold and vestibule of larynx
  - Middle branch to the piriform fossa and mucosa of laryngeal ventricle
  - Lower branch to the mucosa over arytenoid cartilage and transverse arytenoid muscle
  - It ends by piercing inferior constrictor and unites with ascending branch of recurrent laryngeal nerve
  - It also supplies the mucosa and muscular layer of oesophagus and trachea.
- The **external laryngeal nerve**
  - Is smaller branch of superior laryngeal nerve
  - Descends behind the sternohyoid
  - Lies on the inferior constrictor
  - Reaches cricothyroid

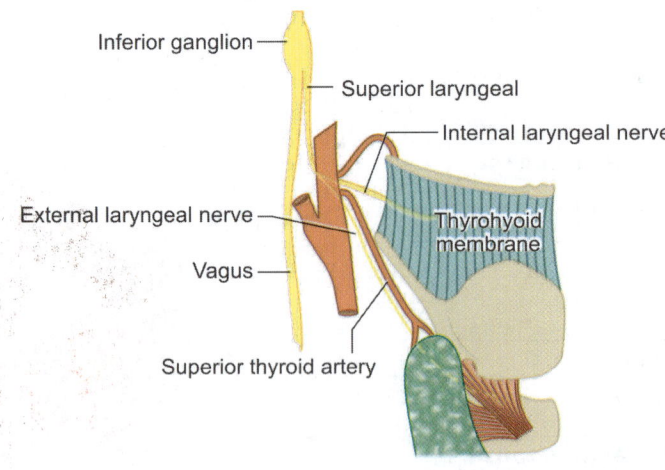

Fig. 33: Superior laryngeal nerve.

- It supplies cricothyroid muscle and gives a twig to inferior constrictor
- Its close relationship with the superior thyroid artery should be considered in thyroid surgeries before clamping the artery.

Applied Anatomy

- The external laryngeal nerve is usually injured during thyroid surgeries. Unilateral lesion results in mild hoarseness and bilateral lesion results in reduction of pitch and loudness
- Bilateral internal laryngeal nerve injury results in aspiration and dysphagia
- In case of foreign particles (fish bone) stuck in piriform fossa, during removal care should be taken to avoid injury to internal laryngeal nerve.

53. Histology of cerebellum.

Refer Short Note 18 – 2004.

54. Muscles of mastication.

Refer Essay Q. No. 7 – 2008.

55. Development of interatrial septum.

Refer Short Note 25 – 2006.

56. Maxillary sinus.

Refer Short Note 25 – 2007.

57. Basilar artery.

- **Formed** by the union of the two vertebral arteries at the lower border of pons
- It is related to basilar sulcus of pons
- It is a content of pontine cistern
- It **terminates** at the upper border of pons into two posterior cerebral arteries.
- **Branches and its distribution:**
  - **Anterior inferior cerebellar artery**—runs along the lower border of pons. The abducent and facial nerves are between the anterior inferior cerebellar and labyrinthine arteries. Supplies anterior part of inferior surface of cerebellum, pons and upper part of medulla oblongata
  - **Pontine branches**—many in number supply pons
  - **Labyrinthine artery**—runs parallel to anterior inferior cerebellar artery, passes through the internal acoustic meatus along with facial and stato acoustic nerves to supply internal ear
  - **Superior cerebellar artery**—given near termination, winds around the cerebral peduncle. The oculomotor and trochlear nerves are in-between the superior cerebellar and posterior

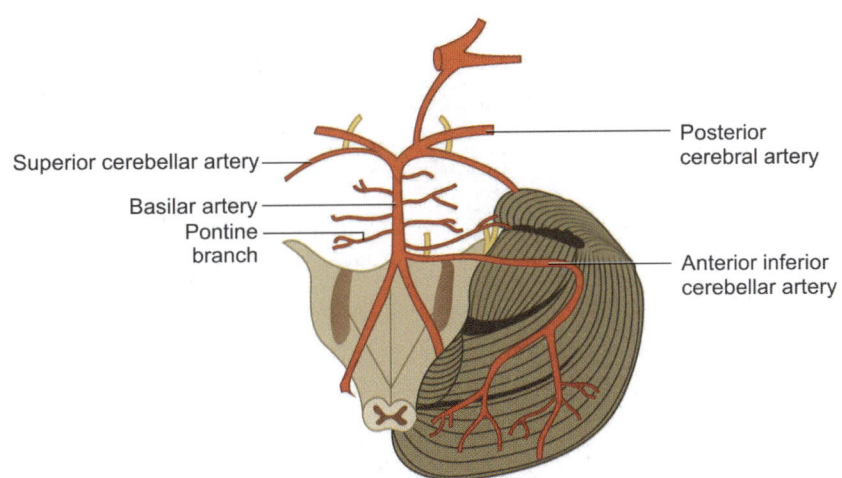

Fig. 34: Basilar artery.

cerebral arteries. Supplies superior surface of cerebellum, pons, pineal gland, take part in the formation of choroid plexus of third ventricle
- **Posterior cerebral artery**—the posterior communicating branch of ICA joins with this. It runs laterally around the cerebral peduncle of midbrain and enters the tentorial surface of cerebrum
- **In the cerebrum it supplies:**
  - **Superolateral surface**—occipital lobe and most of the inferior temporal gyrus
  - **Inferior surface**—uncus, para hippocampal, medial and lateral occipitotemporal gyri
  - **Medial surface**—cuneus, precuneus, lingual gyri. visual area is supplied by this artery
  - **Central branches**—posteromedial/thalamo perforator branches and posterolateral/thalamo geniculate branches supply thalamus, subthalamus, third ventricle, globus pallidus, geniculate bodies, pineal gland.

- **Applied anatomy**
  - Lesion of cortical branches of posterior cerebral artery results in contralateral homonymous hemianopia
  - **Anterior inferior cerebellar syndrome**
    - Affecting the lateral portion of lower part of pons
    - It affects the facial nucleus, cochlear nucleus, vestibular nucleus, spinal tract and nucleus of trigeminal, solitary nucleus and spinothalamic tract
    - It results in vertigo, nausea, nystagmus, loss of taste, lower motor neuron facial palsy, and loss of pain and temperature on face on side of lesion.

58. Vocal cord.

Refer Short Note 33 – 2005.

59. Bell's palsy.

Refer Essay Q. No. 9 – 2007.

60. Bronchopulmonary segments.

Refer Essay Q. No. 3 – 2004.

MBBS Examination 2016

ANSWER ALL QUESTIONS

I. Essay questions   **(15/10 Marks)**

1. Describe commencement, course, parts, relations, branches and termination of axillary artery.
2. Describe external features, relations, ligaments, blood supply and developmental anatomy of urinary bladder. Add a note on its applied anatomy.
3. Situation, capsules, relations, blood supply, and applied anatomy of thyroid gland.
4. Describe in detail parts, muscles, innervations, histology and development of tongue.

II. Short notes   **(5/4 Marks)**

1. Ankle joint.
2. Blood supply and lymphatic drainage of stomach.
3. Sacral plexus.
4. Third part of axillary artery.
5. Fourth ventricle.
6. Azygos vein.
7. Nucleus, course, distribution and applied anatomy of trochlear nerve.
8. Circle of Willis.

III. Short answer questions   **(3/2 Marks)**

1. Epiploic foramen.
2. Thenar space.
3. Oogenesis.
4. Medial plantar nerve.
5. Histology of liver.
6. Trigone of urinary bladder.
7. Deltoid muscle.
8. Bilaminar germ disc.
9. Arterial anastomosis around knee joint.
10. Iliofemoral ligament.
11. Blood supply of long bone.
12. Meckel's diverticulum.
13. Ulnar claw hand.
14. Histology of skeletal muscle.
15. Somites.
16. Branches of posterior cord of brachial plexus.
17. Intercostobrachial nerve.
18. Epo-ophoron and paro-ophoron.
19. Peroneal artery.
20. Sural nerve.
21. Histology of skin.
22. Development of palatine tonsil.
23. Orbicularis oculi.
24. Little's area.
25. Maxillary sinus.
26. Thoracic part of trachea.
27. Left coronary artery.
28. Cross section of midbrain at the level of superior colliculus.
29. Corpus callosum.
30. List out paired dural venous sinuses.
31. Middle meatus of nose.
32. Rathke's pouch.
33. Histology of thyroid gland.
34. Cross sectional diagram at the level of lower pons.
35. Coronary sinus.
36. Recurrent laryngeal nerve.
37. Arch of aorta.
38. Cervical sinus.
39. Boundaries and contents of superior mediastinum.
40. Sternocleidomastoid muscle.

I. ESSAY QUESTIONS

1. **Describe the commencement, course, parts, relations, branches and termination of axillary artery.**

Refer Essay Q. No. 4 – 2007.

2. **Describe external features, relations, ligaments, blood supply and developmental anatomy of urinary bladder. Add a note on its applied anatomy.**

External features, relations, applied anatomy Refer Essay Q. No. 2 – 2003.
Ligaments Refer Essay 4 – 2011.
Blood supply: Refer Essay 3 – 2010.
Development: Refer Short Notes 10 – 2007.

3. **Situation, capsules, relations, blood supply, and applied anatomy of thyroid gland.**

Situation, Capsule, relations Refer Short Notes Q. No. 17 – 2004.
Blood supply, applied anatomy Refer Short Notes 38 – 2008.

4. **Describe in detail the parts, muscles, innervations, histology and development of tongue.**

Parts, Innervation Refer Essay Q. No. 6 – 2007.
Muscles Refer Short Notes 31 – 2005.
Histology Refer Essay Q. No. 7 – 2009.
Development Refer Short Notes 20 – 2003.

II. SHORT NOTES

1. **Ankle joint.**

It is also known as **talocrural** joint.
- **Type:** It is a uniaxial, synovial, modified hinge variety.
- **Bones forming (Fig. 1):**
  - Tibiofibular mortise—formed by the inferior surface of tibia, medial malleolus of tibia and lateral malleolus of fibula
  - Trochlea tali—formed by (i) the trochlear surface of body of the talus, which is pulley shaped related to its upper surface (ii) comma shaped facet for tibial malleolus on the medial side, and (iii) triangular facet for the fibular malleolus on the lateral side.
- **Ligaments:**
  - **Fibrous capsule:**
    - It encloses the joint completely
    - It is thin in front and behind, and thickened at the sides
    - **Attachment:**
      * Above to the margins of tibiofibular mortise close to the articular surfaces
      * Below to the margins of trochlea tali.
  - **Deltoid ligament (Fig. 2A):**
    - It is triangular in shape
    - It is a strong ligament on the medial side

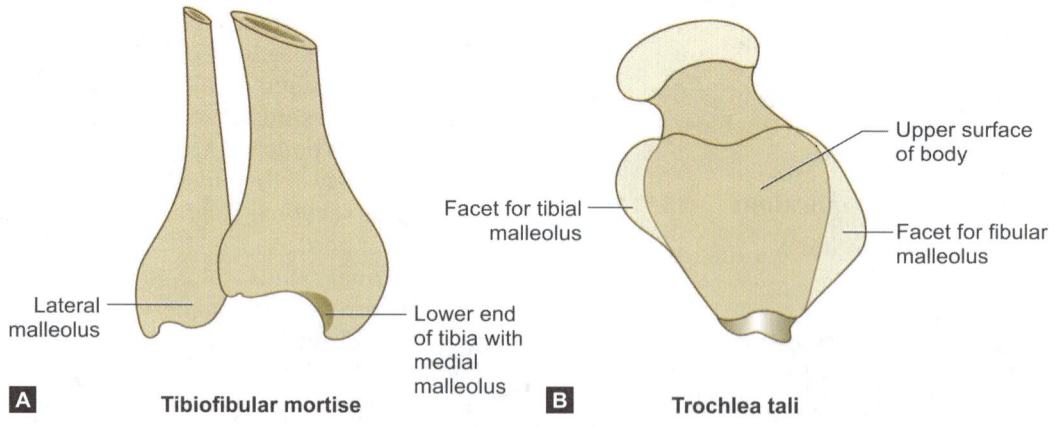

Figs. 1A and B: Bones forming.

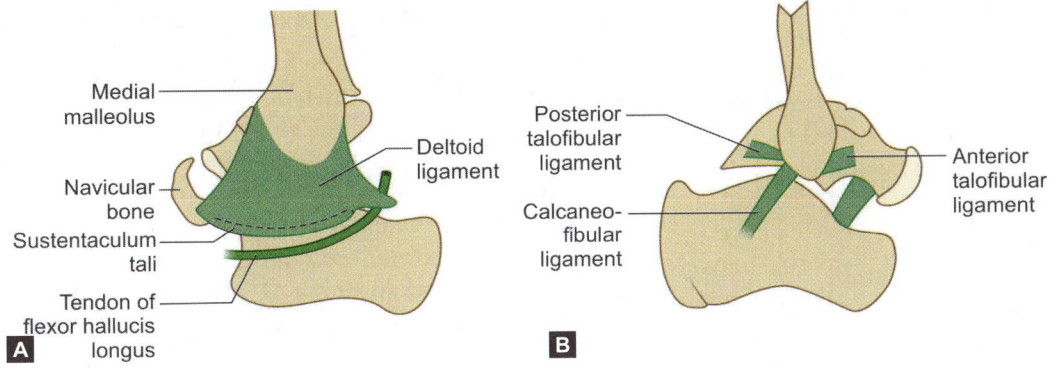

Figs. 2A and B: (A) Deltoid ligament; (B) Lateral ligament.

- It merges with the fibrous capsule
- The tendons of tibialis posterior and flexor digitorum longus cross it superficially
- It has two **parts**—superficial and deep
- **Attachment: Superficial part** is attached **above** to the tip and margins of medial malleolus. **Below** it divides into:
    * An **anterior part** attached to the tuberosity of navicular bone and blends with spring ligament
    * **Intermediate part** attached to the medial surface of sustentaculum tali of calcaneus
    * **Posterior part** to the medial tubercle of talus.
  - **Deep part:** From tip of medial malleolus to the non-articular portion of the medial surface of talus.
  - **Lateral ligaments (Fig. 2B):**
    - **Anterior talofibular ligament**—from anterior margin of lateral malleolus to the lateral side of neck of talus
    - **Posterior talofibular ligament**—from malleolar fossa of lateral malleolus of fibula to the posterior tubercle of talus
    - **Calcaneofibular ligament**—from tip of lateral malleolus to the peroneal tubercle on the lateral surface of calcaneus.
- **Movements and muscles producing:** Movements are dorsiflexion and plantar flexion.
  - **Dorsiflexion**
    - In dorsiflexion the angle between leg and foot is diminished
    - The heel touches the ground
    - The **range of movement** is about 10° when knee is straight and increased to 30° when knee is flexed
    - **Changes occurring** are:
      * During dorsiflexion the trochlear surface of talus comes in contact with the tibiofibular mortise
      * The lower end of fibula is displaced laterally
      * The inferior tibiofibular joint is stretched
      * At the same time the fibula glides upwards at the superior tibiofibular joint
      * The ankle joint becomes close packed, and provides maximum stability.
    - **Muscles producing**—tibialis anterior, extensor digitorum longus, extensor hallucis longus and peroneus tertius
  - **Plantar flexion**
    - In plantar flexion, the angle between the leg and foot is increased.

- Stands on toes
- It helps for forward thrust during locomotion
- The **range of movement** is about 30°, it is increased to 40° with assistance of tarsal joints
- Changes occurring are the joint becomes loose packed
- Space is available between the tibiofibular mortise and trochlear surface of talus
- Hence accessory movements—adduction and abduction are possible
- **Muscles producing** are—gastrocnemius, soleus assisted by tibialis posterior, flexor digitorum longus, flexor hallucis longus.
- **Arterial supply:** Malleolar branches of peroneal and anterior tibial arteries.
- **Nerve supply**
  - Deep peroneal nerve
  - Tibial nerve
  - Saphenous nerve.
- **Applied anatomy**
  - Ankle sprain—injury due to excessive inversion of foot. The anterior talofibular and calcaneofibular ligaments are torn sometimes
  - Ankle fracture usually associated with ligamentous tear. In supinated and adduction force is applied it results in transverse fracture of distal part of fibula and oblique medial malleolar fracture. In pronated and abduction force, transverse medial malleolar and oblique fibular fracture. It is also known as **Pott's fracture.**

2. Blood supply and lymphatic drainage of stomach.

Blood supply Refer Essay Q. No. 2 – 2007.
Lymphatic drainage Refer Short Notes 6 – 2007.

3. Sacral plexus.

Refer Short Notes 7 – 2011.

4. Third part of axillary artery.

Refer Essay Q. No. 4 – 2007.

5. Fourth ventricle.

Refer Short Notes 35 – 2012.

6. Azygos vein.

Refer Short Notes 21 – 2011.

7. Nucleus, course, distribution and applied anatomy of trochlear nerve.

- It is the fourth cranial nerve
- Purely motor
- Supplies the extraocular muscle which is developed from 3rd somitomere
- **Structures supplied:** The nerve supplies the extraocular muscle superior oblique
- **Peculiarities:** Only cranial nerve emerging dorsally—dorsal surface of the midbrain
  - Only cranial nerve which decussate completely
  - Thinnest cranial nerve.
- **Functional component:** Somatic efferent supplying the extraocular muscle which is developed from head somite
- **Nucleus of origin:** Trochlear nucleus is situated in the gray matter around the cerebral aqueduct in the midbrain at the level of inferior colliculus.
- **Course**
  - **Within midbrain (Fig. 3A)**
    - The nerve fibers pass dorsolaterally around the central gray matter
    - Passes medial to the mesencephalic nucleus
    - Decussates before it emerges.
  - **Emergence (Fig. 3B)**
    - Emerges below the inferior colliculus, on either side of frenulum veli.
    - It winds around the cerebral peduncle.
  - **Interpeduncular fossa:**
    - Lateral to the cerebral peduncle
    - Situated between the two arteries posterior cerebral and superior cerebellar arteries.

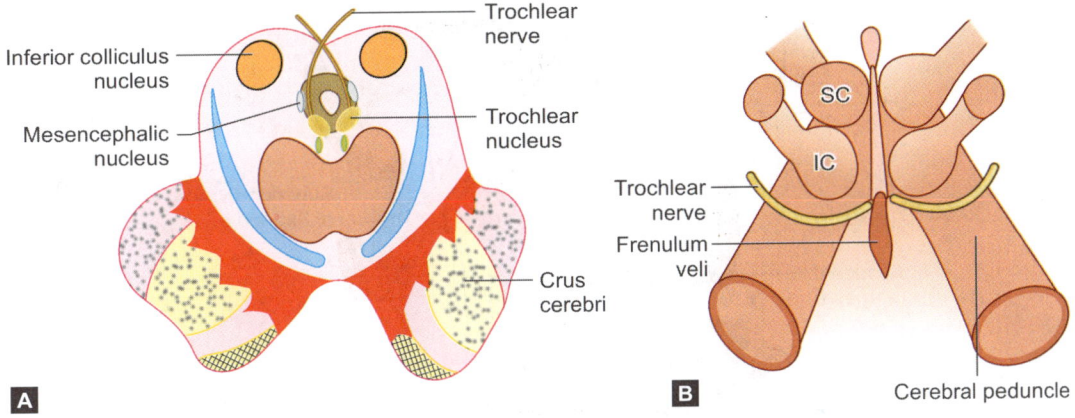

Figs. 3A and B: Course of trochlear nerve: (A) Midbrain inferior colliculus; (B) Dorsal emergence.

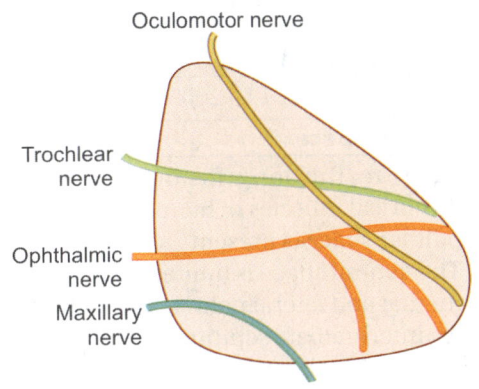

Fig. 4: Lateral wall of cavernous sinus.

- **Intracranial**
  - It runs forward, pierces the dura mater just below the attached border of tentorium cerebelli
  - It reaches the lateral wall of cavernous sinus.
- **Lateral wall of cavernous sinus (Fig. 4)**
  - In the **lateral wall of cavernous sinus,** the trochlear nerve is related below to the ophthalmic and maxillary nerves and above to the oculomotor nerve
  - From lateral wall, it enters the orbit by passing through the superior orbital fissure.

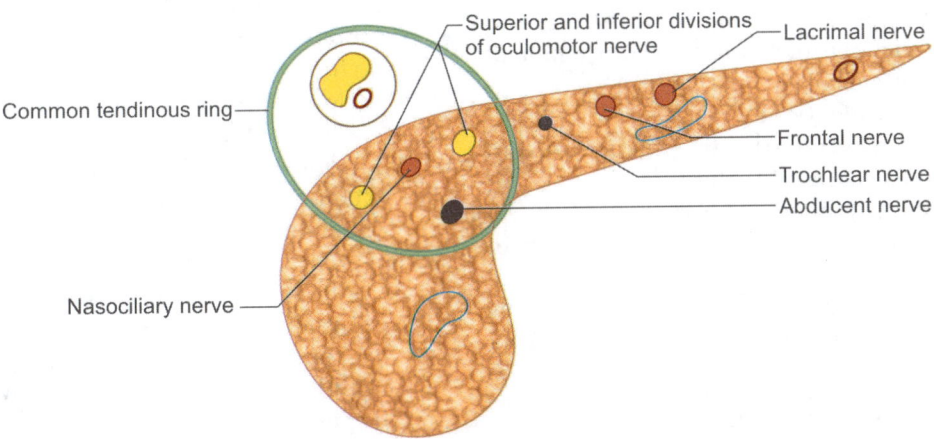

Fig. 5: Superior orbital fissure.

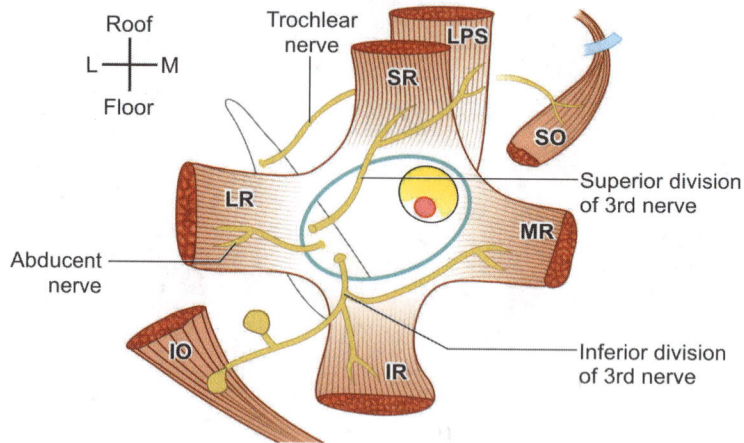

Fig. 6: In the orbit.

- **Superior orbital fissure (Fig. 5)**
  - It passes outside the common tendinous ring through the lateral compartment
  - It is medial to the lacrimal and frontal nerves.
- **In the orbit (Fig. 6):** It passes above the levator palpabrae and superior rectus muscles.
- **Distribution:** Terminates by supplying the ocular surface of superior oblique muscle
- **Connections**
  - Cerebral cortex through corticobulbar fibers
  - To visual cortex
  - Through medial longitudinal fasciculus the nerve is connected to 3rd, 6th, and 8th nerve for coordinated movement of the eyeball.
- **Communications**
  - With sympathetic plexus around internal carotid artery
  - With ophthalmic nerve.
- **Applied anatomy:** Unilateral lesion of trochlear nerve the superior oblique muscle is paralysed. The patient complains of double vision whenever he looks down.

8. Circle of Willis.
Refer Short Notes 24 – 2005.

III. SHORT ANSWER QUESTIONS

1. Epiploic foramen.
Refer Short Answer 14 – 2009.

2. Thenar space.
- Deep to the long flexor tendons and lumbrical muscles of hand, a large central palmar space is present
- The central space is limited at the sides by medial and lateral palmar septae
- An intermediate septum divides the space into a midpalmar space and thenar space.

Thenar Space
- **Shape** is triangular
  - It is situated lateral to midpalmar space.
- **Boundaries (Fig. 7)**
  - In front
    - Muscles of thenar eminence
    - Flexor tendons of the index finger
    - First and the second lumbricals.
  - Behind: Adductor pollicis
  - Laterally:
    - Lateral palmar septum extending from palmar aponeurosis to the first metacarpal bone
    - Tendon of flexor pollicis longus.
  - Medially: The intermediate fibrous septa separating the mid palmar space,

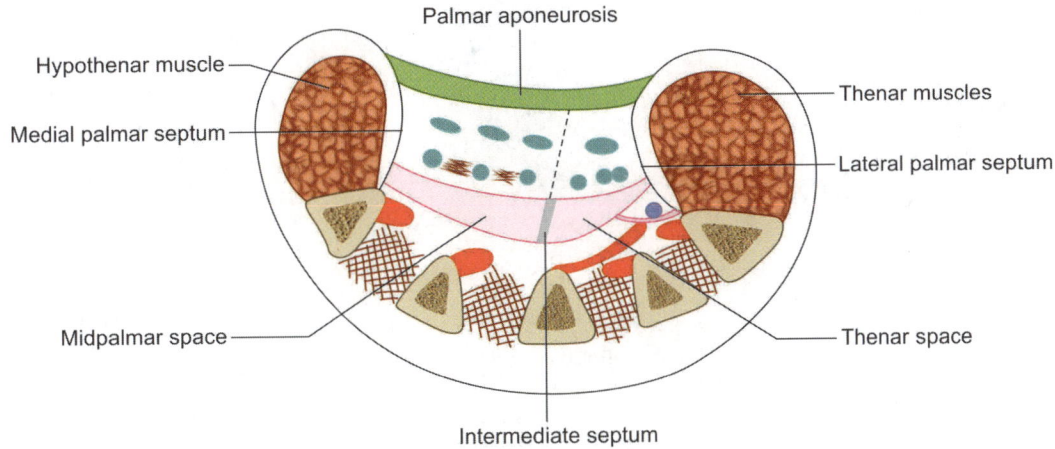

Fig. 7: Fascial spaces of hand.

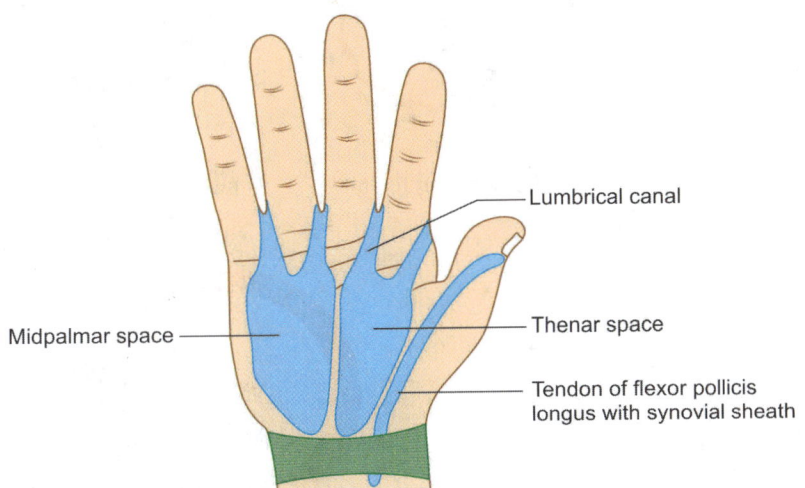

Fig. 8: Communication through lumbrical canal.

extending from fascia covering the undersurface of flexor tendons to the third metacarpal bone
- Proximal—sometimes communicate with space of parona
- Distally—extends as diverticula along the first and second lumbrical tendons to the interdigital clefts.

3. **Oogenesis.**

- The process of maturation of primordial female germ cell from primary oocyte to mature ovum is called oogenesis
- The endodermal cells from hindgut enters the gonadal ridge and give rise to **oogonia**
- Oogonia by end of 3rd month differentiate into **primary oocyte**
- At birth, each ovary consists of 600,000 to 800,000 primary oocytes
- At puberty, it is reduced to 40,000
- The primary oocyte surrounded by a layer of follicular cells forms the **primary ovarian follicle.** The nucleus of oocyte is eccentric and contains **44 + 2X** chromosomes

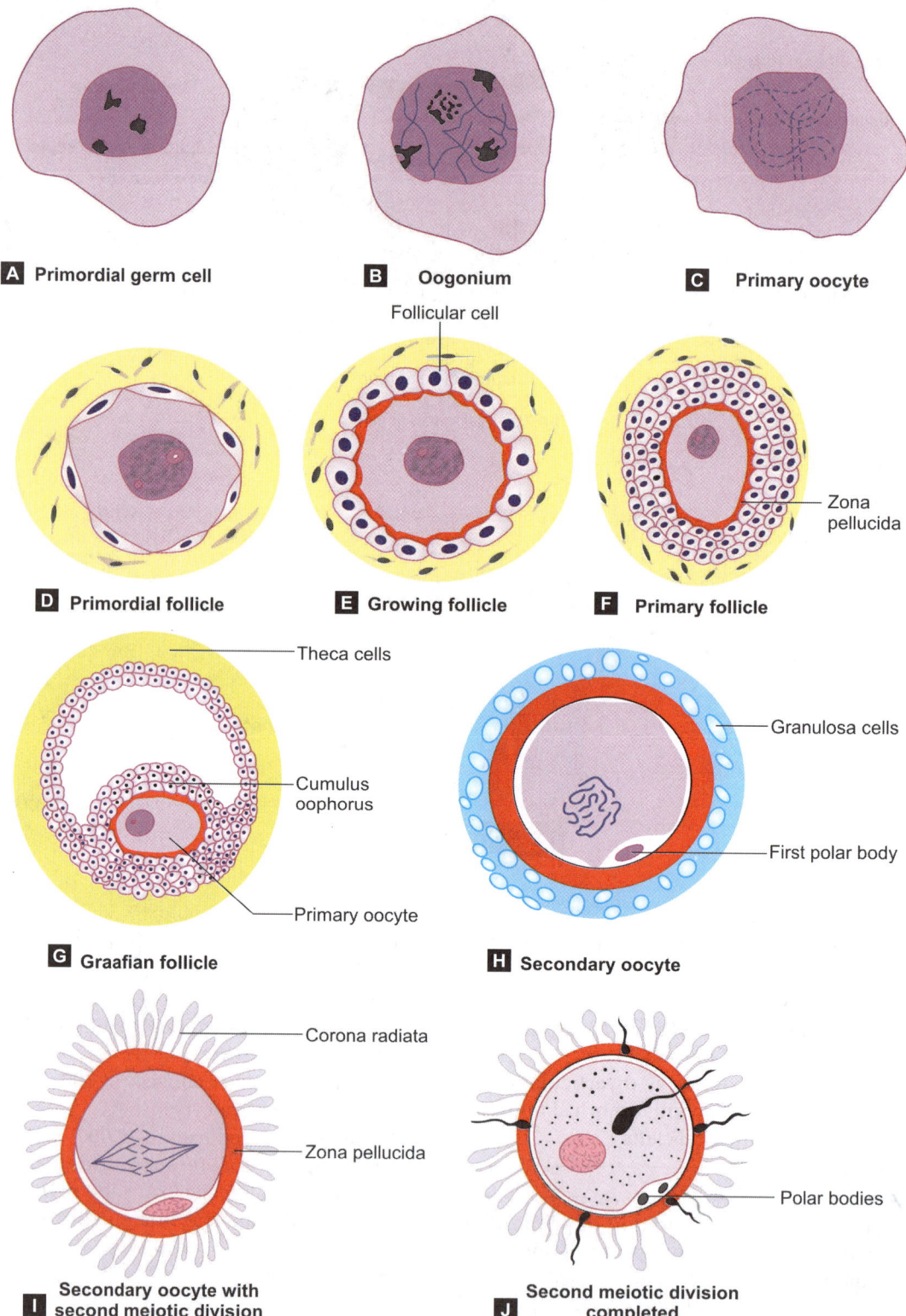

Figs. 9A to J: Stages of oogenesis.

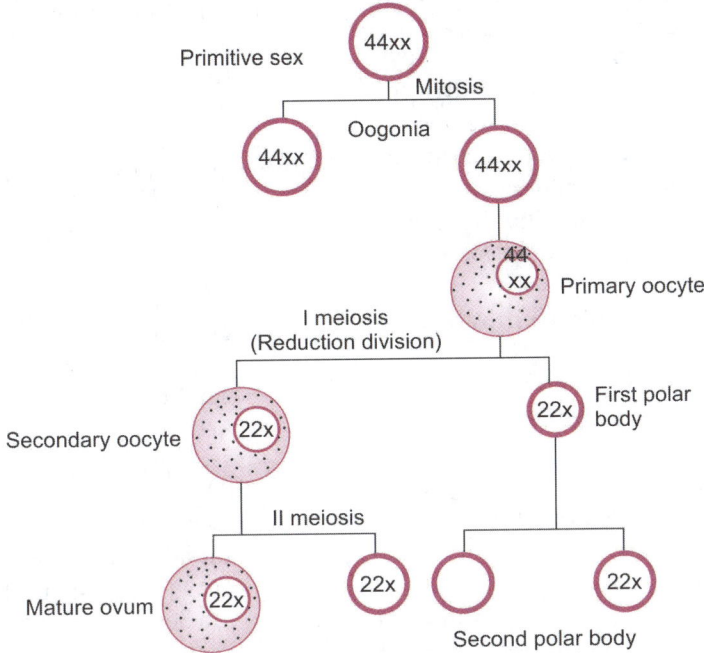

Fig. 10: Oogenesis.

- The follicular cells become cuboidal and form several layers
- Amorphous material accumulates between oocyte and follicular cells, which aggregate to form a membrane called **zona pellucida**
- As follicle enlarges, fluid filled spaces appear. These spaces join to form a cavity known as **antrum folliculi.** The fluid is called liquor folliculi
- Because of formation of antrum folliculi the follicular cells are divided into an outer layer called **stratum granulosum** and an inner layer called **cumulus ovaricus**. The cumulus surrounds the oocyte
- Outside stratum granulosum, stromal cells of ovary form a sheath known as **theca folliculi**. It has an outer fibrous layer—theca externa and inner vascular layer—theca interna
- The primary oocyte completes 1st meiosis. The nuclear division is equal (22+X chromosome), whereas the cytoplasmic division is unequal. The result of this division is a large cell called **secondary oocyte** and smaller cell, the **first polar body**
- The secondary oocyte and the 1st polar body in the perivitelline space is called the **vesicular/Graafian follicle**
- The secondary oocyte enters 2nd meiotic division
- Fully formed graafian follicle rupturing from the surface of ovary is called ovulation. The secondary oocyte with cumulus ovaricus and zona pellucida is shed
- The shed ova enter the fallopian tube by the movement of cilia and contraction of the tube. If fertilization occurs, then the secondary oocyte completes the 2nd meiotic division
- The division is unequal, the large cell with abundant cytoplasm is called **mature ova** (22+X) and smaller is the second polar body. If fertilization does not occur, it begins to degenerate after 24 to 48 hours.

4. **Medial plantar nerve.**
- The tibial nerve passes deep to flexor retinaculum and terminates by dividing into medial and lateral plantar nerves
- The medial plantar nerve is the **largest terminal branch of tibial nerve**
- The nerve is accompanied by the medial plantar artery along the medial side.
- **Course**
  - Enters the sole passing deep to abductor hallucis
  - Then it passes between the abductor hallucis and flexor digitorum brevis muscle.
- **Termination:** It divides into a proper digital nerve and three common plantar digital nerves.
- **Branches:**
  - **From trunk:** Branches to abductor hallucis and flexor digitorum brevis
  - **Proper digital nerve:**
    - Muscular branch to flexor hallucis brevis
    - Cutaneous branch to skin of medial side of great toe.
  - **Three common plantar digital nerves**
    1. The first branch supplies skin of adjacent sides of great and second toe, and it also supplies first lumbricals
    2. The second branch supplies skin of adjacent sides of second and third toes
    3. The third branch supplies skin of adjacent sides of third and fourth toe, and communicates with lateral plantar nerve
    - Dorsal branches supply skin around nail bed
    - Articular branches to interphalangeal joints.
- **Applied anatomy**
  - **Entrapment syndromes**
    - Tarsal tunnel syndrome: The tibial nerve may be compressed deep to the flexor retinaculum
    - Entrapment may be due to space occupying ganglion, network of blood vessels, deep fascia of abductor hallucis brevis
    - The nerve can be compressed at Henry's knot (Turner's slip) where the fibers from tendon of flexor

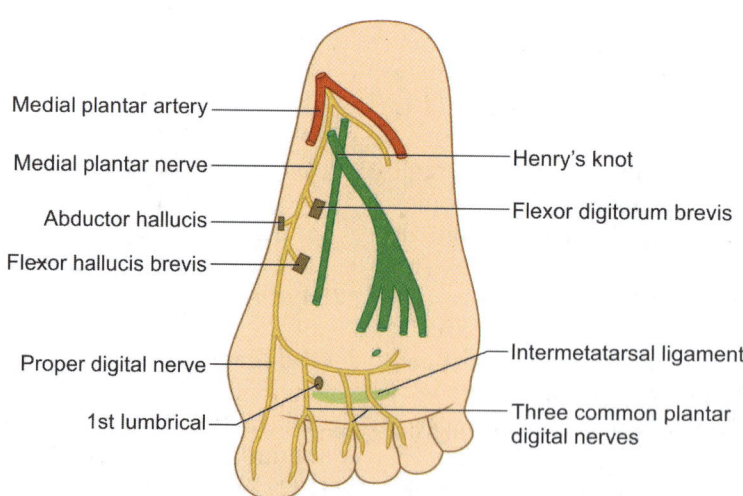

Fig. 11: Medial plantar nerve.

hallucis longus pass deep to the flexor digitorum longus
- Entrapment of the common digital nerves as they pass deep to the intermetatarsal ligament can result in Morton's neuroma.

5. Histology of liver.

- Liver is covered by a **capsule** made of connective tissue called Glisson's capsule
- Septae extends from capsule into the liver substance dividing into hepatic lobules
- **Hepatic lobules** are hexagonal in shape
- Each lobule is made up of plates of hepatocytes and central vein in the center of each lobule
- The **hepatocytes** are large cells with rounded nucleus in the center. The cytoplasm contains numerous mitochondria, roughened endoplasmic reticulum, golgi complex, lysosomes and vacuoles containing enzymes
- The hepatocytes are highly active and store glycogen, lipids and iron
- The hepatocytes are arranged in the form of anastomosing plates (one cell thick)
- Spaces in between hepatocytes are occupied by sinusoids
- The sinusoids open into a central vein
- **The sinusoids** are lined by discontinuous endothelial cells and **Kupffer cells** which are the hepatic macrophages
- **Portal canals** are at angular intervals seen at the periphery of the lobules
- Each portal canal contains **portal triad** formed by a) a branch of the portal vein, b) a branch of the hepatic artery and c) an interlobular bile duct
- **Space of Mall** is seen surrounding the portal triad
- **Perisinusoidal space of Disse** is space between sinusoids and hepatocytes. Microvilli of hepatocytes extend into this space
- **Ito/hepatic stellate cells** are present in perisinusoidal space which helps in hepatic fibrosis
- **Portal lobule** containing portal triad at center and central veins at angles is triangular in shape
- **Portal acinus** is the area of liver tissue supplied by a hepatic arteriole, seen between junction of two hepatic lobules.

6. Trigone of urinary bladder.

Refer Essay Q. No. 2 – 2003.

7. Deltoid muscle.

Refer Short Notes 11 – 2012.

8. Bilaminar germ disc.

- After fertilization, the cell division starts
- It divides into 2 cell, 4 cell, 16 cell stage called the morula
- The morula is converted to blastocyst stage by the entry of fluid from the uterine cavity
- By the formation of blastocele the cells are differentiated into an inner cell mass

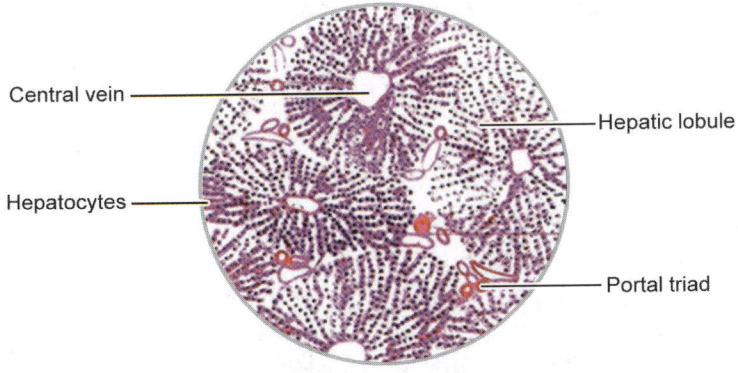

Fig. 12: Histology of liver.

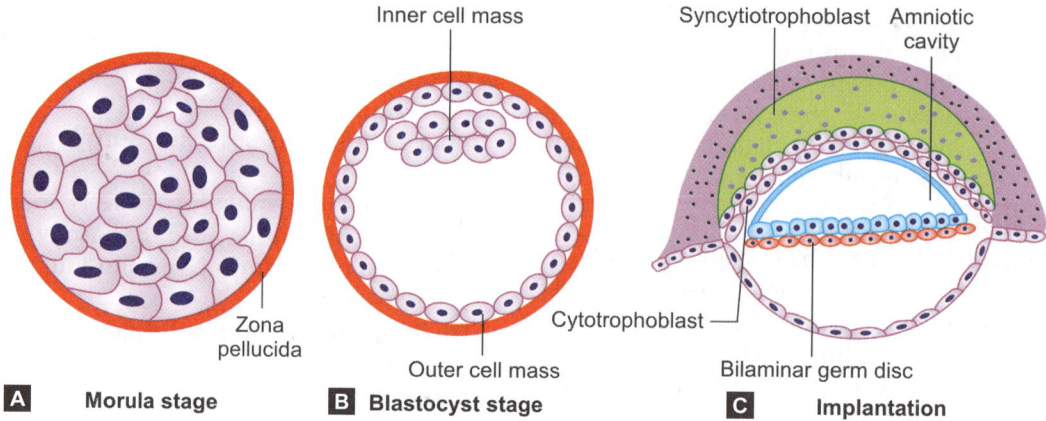

Figs. 13A to C: Formation of amniotic and primary yolk sac cavities.

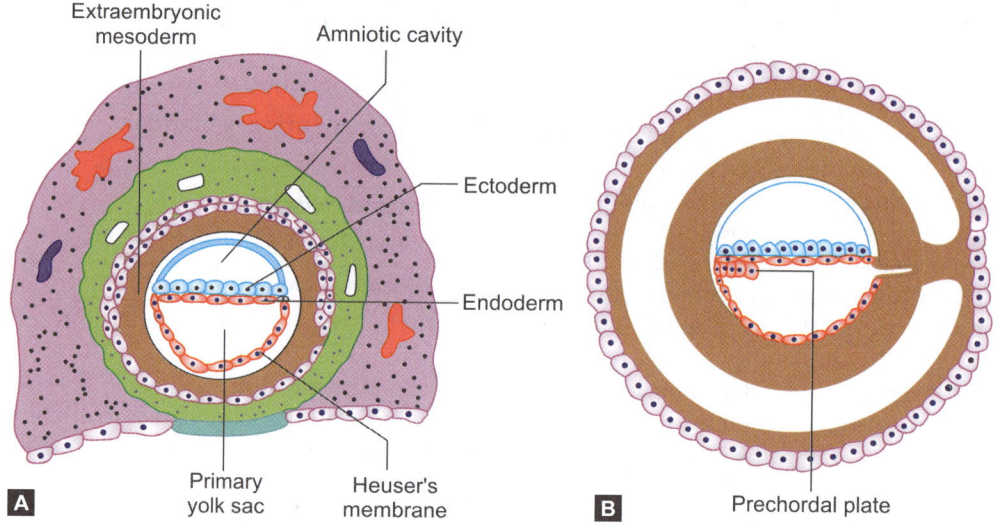

Figs. 14A and B: Formation of bilaminar germ disc.

called embryoblast and outer cell mass the trophoblast
- At the eighth day, the blastocyst is partially embedded in the endometrial stroma
- The trophoblast differentiates into inner **cytotrophoblast** and multinucleated syncytium or **syncytiotrophoblast**
- The inner cell mass differentiates into two layers
- Upper high columnar cells forming **epiblast or primary ectoderm** and lower flattened or cuboidal cells known as **hypoblast or primary endoderm**

- A thin basement membrane intervenes between the two laminae
- The two layers form a flat disc called the **bilaminar germ disc** which gives rise to the development of embryo proper
- A cavity appears related to epiblast enlarges to form the **amniotic cavity**, bounded by the amnioblasts and epiblast layer
- On the ninth day, another cavity the primary yolk sac cavity is formed, by the appearance of the Heuser's membrane
- The first differentiation seen in the germ disc is appearance of **prechordal plate**

- At the cephalic end the endodermal cells are thickened over an oval area and form **prechordal plate**
- The plate establishes the cephalocaudal axis
- The bilaminar germ disc is converted into **trilaminar disc** by the third week by the process of **gastrulation**
- It is formed by the appearance of **secondary intraembryonic mesoderm**, between the ectodermal and endodermal layers.

9. **Arterial anastomosis around knee joint.**
- It is also known as **genicular anastomosis**
- It is on the anterior aspect of the knee
- The **arteries taking part in the anastomosis** are: 1. Superior medial genicular artery, 2. Superior lateral genicular artery, 3. Inferior medial genicular artery, 4. Inferior lateral genicular artery, 5. Descending genicular artery, 6. Descending branch of lateral circumflex artery, 7. Anterior tibial recurrent and 8. Circumflex fibular artery
- The anastomosis is **formed** by the branches of popliteal artery, femoral artery and anterior and posterior tibial arteries
- **Horizontal anastomosis**
  - **Above**—superior medial genicular artery anastomoses with superior lateral genicular artery branches of popliteal artery, descending genicular branch of femoral artery and descending branch of lateral circumflex artery from profunda femoris. This anastomosis is across lower end of femur.
  - **Below**—inferior medial genicular artery anastomoses with inferior lateral genicular artery branches of popliteal artery, the recurrent branch of anterior tibial and circumflex fibular branch of posterior tibial artery, saphenous branch of descending genicular artery. This anastomosis is deep to ligamentum patellae.
- **Vertical anastomosis**
  - **Medially**—superior medial genicular with inferior medial genicular artery
  - **Laterally**—superior lateral genicular with inferior lateral genicular artery.
- **Function:** During flexion of knee joint, the popliteal artery is kinked resulting in sluggish blood flow. This anastomosis is to

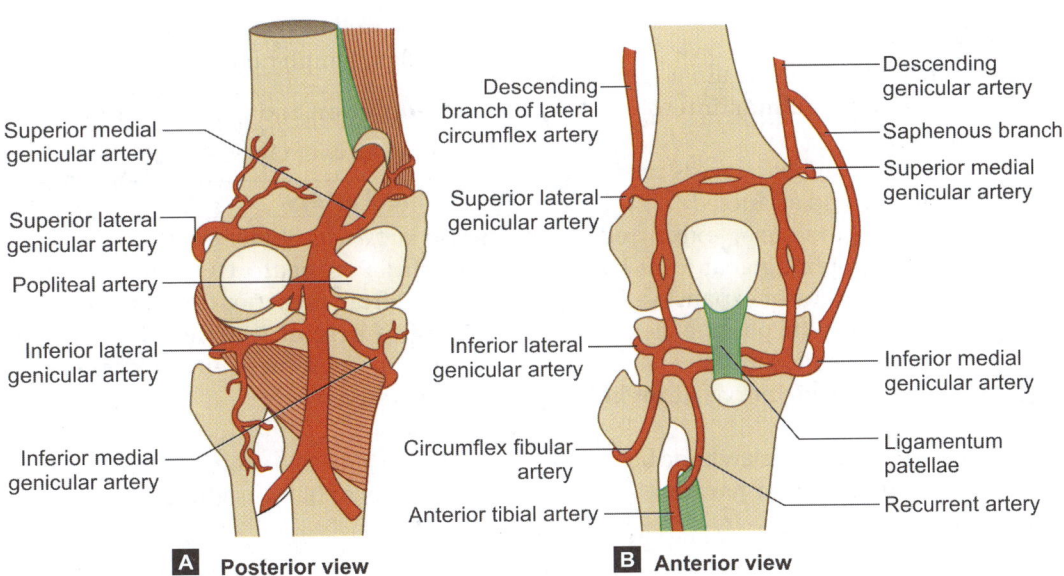

Figs. 15A and B: Anastomosis around knee.

maintain the blood flow to the leg during full knee flexion.

10. Iliofemoral ligament.

Refer Essay Q. No. 1 – 2004.

11. Blood supply of long bone.

Refer Short Notes 2 – 2009.

12. Meckel's diverticulum.

Refer Short Notes 12 – 2005.

13. Ulnar claw hand.

- Ulnar nerve passes superficial to the flexor retinaculum
- Enters the hand by passing through Guyon's canal accompanied by ulnar artery
- The **muscles supplied** by ulnar nerve in hand:
  – Hypothenar muscles
  – 3rd and 4th lumbricals
  – Adductor pollicis
  – All palmar interossei
  – All dorsal interossei.
- **Cause: Injury to ulnar nerve behind medial epicondyle** can result in claw hand
  – **Effect of lesion**: The medial two fingers are extended at metacarpophalangeal joints, and partly flexed at the interphalangeal joints.
  – **Reason for lesion**
    - Due to injury to the ulnar nerve the dorsal and palmar interossei are paralyzed
    - Hence the medial fingers cannot be abducted and adducted
    - The fingers are extended at metacarpophalangeal joint by the action of extensor expansion
    - This results in passive flexion at interphalangeal joint
    - Injury to ulnar nerve **at or below wrist**.
  – **Effect of lesion**: The claw hand becomes more marked—**ulnar paradox**

– **Reason for lesion**
  - The nerve supply to the flexor digitorum profundus is spared
  - Hence the extension at metacarpophalangeal joints is associated with active flexion at interphalangeal joints of the medial two fingers.

14. Histology of skeletal muscle.

Refer Short Answer Questions 26 – 2010.

15. Somites.

Refer Short Answer Questions 3 – 2014.

16. Branches of posterior cord of brachial plexus.

Refer Short Answer Questions 4 – 2008.

17. Intercostobrachial nerve.

- The lateral branch of second intercostal nerve is known as intercostobrachial nerve
- The lateral cutaneous branch of second intercostal nerve remains undivided.
- The structure **supplied** by the intercostobrachial nerve is the skin of floor of axilla and upper medial part of arm
- It **is connected** with:
  – Medial cutaneous nerve of arm from brachial plexus
  – Posterior cutaneous nerve of radial nerve.
- **Situation**: It lies among the central group of axillary lymph nodes.

18. Epo-ophoron and paro-ophoron.

Refer Short Answer Questions 20 – 2011.

19. Peroneal artery.

It is also known as fibular artery.
- **Origin**: Peroneal artery is the largest branch from posterior tibial artery
  Level of origin: It arises about 2.5 cm below the commencement of posterior tibial artery.
- **Course**
  – Descends between tibialis posterior and flexor hallucis longus muscles

- Runs along the medial crest of fibula
- Passes behind the inferior tibiofibular joint.
- **Termination:** The peroneal artery is continued as lateral calcaneal artery.
- **Branches**
  - Nutrient artery to fibula
  - Muscular branches to posterior compartment muscles
  - Communicating branch to join posterior tibial artery
  - Perforating branch pierces the interosseous membrane to take part in lateral malleolar network by anastomosing with dorsalis pedis and anterior tibial arteries
  - Lateral calcaneal branch.

20. Sural nerve.

- The sural nerve is a cutaneous **branch of** tibial nerve
- It is also called as **medial sural cutaneous nerve**
- **Course**
  - The nerve descends between the medial and lateral heads of gastrocnemius muscle
  - Pierces the deep fascia in the upper part of leg
  - Joins with the sural communicating branch from common peroneal nerve
  - Passes lateral to calcanean tendon
  - Then it runs along the lateral side of the foot and little toe
  - Between lateral malleolus and calcaneus, the nerve is **related** to short saphenous vein.
- **Areas supplied**
  - Skin of distal third of Posterior surface of the leg
  - Skin of distal third of lateral surface of the leg
  - Skin of lateral side of foot and little toe.
- **Applied anatomy**
  - Injury to sural nerve can result in painful neuromas
  - The nerve is used for graft as it is purely sensory and as it is superficial it is easily identified.

21. Histology of skin.

Refer Short Notes 20 – 2011.

22. Development of palatine tonsil.

Refer Short Notes 34 – 2005.

23. Orbicularis oculi.

Refer Short Answer Questions 41 – 2014.

24. Little's area.

Refer Short Answer Questions 39 – 2015.

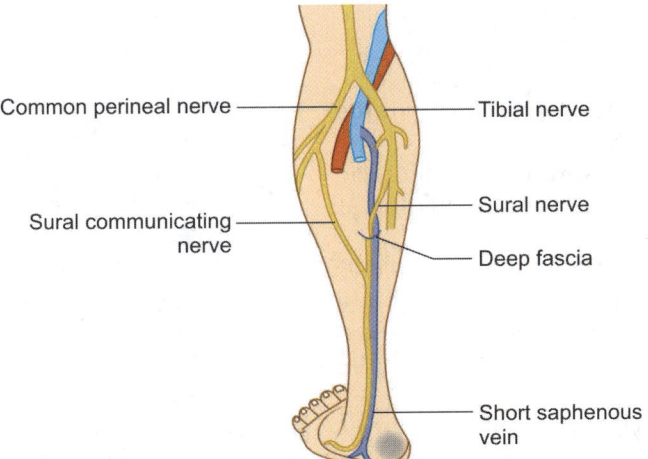

Fig. 16: Sural nerve.

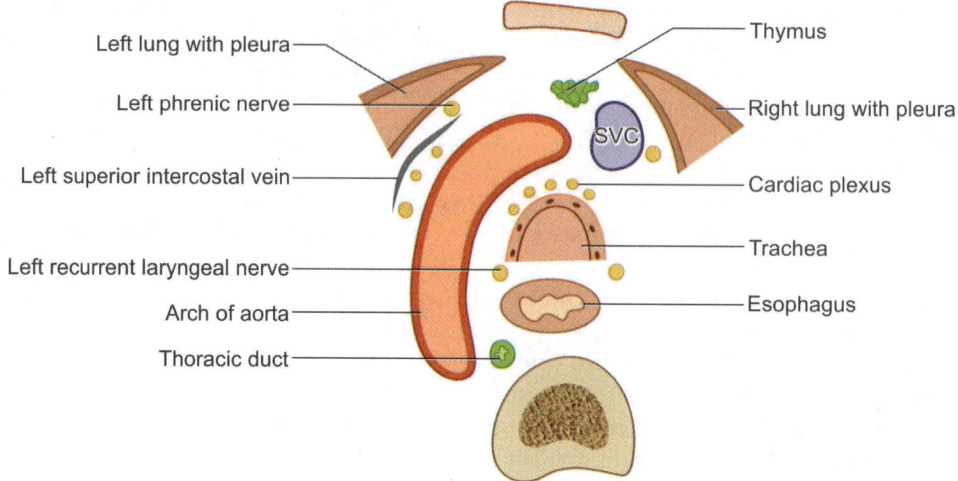

Fig. 17: Relations of trachea in superior mediastinum.

25. Maxillary sinus.
Refer Short Answer Questions 25 – 2007.

26. Thoracic part of trachea.

- Trachea commences from the lower border of cricoid cartilage at the level of C6
- It passes through neck and enters the superior mediastinum
- The thoracic part is 5 – 6 cm long
- In the superior mediastinum, it lies in median plane.
- **Termination**
  - Opposite to sternal angle divides into right and left bronchi
  - The bifurcation corresponds to T4 level.
  - Towards termination it deviates towards right side.
- **Relations (Figs. 17 and 18):** The thoracic part of trachea is surrounded by blood vessels.
  - **In front**
    - Manubrium sterni
    - Origins of sternothyroid and sternohyoid muscles
    - Pretracheal fascia
    - Thyroidea ima artery
    - Left brachiocephalic vein crosses
    - Brachiocephalic trunk
    - Left common carotid artery
    - Deep cardiac plexus
    - Arch of aorta.
  - **Behind:**
    - Esophagus
    - Left recurrent laryngeal nerve in tracheoesophageal groove.
  - **Right side:**
    - Right lung and pleura
    - Right vagus nerve
    - Arch of azygos.
  - **Left side**
    - Left lung
    - Arch of aorta
    - Left common carotid artery.
- **Structure**
  - Trachea is made of incomplete C shaped cartilaginous rings
  - The last ring is triangular in shape called carina
  - The interior of carina presents a ridge and acts as a guide for surgeons during bronchoscopy.
- **Blood supply:** Inferior thyroid artery and bronchial arteries
- **Lymphatic drainage:** Pretracheal and paratracheal nodes

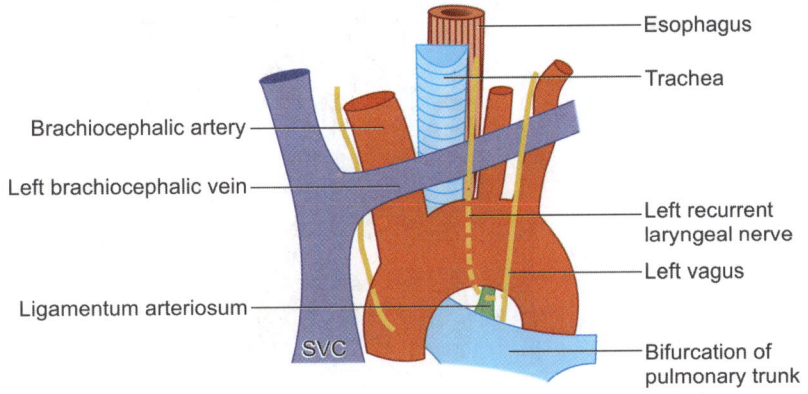

Fig. 18: Relation of trachea.

- **Nerve supply**
  - Parasympathetic—both vagi and recurrent laryngeal nerves
  - Sympathetic—T1 - T5 thoracic segments of spinal cord.
- **Development**
  - Developed from intermediate part of laryngotracheal tube
  - The laryngotracheal tube is from the ventral wall of the pharyngeal part of foregut.
  - The cartilaginous rings are developed from mesoderm of 6th pharyngeal arch.
- **Congenital anomaly:** Tracheoesophageal fistula—distal part of esophagus is connected to the trachea by a narrow canal just above bifurcation
- **Applied anatomy**: The trachea is compressed sometimes by the enlargement of thymus, arch of aorta or lymph nodes. Compression of trachea results in dyspnea (difficulty in breathing), irritative cough.

27. Left coronary artery.
Refer Essay Q. No. 5 – 2005.

28. Cross section of midbrain at the level of superior colliculus.
Refer Short Notes 40 – 2009.

29. Corpus callosum.
Refer Short Notes 25 – 2011.

30. List out paired dural venous sinuses.
Refer Essay Q. No. 5 – 2015.

31. Middle meatus of nose.
Refer Short Notes Q. No. 16 – 2004.

32. Rathke's pouch.
Refer Short Answer Questions 42 – 2012.

33. Histology of thyroid gland.
Refer Essay Q. No. 8 – 2007.

34. Cross sectional diagram at the level of lower pons.
Refer Short Notes 13 – 2004.

35. Coronary sinus.
Refer Essay Q. No. 5 – 2005.

36. Recurrent Laryngeal nerve.

- The recurrent laryngeal nerve is branch from vagus, and the origin of the branch differ on either side.
- **Origin**
  - **Right recurrent laryngeal nerve**
    - The right recurrent laryngeal nerve is given by right vagus in front of the right subclavian artery
    - Descends, and winds around the 1st part of subclavian artery and runs upwards.
  - **Left recurrent laryngeal nerve (Fig. 19):**

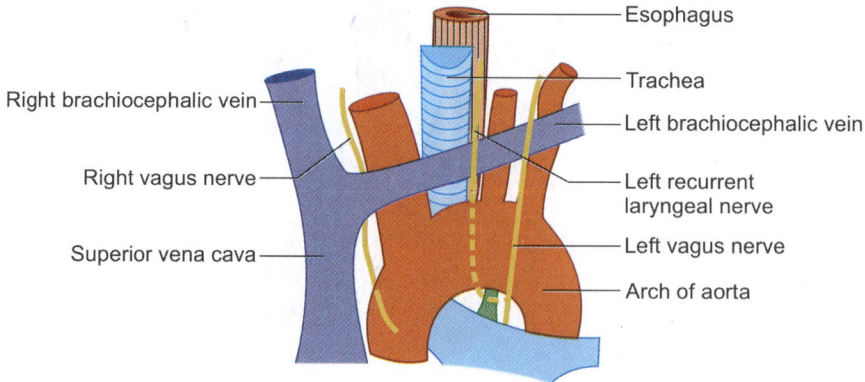

Fig. 19: Recurrent laryngeal nerve—Left.

- The left recurrent laryngeal nerve is from left vagus in the thorax
- It is given inferolateral to the arch of aorta
- Passes inferior to the arch and posterior to the ligamentum arteriosum.
– **Course in the neck—for both nerves**
  - The nerve passes close to the lower pole of lateral lobe of thyroid, and is closely related to the inferior thyroid artery
  - The nerve may pass between the branches of artery or in front or behind the artery
  - Ascends upwards in the tracheo-esophageal groove
  - Passes below the lower border of inferior constrictor
  - The nerve enters the larynx behind the articulation of inferior horn of thyroid cartilage with cricoid cartilage
  - It terminates within the submucosa of the larynx.
- **Distribution:**
  – All the intrinsic muscles of the larynx except cricothyroid
  – Sensory to larynx below the level of vocal cords
  – Cardiac branches to deep cardiac plexus
  – Branches to trachea and esophagus
  – To inferior constrictor of pharynx.
- **Applied anatomy:** During thyroidectomy, the recurrent laryngeal nerve may be injured as they are closely related to inferior thyroid artery resulting in hoarseness of voice. Injury to nerve can be avoided by ligating the artery away from the gland.

37. Arch of aorta.
Refer Short Notes 11 – 2004.

38. Cervical sinus.
- The depression below the second arch is known as cervical sinus
- Four ectodermal clefts are present in the ectodermal layer of the pharyngeal apparatus
- Later the first cleft alone persists and other clefts disappear

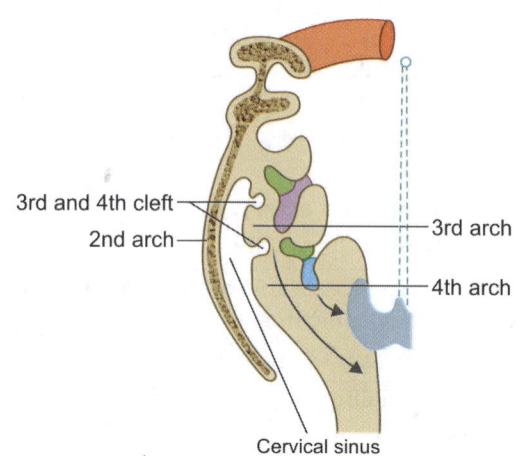

Fig. 20: Branchial clefts.

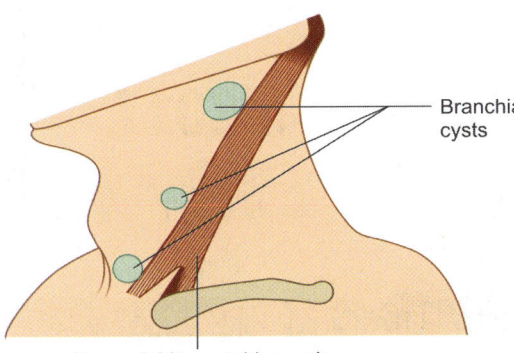

Fig. 21: Sites of branchial cysts.

- The active proliferation of the mesodermal cells of second arch overgrows the 3rd and 4th arches
- The second arch proliferation fuses with the epicardial ridge
- By this the second, third, fourth clefts get submerged, and contact with surface is lost
- The space between the clefts and the proliferation of second arch is called cervical sinus
- The clefts later burrow into the mesoderm and form placodal vesicles
- The sinus is closed and smooth concavity of the neck is restored
- The closure of the sinus is either by proliferation of the second arch or by gradual exteriorization of the third and fourth arches.

Congenital Anomalies

- **Branchial cyst (Fig. 21)**
  - Cystic swelling seen along the anterior border or deep to sternocleidomastoid muscle
  - It is usually situated close to angle of mandible
  - It is a painless cystic swelling
  - Usually not present at birth
  - It is due to failure of complete obliteration of cervical sinus.
- **Branchial fistula**
  - Fistulas are due to failure of second branchial arch to grow over the third and fourth arches
  - It leads to remnant of the second, third, and fourth clefts in contact with the surface
  - May be with external communication, with internal communication, or complete communication
  - Internal fistulas are rare
  - The sinus will be connected to the pharynx and usually in the tonsillar region.

39. Boundaries and contents of superior mediastinum.

Refer Short Notes 38 – 2012.

40. Sternocleidomastoid muscle.

Refer Short Notes 31 – 2006.

MBBS Examination 2017

ANSWER ALL QUESTIONS

I. Essay questions (15/10 Marks)

1. Discuss in detail about portal vein under the following headings: (a) Formation, course and termination, (b) Relations and tributaries, (c) Sites of portosystemic anastomosis and (d) Clinical anatomy.
2. Describe parotid gland in detail. Add a note on its applied aspects.
3. Describe the shoulder joint in detail. Add a note on its applied aspect.
4. Describe in detail about the blood supply of heart. Add a note on its applied anatomy.

II. Short notes (5/4 Marks)

1. Brachial artery.
2. Medial longitudinal arch of foot.
3. Supports of uterus.
4. Clinical anatomy of palmar spaces.
5. Histology of stomach.
6. Popliteal fossa.
7. Descent of testis.
8. Inferior mesenteric artery.
9. Great saphenous vein.
10. Histology of spleen.
11. Bronchopulmonary segments.
12. Blood supply of heart.
13. Third ventricle.
14. Transverse section of midbrain at the level of inferior colliculus with a labelled diagram.
15. Torticollis.
16. Suboccipital triangle.
17. Microstructure of cornea.
18. Cutaneous innervation of face.
19. Pleural recesses.
20. Transverse section of pons at the facial colliculus with labelled diagram.

III. Short answer questions (3/2 Marks)

1. Name the structures present in the free border of lesser omentum.
2. Notochord.
3. Name the structures undercover of flexor retinaculum of foot.
4. Pivot joints.
5. Nutrient artery.
6. Interior of second part of duodenum.
7. Branches of radial nerve in spiral groove.
8. Microanatomy of spleen-labeled diagram only.
9. Cephalic vein.
10. Branches of internal pudendal artery.
11. Layers of scrotum.
12. Pouch of Douglas.
13. Ligaments related to liver.
14. Taenia coli.
15. Erb's palsy.
16. Development of pancreas.
17. Foot drop.
18. Mallet finger.
19. Contents of adductor canal.
20. Guy rope muscles.
21. Pericardial sinuses.
22. Epistaxis.
23. Sibson's fascia.
24. Fallot's tetralogy.
25. Development of tongue.
26. Histology of cerebrum.
27. Enumerate the nuclei of cerebellum.
28. Deep cardiac plexus.

29. Formation and contents of carotid sheath.
30. Bell's palsy.
31. Interpeduncular fossa.
32. Ansa cervicalis.
33. Branches of first part of subclavian artery.
34. Contents of superior mediastinum.
35. Lateral relations of cavernous sinus.
36. Brachiocephalic vein.
37. Name the two sources of the development of pituitary.
38. Piriform fossa.
39. Thyroglossal fistula.
40. Oblique sinus of pericardium.

I. ESSAY QUESTIONS

1. **Discuss in detail about Portal vein under the following headings: (a) Formation, course and termination. (b) Relations and tributaries. (c) Sites of portosystemic anastomosis and (d) Clinical anatomy.**

(b) Relations Refer Essay Q. No. 5 – 2006.
(a, b) tributaries, (c, d) Refer Short Notes 6 – 2004.

2. **Describe parotid gland in detail. Add a note on its applied aspects.**

Refer Essay on Q. No. 4 – 2004.

3. **Describe the shoulder joint in detail. Add a note on its applied aspect.**

Refer Essay Q. No. 2 – 2006.

4. **Describe in detail about the blood supply of heart. Add a note on its applied anatomy.**

Refer Essay on Q. No. 5 – 2005.

II. SHORT NOTES

1. **Brachial artery.**

Refer Short Notes Q. No. 3 – 2003.

2. **Medial longitudinal arch of foot.**

Refer Essay Q. No. 1 – 2003.

3. **Supports of uterus.**

Refer Essay Q. No. 2 – 2004.

4. **Clinical anatomy of palmar spaces.**

Refer Short Notes 5 – 2014, and Short Answer Questions 2 – 2016.

5. **Histology of stomach.**

Refer Essay Q. No. 2 – 2007.

6. **Popliteal fossa.**

Refer Short Notes 8 – 2009.

7. **Descent of testis.**

Refer Short Notes 8 – 2007.

8. **Inferior mesenteric artery.**

Refer Short Notes 13 – 2005.

9. **Great saphenous vein.**

Refer Short Notes 14 – 2005.

10. **Histology of spleen.**

Refer Short Notes 3 – 2005.

11. **Bronchopulmonary segments.**

Refer Essay Q. No. 3 – 2004.

12. **Blood supply of heart.**

Refer Essay Q. No. 5 – 2005.

13. **Third ventricle.**

Refer Short Notes 12 – 2003.

14. **Transverse section of midbrain at the level of inferior colliculus with a labelled diagram.**

- Interior of midbrain is divided by the cerebral aqueduct into a ventral part called **cerebral peduncle** and a dorsal part the **tectum**
- The cerebral peduncle includes 1. **Crus cerebri** which is a divided part, 2. United **tegmental part** and 3. **Substantia nigra** which is in between the two parts (**Fig. 1**).
- **The crus cerebri (Basis pedunculi)**
  - Consists of bundles of corticospinal and corticobulbar fibers occupying middle two-third
  - The corticobulbar fibers are for cranial nerve nuclei and corticospinal the pyramidal tract from motor area
  - Medial one-sixth frontopontine fibers
  - Lateral one-sixth by temperopontine and parieto, occipitopontine fibers

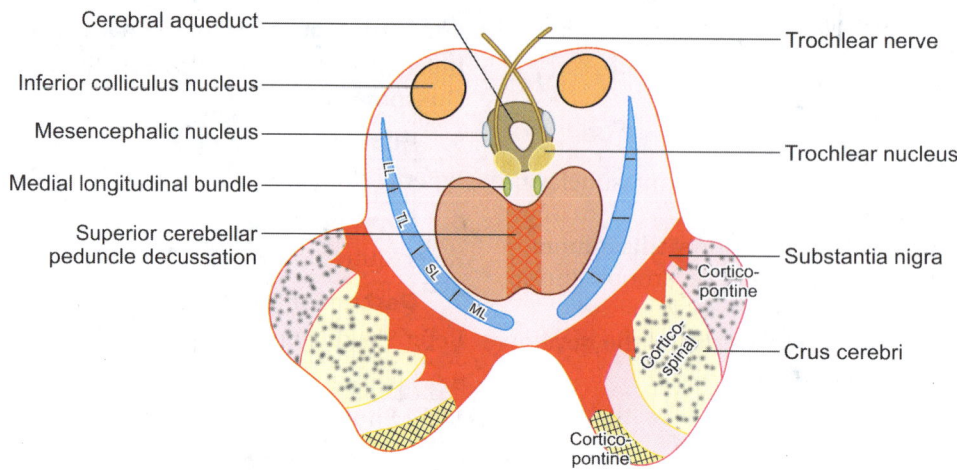

Fig. 1: Section of midbrain—inferior colliculus.
(LL, lateral lemniscus; TL, trigeminal lemniscus; SL, spinal lemniscus; ML, medial lemniscus).

- The pontine fibers arise from area 4 and 6 of cerebral cortex.
- **Tegmentum**
  - Gray matter
  - Periaqueductal gray matter is present
  - The **trochlear nucleus** is situated in it. The trochlear nucleus supplies lateral rectus muscle
  - The trochlear nerve passes dorsolateral and emerges below the inferior colliculus
  - **Mesencephalic nucleus of trigeminal is** dorsolateral in the gray matter. It receives proprioceptive impulses from muscles of mastication, ocular and facial muscles.
- **White matter**:
  - **Decussation** of the superior cerebellar peduncle
  - **Medial longitudinal fasciculus** is ventral to trochlear nucleus
  - The **lemnisci**—medial, spinal, trigeminal and lateral are present. The medial lemniscus is crossed posterior column of spinal cord. The spinal lemniscus is crossed lateral spinothalamic tract and trigeminal lemniscus is crossed fibers carrying sensation from one half of face. The lateral lemniscus carries crossed auditory fibers and end in the nucleus of inferior colliculi and medial geniculate bodies.
- **Substantia nigra** is connected to basal ganglia.
  - It is divided into—i) dorsal pars compacta and ii) ventral pars reticulate
  - Dopamine is secreted by it
  - Degeneration of the substantia nigra results in decrease in the dopamine level leading to Parkinson's diseases
  - **Cerebral aqueduct** is the cavity of midbrain.
- **Tectum:** Nucleus of inferior colliculus is present.

15. Torticollis.

- Torticollis is a condition in which the neck is tilted and slanting of head is produced
- It is due to contraction or shortening of the neck muscles
- Two types are seen—congenital and spasmodic torticollis
  1. **Congenital torticollis**
     - Usually it will be unilateral
     - It is also known as **wry neck**
     - **Due** to spasm of sternocleidomastoid muscle.

- **Reasons** are a. fibrous tissue tumor in the muscle, b. breech delivery, c. hematoma that encloses spinal accessory nerve
- The fibrosis produces shortening of SCM muscle and tilting of head
- Treatment is surgical release of the clavicular or sternal attachment of the muscle.

2. **Spasmodic torticollis**
   - Usually bilateral
   - Due to abnormal tone of the neck muscles more commonly sternocleidomastoid and trapezius muscles
   - The shoulder is elevated and pushed forwards on the side to which the chin is turned.

16. Suboccipital triangle.

Refer Short Answer Questions 46 – 2014.

17. Microstructure of cornea.

Refer Short Notes 35 – 2009.

18. Cutaneous innervation of face.

- Forehead is common to face and scalp
- The face is supplied by cranial and spinal nerves
- The cranial nerve is trigeminal
- The spinal nerve is VR C2,3.

Trigeminal Nerve

The areas supplied by trigeminal are:
- **Ophthalmic division**: The areas supplied by ophthalmic division is forehead, upper eyelid, side and tip of nose
  - Supratrochlear of frontal nerve supplies the skin of medial part of forehead
  - Supraorbital from frontal supply the lateral part of forehead and scalp upto vertex
  - Infratrochlear nerve branch of nasociliary supplies skin of side of nose close to medial angle of eye, medial half of upper eyelid, lacrimal sac
  - External nasal is continuation of anterior ethmoidal nerve supply tip of nose
  - Palpabral branch of lacrimal nerve supply lateral half of upper eyelid.
- **Maxillary division**: Maxillary nerve supplies the lower eyelid, ala of nose, upper lip, prominent part of cheek, anterior part of temple.
  - Infraorbital is continuation of maxillary nerve. It emerges through infraorbital foramen, divides into labial, palpabral and nasal branches:
    - Labial branch supply upper lip
    - Palpabral supply lower eyelid
    - Nasal skin of ala of nose.

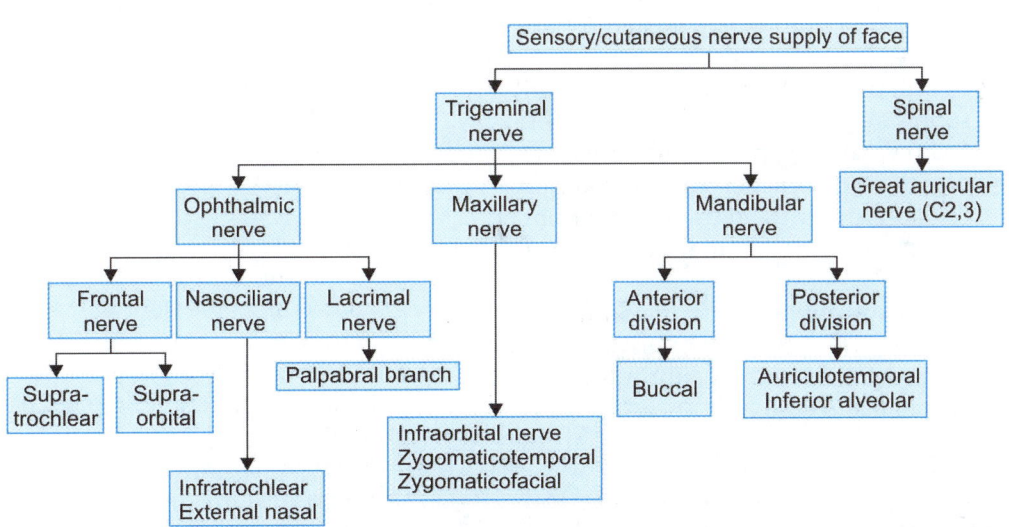

Fig. 2: Trigeminal nerve divisions supplying face.

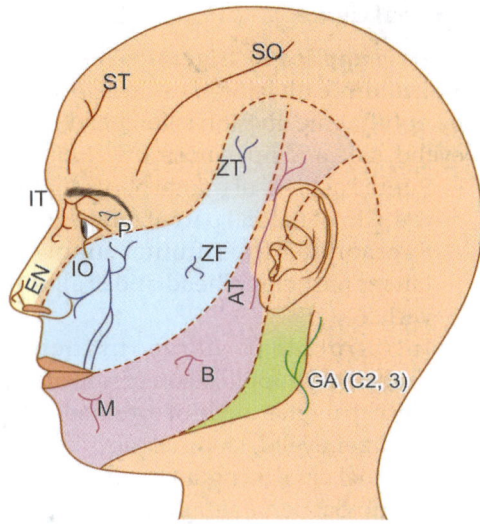

Fig. 3: Cutaneous nerve supply of face.

(ST, supratrochlear; SO, supraorbital; ZT, zygomaticofacial; IT, infratrochlear; IO, infraorbital; EN, external nasal; AT, auriculotemporal; GA, great auricular nerve; P, palpebral branch; M, Mental branch; B, buccal branch).

- Zygomaticotemporal nerve branch of temporal nerve supply skin of anterior part of temple (non-hairy part)
- Zygomaticofacial from zygomatic nerve supply skin covering the prominent part (bony part) of cheek.
- **Mandibular division:** Mandibular nerve supply lower lip, chin, soft part of cheek, tragus, skin in front of ear, posterior part of temple.
  - Buccal branch from anterior division supply skin over the soft part of cheek (skin over anterior portion of buccinator)
  - Auriculotemporal nerve from posterior division supply tragus, portion in front of ear, the posterior part (hairy part) of temple
  - Inferior alveolar nerve is continued as mental nerve. It emerges through mental foramen and supply skin of lower lip and chin.

Spinal Nerve

Great auricular nerve (C2, 3) from cervical plexus supply the skin over the angle of mandible.

Applied Anatomy

Trigeminal neuralgia (Tic douloureux): The patient complains of intense stabbing pain over the area of distribution of one of the division of trigeminal nerve. Usually the maxillary division is often involved. Treatment is cutting or transection of the spinal trigeminal tract. Transection of single division of trigeminal nerve is possible.

19. Pleural recesses.

Refer Essay Q. No. 3 – 2003.

20. Transverse section of pons at the facial colliculus with labelled diagram.

Refer diagram Short Notes Q. No. 13 – 2004.
- The interior of pons is divided into two parts
- The ventral part is larger called **basilar part**, and dorsal **tegmental part**.
- **Basilar part:**
  - It is continuous with pyramids of medulla oblongata, and is continued as middle cerebellar peduncle
  - Bundles of corticospinal, corticobulbar and corticopontine fibers form the longitudinal bundles
  - Pontine nuclei are scattered between the transverse and longitudinal fibers
  - The corticopontine fibers from cerebral cortex end in the pontine nuclei
  - The second order of neuron from pontine nuclei form transverse fibers, and cross to opposite side to reach cerebellum through middle cerebellar peduncle.
- **Tegmental part:** Contains gray and white matter
  - **Gray matter** –
    - Abducent nucleus below the facial colliculus in the floor of the fourth ventricle
    - Motor nucleus of facial nerve situated ventrolateral to the abducent nucleus
    - Parasympathetic superior salivatory, inferior salivatory and lacrimatory nuclei are close to the facial nucleus

- Nucleus tractus solitarius lateral to salivatory nuclei
- Spinal nucleus and tract of trigeminal nerve in the lateral part of reticular formation
- Vestibular nuclei lateral and superior situated close to inferior cerebellar peduncle
- Dorsal and ventral cochlear nuclei situated on the corresponding surfaces of inferior cerebellar peduncle.

– **White matter:**
- The abducent nerve from the nucleus pass ventrally to emerge through lower border of pons
- The motor root of facial nerve pass dorsomedially and loops around the abducent nucleus. The unusual course is due to neurobiotaxis
- Trapezoid body dorsal to the basilar part formed by decussating fibers from dorsal and ventral cochlear nuclei of either side
- Medial longitudinal bundle (MLB) ventral to abducent nucleus
- Tectospinal tracts ventral to MLB
- Medial lemnicus contains crossed posterior column fibers. As it ascends from medulla, it rotates to be arranged horizontally and the arrangement of fibers are neck, arm, trunk and leg from medial to lateral
- Trigeminal, spinal and lateral lemnici are seen.

III. SHORT ANSWER QUESTIONS

1. Name the structures present in the free border of lesser omentum.

Refer Short Answers Q. No. 7 – 2008.

2. Notochord.

Refer Short Notes 15 – 2005.

3. Name the structures undercover of flexor retinaculum of foot.

- Flexor retinaculum extends from tip of medial malleolus of tibia to the medial process of calcaneus and plantar aponeurosis
- It bridges over the grooves between the two bones and forms a tunnel called **tarsal tunnel**
- The structures passing deep to it from medial to lateral are:
  – Tendon of tibialis posterior
  – Tendon of flexor digitorum longus
  – Posterior tibial artery and vein
  – Tibial nerve
  – Tendon of flexor hallucis longus.
- **Applied anatomy:** Tarsal tunnel syndrome in which there is compression of tibial

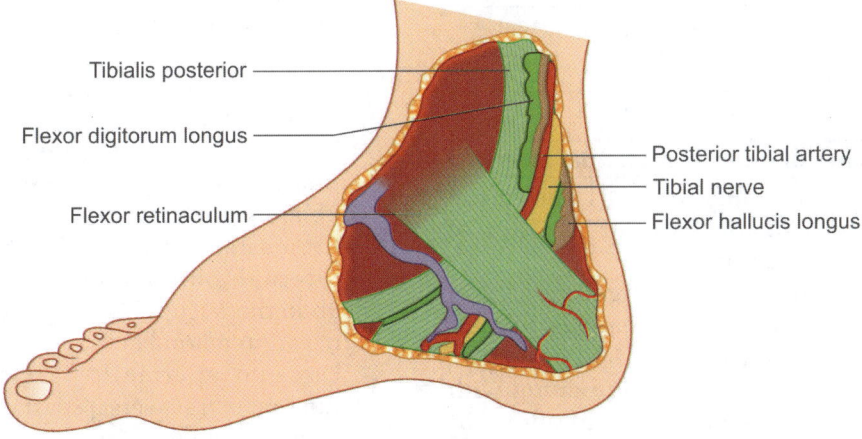

Fig. 4: Flexor retinaculum of foot.

nerve and results in pain and tingling in the sole region. To relieve the pain the retinaculum is divided.

4. Pivot joints.

- It is one variety of synovial joint
- It is an uniaxial joint
- Movement – rotatory, the pivot (part of bone) rotates within an osseoligamentous ring or the ring rotates around the pivot
- The axis of the movement is vertical, around the axis of the pivot alone, e.g.
  - **Superior radioulnar joint:** The ring is formed by the annular ligament and radial notch of ulna, and pivot is the head of radius which rotates within the ring
  - **Median atlantoaxial joint:** The pivot is the dens of axis and the ring is formed by the anterior arch of atlas and transverse ligament which rotates around the pivot.

5. Nutrient artery.
Refer Short Notes 2 – 2009.

6. Interior of second part of duodenum.
Refer Short Notes 13 – 2006.

7. Branches of radial nerve in spiral groove.
Refer Short Answer Q. No. 22 – 2014.

8. Microanatomy of spleen-labeled diagram only.
Refer Short Notes 3 – 2005.

9. Cephalic vein.
Refer Short Notes 7 – 2012.

10. Branches of internal pudendal artery.

- Internal pudendal artery is one of the branch from the anterior division of internal iliac artery
- It leaves the pelvis through the greater sciatic foramen and reaches gluteal region
- It crosses the ischial spine along with pudendal nerve and nerve to obturator internus
- Passes through the lesser sciatic foramen to reach perineum
- Becomes a content of pudendal (Alcock's) canal along the anterolateral wall of ischiorectal fossa
- It terminates by dividing into deep and dorsal artery of penis/clitoris
- **Branches:**
  - Perineal branch to supply scrotum/labium through posterior scrotal/labial branches, muscular branches to perineal muscles, perineal body
  - Artery to bulb of penis in male and bulb of vestibule in female
  - Deep artery of penis/clitoris
  - Dorsal artery of penis/clitoris.

11. Layers of scrotum.

- The scrotum is a sac made of fibrous and muscular tissue
- It contains testis and spermatic cord
- The layers of scrotum is considered as extrinsic coverings of testis
- Formed by six layers which constitute the layers of scrotum. From outer to inner are (**S**ome **D**ame **E**nglish **C**alled **I**t **T**estis):
  - **S**kin is thin, contains hair follicles with sebaceous and sweat glands. The subcutaneous adipose tissue is absent. The rugae are seen in the skin produced by the contraction of dartos. The anterior ⅓ skin is supplied by ilioinguinal and genitofemoral nerves (L1), and posterior ⅔ skin by posterior scrotal nerves and perineal branch of posterior cutaneous nerve of thigh (S3)
  - **D**artos muscle—subcutaneous smooth muscle, helps to maintain the temperature
  - **E**xternal spermatic fascia—continuation of aponeurosis of external oblique
  - **C**remaster muscle and fascia—from internal oblique and transversus abdominis, supplied by genital branch of genitofemoral nerve
  - **I**nternal spermatic fascia—continuation of transversalis fascia
  - **T**unica vaginalis (parietal layer).

12. Pouch of Douglas.
Refer Short Answer Q. No. 15 – 2009.

13. Ligaments related to liver.
Refer Short Notes 6 – 2008.

14. Taenia coli.
- The longitudinal muscular coat is arranged as longitudinal bands in the large intestine and are known as taenia coli
- They are three in number, and named as taenia libera, taenia omentalis, and taenia mesocolica
- They are seen deep to the serosal layer
- Extends from cecum to distal sigmoid colon
- At the base of the appendix the three taeniae converge to form longitudinal coat, acts as a guide
- From the level of distal sigmoid colon and rectosigmoid junction the taenia is seen as two broad bands on anterior and posterior surfaces
- In the rectum the two bands unite to form complete longitudinal coat
- The width of the taenia is uniform throughout the colon
- The length of taenia is less than the length of large intestine, hence the sacculations present in the colon.

15. Erb's palsy.
Refer Essay Q. No. 3 – 2005.

16. Development of pancreas.
Refer Short Notes 6 – 2005.

17. Foot drop.
- Foot drop is due to injury to common peroneal nerve
- Level of lesion is usually at neck of fibula as the nerve winds around it
- Usually it is painless
- The anterior and lateral compartments muscles of leg are affected.
- **Cause of injury**
  - Compression of nerve by the plaster cast
  - Ganglion
  - Entrapment of the nerve between the origin of peroneus longus from head and shaft of fibula
  - Dislocation of lateral part of knee due to traction.
- **Effects of lesion**
  - Weakness of dorsiflexion, and normal plantar flexion
  - Weakness of eversion and normal inversion
  - Ankle reflex is normal.
- **Reasoning**: Injury to common peroneal nerve results in:
  - Weakness of the evertors—peroneus longus and brevis supplied by superficial peroneal nerve
  - Weakness of dorsiflexors—extensor digitorum and hallucis longus supplied by deep peroneal nerve

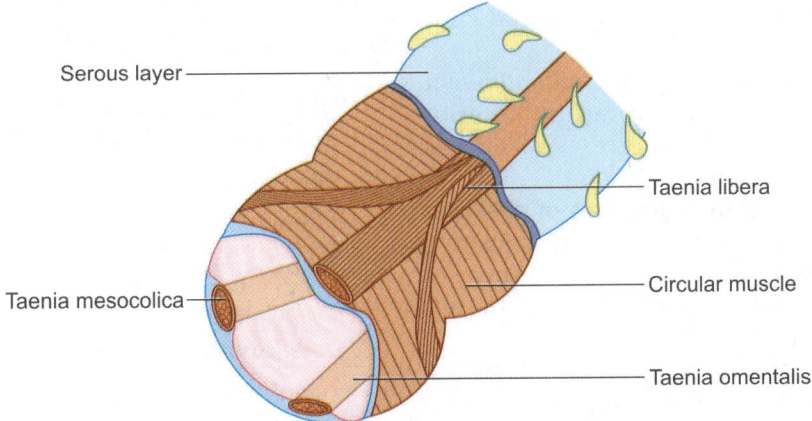

Fig. 5: Taenia coli.

- Plantar flexion and inversion is preserved as the muscles responsible are supplied by the tibial nerve.
- **Position of foot:** Ankle is plantar flexed, foot is inverted and adducted.

18. Mallet finger.

- It is also known as **baseball finger**.
- Causes:
  - Traumatic rupture or laceration or avulsion of the distal attachment of tendon of extensor through dorsal digital expansion to the distal phalanx
  - The terminal phalanx of an extended finger is forcefully flexed
  - Sudden severe degree of tension on the extensor tendon.
- Position of digit:
  - Flexion of the distal phalanx in a fully extended finger. Cannot extend the distal phalanx
  - The position of the finger resembles a mallet and hence called mallet finger.

19. Contents of adductor canal.

Refer Short Notes 3 – 2006.

20. Guy rope muscles.

Girl between two soldiers
- The three muscles inserted to the upper part of medial surface of tibia together form the guy ropes
- They are sartorius, gracilis, semitendinosus
- **Sartorius** is a muscle of anterior compartment of thigh, supplied by femoral nerve, flexes both hip and knee joints
- **Gracilis** is a muscle in the medial adductor compartment, innervated by anterior division of obturator nerve, adductor and medial rotator of the hip joint
- **Semitendinosus** is a muscle of posterior compartment and it belongs to hamstring group, supplied by tibial component of sciatic nerve, extends the hip and flexes the knee joint
- These three muscles arises from the three parts of hip bone namely, sartorius from anterior superior iliac spine (ilium), semitendinosus from ischial tuberosity (ischium), and gracilis from body and ramus of pubis (pubis)
- They taper down to be inserted to the upper part of medial surface of tibia
- These attachments acts as strings and stabilize the pelvis on the femur hence called as **guy ropes**
- A bursa is situated between the tibial collateral and these three tendons called **bursa anserine**, which communicates with the joint cavity of knee joint.

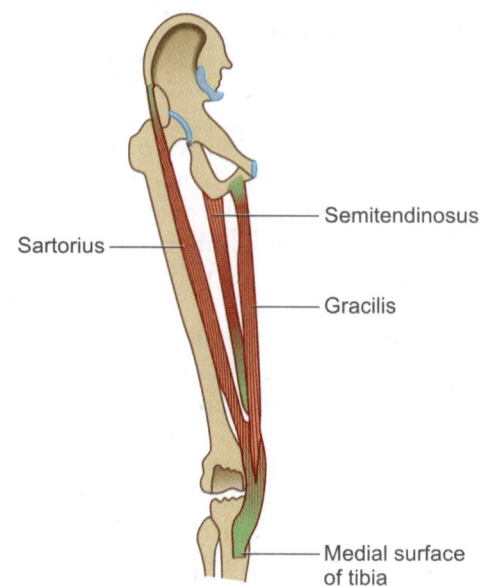

Fig. 6: Guy rope muscles.

21. Pericardial sinuses.

Refer Short Notes 32 – 2007.

22. Epistaxis.

Refer Short Answer Q. No. 39 – 2015.

23. Sibson's fascia.

Refer Short Answer Q. No. 38 – 2009.

24. Fallot's tetralogy.

Refer Essay Q. No. 6 – 2010.

25. Development of tongue.

Refer Short Notes 20 – 2003.

26. Histology of cerebrum.

Refer Short Notes 18 – 2003.

27. Enumerate the nuclei of cerebellum.
Refer Short Answer Q. No. 37 – 2012.

28. Deep cardiac plexus.
Refer Short Notes 17 – 2007.

29. Formation and contents of carotid sheath.
Refer Short Notes 40 – 2010.

30. Bell's palsy.
Refer Essay Q. No. 9 – 2007.

31. Interpeduncular fossa.
Refer Short Notes 33 – 2009.

32. Ansa cervicalis.
Refer Short Notes 26 – 2008.

33. Branches of first part of subclavian artery.

- Subclavian artery supplies head and neck and brain
- **Origin**
  - On the right side it is a branch of brachiocephalic trunk
  - On the left side it is direct branch from arch of aorta
- The artery is crossed by scalenus anterior muscle and divides it into three parts
- **Extent of 1st part**
  - On the right side from the sternoclavicular joint to the inner border of scalenus anterior muscle.
  - On the left side from arch of aorta (intervertebral disc of T3 – T4) to the inner border of scalenus anterior muscle
  - The artery arches over the apex of the lung and cervical pleura.
- **Branches**
  - Vertebral artery—enters the cranial cavity and forms part of vertebrobasilar system and supply brain
  - Internal thoracic artery—supply the wall of thorax, mammary gland, and anterior wall of abdomen
  - Thyrocervical trunk—divides into three branches—(i) inferior thyroid (ii) suprascapular (iii) transverse cervical.
- **Applied anatomy:** Obstruction of the subclavian artery proximal to the origin of vertebral artery may lead to retrograde flow of blood from the brain to the affected side of vertebral artery. This condition is called **subclavian steal syndrome.**

34. Contents of superior mediastinum.
Refer Short Notes Q. No. 38 – 2012.

35. Lateral relations of cavernous sinus.
Refer Essay Q. No. 5 – 2008.

36. Brachiocephalic vein.
Refer Short Notes 29 – 2011.

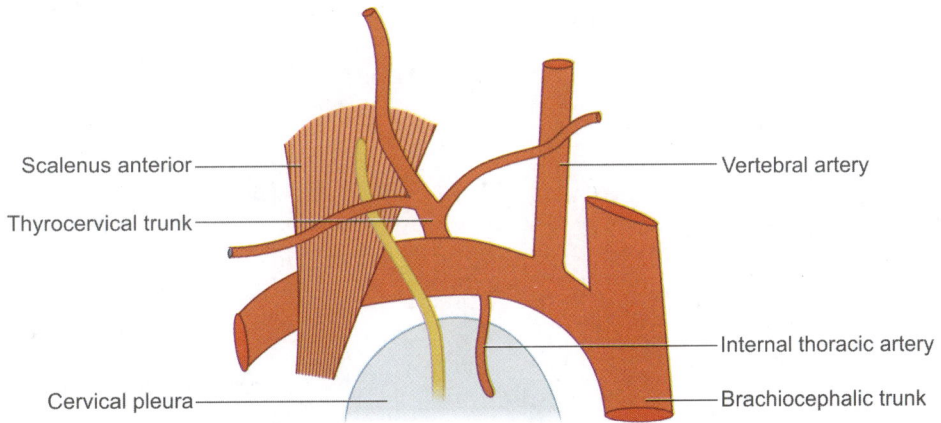

Fig. 7: First part of subclavian artery.

37. Name the two sources of the development of pituitary.

Refer Short Answer Q. No. 42 – 2012.

38. Piriform fossa.

Refer Short Answer Q. No. 32 – 2009.

39. Thyroglossal fistula.

- The downward growth of median thyroid rudiment is called the **thyroglossal duct**
- It extends from root of tongue to the upper part of trachea
- It terminates by dividing into two in front of upper part of trachea
- The two divisions give rise to isthmus and lateral lobes of thyroid gland
- The thyroglossal duct disappears leaving the upper end as **foramen cecum**
- Persistence of the duct undergoes cystic changes and form **thyroglossal cyst**
- Cyst is seen in midline of neck and moves with deglutition
- **Thyroglossal fistula:** Incision or rupture of thyroglossal cyst results in fistula.

40. Oblique sinus of pericardium.

Refer Short Notes 32 – 2007.

MBBS Examination 2018

ANSWER ALL QUESTIONS

I. Essay questions   **(15/10 Marks)**
1. Describe knee joint in detail. Add a note on its applied aspects.
2. Describe uterus in detail. Add a note on its applied aspects.
3. Classify white fibers of cerebrum with examples. Describe internal capsule in detail.
4. Describe the facial nerve under the following headings:
    a. Nuclei of origin and functional components.
    b. Course and emergence.
    c. Branches and its distribution.
    d. Clinical anatomy.

II. Short notes   **(5 Marks)**
1. Cubital fossa.
2. Lymphatic drainage of breast.
3. Rotation of midgut.
4. Internal iliac artery.
5. Structures undercover of gluteus maximus.
6. Flexor retinaculum of upper limb.
7. Supination and pronation.
8. Femoral triangle.
9. Adductor magnus.
10. Porto-caval anastomosis.
11. Thoracic duct.
12. Secretomotor pathway of parotid gland.
13. Draw and label the transverse section of thorax at T4 level.
14. Infrahyoid muscles of neck.
15. Interior of right atrium.
16. Carotid triangle.
17. Features of left ventricle.
18. Histology of cerebrum.
19. Esophagus:
    a. Commencement termination
    b. Blood supply
    c. Lymphatic
    d. Congenital anomalies
20. Hilum of lungs with labeled diagram.

III. Short answer questions   **(3/2 Marks)**
1. Dartos muscle.
2. Trochanteric anastomosis.
3. Superficial inguinal ring.
4. Contents of superficial perineal pouch.
5. Histology of liver.
6. Urachus.
7. Structures passing through fourth compartment of extensor retinaculum of upper limb.
8. Kehr's sign.
9. Wrist drop.
10. Radial bursa.
11. Anatomical snuff box.
12. Structures piercing clavipectoral fascia.
13. Triceps surae.
14. Pes planus.
15. Contents of spermatic cord.
16. Histology of lymph node.
17. Derivatives of midgut.
18. Blood supply of left suprarenal gland.
19. Saphenous nerve.
20. Erb's palsy.
21. Wharton's duct.
22. Waldeyer's ring.
23. Structures related to lateral wall of cavernous sinus.
24. Mention the branches of ophthalmic nerve.
25. Histology of retina.

26. Thyroglossal duct.
27. Name the branches of facial artery in face.
28. Tonsillar bed.
29. Pleural recesses.
30. Millard-Gubler syndrome.
31. Modifications of cranial pia mater.
32. Formation and termination of external jugular vein.
33. Development of thyroid gland.
34. Nerve supply of pinna.
35. Superior orbital fissure.
36. Branches of internal carotid artery.
37. Dangerous area of face.
38. Trigeminal neuralgia.
39. Intrinsic muscles of larynx and nerve supply.
40. Parotid duct.

I. ESSAY QUESTIONS

1. **Describe knee joint in detail. Add a note on its applied aspects.**

- **Type:**
  Synovial
  Modified hinge variety with three joints
  – Two condylar joints between the femur and the tibia – tibiofemoral
  Saddle joint between the femur and patella - patellofemoral
- **Articular surfaces (Fig. 1):**
  – The femoral condyles articulate with the tibial condyles below and behind and with patella in front
  – *Condyles of femur*: The articular surface cover inferior and posterior surface of the two condyles. The surface over lateral condyle is short and the surface over medial is longer and convexity directed medially. The tibial surface is continuous with patellar surface anteriorly
  – *Patellar articular surface (Trochlear surface of femur)*: Extends more on the lateral than on medial side. A vertical groove between the two condyles. Faint grooves separate the tibial and patellar surfaces
  – *Posterior surface of patella:* Articulates with patellar/trochlear articular surface of femur. The lateral area is larger than the medial area of articular surface
  – *Condyles of tibia:* The medial condyle is larger and articulates with medial condyle of femur. The articular surface is oval. The central part is concave and periphery is flat. Meniscus separates the femoral condyle and tibial condyle. Lateral condyle is nearly circular and articulate with lateral condyle of femur
- **Ligaments of knee joint:** Refer Short Notes/Notes on Q. No. 10 – 2014
- **Bursae:** Refer Short Notes/Notes/Answer on Q. No. 14 – 2012
- **Movements:**
  1. Flexion and extension are the chief movements. The range of movement is extension 5 – 10 degree, flexion 120 degree with hip extended and 140

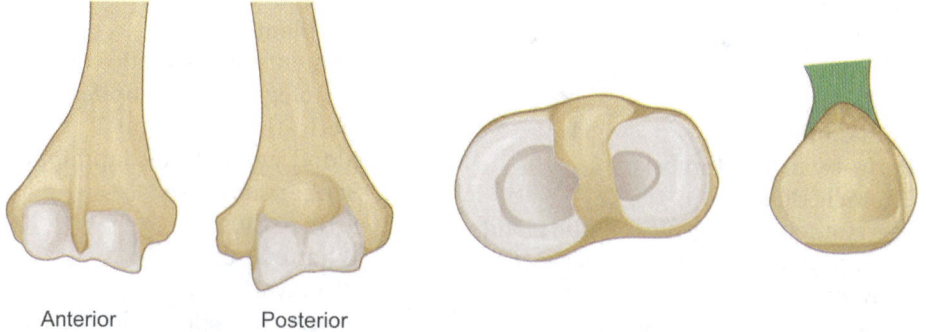

Fig. 1: Articular surfaces.

degree when it is flexed. The muscles producing flexion – biceps femoris, semimembranosus and semitendinosus. Extension by quadriceps femoris assisted by tensor fasciae latae

2. Medial and lateral rotation are combined with flexion and extension. When the foot is on the ground and standing erect as in position of attention, medial rotation of femur occurs during last 30 degree of extension. There is lateral rotation of femur in stand at ease position

3. Locking and unlocking movement (Refer Short Notes/Notes on Q. No. 4 – 2011)

- **Nerve supply:**
  - Femoral nerve through its branch to vastus medialis
  - Sciatic nerve through genicular branches of tibial and common peroneal nerves
  - Posterior division of obturator nerve
- **Applied anatomy:**
  - *Housemaid's knee*: Inflammation of subcutaneous prepatellar bursa
  - *Clergyman's knee*: Inflammation of infrapatellar bursa
  - *Baker's cyst*: Posteriorly a cystic swelling seen in the center of knee joint. The synovial membrane protrudes through a hole in the capsule of knee joint
  - Bucket handle tear (Refer Short Notes/Notes/Answer on Q. No. 20 – 2010).
  - *Unhappy triad*: (Refer Short notes/notes on Q. No. 2 – 2007).

2. **Describe uterus in detail. Add a note on its applied aspects.**

Refer Essay Q. No. 2 – 2004.

3. **Classify white fibers of cerebrum with examples. Describe internal capsule in detail.**

Refer White fibers of cerebrum Essay Q. No. 5 – 2012.
Refer Internal capsule Essay Q. No. 7 – 2005.

4. **Describe the facial nerve under the following headings.**

a. Nuclei of origin and functional components.
b. Course and emergence.
c. Branches and its distribution.
d. Clinical anatomy.

a,b,c Refer Short Notes 15 – 2003
Branches in face & d Refer Essay No 9 – 2007

II. SHORT NOTES

1. **Cubital fossa.**

Refer Short Notes/Notes on Q. No. 16 – 2008.

2. **Lymphatic drainage of breast.**

Refer Short Notes/Notes on Q. No. 19 – 2005.

3. **Rotation of midgut.**

Refer Short Notes/Notes on Q. No. 2 – 2005.

4. **Internal iliac artery (Fig 2).**

- **Origin:** Internal iliac artery is a branch of common iliac artery
- **Level of formation:** At the level with the lumbosacral intervertebral disc
- **Course:** It passes along the superior margin of the greater sciatic foramen
- **Termination:** It divides into an anterior trunk, and a posterior trunk
- **Relations:** Anteriorly—the ureter and, in females the ovary, fimbriated end of the uterine tube
- **Inferior:** The internal iliac vein, lumbosacral vein, obturator nerve
- **Embryological:**
  - In the fetus, the internal iliac artery is a direct continuation of the common iliac artery
  - It runs upwards on the anterior abdominal wall to the umbilicus, and the two arteries enter the umbilical cord as the umbilical arteries
  - After birth only the pelvic segment remains patent as the **internal iliac artery** and part of the **superior vesical artery**
  - The remaining part becomes a fibrous medial umbilical ligament
  - In male, the patent part is the superior vesical artery gives off an artery to the vas deferens
- **Branches**
  - **Anterior trunk:** Supplies the pelvic organs

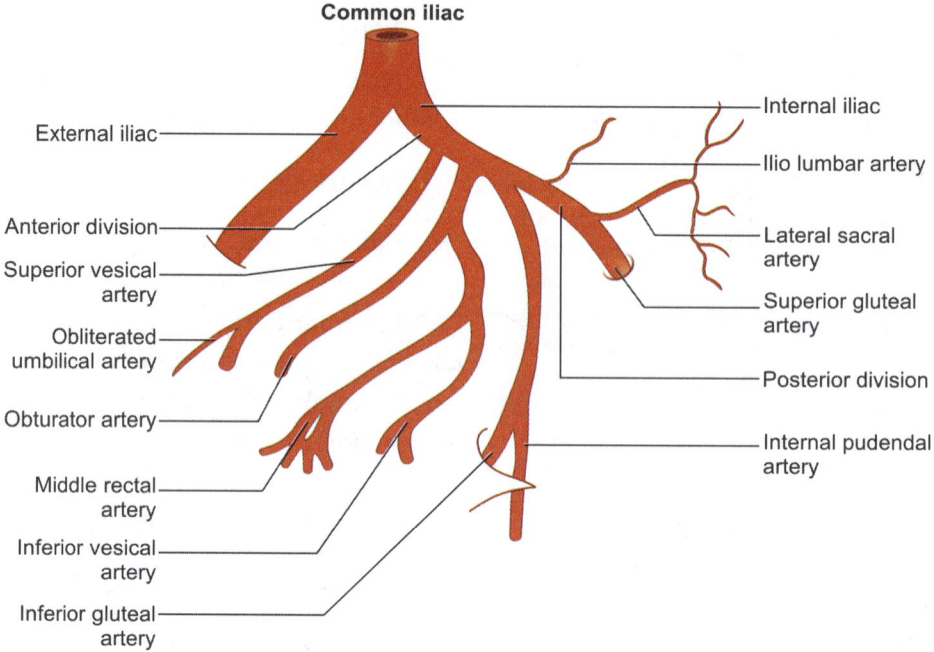

Fig. 2: Branches of internal iliac artery.

1. Superior vesical artery
2. Inferior vesical artery
3. Middle rectal artery
4. Vaginal artery
5. Uterine artery
6. Obturator artery
7. Internal pudendal artery
8. Inferior gluteal artery
- **Posterior trunk:** Supplies muscles in the hip and back.
  1. Ilio lumbar artery
  2. Superior gluteal artery
  3. Lateral sacral artery

5. Structures undercover of gluteus maximus.
Refer Short Notes/Notes on Q. No. 25 – 2013.

6. Flexor retinaculum of upper limb.
Refer Short Notes/Notes on Q. No. 12 – 2012.

7. Supination and pronation.
Refer Short Notes/Notes on Q. No. 7 – 2005.

8. Femoral triangle.
Refer Essay Q. No. 3 – 2012.

9. Adductor magnus.
- It is a muscle of medial compartment of thigh
- Hybrid muscle
- Two parts – adductor & hamstring parts
- Origin – **(Fig. 3)**
  - *Adductor part*: Inferior ramus of the pubis, from the conjoined ischial ramus
  - *Hamstring part*: Inferolateral aspect of the ischial tuberosity.
- **Insertion:**
  - Adductor part
    Inserted into the shaft of femur along medial margin of gluteal tuberosity, medial lip of linea aspera, medial supra condylar line. The pubic fibers are horizontal and are called as adductor minimus
  - Hamstring part
    Are vertical end in tendon inserted to the adductor tubercle. The lower part degenerates as tibial collateral ligament

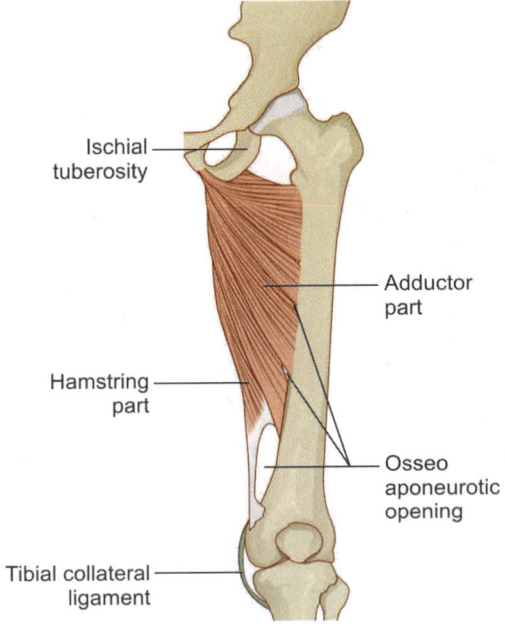

- The muscle is interrupted by a series of osseoaponeurotic openings. The upper four are small and the perforating branches and the termination of the profunda femoris artery pass. The lowest is large and allows the femoral vessels to be continued as popliteal artery.
- **Nerve supply**
  - Adductor part – obturator nerve
  - Hamstring part – tibial component of sciatic nerve
- **Action:**
  - Adductor part – adducts the thigh
  - Hamstring part – flexion of knee

Fig. 3: Adductor magnus.

10. Porto-caval anastomosis.
Refer Short Notes/Notes on Q. No. 6 – 2004.

11. Thoracic duct.
Refer Short Notes/Notes on Q. No. 51 – 2013.

12. Secretomotor pathway of parotid gland.
Refer Essay Q. No. 4 – 2004.

13. Draw and label the transverse section of thorax at T4 level.

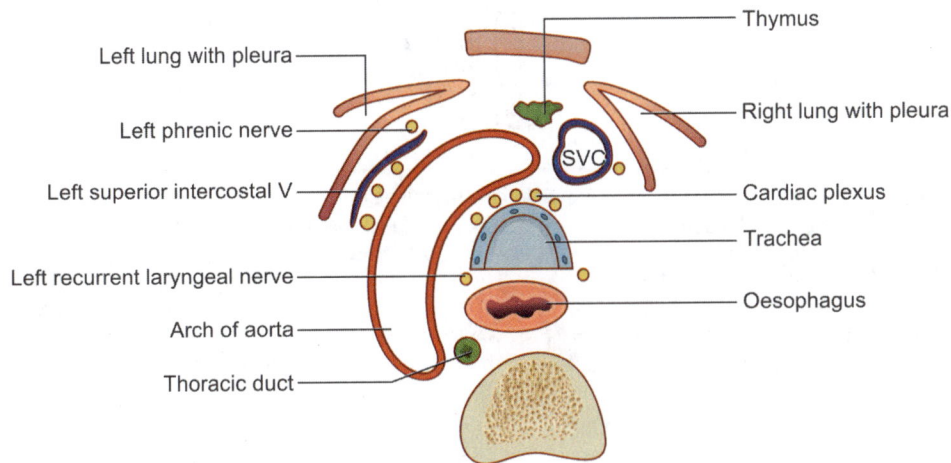

Fig. 4: TS at the level of T4 level.

14. Infrahyoid muscles of neck.

The infrahyoid muscles are strap/ribbon muscles. The muscles help in movements of the hyoid bone and thyroid cartilage during speech, swallowing and mastication. They are sternohyoid, omohyoid, sternothyroid and thyrohyoid.

S.No.	Name of muscle	Attachments (Fig. 5)		Nerve supply	Action
		Origin	Insertion		
1.	Sternohyoid	Posterior surface of the medial end of the clavicle, the posterior sterno clavicular ligament and the upper posterior aspect of the manubrium	Inferior border of the body of hyoid bone	Ansa cervicalis	Depresses the hyoid bone
2.	Omohyoid	• Inferior belly upper border of the scapula, near the scapular notch, the superior transverse scapular ligament • Superior belly Intermediate tendon	• To the intermediate tendon • Inferior border of hyoid bone • At the level of arch of cricoid cartilage (C6). The investing layer of deep cervical fascia forms a sling and attaches it to clavicle and first rib	• From loop of ansa cervicalis (C1, 2, 3) • Superior ramus of ansa cervicalis (C1)	Depresses the hyoid bone

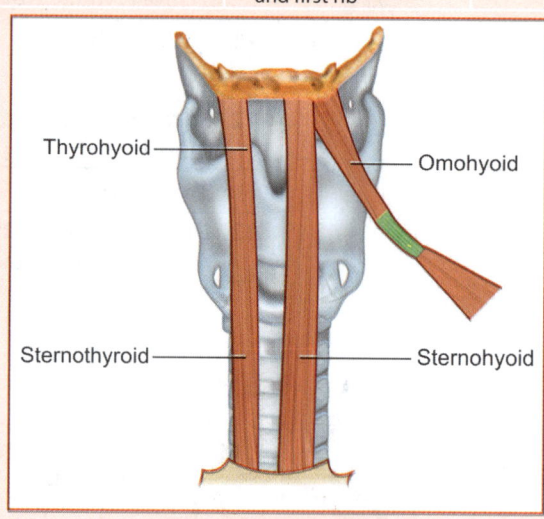

Fig. 5: Infrahyoid muscles.

3.	Sternothyroid	Posterior surface of manubrium sterni and cartilage of first rib	Oblique line of lamina of the thyroid cartilage	Ansa cervicalis	After swallowing the larynx is pulled downwards
4.	Thyrohyoid	Oblique line of lamina of thyroid cartilage	Lower border of greater horn of hyoid bone	Branch from hypoglossal nerve (C1)	Depresses the hyoid bone in early phase of swallowing

15. Interior of right atrium.
Refer Essay Q. No. 7 – 2006.

16. Carotid triangle.
Refer Essay Q. No. 8 – 2011.

17. Features of left ventricle.
Refer Essay Q. No. 7 – 2006.

18. Histology of cerebrum.
Refer Short Notes/Notes on Q. No. 18 – 2003.

19. Esophagus:
a) Commencement termination
b) Blood supply
c) Lymphatic
d) Congenital anomalies

a. **Commencement and termination (Fig. 6).**
   - It is continuation of pharynx from the level of lower border of cricoid cartilage-C6
   - It passes through the Esophageal orifice of diaphragm at T10 and is continued as stomach

b. **Blood supply**
   - Arterial supply
     - Cervical part: Inferior thyroid artery
     - Thoracic part: Bronchial and Esophageal branches from descending thoracic aorta
   - Venous drainage
     - Cervical: Inferior thyroid vein
     - Thoracic: Azygos, intercostal and bronchial veins

c. **Lymphatic drainage**
   - *Cervical part*: Deep cervical nodes
   - *Thoracic part*: Posterior mediastinal nodes

d. **Congenital anomalies**
   - *Tracheoesophageal fistula*: Commonest deformity the esophagus will be connected to the trachea by a canal
   - Oesophageal stenosis

20. Hilum of lungs with labeled diagram.
Refer Essay Q. No. 3 – 2004.

III. SHORT ANSWER QUESTIONS

1. Dartos muscle.
- It is the second layer of scrotum (Skin, Dartos muscle, External spermatic fascia, Cremaster muscle and fascia, Internal spermatic fascia, Parietal layer of tunica vaginalis)
- It is a subcutaneous smooth muscle layer
- It is continuous with colles fascia, Scarpa's fascia, dartos fascia of penis
- It helps to maintains the temperature

2. Trochanteric anastomosis.
Refer Short Notes/Notes/Answer on Q. No. 19 – 2009.

3. Superficial inguinal ring.
Refer Short Notes/Notes on Q. No. 20 – 2008.

4. Contents of superficial perineal pouch.
Refer Short Notes/Notes on Q. No. 15 – 2009.

5. Histology of liver.
Refer Short Notes/Notes on Q. No. 5 – 2016.

6. Urachus.
Refer Short Notes/Notes on Q. No. 10 – 2007.

7. Structures passing through fourth compartment of extensor retinaculum of upper limb.
Four structures pass deep to fourth compartment of extensor retinaculum (**Fig. 7**)
- Tendon of extensor digitorum
- Tendon of extensor indices
- Posterior interosseous nerve
- Anterior interosseous artery

8. Kehr's sign.
- The smaller branches of splenic artery are end arteries.
- The obstruction of the arteries results in infarction of spleen

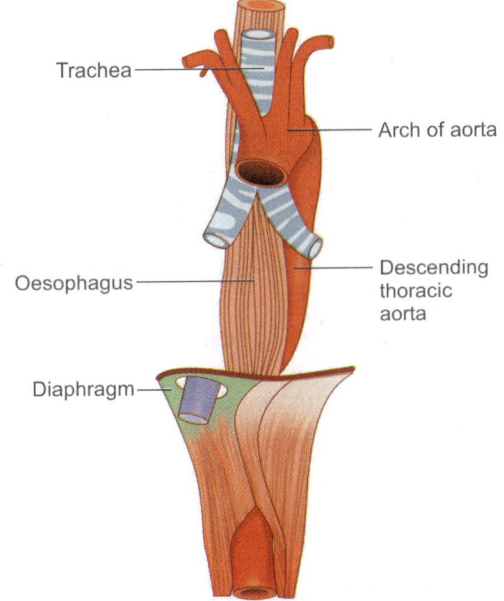

Fig. 6: Esophagus.

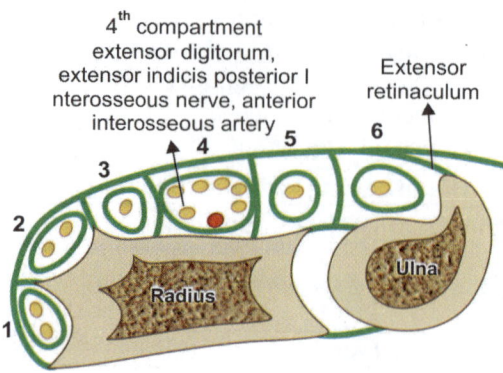

Fig. 7: Extensor retinaculum.

- This causes referred pain to left shoulder known as Kehr's sign

9. Wrist drop.
Refer Short Notes/Notes on Q. No. 4 – 2014.

10. Radial bursa (Fig. 8).
- The synovial sheath of the tendon of flexor pollicis longus in the hand is known as radial bursa
- This sheath is usually separate but may communicate with the common sheath behind the retinaculum
- Extent: Superiorly, it is with the common sheath and inferiorly it extends up to the distal phalanx of the thumb

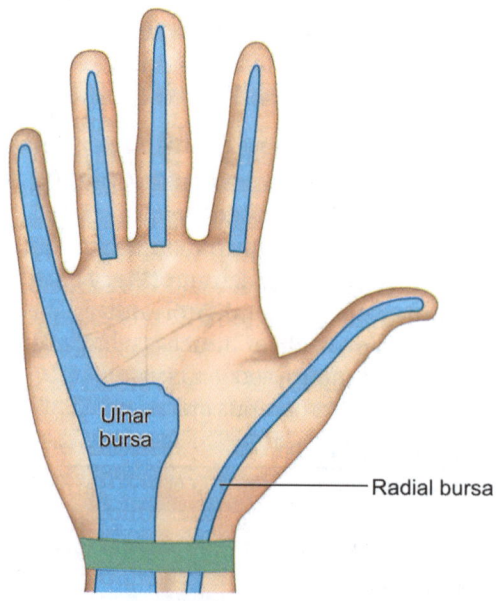

Fig. 8: Radial bursa.

11. Anatomical snuff box.
Refer boundaries, content, applied anatomy Short Notes/Answers on Q. No. 8 – 2013.
  Roof is formed by skin, superficial branch of radial nerve and cephalic vein

12. Structures piercing clavipectoral fascia.
Refer Short Notes/Notes on Q. No. 5 – 2006.

13. Triceps surae.
Refer Short Notes/Notes on Q. No. 25 – 2013.

14. Pes planus.
- Pes planus is excessive flat foot
- It may be physiological or pathological
- Physiological condition usually in pre-school children in the age group of 2 – 6.
- In Pathological condition, there will be stiffness and pain
- Causes of pathological pes planus include tarsal coalition, disruption of the tendon of tibialis posterior, rupture of the spring ligament, tarsometatarsal arthritis, degenerative or inflammatory arthritis.
- Windlass test done and in pathological condition no prominence of the arch.

15. Contents of spermatic cord.
Refer Short Notes/Notes/Answers on Q. No. 1 – 2009.

16. Histology of lymph node.
Refer Short Notes/Notes/Answers on Q. No. 19 – 2011.

17. Derivatives of midgut.
Refer Short Notes/Notes/Answers on Q. No. 25 – 2012.

18. Blood supply of left suprarenal gland (Fig. 9).
- **Arterial supply:** Three arteries supply the suprarenal gland
  - Superior suprarenal artery from inferior phrenic artery
  - Middle suprarenal artery from abdominal aorta
  - Inferior suprarenal artery from renal artery
- **Venous drainage:** single vein emerges from hilum of the gland and drains to left renal vein

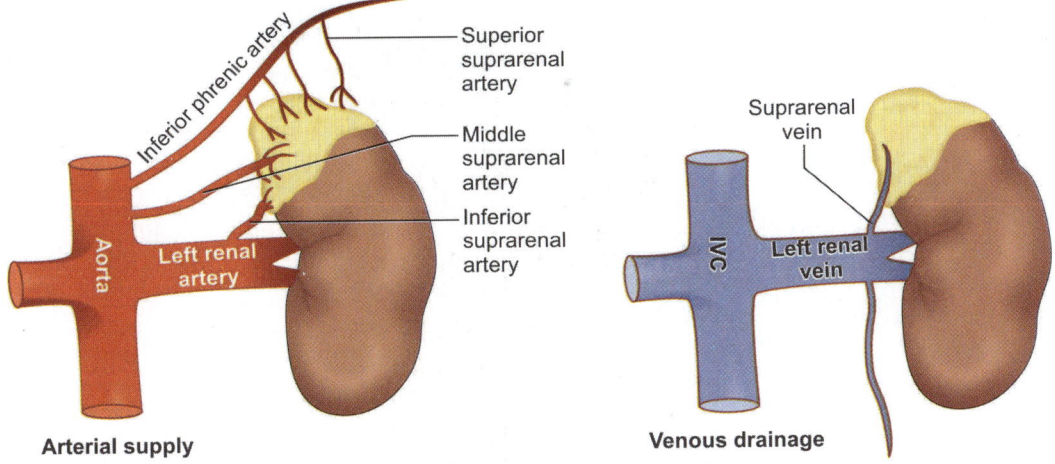

Fig. 9: Blood supply of left suprarenal.

19. Saphenous nerve.

- The saphenous nerve is the largest and longest cutaneous branch in the body
- It is branch from posterior division of femoral nerve
- **Course:** Situated lateral to femoral artery in the femoral triangle. It crosses anterior to the artery in the adductor canal from lateral to medial. It leaves the canal by accompanying saphenous branch of descending genicular artery. It descends along the medial border of the tibia accompanied by great saphenous vein. It passes in front of ankle and extends up to first metatarsophalangeal joint.
- **Branches:** Infrapatellar branch to take part in peripatellar plexus
  - Skin in front of patella
  - Skin along the medial border of foot up to first metatarsophalangeal joint.

20. Erb's palsy.
Refer Essay Q. No. 3 – 2005.

21. Wharton's duct.
Refer Short Notes/Notes on Q. No. 14 – 2003.

22. Waldeyer's ring.
Refer Short Notes/Notes/Answers on Q. No. 35 – 2011.

23. Structures related to lateral wall of cavernous sinus.
Refer Short Notes/Notes/Answers on Q. No. 22 – 2009.

24. Mention the branches of ophthalmic nerve.

- Ophthalmic nerve is a branch from trigeminal ganglion given in the middle cranial fossa
- It runs forward and enters the lateral wall of cavernous sinus
- It divides into three branches – frontal, nasociliary, and lacrimal **(Fig. 10)**
- The frontal nerve enters the orbit through lateral compartment of superior orbital fissure and divides into supratrochlear and supraorbital. It supplies the skin of forehead
- The nasociliary nerve enters orbit through middle compartment (within common tendinous ring) of superior orbital fissure and crosses the optic nerve from lateral to medial.
- It gives of anterior and posterior ethmoid nerves, infratrochlear, ciliary branches and a communicating branch to ciliary ganglion.
- The **lacrimal nerve** enters orbit outside common tendinous ring and supply conjunctive, skin of lateral half of upper eyelid, and lacrimal gland through its

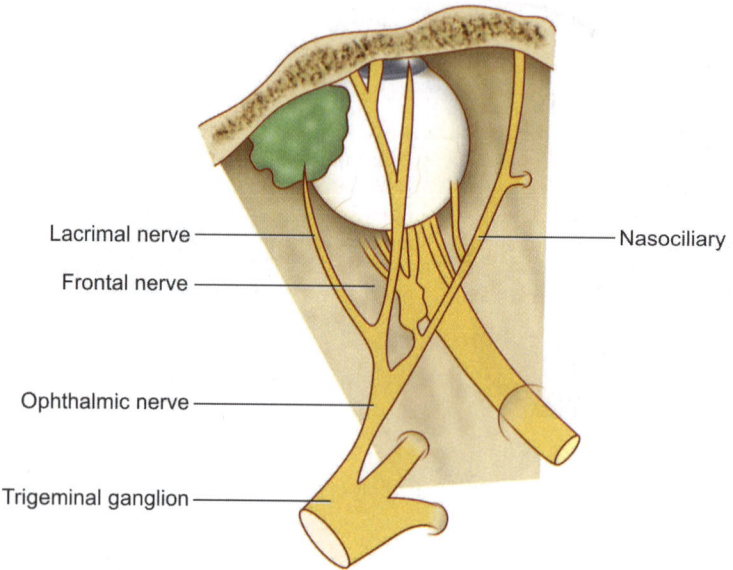

Fig. 10: Branches of ophthalmic nerve.

communication with zygomatic branch of maxillary nerve

25. Histology of retina.
Refer Short Notes/Notes on Q. No. 24 – 2008.

26. Thyroglossal duct.
Refer Essay Q. No. 8 – 2007.

27. Name the branches of facial artery in face.
Refer Short Notes/Notes on Q. No. 26 – 2007.

28. Tonsillar bed.
Refer Short Notes/Notes on Q. No. 32 – 2008.

29. Pleural recesses.
Refer Essay Q. No. 3 – 2003.

30. Millard-Gubler syndrome (Fig. 11).
- It is also known as alternating facial hemiplegia
- It is due to occlusion of branches of basilar artery to pons
- The structures affected are facial nerve and corticospinal tract
- The effect of lesion are a) facial nerve – ipsilateral Bell's palsy, hyperacusis

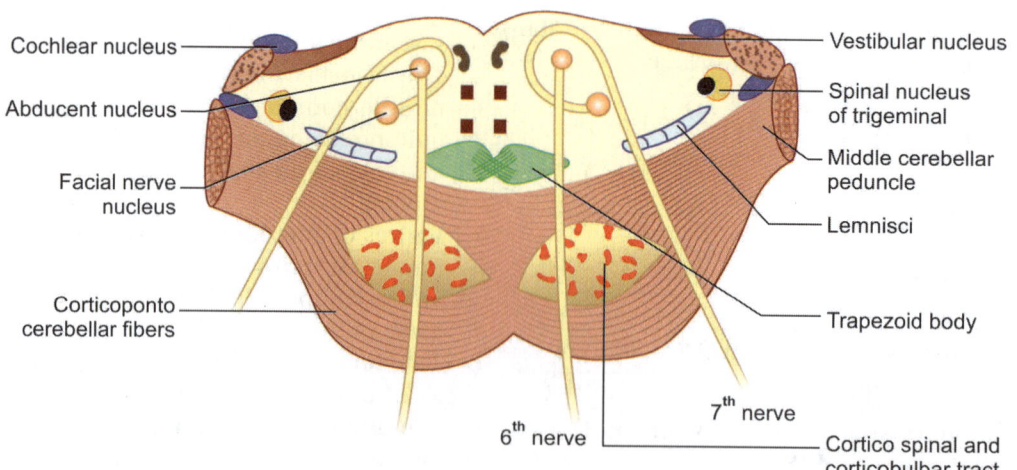

Fig. 11: Section of lower pons.

and loss of taste, b) corticospinal tract – contralateral hemiplegia

31. Modifications of cranial pia mater.
- Pia mater is the inner layer deep to arachnoid mater
- It has two layers, outer epi pia and inner pia glial
- Pia mater covers the surface of brain
- It dips into the concavities, fissures and sulci of brain
- It surrounds the blood vessels and is connected to perivascular space (Virchow Robin)
- Double layer of (fold of) pia mater is called tela choroidea
- Tela choroidea with ependyma, blood vessels form choroid plexus

32. Formation and termination of external jugular vein.
Refer Short Notes/Notes on Q. No. 29 – 2006.

33. Development of thyroid gland.
Refer Essay Q. No. 8 – 2007.

34. Nerve supply of pinna.
It is also known as auricle
- Parts of the pinna are: helix, crus of helix, auricular tubercle, anti helix, crura of antihelix, triangular fossa, scaphoid fossa, concha of auricle, external acoustic meatus, tragus, antitragus, intertragic notch, lobule of auricle
- Muscles are extrinsic and intrinsic – extrinsic are auricularis anterior, posterior and superior
- Intrinsic are halicis major, minor, tragicus, antitragicus, transversus and obliqus auriculare

Sensory nerve supply
- Helix, antihelix, lobule (Cranial surface) – most of cranial and posterior part of lateral surface by great auricular nerve and upper part by lesser occipital nerve
- Concavity of concha – auricular branch of vagus
- Tragus, crus of helix – auriculotemporal nerve
- Small area on both surface of auricle and depression of concha – facial nerve through auricular branch of vagus

Motor nerve supply
Extrinsic and intrinsic muscles - Temporal branch and posterior auricular branch of facial nerve

35. Superior orbital fissure.
- Superior orbital fissure is present in the sphenoid bone contributed by body of sphenoid medially, lesser wing above and greater wing below
- It is retort shaped broader medially and narrower laterally
- It is divided into three compartments by the common tendinous ring
- Communication – connects middle cranial fossa with orbit
- Structures passing **(Fig. 13)**
  - Medial compartment – inferior ophthalmic vein
  - Intermediate compartment – two divisions of oculomotor nerve, nasociliary nerve, abducent nerve
  - Lateral compartment – lacrimal, frontal branches from ophthalmic nerve and trochlear nerve, superior ophthalmic vein, recurrent meningeal branch from lacrimal artery, orbital branch of middle meningeal artery.

36. Branches of internal carotid artery.
- The internal carotid artery is branch from common carotid artery given at the level of upper border of thyroid cartilage

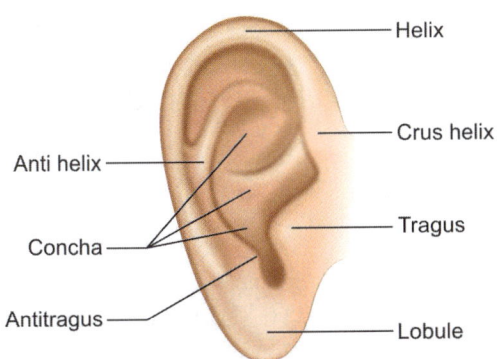

Fig. 12: Parts of pinna.

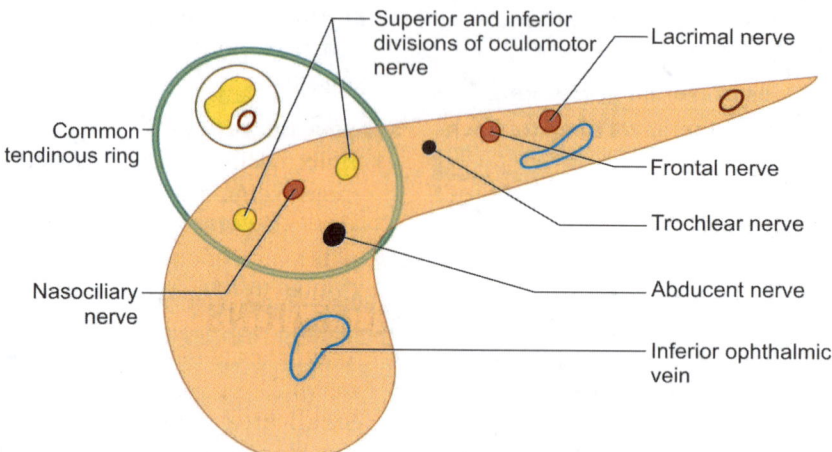

Fig. 13: Superior orbital fissure.

- It ascends upwards in the neck and enters the cranial cavity through carotid canal, runs within petrous part of temporal bone, crosses the foramen lacerum and enters the cavernous sinus. It pierces the roof of the sinus and reaches anterior perforated substance and terminates lateral to optic chiasma as middle and anterior cerebral branches
- The course is divided into cervical, petrous, cavernous and cranial parts
- Branches:
  - Cervical part—no branch given
  - Petrous part—caroticotympanic branch, pterygoid artery
  - Cavernous part—branch to trigeminal ganglion, cavernous sinus, hypophyseal branches.
  - Cranial part—ophthalmic artery, anterior cerebral, middle cerebral, anterior choroidal and posterior communicating artery

37. Dangerous area of face.
Refer Short Notes/Notes/Answer on Q. No. 37 – 2009.

38. Trigeminal neuralgia.
Refer Short Notes/Notes on Q. No. 18 – 2017.

39. Intrinsic muscles of larynx and nerve supply.
Refer Short Notes/Notes on Q. No. 28 – 2012.

40. Parotid duct.
Refer Essay Q. No. 4 – 2004.

MBBS Examination 2019

ANSWER ALL QUESTIONS

I. Essay questions (15/10 Marks)

1. Describe, in detail, about brachial plexus including its formation, branches, and its distribution. Add a note on its applied anatomy.
2. Describe the structure, blood supply, lymphatic drainage and applied aspects of mammary gland.
3. Describe, in detail, about the parotid gland. Add a note on its applied anatomy
4. Describe, in detail, about the lung under the following headings:
   a. Coverings.
   b. Surfaces and borders.
   c. Difference between right and left lung.
   d. Blood supply, nerve supply and lymphatic drainage. Add a note on its applied anatomy.

II. Short notes (5 Marks)

1. Inguinal canal.
2. Development and microstructure of urinary bladder.
3. Dorsalis pedis artery.
4. Inversion and eversion of foot.
5. Lobes of prostate and its applied anatomy.
6. Femoral hernia.
7. Male urethra.
8. Blood supply of stomach.
9. Anastomosis around scapula and collateral circulation.
10. Arches of foot.
11. Cavernous sinus.
12. Microstructure of tongue.
13. Intercostal space.
14. Recurrent laryngeal nerve.
15. Relations of thyroid gland.
16. Section of medulla oblongata at sensory decussation level with labelled diagram.
17. Microstructure of thyroid gland.
18. Extra-ocular muscles.
19. Venous drainage of heart.
20. Development of face.

III. Short answer questions (3/2 Marks)

1. Fibrous joint.
2. Superficial palmar arch.
3. Boundaries of femoral triangle.
4. Cutaneous innervation of sole of foot.
5. Parts of uterine tube.
6. Varicocele.
7. Flexor retinaculum of leg.
8. Space of Retzius.
9. Shoemakers line.
10. Contents of rectus sheath.
11. Hilton's law.
12. Muscles involved in the movements of wrist joint.
13. Nutrient artery.
14. Micro anatomy of spleen labelled diagram only.
15. Trendelenburg's sign.
16. Derivatives of ectoderm.
17. Cremastric muscle.
18. Carrying angle.
19. Perineal membrane
20. Branches of internal thoracic artery.
21. Wallenberg syndrome.
22. Contents of posterior mediastinum.
23. Pterygopalatine ganglion.
24. Formation of superior vena cava.

25. Bell's Palsy.
26. Derivatives of second pharyngeal arch.
27. Structures forming limbic system.
28. Development of pituitary gland.
29. Transverse sinus of pericardium.
30. Superior orbital fissure.
31. Enumerate nuclei of cerebellum.
32. Components of basal ganglia.
33. Waldeyer's ring.
34. Structures inside parotid gland.
35. Pterion.
36. Wry neck.
37. Name any four branches of external carotid artery.
38. Killian's dehiscence.
39. Fibrous skeleton of heart.

c. Difference between right and left lung
d. Nerve supply
   - Autonomic nerves
     - *Parasympathetic*: Pulmonary plexus formed by vagi
     - *Sympathetic*: Cervical cardiac nerves through superficial cardiac plexus
d. Lymphatic drainage
   - Superficial and deep plexus
   - Superficial – from margins of lung and fissures to bronchopulmonary nodes
   - Deep – from bronchiolar level and drain to bronchopulmonary nodes

I. ESSAY QUESTIONS

1. **Describe, in detail, about brachial plexus including its formation, branches, and its distribution. Add a note on its applied anatomy.**
Refer Essay Q. No. 3 – 2005.

2. **Describe the structure, blood supply, lymphatic drainage and applied aspects of mammary gland.**
Refer Essay Q. No. 4 – 2006.
Refer Lymphatic drainage—Short Notes Q. No. 19 – 2005.

3. **Describe, in detail, about the parotid gland. Add a note on its applied anatomy.**
Refer Essay Q. No. 4 – 2004.

4. **Describe, in detail, about the lung under the following headings:**
   a. **Coverings.**
   b. **Surfaces and borders.**
   c. **Difference between right and left lung.**
   d. **Blood supply, nerve supply and lymphatic drainage. Add a note on its applied anatomy.**
Refer A. Coverings—Essay Q. No. 3 – 2005.
Refer B. Surfaces, borders, d. Applied anatomy—Essay Q. No. 3 – 2004.
Refer d. Blood supply—Short Notes/Notes/Answer on Q. No. 49 – 2013.

II. SHORT NOTES

1. **Inguinal canal.**
Refer Short Notes/Notes on Q. No. 20 – 2008.

2. **Development and microstructure of urinary bladder.**
Refer development—Short Notes/Notes on Q. No. 10 – 2007.
Refer Histology—Essay Q. No. 3 – 2010.

3. **Dorsalis pedis artery.**
Refer Short Notes/Notes on Q. No. 19 – 2008.

4. **Inversion and eversion of foot.**
Refer Short Notes/Notes on Q. No. 6 – 2013.

5. **Lobes of prostate and its applied anatomy.**
Refer Essay Q. No. 4 – 2008.

6. **Femoral hernia.**
- The femoral hernia **protrudes** through the femoral ring into the femoral canal, then through saphenous opening towards inguinal ligament.
- The femoral canal is the medial compartment of femoral sheath. It is a dead space containing loose areolar tissue and lymph node (Cloquet/Rosenmuller)
- The **direction** of the hernia is downwards, forwards and then upwards
- The **coverings** of the hernia are:
  - Peritoneum, femoral septum, anterior wall of femoral sheath, cribriform fascia, superficial fascia and skin

Essay 4. C Difference between right and left lung

Topics	Right lung	Left lung
Size and shape	Shorter and broader	Longer and narrower
Weight	625 gm	565 gm
Fissures	2. Oblique and horizontal	1. Oblique
	(Diagram showing right lung with Oblique fissure and Horizontal fissure labeled)	*(Diagram showing left lung with Cardiac notch labeled)*
Lobes	3. superior, middle and inferior	2. superior and inferior
Borders - anterior	Corresponds to costomediastinal reflexions of pleura	Cardiac notch present below the forth costal cartilage
Surface – mediastinal surface hilum and impressions	*(Diagram of right lung mediastinal surface with labels: Scalenus anterior, Brachiocephalic trunk, Superior vena cava, Right phrenic nerve, Cardiac impression, Trachea, Right vagus nerve, Azygos arch, Esophagus, Inferior vena cava)*	*(Diagram of left lung mediastinal surface with labels: Left subclavian artery, Arch of aorta, Pulmonary trunk, Cardiac impression, Esophagus, Thoracic duct, Descending thoracic aorta)*

(Contd...)

Topics	Right lung	Left lung
Roots of the lung	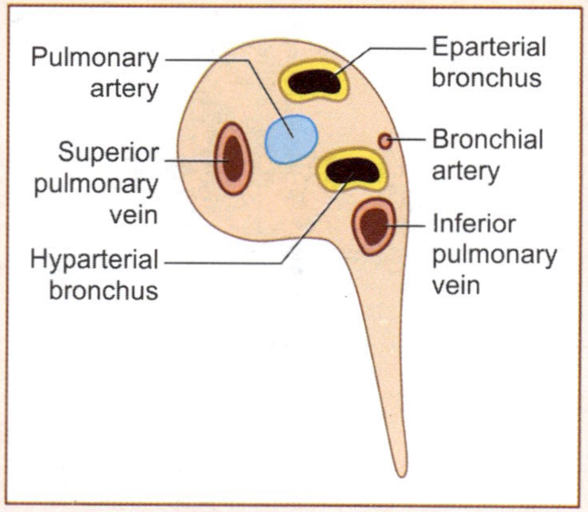 Eparterial bronchus, Bronchial artery, Inferior pulmonary vein, Pulmonary artery, Superior pulmonary vein, Hyparterial bronchus	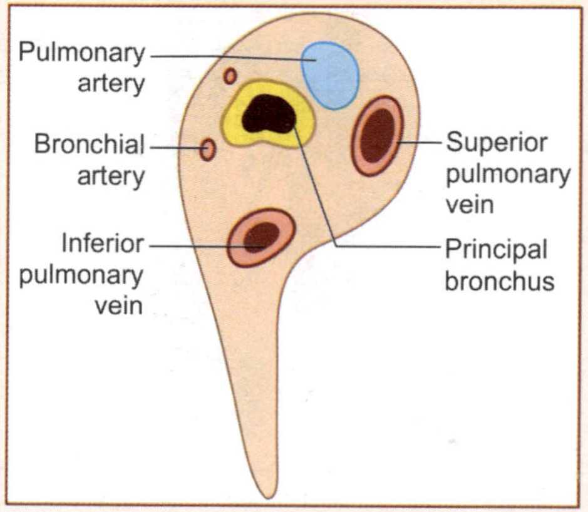 Superior pulmonary vein, Principal bronchus, Pulmonary artery, Bronchial artery, Inferior pulmonary vein
Broncho pulmonary segments	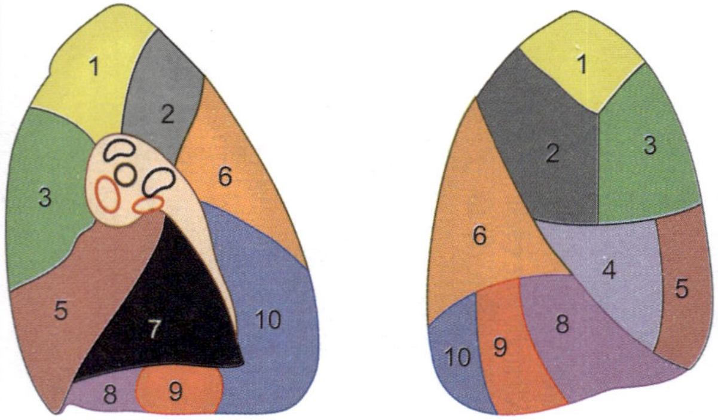 Upper lobe: 1 – Apical segment of upper lobe, 2 – Posterior, 3 – Anterior Middle lobe: 4 – Lateral, 5 – Medial Lower lobe: 6 – Apical segment of lower lobe, 7 – Medial basal, 8 – Anterior basal, 9 – Lateral basal, 10 – Posterior basal	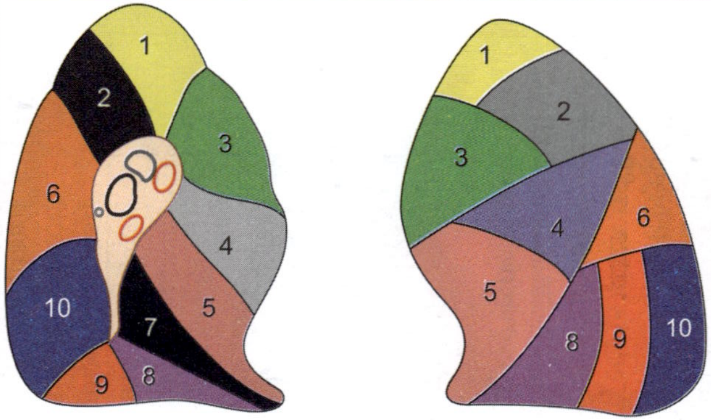 Upper lobe: 1 – Apical segment of upper lobe, 2 – Posterior, 3 – Anterior, 4 – Superior lingula, 5 – Inferior lingula Lower lobe: 6 – Apical segment of lower lobe, 7 – Medial basal (occasional), 8 – Anterior basal, 9 – Lateral basal, 10 – Posterior basal

- In the **treatment** of strangulated hernia, the lacunar ligament may be incised. Sometimes abnormal obturator artery may be present

7. Male urethra.
Refer Essay Q. No. 2 – 2011.

8. Blood supply of stomach.
Refer Essay Q. No. 2 – 2007.

9. Anastomosis around scapula and collateral circulation.

- Anastomosis around scapula is seen over acromion process and the fossae **(Fig. 1)**.
- **Over acromion process**: Acromion branch of suprascapular artery branch from subclavian artery with acromial branch of thoraco acromial and posterior circumflex humeral arteries from axillary artery
- **In the scapular, supraspinous and infraspinous fossae**: Suprascapular and deep branch of transverse cervical artery branch of thyrocervical trunk from subclavian artery with circumflex scapular artery branch of subscapular from third part of axillary artery
- **Collateral circulation:** Between branches of first part of subclavian artery and third part of axillary artery

10. Arches of foot.
Refer Essay Q. No. 1 – 2003.

11. Cavernous sinus.
Refer Essay Q. No. 5 – 2008.

12. Microstructure of tongue.
Refer Essay Q. No. 7 – 2009.

13. Intercostal space
Refer Essay Q. No. 6 – 2009.

14. Recurrent laryngeal nerve.
Refer Short Notes/Notes on Q. No. 36 – 2016.

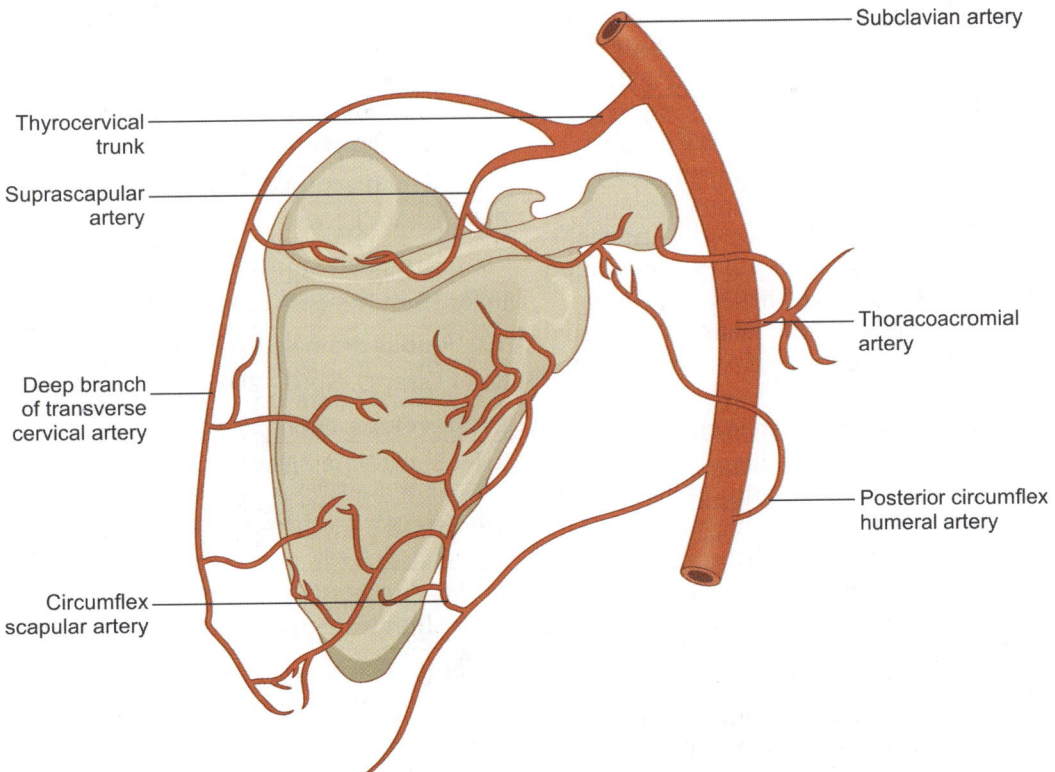

Fig. 1: Anastomosis around scapula.

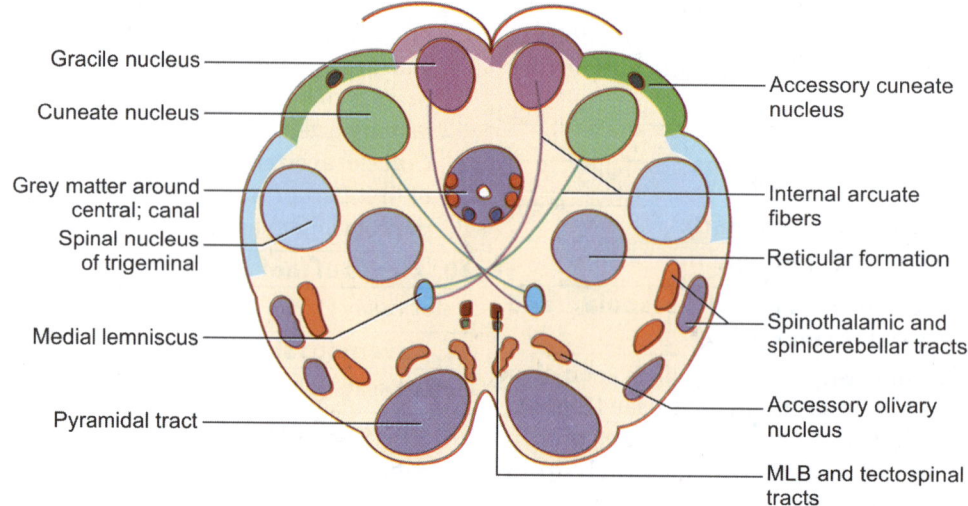

Fig 2: Section of medulla oblongata at sensory decussation.

15. Relations of thyroid gland.
Refer Short Notes/Notes on Q. No. 17 – 2004.

16. Section of medulla oblongata at sensory decussation level with labelled diagram.
- This section is in closed part of medulla oblongata
- Features
- White matter
  - Deep to pyramid bundle of corticospinal tract
  - Medial longitudinal bundle and tectospinal tract are ventral to decussation of internal arcuate fibres
  - Reticular formation is lateral to internal arcuate fibers
- Gray matter
  - Deep to gracile tubercle nucleus gracilis with fasciculus gracilis
  - Deep to cuneate tubercle nucleus cuneatus and fasciculus cuneatus
  - The fibers end in the corresponding nuclei, second order of neuron starts called internal arcuate fibers which decussate ventral to central canal to be continued as medial lemnisci.
  - Accessory cuneate nucleus situated dorsal to cuneate nucleus. The posterior external arcuate/cuneocerebellar tract arises and reach cerebellum
  - Deep to tuberculum cinerium the spinal nucleus of trigeminal nerve
  - Medial and dorsal accessory olivary nuclei dorsal to pyramidal tract
  - Central canal is pushed dorsally surrounded by gray matter
  - Appearance of hypoglossal, vagal and nucleus solitarius in the gray matter around central canal

17. Microstructure of thyroid gland.
Refer Essay Q. No. 8 – 2007.

18. Extra-ocular muscles.
Refer Short Notes/Notes on Q. No. 25 – 2009.

19. Venous drainage of heart.
Refer Essay Q. No. 5 – 2005.

20. Development of face
Refer Short Notes/Notes on Q. No. 22 – 2007.

III. SHORT ANSWER QUESTIONS

1. Fibrous joint.
Refer Short Notes/Notes on Q. No. 12 – 2014.

2. Superficial palmar arch.
Refer Short Notes/Notes/Answers on Q. No. 4 – 2011.

3. Boundaries of femoral triangle.
Refer Essay Q. No. 3 – 2012.

4. Cutaneous innervation of sole of foot.

Refer Short Notes/Notes on Q. No. 8 – 2005.

5. Parts of uterine tube.

Refer Short Notes/Notes/Answers on Q. No. 17 – 2010.

6. Varicocele.

The Pampiniform plexus of veins of the testis become dilated and tortuous producing varicocele

- It feels like a bag of worm
- Becomes prominent when the person stands or strains
- Reason is due to defective valves in the testicular vein and also due to problems in kidney or testicular vein
- More common on the left side as it drains to left renal vein at 90 degree

7. Flexor retinaculum of leg.

Refer Short notes/Notes/Answers on Q. No. 3 – 2017.

8. Space of Retzius.

- It is a retropubic space
- It is filled with retropubic fat and venous plexus
- The adipose tissue in this space separates the anterior surface of urinary bladder from transversalis fascia
- In male, the prostatic venous plexus is situated in this space
- Upper part of pubic symphysis joint is separated from the inferolateral surface of bladder by this space, and the prostatic venous plexus separates the lower part of joint

9. Shoemakers line.

- A line is drawn on each side of the body from the greater trochanter beyond anterior superior iliac spine
- Normal - The two lines meet in the midline at or above the umbilicus.
- If one femur is displaced upwards the lines meet away from the midline.
- If both are displaced upwards the lines meet below the umbilicus

10. Contents of rectus sheath.

Refer Short Notes/Notes on Q. No. 6 – 2003.

11. Hilton's law.

A nerve which supplies the muscle, the joint on which the muscle acts and the skin covering the joint is known as Hilton's law. Ex – axillary nerve

12. Muscles involved in the movements of wrist joint.

- Flexion—flexor carpi radialis, ulnaris and palmaris longus. Assisted by flexor digitorum superficialis and profundus
- Extension—extensor carpi radialis longus, brevis and ulnaris. Assisted by extensor

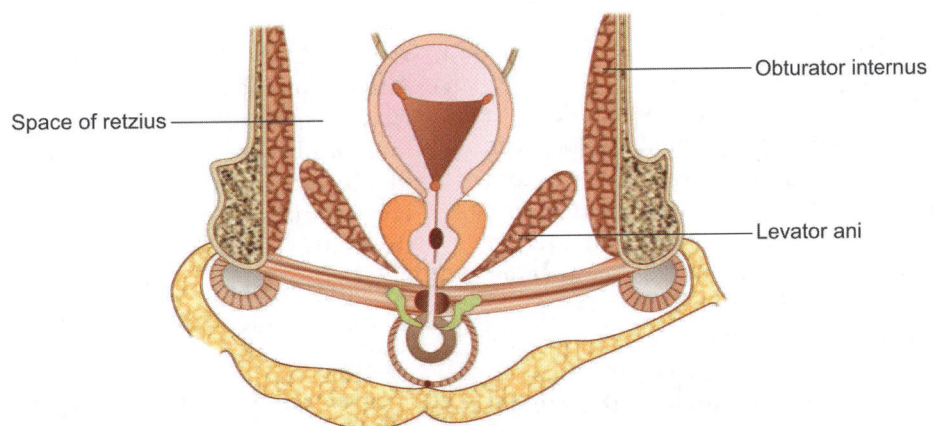

Fig. 3: Space of Retzius.

digitorum, indicis, digiti minimi and pollicis longus
- Adduction (ulnar deviation)—flexor and extensor carpi ulnaris
- Abduction (radial deviation)—Flexor carpi radialis, extensor carpi radialis longus and brevis. Associated with abductor pollicis longus and extensor pollicis brevis.

13. Nutrient artery.
Refer Short notes/Notes on Q. No. 2 – 2009

14. Micro anatomy of spleen labelled diagram only.
Refer Short Notes/Notes/Answer on Q. No. 3 – 2005.

15. Trendelenburg's sign.
Refer Short Notes/Notes on Q. No. 9 – 2013.

16. Derivatives of ectoderm.
Refer Short notes/Notes/Answer on Q. No. 10 – 2009.

17. Cremastric muscle.
- It forms one of the covering of testis deep to external spermatic fascia
- Attachment: Arched fibers of internal oblique and transversus abdominis and fibers from inguinal ligament form the **cremaster muscle**
- It loops around the spermatic cord or round ligament of uterus
- Nerve supply: Genital branch of genitofemoral nerve
- Action: Pulls the testis upwards to superficial inguinal ring

18. Carrying angle.
- When the elbow is fully extended with forearm and hand supinated, the long axis of humerus makes an angle with long axis of ulna called the carrying angle
- The angle is 165° in male and 175° in female. It is more in female due to wider pelvis
- The angle disappears when the forearm is fully pronated and in full elbow flexion
- The reason for the angle is the medial flange of trochlea of humerus extends 6 mm below the lateral margin
- The use of the angle: It helps to carry the things carried by the hand without any contact of the ulnar border of forearm with lateral surface of thigh

19. Perineal membrane.
Refer Short notes/Notes on Q. No. 9 – 2005.

20. Branches of internal thoracic artery.
Refer Short Notes/Notes/Answer on Q. No. 24 – 2014.

21. Wallenberg syndrome.
Refer Short Notes/Notes/Answer on Q. No. 38 – 2009.

22. Contents of posterior mediastinum.
Refer Essay Q. No. 6 – 2012.

23. Pterygopalatine ganglion.
Refer Short Notes/Notes/Answer on Q. No. 23 – 2012.

24. Formation of superior vena cava.
Refer Short Notes/Notes/Answer on Q. No. 11 – 2003.

25. Bell's Palsy.
Refer Essay Q. No. 9 – 2007.

26. Derivatives of second pharyngeal arch.
Refer Short Notes/Notes/Answer on Q. No. 27 – 2005.

27. Structures forming limbic system.
The components of limbic system are
- Olfactory pathway—olfactory nerves, olfactory bulb, anterior olfactory nucleus, olfactory tracts
- Piriform lobe
- Amygdaloid body
- Hippocampal formation
- Limbic lobe—septal area, cingulate gyrus, parahippocampal gyrus
- Hypothalamus, anterior nucleus of thalamus, habenular nucleus

28. Development of pituitary gland.
Refer Short Notes/Notes/Answer on Q. No. 42 – 2012.

29. Transverse sinus of pericardium.
Refer Short Notes/Notes/Answer on Q. No. 32 – 2007.

30. Superior orbital fissure.
Refer Short Notes/Notes/Answer on Q. No. 35 – 2018)

31. Enumerate nuclei of cerebellum.
Refer Short Notes/Notes/Answer on Q. No. 37 – 2012.

32. Components of basal ganglia.
Refer Short Notes/Notes/Answer on Q. No. 37 – 2011.

33. Waldeyer's ring.
Refer Short Notes/Notes/Answer on Q. No. 35 – 2011.

34. Structures inside parotid gland.
Refer Essay Q. No. 4 – 2004.

35. Pterion.
Refer Short Notes/Notes/Answer on Q. No. 31 – 2012.

36. Wry neck.
Refer Short Notes/Notes/Answer on Q. No. 15 – 2017.

37. Name any four branches of external carotid artery.
Refer Short Notes/Notes/Answer on Q. No. 39 – 2012.

38. Killian's dehiscence.
Refer Essay Q. No. 8 – 2006.

39. Fibrous skeleton of heart.
Refer Essay Q. No. 7 – 2006.

MBBS Examination 2020

ANSWER ALL QUESTIONS

I. Essay questions (1 × 10 = 10)

1. Write, in detail, about the femoral artery under the following headings: Origin, course, termination, relations, branches. Add a note on applied anatomy.
2. Write, in detail, about the shoulder joint under the following headings: Type and articular surfaces, ligaments, relations, movements and muscles involved, blood and nerve supply. Add a note on applied anatomy.
3. Write, in detail, about the thyroid gland under the following headings: Situation, lobes, coverings, relations, blood supply. Add a note on applied anatomy.
4. Describe, in detail, about lateral wall of nose under the following headings: Formation, nasal conchae and meatuses, blood supply, nerve supply. Add a note on paranasal air sinuses.

II. Short notes (5 × 4 = 20)

1. Microanatomy of hyaline cartilage.
2. Lymphatic drainage of mammary gland.
3. Thoracolumbar fascia.
4. Inguinal canal.
5. Fascial spaces of hand.
6. Inguinal lymph nodes.
7. Sacral plexus.
8. Histology of elastic artery.
9. Portal vein.
10. Ischiorectal fossa.
11. Sinuses of pericardium.
12. Nasal septum.
13. Cerebellar peduncles.
14. Histology of cornea
15. Hyoglossus.
16. Internal thoracic artery.
17. Orbicularis oris.
18. Tympanic membrane.
19. Draw T.S of spinal cord at thoracic level.
20. Histology of pituitary gland.

III. Short answer questions (10 × 2 = 20)

1. Parts of uterine tube.
2. Sesamoid bones.
3. Saturday night palsy.
4. Caput medusae.
5. Perineal body.
6. Juxta glomerular apparatus.
7. Down's syndrome.
8. Structures piercing clavipectoral fascia.
9. Suprapubic cystostomy.
10. Contents of lesser omentum.
11. Conjoint twins.
12. Claw hand.
13. Superficial inguinal ring.
14. Pneumatic bones.
15. Rectouterine pouch.
16. Derivatives of midgut.
17. Club foot.
18. Meckel's diverticulum.
19. Erythroblastosis foetalis.
20. Triangle of auscultation.
21. Fallot's tetralogy.
22. Pleural recesses.
23. Corpus callosum.
24. Auditory tube.
25. Ligamentum arteriosum.
26. Paratonsillar abscess.
27. Weber's syndrome.
28. Ciliary ganglion.

29. Tendon of todaro.
30. Reticular formation.
31. Flial chest.
32. Phernic nerve.
33. Tracheoesophageal fistula.
34. Muscles supplied by ansa cervicalis.
35. Name the structures derived from first pharyngeal arch cartilage.
36. Palatine muscles.
37. Superior vena cava.
38. Charcot's artery of hemorrhage.
39. Interpeduncular fossa.
40. Cerebral aqueduct.

I. ESSAY QUESTIONS

1. **Write, in detail, about the femoral artery under the following headings: Origin, course, termination, relations, branches. Add a note on applied anatomy.**

Refer Short Notes/Notes on Q. No. 2 – 2014.

2. **Write, in detail, about the shoulder joint under the following headings: Type and articular surfaces, ligaments, relations, movements and muscles involved, blood and nerve supply. Add a note on applied anatomy.**

Refer Essay Q. No. 2 – 2006.

Relations: (Fig. 1)
- Above—supraspinatus, supraspinatus bursa, coracoacromial arch
- Below—long head of triceps, quadrangular space, axillary nerve and posterior circumflex humeral vessels
- Anterior—subscapularis, coracobrachialis, short head of biceps
- Posterior—infraspinatus and teres minor
- All around—deltoid
- Blood supply—suprascapular, anterior and posterior circumflex humeral arteries
- Nerve supply—**capsule** is supplied by axillary, suprascapular and lateral pectoral nerves
- The **joint** is supplied by subscapular nerves

3. **Write, in detail, about the thyroid gland under the following headings: Situation, lobes, coverings, relations, blood supply. Add a note on applied anatomy.**

Refer Short Notes/Notes on Q. No. 17 – 2004.
Refer Applied Anatomy—Essay Q. No. 8 – 2007.

4. **Describe, in detail, about lateral wall of nose under the following headings: Formation, nasal conchae and meatuses, blood supply, nerve supply. Add a note on paranasal air sinuses.**

Refer Short Notes/Notes on Q. No. 16 – 2004.

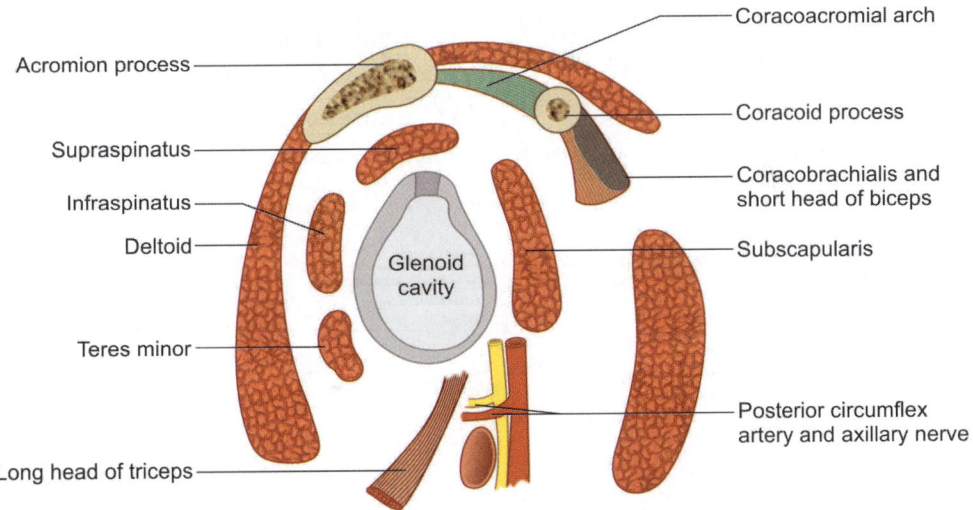

Fig. 1: Relations of shoulder joint.

Refer Paranasl Air Sinuses—Short Notes/Notes on Q. No. 37 – 2008.

II. SHORT NOTES

1. **Microanatomy of hyaline cartilage.**
Refer Short Notes/Notes on Q. No. 1 – 2006.

2. **Lymphatic drainage of mammary gland.**
Refer Short Notes/Notes on Q. No. 19 – 2005.

3. **Thoracolumbar fascia.**
Refer Short Notes/Notes on Q. No. 5 – 2009.

4. **Inguinal canal.**
Refer Short Notes/Notes on Q. No. 20 – 2008.

5. **Fascial spaces of hand.**
Refer midpalmar space—Short Notes on Q. No. 5 – 2014, & thenar space—Short Answers on Q. No. 2 – 2016.

Pulp space (Fig. 2)
- It is space between palmar skin and distal phalanges of all digits of the hand
- It lies distal to the fibrous sheath of flexor tendons
- The skin of the distal phalanx is connected to the periosteum by many fibrous septae in the pulp space
- So the space is divided into numerous compartments
- The compartments are very tight
- They contain subcutaneous fat and blood vessels
- The distal four- fifth (4/5) of the phalanx receive blood supply from the digital arteries
- These arteries pierces the fibrous septae
- The proximal part (1/5) get separate blood supply without passing through the septa
- Applied anatomy – infection of the pulp space is known as whitlow. There will be severe pain. If not treated it can result in avascular of the distal 4/5 of the distal phalanx

6. **Inguinal lymph nodes.**
Refer Short Notes/Notes on Q. No. 5 – 2004.

7. **Sacral plexus.**
Refer Short Notes/Notes on Q. No. 7 – 2011.

8. **Histology of elastic artery.**
Refer Short Notes/Notes on Q. No. 23 – 2012.

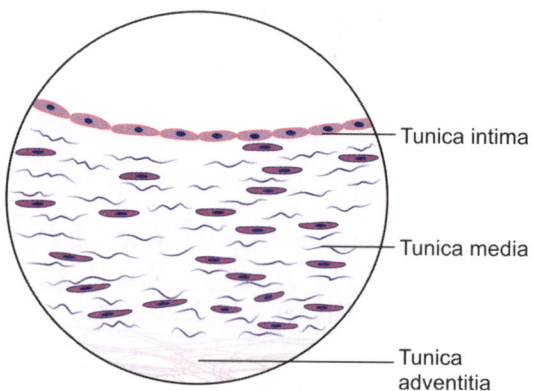

Fig. 3: Histology of elastic artery/aorta.

9. **Portal vein.**
Refer Short Notes/Notes on Q. No. 6 – 2004.

10. **Ischiorectal fossa.**
Refer Short Notes/Notes on Q. No. 8 – 2003.

11. **Sinuses of pericardium.**
Refer Short Notes/Notes on Q. No. 32 – 2007.

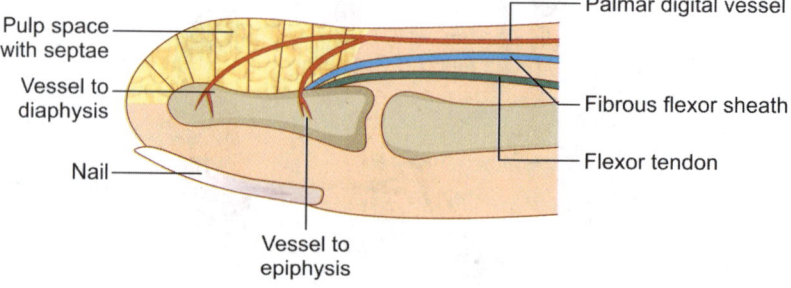

Fig. 2: Pulp space.

12. Nasal septum.
Refer Short Notes/Notes on Q. No. 17 – 2003.

13. Cerebellar peduncles.
Refer Short Notes/Notes on Q. No. 20 – 2006.

14. Histology of cornea.
Refer Short Notes/Notes on Q. No. 35 – 2009.

15. Hyoglossus.
Refer Short Notes/Notes on Q. No. 15 – 2004.

16. Internal thoracic artery.
Refer Short Notes/Notes on Q. No. 24 – 2014.

17. Orbicularis oris.
- It is a muscle of facial expression
- Attachment: It has an extrinsic and an intrinsic parts
- Extrinsic part—contributed by the other muscles of facial expressions – zygomaticus major and minor, levator and depressor anguli oris, levator labii superioris, levator labii superioris alaeque nasi, depressor labii inferioris, buccinator, risorius and mentalis. These muscles produce a thickening called **modiolus**
- Intrinsic part—upper fibers arise from incisive fossa of maxilla above the eminence of lateral incisors, lower fibers from incisive fossa of mandible below the eminence of lateral incisors. They converse at modiolus
- Nerve supply—buccal and marginal mandibular branches of facial nerve
- Actions—various movements of the lip
- Applied anatomy—in Bell's palsy injury to facial nerve results in paralysis of the muscle. The effect of lesion is deviation of the angle of the mouth to the normal side and drooling of saliva.

18. Tympanic membrane.
Refer Short Notes/Notes on Q. No. 26 – 2005.

19. Draw T.S of spinal cord at thoracic level.
Refer Essay Q. No. 11 – 2013.

20. Histology of pituitary gland.
Refer Short Notes/Notes on Q. No. 23 – 2005.

III. SHORT ANSWER QUESTIONS

1. Parts of uterine tube.
Refer Short Notes/Notes Q. No. 17 – 2010.

2. Sesamoid bones.
Refer Short Notes/Notes/Answers Q. No. 4 – 2007.

3. Saturday night palsy.
Refer Essay Q. No. 2 – 2010.

4. Caput medusae.
Refer Short Notes/Notes/Answer on Q. No. 6 – 2004.

5. Perineal body.
Refer Short notes/Notes/Answer on Q. No. 8 – 2004.

6. Juxta glomerular apparatus.
Refer Short Notes/Notes/Answer on Q. No. 12 – 2013.

7. Down's syndrome.
Refer Short notes/Notes/Answer on Q. No. 22 – 2005.

8. Structures piercing clavipectoral fascia.
Refer Short Notes/Notes/Answer on Q. No. 5 – 2006.

9. Suprapubic cystostomy.
- The urinary bladder is punctured above pubic symphysis without traversing

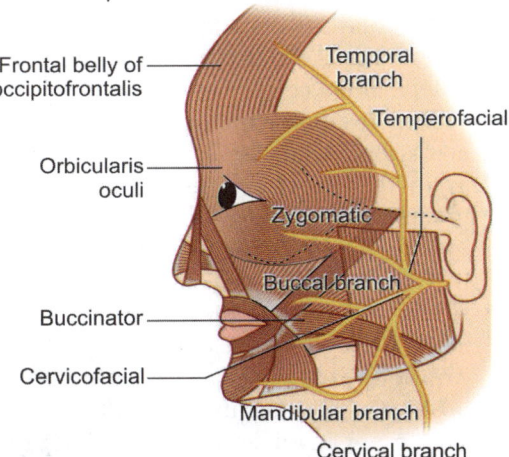

Fig. 4: Orbicularis oris.

peritoneum is called suprapubic cystostomy
- When the bladder is distended it becomes ovoid in shape
- It extend upwards in the suprapubic region, in the extraperitoneal fatty tissue of anterior abdominal wall
- The infrolateral surface of the bladder become anterior and lies directly in contact with anterior abdominal wall without intervention of peritoneum

10. Contents of lesser omentum.
Refer Essay Q. No. 2 – 2007.

11. Conjoint twins.
- The conjoint twin is due to defect in splitting of Henson's node and primitive streak
- The classification is based on the union
- The type of twin depends on the extent of defect of the Henson's node and primitive streak
- Monozygotic twins are rare and connected by skin or common liver
- The types of conjoint twin are a) Thoracopagus – united in the chest, b) Pygopagus – united in the sacral region, c) Craniopagus – joined at head

12. Claw hand.
Refer Short Notes/Notes/Answer on Q. No. 22 – 2013.

13. Superficial inguinal ring.
Refer Short Notes/Notes/Answer on Q. No. 20 – 2008.

14. Pneumatic bones.
- Bones containing space filled with air are called pneumatic bone
- Some bones in the skull are filled with air. Example- Mastoid process of temporal bone, sphenoid, ethmoid, maxilla and frontal bones
- The bones present close to nasal cavity form paranasal air sinuses filled with air, namely sphenoid, ethmoid, maxilla and frontal bones
- The amount of air present varies
- Function- Help in resonance of voice, and the temperature of the inhaled air is made optimum.

15. Rectouterine pouch.
Refer Short Notes/Notes/Answer on Q. No. 15 – 2009.

16. Derivatives of midgut.
Refer Short Notes/Notes/Answer on Q. No. 25 – 2012.

17. Club foot.
- The club foot is also known as Talipes
- It may be congenital or acquired
- Types of club foot are
  1. Talipes equinus – Foot is flexed in plantar flexed position and the toes are towards ground
  2. Talipes calcaneus – Heel rest on ground, toes upturned and the position of the foot is dorsiflexed
  3. Talipes varus – The foot is inverted and adducted. The deformity is in subtalar and talocalcaneo-navicular joints
  4. Talipes valgus – The foot is everted and abducted
  5. Talipes equinovarus – Combination of primary deformities

18. Meckel's diverticulum.
Refer Short Notes/Notes/Answer on Q. No. 12 – 2005.

19. Erythroblastosis foetalis.
- It is also known as hemolytic disease of newborn as the maternal antibodies hemolyze fetal red blood cells
- It is called erythroblastosis foetalis because erythroblasts occurs due to the hemolysis of blood cells which stimulate an increase in fetal blood cells
- This is due to escape of fetal blood cells across placental barrier, which causes an antibody by the mother's immune system in return
- This response is known as isoimmunization
- In fetal hydrops, the anemia becomes severe and the fetus dies
- Severe cases are caused by D/ Rh antigen
- Antibody response occurs when Rh is positive in fetus and mother is Rh negative
- Treatment involves with anti D immunoglobulin to the mother, intrauterine or postnatal transfusion for fetus

20. Triangle of auscultation.
Refer Short Notes/Notes/Answer on Q. No. 25 – 2011.

21. Fallot's tetralogy.
Refer Essay Q. No. 6 – 2010.

22. Pleural recesses.
Refer Essay Q. No. 3 – 2003.

23. Corpus callosum.
Refer Short Notes/Notes/Answer on Q. No. 25 – 2011.

24. Auditory tube.
Refer Short Notes/Notes/Answer on Q. No. 15 – 2014.

25. Ligamentum arteriosum.
Refer Short Notes/Notes/Answer on Q. No. 31 – 2009.

26. Peritonsillar abscess.
- It is one of the complication of untreated tonsillitis
- There is collection of pus between superior constrictor and tonsillar hemicapsule
- Tonsil is sometimes removed to treat the abscess
- It is commonly seen in children, adolescent

27. Weber's syndrome.
- Due vascular lesion affecting mid brain the oculomotor nerve fiber, corticospinal tract will be affected resulting in oculomotor syndrome and contralateral hemiplegia.
- Oculomotor syndrome—injury to oculomotor nerve results in
  a. Ptosis—due to paralysis of levator palpabrae superioris
  b. Lateral squint—due to unopposed action of lateral rectus
  c. Dilated pupil—due to paralysis of sphincter pupillae
  d. Enophthalmos—as most of the extra ocular muscles are paralyzed
  e. Loss of accommodation—due to paralysis of ciliaris

28. Ciliary ganglion.
Refer Short Notes/Notes/Answer on Q. No. 31 – 2009.

29. Tendon of todaro.
- Tendon of todaro is present in the septal wall of right atrium
- It is a collagenous subendocardial tendon
- It is palpable and round in shape
- It forms a boundary for the triangle of Koch, which is situated anteroinferiorly bounded by septal leaflet of tricuspid valve, tendon of todaro and coronary sinus opening. AV node is situated in it.

30. Reticular formation.
- It is formed by network of fibres and the scattered neurons are situated
- It extends throughout the length of spinal cord and brainstem
- In spinal cord, there is intermingling of white and gray matter, on the lateral side of dorsal column
- In the medulla, it is dorsal to the inferior olivary nucleus
- In the pons lies in the dorsal part

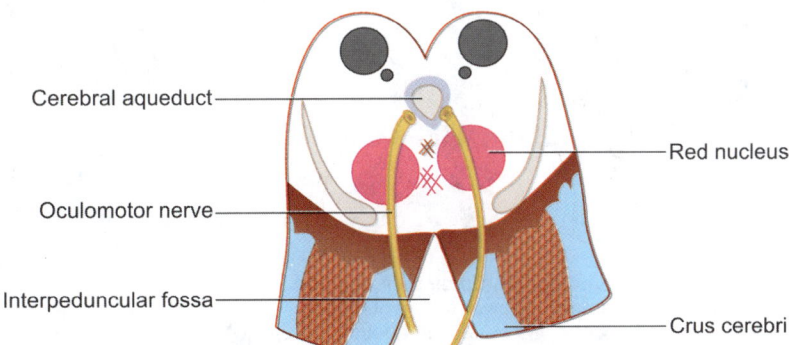

Fig. 5: Section of midbrain at superior colliculus.

- In the midbrain in the tegmentum
- A number of ill-defined nuclei are present
- The pathways include ascending, descending, crossed, uncrossed, somatic and visceral
- It has an important regulatory role- facilitatory and inhibitory

31. Flail chest.

- It is due to injury to chest after blunt trauma
- There will be fracture of many ribs
- Fracture in a rib can be two or more sites
- During inspiration the flail segment will be sucked in and pushed out in expiration producing paradoxical respiratory movement

32. Phernic nerve.

Refer Short Notes/Notes/Answer on Q. No. 45 – 2013.

33. Tracheoesophageal fistula.

- Trachea and Esophagus are developed from proximal part of foregut
- They are separated by tracheoesophageal septum as ventral respiratory part and dorsal Esophagus
- The defective division by the septum results in the tracheoesophageal fistula
- The upper end of Esophagus communicates with trachea and lower end as blind sac **(Fig. 6A)**.
- Esophagus divided into upper and lower part and both ends do not communicate with trachea **(Fig. 6B)**.
- The commonest tracheoesophageal fistula is proximal part of Esophagus ends as blind sac and the distal part is connected to trachea just above bifurcation **(Fig. 6C)**.

34. Muscles supplied by ansa cervicalis.

Refer Short Notes/Notes/Answer on Q. No. 26 – 2008.

35. Name the structures derived from first pharyngeal arch cartilage.

Refer Short Notes/Notes/Answer on Q. No. 24 – 2007.

36. Palatine muscles.

Refer Short Notes/Notes/Answer on Q. No. 41 – 2011.

37. Superior vena cava.

Refer Short Notes/Notes/Answer on Q. No. 11 – 2003.

38. Charcot's artery of hemorrhage.

- The blood supply of the internal capsule of brain is from the central branches of circle of Willis
- They are end arteries
- 6 sets of central branches are from the arterial circle
- The anterolateral set is from anterior cerebral and middle cerebral artery
- The branches from middle cerebral artery is known as lateral striate or lenticulostriate branches

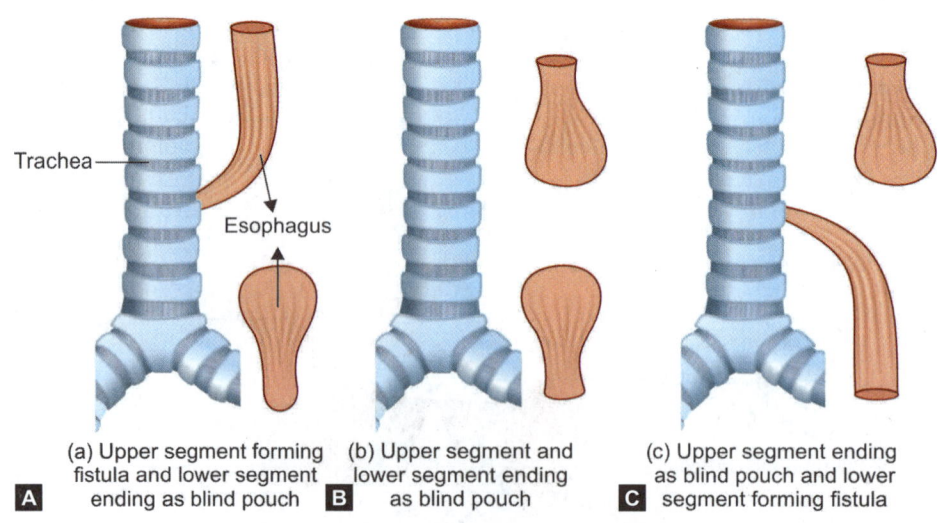

(a) Upper segment forming fistula and lower segment ending as blind pouch
(b) Upper segment and lower segment ending as blind pouch
(c) Upper segment ending as blind pouch and lower segment forming fistula

Figs. 6A to C: Types of tracheoesophageal fistulas.

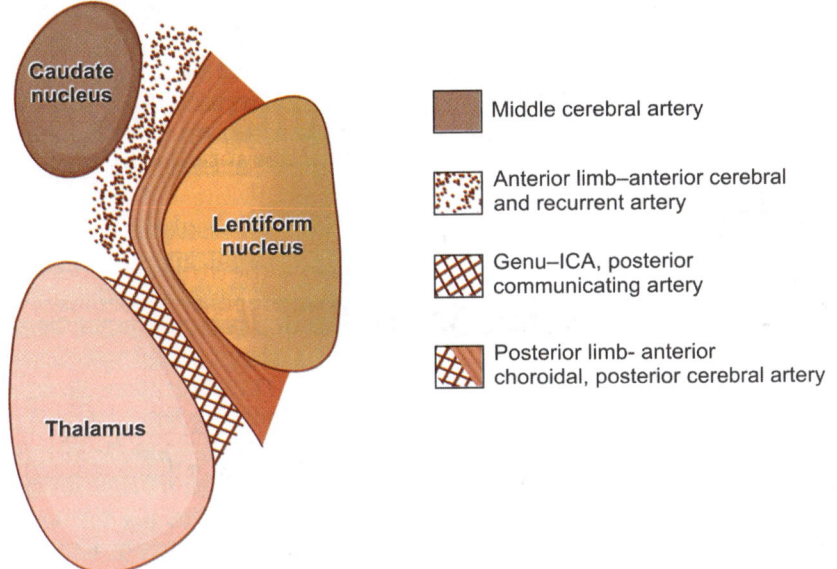

Fig. 7: Blood supply of internal capsule.

- The branches from middle cerebral is also known as Charcot's artery of cerebral hemorrhage
- They pierce through the anterior perforated substance and supply the corpus striatum, the anterior limb, genu and posterior limb of the internal capsule **(Fig. 7)**.
- Lesion of lenticulostriate branches leads to contralateral hemiplegia as it supplies corticospinal tract

39. Interpeduncular fossa.

Refer Short Notes/Notes/Answer on Q. No. 33 – 2009.

40. Cerebral aqueduct.

- It is the cavity of midbrain present in both inferior and superior colliculi levels
- It connects the third and fourth ventricles of brain
- It is developmentally cavity of mesencephalon
- It is surrounded by peri aqudactal gray matter and the cranial nerve nuclei present in it are oculomotor, trochlear, mesencephalic nucleus of trigeminal.

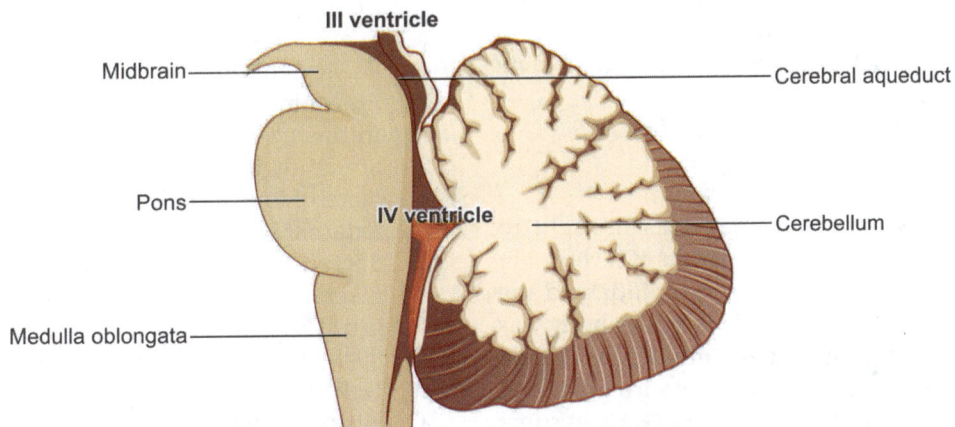

Fig. 8: Median section through brain stem and cerebellum.

MBBS Examination 2021

ANSWER ALL QUESTIONS

I. Essay questions

1. Describe mammary gland under the following headings: Extent, Relations, Blood Supply, Lymphatic Drainage and Clinical Anatomy.
2. Discuss the uterus under the following headings: Position, Parts, External Features, Relations, Blood Supply, Lymphatic Drainage and Clinical Anatomy.
3. Describe pancreas under the following headings:
   a. Parts and relations.
   b. Blood supply.
   c. Development.
4. Explain the formation of lumbar plexus. Add a brief note on sciatic nerve.
5. Describe, in detail, about blood supply of heart and its clinical anatomy.
6. Discuss the pharynx under the following headings: Extent, Parts, Features, Blood Supply, Muscles forming it and its clinical anatomy.
7. Describe pharynx under the following headings:
   a. Extent and Subdivisions.
   b. Pharyngeal Muscles.
   c. Applied Anatomy.
8. A 55-year-old man was brought to hospital with complaints of severe pain in retrosternal area radiating to the medial side of left arm. His body was profusely sweating and he was found to be restless. Pulse was irregular and heart beat was rapid. ECG shows some changes
   a. What will be the probable diagnosis?
   b. Write, in detail, about blood supply of heart.

II. Short notes $(10 \times 5 = 50)$

1. Structures under cover of gluteus maximus.
2. Great saphenous vein.
3. Femoral triangle.
4. Adductor magnus.
5. Ligaments of knee joint.
6. Rectus sheath.
7. Erb's point.
8. Rotator cuff muscles.
9. Microstructure of Esophagus.
10. Development of pancreas.
11. Microscopic anatomy of compact bone.
12. Cubital fossa.
13. Trigone of bladder.
14. Axillary nerve.
15. Coeliac trunk.
16. Spermatic cord.
17. Pelvic diaphragm.
18. Anastomosis around knee joint.
19. Intrinsic muscles of hand.
20. Structures in lateral compartment of leg
21. Floor of fourth ventricle.
22. External jugular vein.
23. Secretomotor innervation of parotid gland.
24. Cartilages of larynx.
25. Superior mediastinum.
26. Development of face.
27. Histology of thymus.
28. Pleura.

29. Falx cerebri.
30. Circle of willis.
31. Lateral wall of nasal cavity.
32. Karyotyping.
33. Derivatives of endodermal pouches.
34. Microscopic anatomy of trachea.
35. Sulci and gyri in the medial surface of brain.
36. Posterior triangle of neck.
37. Temporomandibular joint.
38. Medial surface of left lung.
39. Spinal meninges and its modifications.
40. Thoracic part of Esophagus.

III. Multiple Choice Questions (20 × 1 = 20)

I. ESSAY QUESTIONS

1. **Describe mammary gland under the following headings: Extent, Relations, Blood Supply, Lymphatic Drainage and Clinical Anatomy.**

Refer Essay Q. No. 4 – 2006.

2. **Discuss the uterus under the following headings: Position, Parts, External Features, Relations, Blood Supply, Lymphatic Drainage and Clinical Anatomy.**

Refer Essay Q. No. 2 – 2004.
Refer Blood supply—Arterial supply Essay Q. No. 3 – 2006, Venous drainage—Essay Q. No. 1 – 2009.

Lymphatic drainage (Fig. 1)

- From upper part of body of uterus, fundus – i) lymphatics follow the lymphatics of ovary and end in the pre- and para-aortic nodes ii) lymphatics from lateral cornu where the intramural part of uterine tube is attached to superficial inguinal nodes

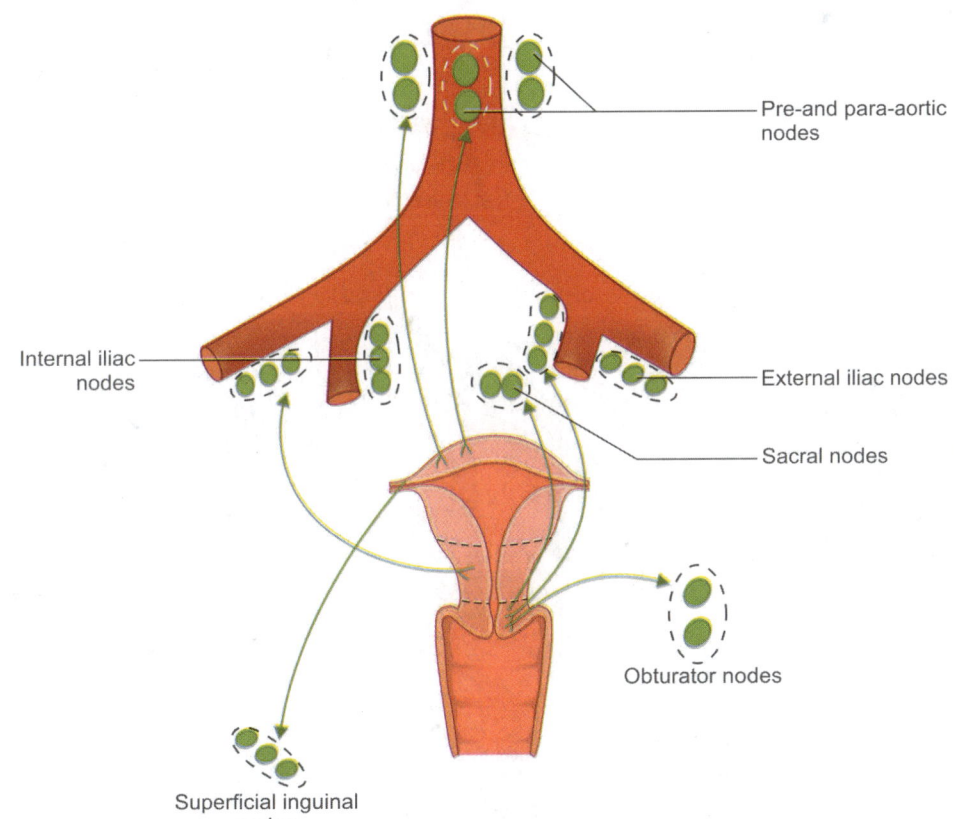

Fig. 1: Lymphatic drainage of uterus.

- From middle of body—to external iliac nodes
- From cervix—to external, and internal iliac nodes, sacral nodes, few to obturator nodes.

3. **Describe pancreas under the following headings:**
   a. **Parts and relations.**
   b. **Blood supply.**
   c. **Development.**

Refer (a) Parts and relations—Essay Q. No. 1 – 2006.
Refer (b) Blood supply—Essay Q. No. 2 – 2008.
Refer (c) Development—Short Notes on/Notes on Q. No. 6 – 2005.

4. **Explain the formation of lumbar plexus. Add a brief note on sciatic nerve.**

Refer Sciatic nerve—Essay Q. No. 5 – 2007.

Lumbar Plexus Formation

- The plexus is formed by VR of upper four lumbar nerves within the substance of psoas major
- The L4 is called as nervus furcalis, as it divides to take part in lumbar and sacral plexus
- **Types** – **Prefixed** if the L3 nerve divides and form nervus furcalis instead of L4. **Postfixed** in which the L5 divides instead of L4

Mode of Formation (Fig. 2)

- L1 receives small twig from T12 (Dorsolumbar nerve) and divides into a larger upper and smaller lower divisions. L2 divides into a smaller upper and larger lower divisions
- The larger upper of L1 gives of iliohypogastric (L1) and ilioinguinal (L1)
- The smaller lower division of L1 unite with smaller upper division of L2 to form genitofemoral nerve (L1, 2)
- The L4 divides into a larger upper and smaller lower divisions.
- The larger lower division of L2, entire L3, and larger upper division of L4 each splits into a dorsal and a ventral branch

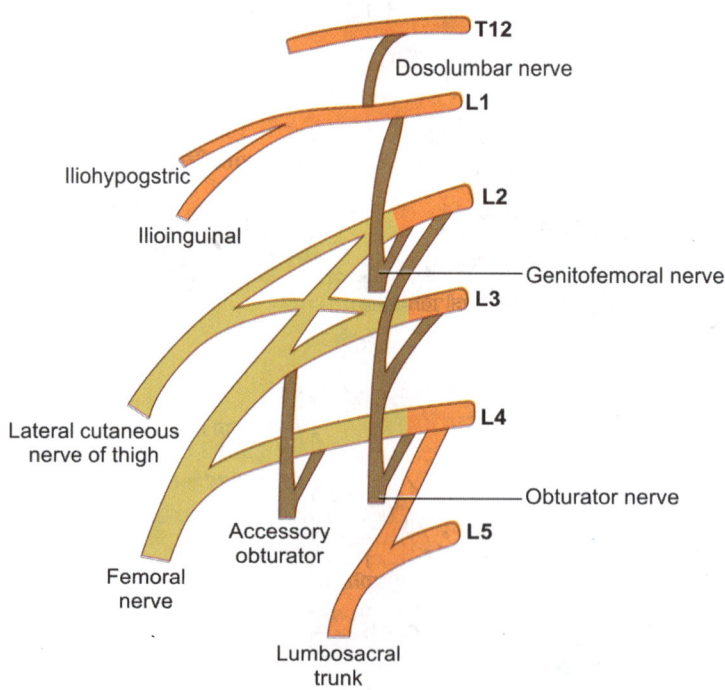

Fig. 2: Lumbar plexus.

- The dorsal branches of L2, 3 join to form lateral cutaneous nerve of the thigh
- The dorsal branches of L2, 3, 4 join to form the femoral nerve
- The ventral branches of L3, 4 join to form accessory obturator nerve
- The ventral branches of L2, 3, 4 join to form obturator nerve

5. **Describe, in detail, about blood supply of heart and its clinical anatomy.**

Refer Essay Q. No. 5 – 2005.

6. **Discuss the pharynx under the following headings: Extent, Parts, Features, Blood Supply, Muscles forming it and its clinical anatomy.**

Refer Essay Q. No. 8 – 2006.

Blood supply:
- Arterial supply
  - Ascending pharyngeal artery
  - Ascending palatine and tonsillar branch from facial artery
  - Greater palatine, pharyngeal and artery of pterygoid canal from maxillary artery
  - Dorsal lingual from lingual artery
- Venous drainage
  - By the pharyngeal plexus of vein drain into the internal jugular vein and facial vein. The plexus communicate with pterygoid venous plexus

7. **Describe pharynx under the following headings:**
   a. **Extent and Subdivisions.**
   b. **Pharyngeal Muscles.**
   c. **Applied Anatomy.**

Refer Essay Q. No. 8 – 2006.

8. **A 55-year-old man was brought to hospital with complaints of severe pain in retrosternal area radiating to the medial side of left arm. His body was profusely sweating and he was found to be restless. Pulse was irregular and heart beat was rapid. ECG shows some changes**
   a. **What will be the probable diagnosis?**
   b. **Write, in detail, about blood supply of heart.**

a. The diagnosis is myocardial infarction due to block in coronary arteries.
b. Refer Essay Q. No. 5 – 2005.

II. SHORT NOTES

1. **Structures under cover of gluteus maximus.**

Refer Short Notes/Notes on Q. No. 25 – 2013.

2. **Great saphenous vein.**

Refer Short Notes/Notes on Q. No. 14 – 2005.

3. **Femoral triangle.**

Refer Essay Q. No. 3 – 2012.

4. **Adductor magnus.**

Refer Short Notes/Notes on Q. No. 9 – 2018.

5. **Ligaments of knee joint.**

Refer Short Notes/Notes on Q. No. 10 – 2014.

6. **Rectus sheath.**

Refer Short Notes/Notes on Q. No. 6 – 2003.

7. **Erb's point.**

Refer Short Notes/Notes on Q. No. 6 – 2009.

8. **Rotator cuff muscles.**

Refer Short Notes/Notes on Q. No. 4 – 2003.

9. **Microstructure of Esophagus.**

Refer Short Notes/Notes on Q. No. 31 – 2008.

10. **Development of pancreas.**

Refer Short Notes/Notes on Q. No. 6 – 2005.

11. **Microscopic anatomy of compact bone.**

Refer Short Notes/Notes on Q. No. 1 – 2003.

12. **Cubital fossa.**

Refer Short Notes/Notes on Q. No. 16 – 2008.

13. **Trigone of bladder.**

Refer Essay Q. No. 2 – 2003.

14. Axillary nerve.
Refer Short Notes/Notes on Q. No. 2 – 2013.

15. Coeliac trunk.
Refer Short Notes/Notes on Q. No. 10 – 2009.

16. Spermatic cord.
Refer Short Notes/Notes on Q. No. 12 – 2015.

17. Pelvic diaphragm.
Refer Short Notes/Notes on Q. No. 18 – 2005.

18. Anastomosis around knee joint.
Refer Short Notes/Notes on Q. No. 9 – 2016.

19. Intrinsic muscles of hand.

S. No.	Name of the muscles	Attachment		Nerve supply	Action
		Origin	Insertion		
1.	Thenar muscles				
	Abductor pollicis brevis	Tubercle of scaphoid, crest of trapezium, flexor retinaculum	Lateral side of base of proximal phalanx of thumb	Median nerve	Abduction of thumb
	Flexor pollicis brevis	Tubercle of scaphoid, flexor retinaculum	Lateral side of base of proximal phalanx of thumb	Median nerve	Flexion of thumb
	Opponens pollicis	Crest of trapezium, flexor retinaculum	Lateral half of palmar surface of shaft of first metacarpal	Median nerve	Opposition of tip of thumb with tips of other fingers
2.	Hypothenar muscles				
	Abductor digiti minimi	Pisiform, pisohamate ligament and tendon of flexor carpi ulnaris	Medial side of base of proximal phalanx of little finger	Deep branch of ulnar nerve	Abduction of little finger
	Flexor digiti minimi	Hook of hamate and flexor retinaculum	Medial side of base of proximal phalanx of little finger	Deep branch of ulnar nerve	Flexion of little finger
	Opponens digiti minimi	Hook of hamate and flexor retinaculum	Ulnar margin of the shaft of 5th metacarpal	Deep branch of ulnar nerve	Opposition of tip of little finger with thumb
3.	Adductor pollicis	• Oblique head from capitate, hamate, and bases of 2nd and 3rd metacarpals • Transverse head from distal 2/3 of palmar surface of 3rd metacarpal	Medial side of base of proximal phalanx of thumb	Deep branch of ulnar nerve	Adduction of thumb
4.	Lumbricals	Refer Short Notes/Notes on Q. No. 15 – 2008.			

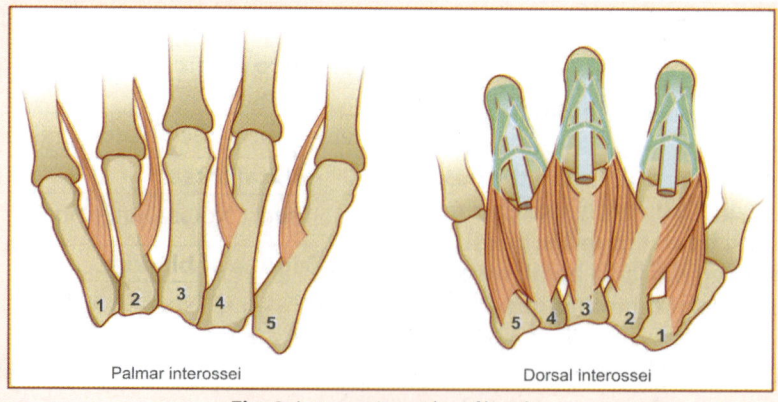

Fig. 3: Interossei muscles of hand.

(Contd...)

(Contd...)

S. No.	Name of the muscles	Attachment		Nerve supply	Action
		Origin	Insertion		
5.	Interossei – palmar and dorsal (Fig. 3)	Palmar interossei – 4 in number and all unipennate. 1. Ulnar side of base of first metacarpal 2. Ulnar side of shaft of second metacarpal 3. Radial side of shaft of fourth metacarpal 4. Radial side of shaft of fifth metacarpal	• Ulnar side of base of proximal phalanx of thumb and extensor expansion • Ulnar side of base of proximal phalanx and extensor expansion • Radial side of base of proximal phalanx and extensor expansion • Radial side of base of proximal phalanx and extensor expansion	• Deep branch of ulnar nerve	• Adduction of fingers towards middle finger
		Dorsal interossei – 4 in number and all bipennate Arises by two heads from the adjoining sides of metacarpals	1. Radial side of base of proximal phalanx of index and extensor expansion 2. Radial side of base of proximal phalanx of middle finger and extensor expansion 3. Ulnar side of base of proximal phalanx of middle finger and extensor expansion 4. Ulnar side of base of proximal phalanx of ring finger and extensor expansion	• Deep branch of ulnar nerve	• Abduction of fingers away from middle finger

20. Structures in lateral compartment of leg.

S. No.	Name of muscle	Attachment (Fig. 4)		Nerve supply	Action
		Origin	Insertion		
1.	Peroneus/ Fibularis longus	Head and proximal 2/3 of lateral surface of shaft of fibula, anterior and posterior intermuscular septae and few fibers from lateral condyle of tibia	Inserted to the lateral surface of base of first metatarsal and medial cuneiform. The tendon passes in the groove behind the lateral malleolus along with brevis, lateral surface of calcaneus below peroneal tubercle, groove in the cuboid	Superficial peroneal/ fibular nerve	Powerful evertors, maintains the lateral longitudinal and transverse arches

(Contd...)

(Contd...)

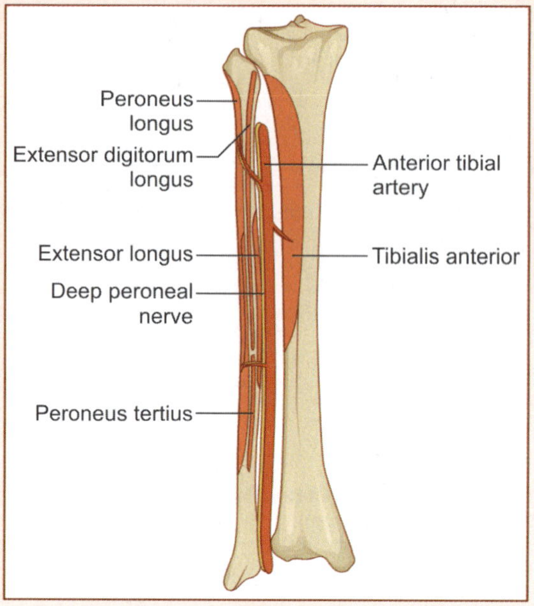

S. No.	Name of muscle	Origin	Insertion	Nerve supply	Action
		Attachment (Fig. 4)			
2.	Peroneus/ Fibularis brevis	Lower 2/3 of lateral surface of shaft of fibula	Tuberosity of base of fifth metatarsal	Superficial peroneal nerve	Powerful evertors

Fig. 4: Attachment of muscles of the lateral compartment of leg.

21. Floor of fourth ventricle.
Refer Short Notes/Notes on Q. No. 21 – 2008.

22. External jugular vein.
Refer Short Notes/Notes on Q. No. 29 – 2006.

23. Secretomotor innervation of parotid gland.
Refer Essay Q. No. 4 – 2004.

24. Cartilages of larynx.
- The cartilages of larynx are classified as paired and unpaired. The paired are arytenoid, cuneiform and corniculate cartilages. The unpaired are thyroid, cricoid and epiglottis
- The thyroid, cricoid and part of arytenoid cartilages are made of hyaline cartilage. The rest are elastic cartilage.
- **Thyroid cartilage (Fig 5)**
  – It is the largest cartilage of larynx
  – It is made of two laminae each with outer and inner surfaces, and four borders – superior, inferior, anterior and posterior

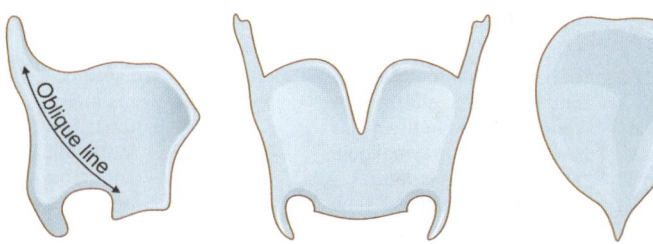 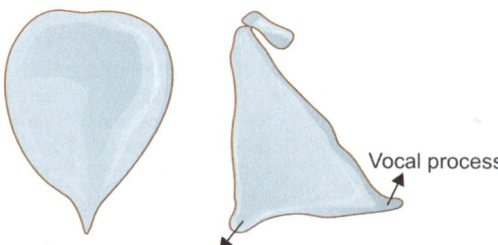

Thyroid cartilage   Epiglottis   Arytenoid cartilage

Fig. 5: Cartilages of larynx.

- The anterior border is united, and the union is at an angle. In male it is 90° and 120° in female
- The posterior border is prolonged above and below as superior and inferior horn.
- The superior border is concave behind and convex in front
- The inferior border is concave and straight in front
- In the outer surface, oblique line of thyroid cartilage is seen and it gives attachment to sternothyroid, thyrohyoid, and inferior constrictor (thyropharyngeus)
- The inner surface covered by mucous membrane

- **Cricoid cartilage**
Refer Short Notes/Notes on Q. No. 32 – 2015.

- **Epiglottis**
  - Leaf shaped, has upper and lower ends, anterior and posterior surfaces, and 2 lateral borders.
  - The narrow lower end is attached by thyroepiglottic ligament to the inner surface of thyroid cartilage just below the thyroid notch
  - The broader upper end is free and directed upwards
  - The anterior surface is attached to the tongue by a median and two lateral glossoepiglottic folds, and below to the hyoid bone by hyoepiglottic ligament
  - The posterior surface is covered by mucous membrane. An eminence is seen called tubercle of epiglottis

- **Arytenoid cartilage:** Pyramidal/ladle shaped, with an apex, base, 3 surfaces- medial, posterior, anterolateral, 2 processes – vocal and muscular

- **Corniculate cartilage:** Articulates with apex of arytenoid cartilage and lie within the aryepiglottic folds

- **Cuneiform cartilage:** Rod shaped, lie in front of corniculate cartilage and lie within the aryepiglottic folds

25. Superior mediastinum.
Refer Short Notes/Notes on Q. No. 38 – 2012.

26. Development of face.
Refer Short Notes/Notes on Q. No. 22 – 2007.

27. Histology of thymus.
Refer Short Notes/Notes on Q. No. 45 – 2014.

28. Pleura.
Refer Essay Q. No. 3 – 2003.

29. Falx cerebri.
Refer Short Notes/Notes on Q. No. 29 – 2007.

30. Circle of willis.
Refer Short Notes/Notes on Q. No. 24 – 2005.

31. Lateral wall of nasal cavity
Refer Short Notes/Notes on Q. No. 16 – 2004.

32. Karyotyping.
Refer Short Notes/Notes on Q. No. 40 – 2008.

33. Derivatives of endodermal pouches.
Refer 3rd and 4th pouches Short Notes/Notes on Q. No. 19 – 2004.
- First pouch—extends laterally and comes in contact with the first cleft, known as **tubo tympanic recess**. The lateral part is broader and forms the tympanic cavity and the medial narrower part the auditory tube. The part in contact with cleft forms the mucous layer of tympanic membrane
- Second pouch—the pouch penetrate into the surrounding mesoderm. Buds develop and enter the mesoderm and form palatine tonsil

34. Microscopic anatomy of trachea.
Refer Short Notes/Notes on Q. No. 32 – 2005.

35. Sulci and gyri in the medial surface of brain.
- The corpus callosum band largest commissural fibers present
  - Sulci **(Fig. 6)**
    - Callosal sulcus—along convex margin of the corpus callosum
    - Cingulate sulcus—above and parallel to the callosal sulcus. The posterior end curves upwards and reaches the superomedial border
    - Suprasplenial sulcus—short sulcus above splenium

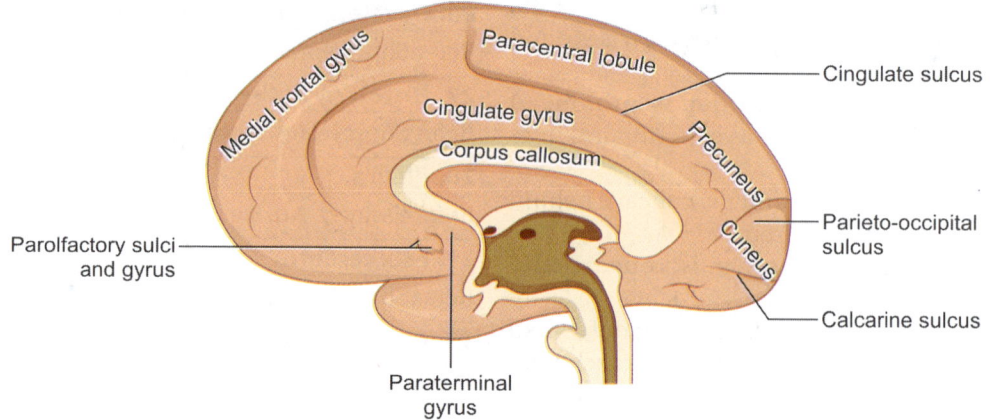

Fig. 6: Sulci, gyri of medial surface of the brain.

- Anterior and posterior parolfactory sulci—short sulci in front of lamina terminalis
- Calcarine sulcus—starts from inferior surface runs backwards above and parallel to medial occipital border it cuts the occipital pole
- Parieto-occipital sulcus—starts from superolateral surface cuts the superomedial border about 5 cm from occipital pole and meets the calcarine sulcus
- Gyri
  - Cingular gyrus—between cingular and callosal sulci
  - Supraspleinal gyrus—between supraspleinal and posterior part of callosal sulci
  - Paraterminal gyrus—between lamina terminalis and posterior parolfactory sulci
  - Parolfactory gyrus/subcallosal area—between anterior and posterior parolfactory sulci
  - Medial frontal gyrus—the portion above cingulate sulcus is divided by a short vertical sulci. The anterior part is medial frontal gyrus
  - Paracentral lobule—the posterior part of the above mentioned. Into this the central sulcus enters
  - Cuneus—between calcarine and parieto-occipital sulci
  - Precuneus—above the supraspleinal sulcus

36. Posterior triangle of neck.

Refer Contents of posterior triangle—Short notes/Notes on Q. No. 27 – 2011.

Boundaries (Fig. 7)

- Anteromedially—posterior border of sternocleidomastoid
- Posterolaterally—anterior border of trapezius
- Base—middle third of superior surface of clavicle
- Apex—by meeting point of sternomastiod and trapezius on the superior nuchal line. Sometimes gap will be seen
- Roof—skin, superficial fascia with platysma, investing layer of deep cervical fascia
- Floor—from above downwards semi-spinalis capitis, splenius capitis, levator scapulae, scalenus posterior, scalenus medius, scalenus anterior, first rib, first digitation of serratus anterior and prevertebral fascia

37. Temporomandibular joint.

Refer Essay Q. No. 4 – 2003.

38. Medial surface of left lung.

Refer Essay Q. No. 3 – 2004.

39. Spinal meninges and its modifications.

Refer Essay Q. No. 11 – 2013.

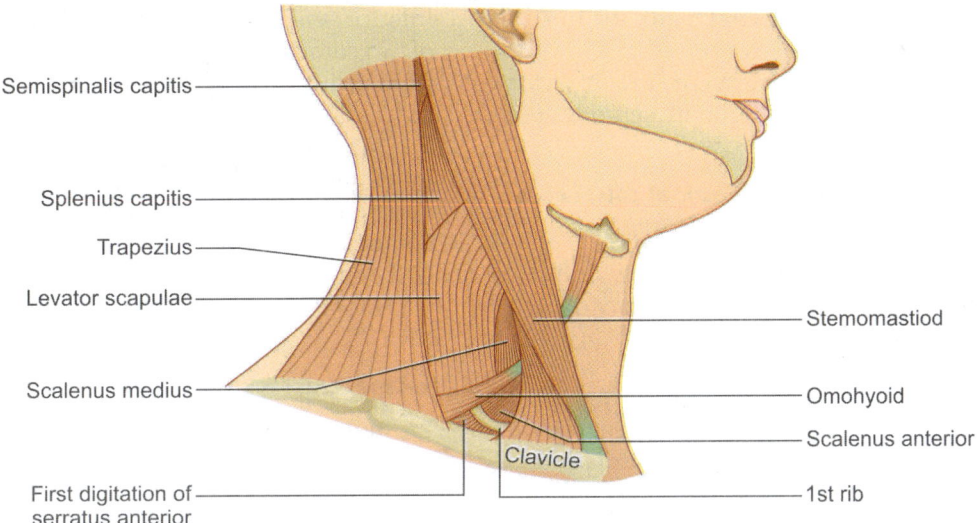

Fig. 7: Boundaries of posterior triangle.

40. Thoracic part of Esophagus.
Refer Short Notes/Notes on Q. No. 16 – 2003.

III. MULTIPLE CHOICE QUESTIONS

1. The bilaminar germinal disc:
A. Consist of epiblast and mesoderm.
B. Is derived from outer cells of morula.
C. Forms the embryo proper.
D. Contributes to the formation of trophoblast.

Ans: C (Refer—Langman's embryology 11th ed. pg. 54).
C. Forms the embryo proper—The cells in the blastocyst are differentiated to inner cell mass/embryoblast and outer cell mass the trophoblast. The embryoblast forms the bilaminar germ disc made of epiblast or ectoderm and hypoblast or endoderm. Later will be converted into trilaminar germ disc by gastrulation with formation of mesoderm. This contributes for the development of entire embryo proper.
A. Consist of epiblast and mesoderm—The bilaminar germinal disc is made of epiblast/ectoderm and hypoblast/endoderm. The mesoderm will be present in trilaminar germ disc
B. Is derived from outer cells of morula—The morula is converted to blastocyst in which cells are differentiated to inner and outer cell mass. The outer cells are called as trophoblast. The placenta is derived from outer cell mass
D. Contributes to the formation of trophoblast—The outer cells are called as trophoblast.

2. The portal vein is formed by the union of following veins:
A. Splenic vein and superior pancreatico duodenal vein.
B. Superior mesenteric vein and superior pancreatico duodenal vein.
C. Superior mesenteric vein and splenic vein.
D. Superior mesenteric vein and inferior mesenteric vein.

Ans: C (Refer—Cunningham Vol. 2 15th ed. pg. 149)
C. Superior mesenteric vein and splenic vein—The superior mesenteric vein draining the entire GI tract except lower part of anal canal joins with splenic vein behind the neck of the pancreas to form portal vein
A. Splenic vein and superior pancreatico duodenal vein—The superior pancreatico duodenal vein is a tributary of superior mesenteric vein
B. Superior mesenteric vein and superior pancreatico duodenal vein—The superior

pancreatico duodenal vein drains to superior mesenteric vein
D. Superior mesenteric vein and Inferior mesenteric vein—inferior mesenteric vein is a tributary of splenic vein

3. Structure present in inguinal canal common to both male and female is:

A. Round Ligament.
B. Spermatic Cord.
C. Ilioinguinal Nerve.
D. Iliohypogastric Nerve.

Ans: C (Refer—Gray's anatomy 41ed. pg. 1079)

C. Ilioinguinal nerve—The ilioinguinal nerve (VR L1) branch from lumbar plexus enters the inguinal canal by piercing the posterior wall of the canal and supplies internal oblique and transversus abdominis and sensory fibers to skin of proximal part of medial side of thigh, root of penis, upper part of scrotum in male and mons pubis and labia majora in female

A. Round ligament—present in female. It extends from anteroinferior to lateral cornua of uterus to labium majus. It traverses the inguinal canal entering through the deep inguinal ring. It splits into many bands after emerging from superficial inguinal ring to be attached to mons pubis and labia majora

B. Spermatic cord—In male, the spermatic cord with the contents vas deferens, vessels, nerves of testis and epididymis, covered by external spermatic fascia, cremaster muscle and fascia and internal spermatic fascia

D. Iliohypogastric nerve—(VR L1) branch from lumbar plexus. It pierces medial to superficial inguinal ring and supplies skin of suprapubic area.

4. Left testicular vein drains into:

A. Inferior Vena Cava.
B. Left Renal Vein.
C. Left Internal Iliac Vein.
D. Left Common Iliac Vein.

Ans: B (Refer—Gray's anatomy 41st ed. pg. 1274)

B. Left renal vein—The left renal vein receives left testicular and left suprarenal veins and then it drains to inferior vena cava

A. Inferior vena cava— It is formed by union of two common iliac veins, terminates into right atrium. The tributaries are lumbar, right gonadal, right suprarenal, hepatic and inferior phrenic veins

C. Left internal iliac vein—the internal iliac vein joins with external iliac to form common iliac vein

D. Left common iliac vein—joins with right common iliac vein to form inferior vena cava

5. Urethral crest is situated in:

A. Prostatic urethra.
B. Membranous urethra.
C. Penile urethra.
D. Bulbar urethra.

Ans: A (Refer—Gray's anatomy 41ed. pg. 1261)

A. Prostatic urethra—A midline ridge is seen known as urethral crest; an elevation at the middle of the crest called verumontanum (colliculus seminalis). In the middle of verumontanum orifice of prostatic utricle and the openings of the ejaculatory ducts which is formed by the union of vas deferens and duct of seminal vesicle are seen. A depression on each side of the crest - called prostatic/urethral sinus; into the sinus about 15 - 20 ducts of prostate gland open

B. Membranous urethra—shortest part, and narrowest part. It extends from prostate to bulb of penis. It pierces the perineal membrane is a content of deep perineal pouch

C. Penile urethra—15 cm in length. A dilatation is seen at glans penis called navicular fossa. At external as seen as a vertical slit, which is the narrowest part of urethra.

D. Bulbar urethra—It is surrounded by bulbospongiosus. It is the widest part of male urethra. The bulbourethral glands open into it.

6. Trigone of urinary bladder develops from:

A. Ectoderm.
B. Endoderm.
C. Mesoderm.
D. Neural Crest Cells.

Ans: C (Refer—Langman's embryology 13th ed. pg. 260)
C. Mesoderm—Trigone is developed from absorbed part of mesonephric duct which is mesodermal in origin
A. Ectoderm—The structures derived from ectoderm are central nervous system, peripheral nervous system, sensory epithelium of nose, ear, eye, epidermis, hair and nails, the glands-mammary, pituitary, subcutaneous glands, enamel of teeth
B. Endoderm—The rest of the part of urinary bladder is from urogenital sinus from post allantoic part of hind gut
D. Neural crest cells are at the lateral ends of neural tube. They migrate to the underlying mesoderm. These cells are important and contribute to many organs and tissues.

7. Craniocaudal axis of embryo is determined by:

A. Primitive Node.
B. Notochord.
C. Primitive Streak.
D. Cloacal Membrane.

Ans: C (Refer—Gray's anatomy 41 ed. pg. 193)
C. Primitive streak—The craniocaudal/cephalocaudal axis is determined by the appearance of primitive streak. The primitive streak is derived from pleuripotent cells of the ectoderm
A. Primitive node—It is also known as Henson's node seen at the proximal end of primitive streak
B. Notochord—Notochord persists (remnant) as nucleus pulposus in the center of intervertebral disc, and apical ligament. It induces differentiation of neural tube from the medullary plate. It also acts as fore runner in development of vertebral column
D. Cloacal membrane—It is formed at the caudal end of the embryonic disc. The ectoderm is adherent to the endoderm without intervention of mesoderm. Later it is divided into anal membrane and urogenital membrane by urorectal septum

8. Somites are derived from:

A. Lateral Plate Mesoderm.
B. Paraxial Mesoderm.
C. Intermediate Mesoderm.
D. Extraembryonic Mesoderm.

Ans: B (Ref—Langman's embryology 13th ed. pg. 92)
B. Paraxial mesoderm—It extends from prochordal plate to primitive streak. It passes on either side of hind brain, close to otic vesicle. The paraxial mesoderm undergoes segmentation to form somites or somitomere. The somites give rise to muscle tissue, dermis, cartilage and bone
A. Lateral plate mesoderm—formation of cavities of the body – pleural, pericardial, peritoneal cavities.
C. Intermediate mesoderm—It gives rise to urogenital system – kidney and gonads and the gonadal ducts
D. Extraembryonic mesoderm—by 11 – 12th day the extraembryonic mesoderm appears which is divide into splanchnopleuric and somatopleuric mesoderm by appearance of the extraembryonic cavity/chorionic cavity

9. Menisci are made up of:

A. Yellow Elastic Cartilage.
B. Fibro Cartilage.
C. Hyaline Cartilage.
D. Collagen.

Ans : B (Refer—Gray's anatomy 41st ed. pg. 83)
B. Fibro cartilage—Fibro cartilage is present in intervertebral disc, menisci, glenoid and acetabular labrum. Perichondrium is absent. The type I collagen fibers are present in bundles with few chondrocytes in rows. The function is, it resists high compression forces
A. Yellow elastic cartilage—Present in external auditory meatus, epiglottis, corniculate and part of arytenoid cartilages. It contains chondrocytes and elastic fibers. It has the capacity of recoiling and vibration (phonation).
C. Hyaline cartilage—It is present in articular cartilages, cartilages of nose, thyroid, cricoid and part of arytenoid cartilages. It contains chondrocytes arranged in groups (cell nest), and type II collagen fiber. It has the property to ossify.

D. Collagen—Collagen are fibers of connective tissue. Different types of collagen fibers present at different structures.

10. Sebaceous gland:

A. Eccrine.
B. Endocrine.
C. Holocrine.
D. Apocrine.

Ans : C (Refer—Gray's anatomy 41st ed. pg. 32)
C. Holocrine—The secretory product fills the cells of the gland. Then the entire cell disintegrate and the product is pushed to the duct or hair follicle. Ex: Sebaceous gland
A. Eccrine—As exudate of ion and water are transported from plasma. These glands are now renamed as merocrine as they secrete some amount of protein. Ex: Sweat glands of skin
B. Endocrine—are ductless gland. The secretions are poured into the interstitial fluid and then to the circulatory system
D. Apocrine—Some portion of cytoplasm at the apex of the gland is shed with the secretion of the gland. Ex: Secretion of milk fat by mammary gland

11. Hepatic macrophages are:

A. Hepatocytes.
B. Kupffer Cells.
C. Ito Cells.
D. Pit Cells.

Ans: B (Ref—Gray's anatomy 41st ed. pg. 1171)
B. Kupffer cells—They are hepatic macrophages. They are derived from monocytes. They are irregular in shape. They lie within the sinusoids, attached to the endothelium. They remove cellular and microbial debris, aged and damaged red blood cells. They secrete cytokines.
A. Hepatocytes—They are polyhedral in shape. They form 60% of the cellular population. The sinusoids are separated from hepatocytes by perisinusoidal space of disse. They secrete bile. They contain vacuoles containing ferritin and hemosiderin, which helps for iron metabolism.
C. Ito cells—They are hepatic stellate cells. Seen in the perisinusoidal space between hepatocytes and sinusoids. They are derived from mesoderm. They contain numerous lipid droplets, secrete collagen type III fibers, and store vitamin A. They are responsible for replacement of the damaged hepatocytes by the collagen fibers.
D. Pit cells—They are lymphoid cells. They are natural killer lymphocyte. Situated in sinusoid attached to it. They have cytotoxicity against tumor cell

12. Centroacinar cells are present in:

A. Pancreas.
B. Gall Bladder.
C. Spleen.
D. Liver.

Ans : A (Refer Gray's anatomy 41st ed. pg. 1185).
A. Pancreas—The intralobular ducts are lined by centroacinar cells. They are cuboidal or flat cells
B. Gallbladder—The epithelium of mucous membrane is columnar cells with microvilli
C. Spleen—Lymphocytes B and T are present in the red and white pulp with sinusoids
D. Liver—Hepatocytes, Kupffer cells, pit cells, Ito cells are present

13. High endothelial venules are found in:

A. Spleen.
B. Thymus.
C. Lymph node.
D. Tonsil.

Ans: C (Refer—Gray's anatomy 41st ed. pg. 74)
C. Lymph node—The lymph node has a cortex, deep cortex the paracortex and medulla. The postcapillary high endothelial venules are present in the paracortex. They are important for extravasation of blood borne lymphocytes into lymphoid tissue.
A. Spleen— It is made of red pulp and white pulp, with sinusoids
B. Thymus— It is made of cortex and medulla. The T lymphocytes are arranged on the

epitheliocytes. The Hassel's corpuscle are present in the medulla

D. Tonsil—Collection of lymphoid tissue deep to mucous membrane of oropharynx. The lining epithelium is stratified squamous epithelium

14. What is the type of joint seen at growth plate?

A. Fibrocartilaginous.
B. Primary Cartilaginous.
C. Secondary Cartilaginous.
D. Gomphoses.

Ans: B (Refer—Gray's anatomy 41st ed. pg. 97)

B. Primary cartilaginous—It is also known as synchondrosis. They are lined by hyaline cartilage. The hyaline cartilage has the capacity to ossify. Hence seen in all growth plates/between epiphysis and diaphysis of the bones, the joint between the basisphenoid and basiocciput, first chondrosternal

A. Fibrocartilaginous—It is secondary cartilaginous joint. It is also known as symphysis. The fibrocartilage is between the bones. Ex: intervertebral disc, pubic symphysis, manubriosternal

C. Secondary Cartilaginous—It is the same fibrocartilaginous joint

D. Gomphoses—It is the joint between teeth and gums

15. Unlocking of knee joint is by contraction of:

A. Quadriceps Femoris.
B. Popliteus.
C. Plantaris.
D. Sartorius.

Ans: B (Refer—Gray's anatomy 41st ed. pg. 1397)

B. Popliteus—It forms the floor of the popliteal fossa. It is tendinous in origin and is intracapsular. Origin from lateral condyle of femur, and is inserted to the posterior surface of tibia above the soleal line. The nerve supply is tibial nerve. Action is unlocking of knee joint

A. Quadriceps Femoris—The three vasti and rectus femoris form the quadriceps. They are extensors of knee joint, present in the anterior compartment of thigh. They are supplied by femoral nerve

C. Plantaris—It is one of the component of triceps surae (gastrocnemius, plantaris, soleus). It has a long tendon inserted to calcaneus or fuses with the tendo achilles/calcaneal tendon

D. Sartorius—Longest muscle in the body. It is also known as tailor's muscle. Origin from anterior superior iliac spine and is inserted to the upper part of medial surface of tibia along with gracilis and semitendinosus. It is supplied by femoral nerve. Its action is flexion of leg and thigh, abduction and lateral rotation of thigh.

16. A 42-year-old women complaint of severe pain in the back of her right thigh radiating to the leg. Which nerve is most likely to be involved:

A. Tibial Nerve.
B. Common Peroneal Nerve.
C. Sciatic Nerve.
D. Deep Peroneal Nerve.

Ans: C (Refer—Keith and Moore 6th ed. pg. 475)

C Sciatic nerve—It is the thickest nerve in the body. It is from sacral plexus (VR L_4, L_5, S_1, S_2, S_3). It has two divisions - tibial component formed by the ventral divisions of anterior primary rami of L_4, L_5, S_1, S_2, S_3 and common peroneal component - formed by the dorsal divisions of anterior primary rami of L_4, L_5, S_1, S_2. It supplies hamstring muscles of back of thigh. The compression of the nerve can result in sciatica. It is pain radiating along the cutaneous distribution of the sciatic nerve – pain is felt in the gluteal region or even higher, radiates along the back of thigh and lateral side of leg, to the dorsum of foot.

A. Tibial nerve—It is formed by the ventral divisions of anterior primary rami of L_4, L_5, S_1, S_2, S_3. It supplies the muscles along the posterior compartment

B. Common peroneal nerve—It is formed by the dorsal divisions of anterior primary rami of L_4, L_5, S_1, S_2. It divides into superficial and deep peroneal nerve.

D. Deep peroneal nerve—It supplies the anterior compartment muscles of leg and skin of first interdigital cleft. Lesion of the nerve results in foot drop.

17. Dorsalis pedis artery is a continuation of:

A. Popliteal Artery.
B. Femoral Artery.
C. Anterior Tibial Artery.
D. Posterior Tibial Artery.

Ans: C (Refer—Gray's anatomy 41st ed. pg. 1444)

C. Anterior tibial artery—Distal to ankle joint the anterior tibial artery is continued as dorsalis pedis artery. It terminates by dipping into the proximal end of first intermetatarsal space and completes the plantar arch. The branches are tarsal arteries, arcuate artery, and first dorsal metatarsal artery

A. Popliteal artery—The femoral artery passes through osseofibrous opening of adductor magnus muscle and is continued as popliteal artery. It terminates by dividing into anterior and posterior tibial arteries

B. Femoral artery—The external iliac artery is continued as femoral artery behind the midinguinal point between anterior superior iliac spine and pubic symphysis. The branches are superficial epigastric, superficial circumflex iliac, superficial external pudendal, deep external pudendal, profunda femoris, and descending genicular artery

D. Posterior tibial artery—It is one of the branch of popliteal artery. It terminates by dividing into medial and lateral plantar arteries.

18. Injury to the long thoracic nerve causes:

A. Poland syndrome.
B. Pronator syndrome.
C. Winging of scapula.
D. Wrist drop.

Ans: C (Refer Keith and Moore 6th ed. pg. 709)

C. Winging of scapula—The long thoracic nerve supplies serratus anterior muscle. Injury to the nerve results in paralysis of the muscle. Action of the muscle is protracts the scapula in pushing and punching movements. The bulk insertion to the lower part pulls the inferior angle of scapula forwards around thorax. The action of serratus anterior is antagonized by retraction of scapula by the rhomboids and middle fibers of trapezius. Because of the unopposed action of paralyzed serratus anterior muscle, the medial border of the scapula is elevated by the actions of rhomboids and middle fibers of trapezius

A. Poland syndrome—The pectoralis major muscle is absent
B. Pronator syndrome—Compression of median nerve at elbow can occur in four areas. i) Struther's ligament ii) Posterior to bicipital aponeurosis iii) Aponeurotic edge of ulnar head of pronator teres iv) Aponeurotic origin of flexor digitorum superficialis from radius. Patient complains of pain in the proximal part of forearm. Pain is increased in pronation of forearm, flexing elbow, flexion of middle finger all against resistance. Sensory impairment on the palm of hand
D. Wrist Drop—due to radial nerve injury. Wrist drops due to paralysis of extensor carpi radialis longus and brevis and extensor carpi ulnaris. Hand drops due to paralysis of extensor digitorum and so there is loss of extension at metacarpo phalangeal joints of fingers. Thumb drops due to paralysis of extensor pollicis longus and brevis a) Loss of extension at metacarpophalangeal joint (finger drop) b) Loss of sensation at the dorsum of hand (base of thumb)

19. Secondary socket for the head of humerus is:

A. Glenoidal Labrum.
B. Coracoacromial Arch.
C. Coraco-Humeral Ligament.
D. Capsule.

Ans: B (Refer—Human anatomy AK Datta Vol. III 4th ed. pg. 120)

B. Coracoacromial arch—It is formed by coracoid process and acromion process of scapula, and coracoacromial ligament. The arch is separated by a bursa from the tendon of supraspinatus. It acts as a sec-

ondary socket for head of humerus and helps in hyper abduction of shoulder joint
A. Glenoidal labrum—It is made of fibrocartilage attached to the margins of glenoid fossa. It deepens the cavity
C. Coraco-Humeral ligament—It extends from coracoid process to anatomical neck of humerus
D. Capsule—It is attached to the margins of glenoid fossa beyond glenoid labrum, laterally to anatomical neck, inferiorly 1 cm below the surgical neck of humerus. The capsule is strengthened by the musculotendinous cuff/rotator cuff.

20. Superior radioulnar joint is:

A. Ellipsoid.
B. Condylar.
C. Pivot Joint.
D. Saddle.

Ans: C (Refer—Gray's anatomy 41st ed. pg. 845, 101)

C. Pivot joint—In pivot joint, the osseous pivot rotates within osteoligamentous ring. In superior radio ulnar joint, the head of the radius rotates within the osteofibrous ring formed by annular ligament and radial notch of ulna. The movement of the joint is supination and pronation
A. Ellipsoid—It is a biaxial joint in which oval, concave surface articulates with ellipsoid convex surface. For example, wrist joint, and metacarpophalangeal joints
B. Condylar—bicondylar hinge variety. Uniaxial, with limited rotatory movement. For example, knee joint
D. Saddle—concave and convex surfaces. For example, carpometacarpal joint of thumb, ankle and calcaneocuboid joint

21. Which part of the structure in a mature spermatozoa is formed by the mitochondria of spermatids?

A. Acrosomic cap.
B. Spiral Sheath around middle piece.
C. Axial Filament.
D. Nucleus.

Ans: B (Refer—Gray's anatomy 41st ed. pg. 1276)

B. Spiral sheath around middle piece—Around the middle piece, the mitochondria aggregate in spiral manner and forms mitochondrial sheath
A. Acrosomic cap—Acrosomal granules of Golgi apparatus join and spread over the anterior pole of nucleus to form head cap. This covers 2/3 of nucleus
C. Axial filament—The centrosome divides into two centrioles. This gives rise to axial filament of the body and tail of the spermatozoa
D. Nucleus—Nucleus occupies the head of the sperm

22. One of the content of rectus sheath is:

A. Superior Epigastric Vessels.
B. Superficial Epigastric Vessels.
C. Superficial Circumflex Iliac Artery.
D. Superficial External Pudendal Artery.

Ans: A (Refer—Keith and Moore 6th ed. pg. 192)

A. Superior epigastric vessels—It is a branch from internal thoracic artery. The vessel contents are superior and inferior epigastric artery. The superior epigastric enters the rectus sheath by passing between the xiphoid process and 7th costal origins of the diaphragm through a gap called space of Larrey. The inferior epigastric artery is branch from external iliac. The artery at the lateral border of rectus abdominis pierces the transversalis fascia and passes deep to the rectus muscle
B. Superficial epigastric vessels—Superficial branch from femoral artery. Runs in the fascia of abdomen up to umbilicus. Supplies inguinal nodes and skin
C. Superficial circumflex iliac artery—Superficial branch from femoral artery passes towards anterior superior iliac spine. Supply the skin and inguinal nodes.
D. Superficial external pudendal artery—Superficial branch from femoral artery, runs medially deep to great saphenous vein and supply the skin of external genitalia

23. Contents of broad ligament are the following, *except*.

A. Uterine Tube.
B. Ligament of Ovary.
C. Ureter.
D. Round Ligament of Uterus.

Ans: C (Refer—Keith and Moore 6th ed. pg. 387)

C. Ureter—In the female, the ureter is posteroinferior to ovary. At the level of ischial spine, it curves and passes beside the lateral fornix of vagina inferior to broad ligament and to the uterine artery.
A. Uterine tube—The infundibulum, ampulla and isthmus parts are along the upper free margin of the broad ligament
B. Ligament of ovary—It is made of connective tissue and smooth muscle. It extends from medial end of ovary to the lateral cornua of uterus
D. Round ligament of uterus—It extends from anteroinferior to lateral cornua of uterus to labium majus. It is a fibromuscular band about 10 – 12 cm long. It passes between the two layers of broad ligament, to the lateral wall of pelvis. Then it traverses the inguinal canal entering through the deep inguinal ring. It splits into many bands after emerging from superficial inguinal ring to be attached to mons pubis and labia majora

24. Following structures form stomach bed, *except*:

A. Splenic Vein.
B. Splenic Artery.
C. Left Kidney.
D. Left Suprarenal.

Ans: A (Refer—Gray's anatomy 41st ed. pg. 1113)

A. Splenic vein—Splenic vein after emerging from hilum of spleen, passes posterior to the pancreas. At the level of neck of pancreas unites with the superior mesenteric vein to form portal vein
B. Splenic artery—It is related to the posteroinferior surface of stomach (Stomach bed). It is a branch from coeliac axis. It is tortuous artery. It runs along the upper border of body and tail of pancreas and enters the hilum of spleen
C. Left kidney—Anterior surface of left kidney is related to the stomach separated by lesser sac
D. Left suprarenal—It is related to the posteroinferior surface of stomach (Stomach bed).

25. Average diameter of ureter is:

A. 3 mm.
B. 5 mm.
C. 7 mm.
D. 9 mm.

Ans: A (Refer—Gray's anatomy 41st ed. pg. 1251, 979, 1174)

A. 3 mm—Ureter, cystic duct, pancreatic duct in the head of the gland.
B. 5 mm—Thoracic duct
C. 7 mm—Common bile duct/bile duct
D. 9 mm—Portal vein

26. During development, the ventral bud of the pancreas gives rise to which of the following part of adult pancreas?

A. Neck of Pancreas.
B. Body of Pancreas.
C. Uncinate Process of Pancreas.
D. Tail of Pancreas.

Ans: C (Refer—Langman's embryology 13th ed. pg. 238)

C. Uncinate process of pancreas—Pancreas is developed in two parts – dorsal bud and ventral bud. Dorsal bud - larger; Ventral bud – smaller. Dorsal bud arises from dorsal wall of primitive duodenum. Ventral bud has two components and is from the bile duct which arises from junction of foregut and midgut. The two components fuse and then undergoes rotation. The second part of duodenum undergoes axial rotation. The ventral and dorsal buds unite to form the pancreas. Ventral bud gives rise to uncinate process and inferior part of head of pancreas. Dorsal bud gives rise to part of the head, neck, body and tail of pancreas
A. Neck of pancreas—from dorsal bud
B. Body of pancreas—from dorsal bud
D. Tail of pancreas—from dorsal bud

27. Remnant of notochord in human adult is:
A. Atlas.
B. Nucleus pulposus.
C. Buccopharyngeal membrane.
D. Cloacal membrane.
Ans: B (Refer—Gray's anatomy 41st ed. pg. 756)
B. Nucleus pulposus—Notochord persists (remnant) as nucleus pulposus in the center of intervertebral disc, and apical ligament. It induces differentiation of neural tube from the medullary plate. It also acts as fore runner in development of vertebral column
A. Atlas—first cervical vertebra. It has no body and spine. It's a ring of bone with anterior and posterior arch. It has foramen transversarium for transmission of vertebral artery
C. Buccopharyngeal membrane—It is made of ectoderm and endoderm. It is future stomodeum
D. Cloacal membrane—It is made of ectoderm and endoderm. It is divided into urogenital and anal membrane by urorectal septum.

28. Primitive streak is a collection of:
A. Ectodermal Cells.
B. Endodermal Cells.
C. Mesodermal Cells.
D. Pluripotent Cells.
Ans: D (Refer—Gray's anatomy 41st ed. pg. 181)
D. Pluripotent cells—The ectoderm is divided into surface ectoderm, neuroectoderm, and pluripotent cells. The pluripotent cells develop into primitive streak and later form notochord
A. Ectodermal cells—The ectoderm is divided into surface ectoderm, neuroectoderm, and pluripotent cells
B. Endodermal cells—It gives rise to gastrointestinal tract
C. Mesodermal cells— Mesodermal cells are divided into paraxial mesoderm, intermediate mesoderm and lateral plate mesoderm

29. The following are the sites of hyaline cartilage, *except***:**
A. Costal Cartilage.
B. Articular Cartilage.
C. Tracheal Rings.
D. Intervertebral Disc.
Ans: D (Refer—Gray's anatomy 41st ed. pg. 83)
D. Intervertebral Disc—fibrous cartilage. Matrix is heterogeneous. It contains collagen type I fibers. The chondrocytes are less in number, and the perichondrium is absent. It is present in secondary cartilaginous joints (symphysis), articular discs, glenoidal labrum and acetabular labrum.
A. Costal Cartilage
B. Articular Cartilage. It is made of hyaline cartilage
C. Tracheal Rings—The cells of hyaline cartilage are arranged in groups (cell nest). The matrix is homogenous. It contains collagen type II fibers. The perichondrium is present. As age advances it gets ossified. It is present in costal cartilage, articular cartilage, thyroid, cricoid, and part of arytenoid cartilages of larynx, trachea, large bronchi, epiphyseal cartilage, and septum of nose.

30. Sensory ganglion contains
A. Unipolar Neurons.
B. Bipolar Neurons.
C. Multipolar Neurons.
D. Both A and B.
Ans: A (Refer—Gray's anatomy 41st ed. pg. 57)
A. Unipolar neurons—The sensory ganglions contain unipolar/pseudounipolar neuron, round in shape arranged in groups. The nucleus is spherical and centrally placed. The neurons are surrounded by capsular/satellite cells. The myelinated and unmyelinated nerve fibers are arranged in bundles
B. Bipolar neurons—It is present in special sensory system. For example, retina, olfactory epithelium
C. Multipolar neurons—It is present in autonomic ganglions (sympathetic and parasympathetic).
D. Both A and B—given in the answer A and B

31. Ito cells are seen in:
A. Spleen.   C. Pancreas.
B. Liver.   D. Gall Bladder.
Ans: B (Refer—Gray's anatomy 41st ed. pg. 1171)
B. Liver—The Ito cells are also known as stellate cells lie within the perisinusoidal

space of disse between the sinusoids and the hepatocyte plates. They are much less in number. They are mesenchymal in origin. They store the fat-soluble vitamin A in their lipid droplets. In response to liver damage, they replace the damaged hepatocytes with collagenous scar tissue. They are source of growth factors involved in liver homeostasis and regeneration

A. Spleen—Lymphocytes B and T are present in the red and white pulp with sinusoids
C. Pancreas—It has exocrine part made of acinar cells, and endocrine part made of islets of Langerhans
D. Gallbladder—The epithelium of mucous membrane is columnar cells with microvilli

32. Lymph from small intestine is dense and milky due to the presence of:

A. Leucocytes.
B. Pigment Granules.
C. Protein molecules.
D. Chylomicrons.

Ans: D (Refer—Gray's anatomy 41st ed. pg. 135)

D. Chylomicrons— Chylomicrons are lipid droplets received from the absorption of fat from mucosal epithelium
A. Leucocytes—Lymphatics carry leukocytes which help defense mechanism
B. Pigment granules—Nissl granules are present in the neurons
C. Protein molecules—Protein are broken into single amino acid and peptides

33. Wharton's jelly is an example for:

A. Loose Areolar Tissue.
B. Dense Connective Tissue.
C. Mucoid Connective Tissue.
D. Adipose Tissue.

Ans: C (Refer—Gray's anatomy 41st ed. pg. 40)

C. Mucoid connective tissue—Wharton's jelly forms the major component of umbilical cord along with vessels. It contains extracellular matrix with fine collagen fibers. Postnatal mucoid tissue is present in vitreous body of eye and pulp of a developing tooth
A. Loose areolar tissue—It consists of collagen and elastic fibers, and connective tissue cells. It binds the structures together
B. Dense connective tissue—Collagen fibers in bundles with few fibroblast. The connective tissue cells are absent
D. Adipose tissue—Adipocytes in the connective tissue with blood vessels. The functions are – thermo regulator, shock absorber, and storage of energy.

34. A nerve that gives articular branch to a joint supplies not only the muscles acting on the joint, but also the skin covering the joint. The statement is represented by:

A. Semon's Law.
B. Henry's Law.
C. Hilton's Law.
D. Courvoisier's Law.

Ans: C (Refer—Gray's anatomy 41st ed. pg. 100)

C. Hilton's Law—Nerves crossing a joint supply the joint, the muscles acting on the joint and the skin overlying the joint. Example: axillary nerve, supplies the deltoid muscle which acts on shoulder joint, supplies the shoulder joint and skin covering the joint (regimental badge area)
A. Semon's Law—Injury to recurrent laryngeal nerve results in paralysis of abductor muscles of vocal cords before the adductors are paralysed
B. Henry's Law—Gas that states that the amount of dissolved gas in a liquid is proportional to its partial pressure above the liquid.
D. Courvoisier's Law—A painless palpably enlarged gallbladder accompanied with mild jaundice is caused only by extrinsic obstruction of bile duct (carcinoma of head of pancreas)

35. Oblique popliteal ligament is a recurrent expansion of the tendon of:

A. Semimembranosus.
B. Semitendinosus.
C. Piriformis.
D. Gracilis.

Ans: A (Refer—Gray's anatomy 41st ed. pg. 1366)

A. Semimembranosus—Insertion of the muscle - the tendon of semimembranosus divides into five slips. It is attached to the tubercle (tuberculum tendinis) on the posterior surface of medial condyle of tibia, medial border of tibia, groove on the posterior surface of medial condyle of tibia, fascia over popliteus, oblique popliteal ligament

B. Semitendinosus—Origin from inferomedial impression of the ischial tuberosity and is inserted to the upper part of medial surface of tibia along with gracilis and sartorius forming guy ropes.

C. Piriformis—Origin from pelvic surface of three pieces of sacrum, and inserted to the apex of greater trochanter of the femur. The nerve supply is VR S1,2

D. Gracilis—It is a weak adductor, flexor and medial rotator of thigh. It is supplied by anterior division of obturator.

36. Which artery is involved in recording of blood pressure in lower limb?

A. Popliteal Artery.
B. Femoral Artery.
C. Tibial Artery.
D. Profunda Femoris Artery.

Ans: A (Refer—Human anatomy B D Chaurasia Vol. II 7th ed. pg. 84)

A. Popliteal artery—It is continuation of femoral artery. In coarctation of the aorta, the popliteal pressure is lower than the brachial pressure.

B. Femoral artery—The external iliac artery is continued as femoral artery at mid inguinal point. The femoral artery is superficial just distal to inguinal ligament and is used for cannulation

C. Tibial artery—The popliteal artery terminates into anterior and posterior tibial arteries which supply the leg region

D. Profunda femoris artery—It is one of the deep branch of femoral artery

37. Superior gluteal nerve supplies all, except:

A. Gluteus Medius.
B. Gluteus Maximus.
C. Gluteus Minimus.
D. Tensor fascia lata

Ans: B (Refer—Gray's anatomy 41st ed. pg. 1374)

B. Gluteus maximus—It is supplied by inferior gluteal nerve VR dorsal branches of L5, S1, 2
A. Gluteus medius
C. Gluteus minimus supplied by superior gluteal nerve VR dorsal branches of L4, 5, S1
D. Tensor fascia lata

38. Anatomical snuff box is related to:

A. Superficial Branch of Ulnar Nerve.
B. Superficial Branch of Radial Nerve.
C. Superficial Branch of Median Nerve.
D. Deep Branch of Ulnar Nerve.

Ans: B (Refer—Gray's anatomy 41st ed. pg. 790)

B. Superficial branch of radial nerve—It is seen in the roof of anatomical snuff box along with cephalic vein. It supplies the skin of lateral three and a half fingers on the dorsal side of hand

A. Superficial branch of ulnar nerve—The ulnar nerve passes through Guyon's canal and reach the palm of hand. It terminates into superficial and deep branch. The superficial branch of ulnar nerve supplies the skin of medial one and a half fingers.

C. Superficial Branch of Median Nerve – The superficial palmar cutaneous branch passes superficial to the flexor retinaculum and supplies thenar and central palmar skin

D. Deep branch of ulnar nerve—It supplies the hypothenar muscles, all interossei, third and fourth lumbricals and adductor pollicis.

39. The structure which divides axillary artery into three parts is:

A. Pectoralis Major.
B. Pectoralis Minor.
C. Teres Major.
D. Teres Minor.

Ans: B (Refer—Gray's anatomy 41st ed. pg. 827)

B. Pectoralis minor—The axillary artery extends from outer border of first rib to lower border of teres major. The pectoralis minor crosses the axillary artery to be attached to the coracoid process of scapula. By crossing, it divides the artery into three parts

A. Pectoralis major—It has clavicular and sternal heads. From origin, it passes to be inserted to the lateral lip of intertubercular sulcus of humerus. It forms anterior axillary fold
C. Teres major—Origin from inferior angle of scapula and inserted to the medial lip of intertubercular sulcus of humerus
D. Teres minor—Origin from upper two third of the dorsal surface of scapula and is inserted to the greater tuberosity of humerus along with supraspinatus and infraspinatus

40. Wrist joint is:

A. Bicondylar.
B. Saddle.
C. Pivot.
D. Ellipsoid.

Ans: D (Refer—Gray's anatomy 41st ed. pg. 872)

D. Ellipsoid—Wrist joint/radiocarpal is synovial, biaxial, and ellipsoid variety. The articular surfaces are distal end of radius and articular disc (elliptical concave), with the carpal bones scaphoid, lunate and triquetrum (oval convex)
A. Bicondylar—bicondylar hinge variety. Uniaxial, with limited rotatory movement, e.g., knee joint
B. Saddle—concave and convex surfaces. For example, carpometacarpal joint of thumb, ankle and calcaneocuboid joint
C. Pivot—uniaxial joint. The osseous pivot rotates within osteoligamentous ring. For example, superior radio ulnar joint, odontoid process of axis with atlas/median atlanto-axial joint

41. Thymus is present in:

A. Superior Mediastinum.
B. Anterior Mediastinum.
C. Middle Mediastinum.
D. Posterior Mediastinum.

Ans: A (Refer—Gray's anatomy 41st ed. pg. 976)

A. Superior mediastinum—The contents of superior mediastinum are thymus, Arch of aorta, Brachiocephalic trunk, Left common carotid artery, Left subclavian artery, Right brachiocephalic veins, Left brachiocephalic veins, Superior vena cava, Left superior intercostal vein, Vagus, Phrenic nerve, Cardiac nerves, Left recurrent laryngeal nerve, origin of sternohyoid, sternothyroid, longus colli, Trachea, esophagus, thoracic duct, Thymus, Tracheo bronchial lymph nodes, Para tracheal lymph nodes
B. Anterior mediastinum—It contains sterno pericardial ligaments, loose connective tissue, few lymph nodes, and mediastinal branches of internal thoracic artery
C. Middle mediastinum—heart and great vessels
D. Posterior mediastinum—Azygos vein, Hemiazygos vein, Accessory azygos vein, Right and left sympathetic chain, Splanchnic nerves, Right and left Vagi, Descending thoracic aorta, Esophagus, Thoracic duct, Posterior mediastinal lymph nodes

42. Arch of aorta ends at the level of:

A. T4
B. T3
C. T5
D. T6

Ans: A (Refer—Gray's anatomy 41st ed. pg. 1024)

A. T4—The beginning and termination of arch of aorta is second costal cartilage/T4 vertebra. The arch of aorta is continued as descending thoracic aorta. Other structures at T4 are the formation of superior vena cava, bifurcation of trachea.
B. T3—Upper margin of arch of aorta
C. T5—The pulmonary trunk terminates into right and left pulmonary arteries, below the arch of aorta
D. T6—Superior margin of left atrium

43. Crista terminalis is a feature of:

A. Right Ventricle.
B. Right Atrium.
C. Left Ventricle.
D. Left Atrium.

Ans: B (Refer—Gray's anatomy 41st ed. pg. 1001)

B. Right atrium—The crista terminalis is a muscular ridge, seperates the rough anterior part and posterior smooth sinus venarum part. It extends from superior vena cava to inferior vena cava. In the upper part, SA node is present.

A. Right ventricle—It is divided into inflow and outflow tracts by supraventricular crest. The inflow tract is rough with ridges, bridges, and 3 papillary muscles
C. Left ventricle—Muscular wall is thick as concerned with systemic circulation. The inflow tract is rough with 2 thick papillary muscles
D. Left atrium—four pulmonary veins open into it. Separated from right atrium by inter atrial septum

44. Conducting tissue of the heart is a modification of:

A. Epicardium.
B. Myocardium.
C. Endocardium.
D. Nerve Fibers.

Ans: B (Refer—Gray's anatomy 41st ed. pg. 1013)
B. Myocardium—The myocytes are specialized for propagation and conduction of heart
A. Epicardium—The visceral layer of serous pericardium
C. Endocardium—The inner lining of heart.
D. Nerve fibers—The heart is supplied by sympathetic from cervical and upper thoracic sympathetic ganglion and parasympathetic from vagus through cardiac plexus

45. The following structures pass along with aorta at the aortic orifice of diaphragm:

A. Vagus Nerve and Hemiazygos Vein.
B. Vagus Nerve and Accessory Hemiazygos Vein.
C. Thoracic Duct and Azygos Vein.
D. Thoracic Duct and Left Phrenic Nerve.

Ans: C (Refer—Gray's anatomy 41st ed. pg. 972)
C. Thoracic duct and azygos vein—pass through aortic orifice along with aorta. The orifice is at T12 level
A. Vagus nerve and hemiazygos vein—Vagus passes through esophageal orifice along with esophagus, gastric nerves and esophageal vessels of left gastric. Hemiazygos occasionally pass through aortic orifice or pierces the left crus
B. Vagus nerve and accessory hemiazygos vein—Accessory hemi azygos vein drains the left 5th – 8th posterior intercostal veins and crosses the seventh vertebra to end in azygos vein
D. Thoracic duct and left phrenic nerve—Thoracic duct through aortic orifice and left phrenic nerve pierces the left cupola.

46. Lining epithelium of lung alveolus is:

A. Simple Columnar.
B. Simple Cuboidal.
C. Simple Squamous.
D. Pseudo Stratified Ciliated Columnar.

Ans: C (Refer—Gray's anatomy 41st ed. pg. 962)
C. Simple squamous—lines the lung alveoli, renal corpuscle, thin segment of renal tubule, and inner ear. The function is diffusion and water across its surface
A. Simple xolumnar—are seen in intestine, gall bladder, PCT, epididymis. The function is absorption and secretion
B. Simple cuboidal—lining the ducts
D. Pseudo stratified ciliated columnar—seen in respiratory tract

47. Pharyngotympanic tube connects the middle ear cavity with:

A. Oropharynx.
B. Nasopharynx.
C. Nasal Cavity.
D. Laryngopharynx.

Ans: B (Refer—Gray's anatomy 41st ed, pg, 574)
B. Nasopharynx—The pharyngotympanic tube has two parts bony and cartilaginous parts. The bony part within the petrous temporal bone and the cartilaginous part opens into nasopharynx and produces an elevation. The function of this connection is it equalizes the pressure on either side of tympanic membrane, and protection from effect of nasopharyngeal environment and sound
A. Oropharynx—The oral cavity is continued as oropharynx through oropharyngeal isthmus
C. Nasal cavity—The para nasal air sinuses open into meatuses of the lateral wall of nasal cavity
D. Laryngopharynx—The inlet of larynx is seen in the upper part of incomplete

anterior wall of laryngopharynx. It is continued as esophagus.

48. The general sensation of anterior two-thirds of the tongue is carried by the following nerve:

A. Hypoglossal Nerve.
B. Lingual Nerve.
C. Chorda Tympani Nerve.
D. Internal Laryngeal Nerve.

Ans: B (Refer—Gray's Anatomy 41st ed. pg. 514)
B. Lingual nerve—It is a branch from posterior division of mandibular nerve, supplies the mucous membrane of anterior two-third of tongue. It carries general sensation from anterior two-third excluding circumvallate papillae
A. Hypoglossal nerve—Nerve supplies all the muscles of the tongue except palatoglossus.
C. Chorda tympani nerve—It is a branch from facial nerve supplies mucous membrane of anterior two-third of tongue. It carries taste sensation from anterior two-third excluding circumvallate papillae
D. Internal laryngeal nerve—branch from superior laryngeal nerve of vagus. It supplies the mucous membrane of larynx above vocal cord, vallecula of epiglottis, piriform fossa.

49. Which of the following lymph nodes are called virchow nodes?

A. Right Supraclavicular.
B. Left Supraclavicular.
C. Right Infraclavicular.
D. Left Infraclavicular.

Ans: B (Refer—Text Book of Anatomy Vishram Singh Vol. III 3rd ed. pg. 86)
B. Left supraclavicular—are named as Virchow's node. The node will be enlarged in metastasis from cancer of stomach, testis, and other abdominal organs
A. Right supraclavicular—The supraclavicular nodes are involved in tuberculosis, Hodgkin disease, and cancer breast
C. Right infraclavicular few lymph vessels of upper limb instead of draining to axillary nodes end

D. Left infraclavicular in infraclavicular nodes

50. The ligament of Berry fixes the thyroid gland to:

A. Thyroid Cartilage.
B. Conus Elasticus.
C. Cricoid Cartilage.
D. Hyoid Bone.

Ans: C (Refer—Text Book of Anatomy Vishram Singh Vol. III 3rd ed, pg 156)
C. Cricoid cartilage—The false capsule of thyroid gland is formed by pretracheal layer of deep cervical fascia. It is attached posteriorly to the arch of cricoid cartilage which is thickened to form Berry ligament
A. Thyroid cartilage—The false capsule is attached to the oblique line of thyroid cartilage
B. Conus elasticus—Extrinsic ligament of larynx. It is formed by cricothyroid ligament lateral part
D. Hyoid bone—The false capsule is attached to the body of hyoid bone in midline.

51. All are tributaries of internal jugular vein, *except*:

A. Inferior petrosal sinus.
B. External Jugular Vein.
C. Lingual Vein.
D. Pharyngeal Vein.

Ans: B (Refer—Gray's anatomy 41st ed. pg. 460)
B. External jugular vein—External jugular vein drains to subclavian vein. It is formed by union of posterior auricular vein with posterior division of retromandibular vein
A. Inferior petrosal sinus—It is the only cranial tributary draining to internal jugular vein.
C. Lingual vein—Tributary of internal jugular vein
D. Pharyngeal vein—Tributary of internal jugular vein

52. Killian's dehiscence is seen in the posterior wall of:

A. Oropharynx.
B. Larynx.

C. Nasopharynx.
D. Laryngopharynx.
Ans: D (Refer—Gray's anatomy 41st ed. pg. 582)
D. Laryngopharynx—Killian's dehiscence is the weak point. Killian's dehiscence (or Killian's triangle) is the weaker area between the oblique and transverse parts of cricopharyngeus
A. Oropharynx—It is related to the superior constrictor of pharynx
B. Larynx—form anterior wall of laryngopharynx
C. Nasopharynx—It is related to the superior constrictor of pharynx

53. Which of the following is not supplied by the anterior division of mandibular nerve (V3)?

A. Temporalis.
B. Medial Pterygoid.
C. Lateral Pterygoid.
D. Masseter.
Ans: B (Refer—Gray's anatomy 41st ed. pg. 550)
B. Medial pterygoid muscle is supplied by branch from trunk of the mandibular nerve
A. Temporalis
C. Lateral pterygoid } are supplied by branch from anterior division of the mandibular
D. Masseter nerve

54. Only abductor of the vocal cord is:

A. Posterior Cricoarytenoid.
B. Inter Arytenoid.
C. Lateral Cricoarytenoid.
D. Cricothyroid.
Ans: A (Refer—Gray's anatomy 41st ed. pg. 595)
A. Posterior cricoarytenoid—abductor of vocal cord. It is also known as safety muscle of larynx
B. Inter arytenoid—adducts the vocal cord
C. Lateral cricoarytenoid—adducts the posterior cartilaginous part of vocal cord
D. Cricothyroid—tensor of vocal cord

55. The spinal cord ends in a tapering extremity. It is called as:

A. Filum Terminale.
B. Cauda Equina.
C. Conus Medullaris.
D. Spinal Canal.
Ans: C (Refer—Gray's anatomy 41st ed. pg. 291)
C. Conus medullaris—The lower tapering end extends upto L1 vertebra in adults.
A. Filum terminale—Below conus medullaris the piamater is continued as filum terminale. Upper 15 cm of the filum terminale is covered by arachnoid and subarachnoid space, (L1 – S2) called filum terminale interna. The lower 5 cm named filum terminale externa is ensheathed by duramater and extends from S2 to posterior surface of coccyx vertebra. It is also called as coccygeal ligament
B. Cauda equina—The lower end of spinal cord below L1 vertebra resembles a horse tail and is known as cauda equina. The structures forming it are i) filum terminale, ii) coccygeal nerves, iii) S1 – S5 nerves, iv) L2 to L5 lumbar nerves
D. Spinal canal—The spinal canal is situated in the central commissure of gray matter. It is more anterior in cervical and thoracic spinal segments. In lumbar segment, it is middle

56. The major neurotransmitter secreted in substantia nigra is:

A. Dopamine.
B. Serotonin.
C. Noradrenalin.
D. Gamma-Aminobutyric Acid
Ans: A (Refer—Gray's anatomy 41st ed. pg. 323)
A. Dopamine—The substantia nigra is in-between the crus cerebri and tegmentum of midbrain. The pigmented neurons synthesize dopamine which is a neurotransmitter
B. Serotonin—It is synthesized in raphe nucleus of brainstem
C. Noradrenalin—It is present in sympathetic ganglion neurons present in various tissues
D. Gamma-Aminobutyric Acid—seen in the vesicles at synapse of the neurons, are

released into the synaptic clefts. It is an inhibitory transmitter

57. Barr bodies are most commonly situated at the:
A. Centre of Nucleus.
B. Outside the Nucleus.
C. Periphery of Nucleus.
D. In the cytoplasm.
Ans: C (Refer—Text Book of Genetics Dr. S N Chugh 1st revised ed. pg. 17)
C. Periphery of nucleus—sex chromatin is Barr body attached to the nuclear membrane
A. Centre of nucleus—the chromosomes are present
B. Outside the nucleus—cytoplasm will be present
D. In the cytoplasm—cellular organelles will be present

58. The paracentral lobule is supplied by:
A. Middle Cerebral Artery.
B. Anterior Cerebral Artery.
C. Both Anterior and Middle Cerebral Artery.
D. Heubner's Artery.
Ans: B (Refer—Gray's anatomy 41st ed. pg. 283)
B. Anterior cerebral artery—It supplies major part of medial surface, small portion along superomedial border of cerebrum
A. Middle cerebral artery—Supply major part of superolateral surface of cerebrum
C. Both anterior and middle cerebral artery—supply medial and superolateral surfaces
D. Heubner's artery—It is medial striate branches from anterior cerebral artery. It supplies the anterior limb of internal capsule.

59. Mossy fibers are seen in:
A. Cerebrum.
B. Cerebellum.
C. Spinal Cord.
D. Pons.
Ans: B (Refer—Gray's anatomy 41st ed. pg. 335)
B. Cerebellum—the afferent fibers are mossy fibers, climbing fibers
A. Cerebrum—the white matter contains the afferent and efferent fibers

C. Spinal cord—The axons in the white matter are seen grouped as tracts as ascending and descending
D. Pons—Contains white matter and gray-matter

60. All of the following are the fibers of corpus callosum, *except*:
A. Forceps Major.
B. Tapetum.
C. Forceps Minor.
D. Corona Radiata.
Ans: D (Refer—Gray's anatomy 41st ed. pg. 393)
D. Corona radiata— Corona radiata are projection fibers which intersect with fibers from trunk of corpus callosum
A. Forceps major—The fibers from splenium curve behind to the occipital lobe called forceps major
B. Tapetum—The fibers from trunk form the roof and lateral wall inferior horn of lateral ventricle called tepetum
C. Forceps minor—The fibers from genu form the forceps minor. They connect the medial and superolateral surfaces of frontal lobe

61. The giant pyramidal cells of Betz are located in which layer of cerebral cortex.
A. Outer Pyramidal Layer.
B. Molecular Layer.
C. Inner Pyramidal Layer.
D. Pleomorphic Layer.
Ans: C (Refer—Gray's anatomy 41st ed. pg. 374)
C. Inner pyramidal layer—The cerebral cortex is made of six layers: 1) Outer molecular layer, 2) Outer granular layer, 3) Outer pyramidal layer, 4) Inner granular layer, 5) Inner pyramidal layer, and 6) Pleomorphic layer. Inner pyramidal layer forms the fifth layer of cerebral cortex. Large pyramidal neurons called Betz cells are present
A. Outer pyramidal layer—Small and medium sized pyramidal cells and less number of granule cells
B. Molecular layer—It consists of horizontal cells of Cajal, axons of stellate cells, Martinoti cells, dendrites of pyramidal cells

D. Pleomorphic layer—It contains multipolar neurons, which are modified pyramidal cells. Cells of Martinoti are more in this layer

62. Deep cerebellar nuclei include all, except:

A. Dentate Nucleus.
B. Emboliform Nucleus.
C. Nucleus Globosus.
D. Lentiform Nucleus.

Ans: D (Refer—Gray's anatomy 41st ed. pg. 336)

D. Lentiform nucleus—It is a mass of gray matter. It forms part of basal ganglia. It is divided into globus pallidus and putamen. It forms lateral boundary for internal capsule
A. Dentate nucleus—nucleus of neocerebellum. Its connections are cortico pontine and is mainly concerned with the regulation of fine movements of the body
B. Emboliformis nucleus—of paleo cerebellum. Its connections are chiefly spinocerebellar and it controls tone, posture and crude movements of the limbs.
C. Nucleus globosus—nucleus of paleo cerebellum. Its connections are chiefly spinocerebellar and it controls tone, posture and crude movements of the limbs.

63. The substantia related to gray matter of spinal cord is:

A. Substantia Nigra.
B. Substantia Propria.
C. Substantia Gelatinosa.
D. Substantia Innominata.

Ans: C (Refer—Gray's anatomy 41st ed. pg. 294)

C. Substantia gelatinosa—It covers the apex of the posterior horn of spinal cord. Present throughout the spinal cord. Above it is continuous with spinal nucleus of trigeminal. It is concerned with pain and temperature
A. Substantia nigra— It is a sheet of pigmented nerve cells. It is present in midbrain. It is situated between crus cerebri and tegmentum of midbrain. It contains iron, dopaminergic neurons rich in neuromelanin
B. Substantia propria—It's a layer in cornea 1. Corneal epithelium, 2. Anterior limiting lamina (Bowman's layer), 3. Substantia propria (Corneal stroma), 4. Posterior limiting lamina (Descemet's membrane), and 5. Endothelium.
D. Substantia innominata—layers in the brain containing partly of gray and white matter, situated within the anterior perforated substance and contains the acetylcholine-rich basal nucleus of Meynert.

64. The fibers of the spinal lemniscus terminate in which group of thalamic nuclei:

A. Ventral Posterior Nucleus.
B. Ventral Anterior Nucleus.
C. Anterior Nuclear Group.
D. Medial Geniculate Bodies.

Ans: A (Refer—Gray's anatomy 41st ed. pg. 352)

A. Ventral posterior nucleus—Nuclear mass in the thalamus. It is subdivided into ventropostero-lateral (VPL) and ventropostero media (VPM). Ventropostero lateral receives medial lemniscus and spinal lemniscus fibers. Ventroposteromedial receives trigeminothalamic and solitariothalimic tracts
B. Ventral anterior nucleus—It is connected to premotor cortex (area 6). It conveys information to motor cortex from corpus striatum and substantia nigra
C. Anterior nuclear group—It is connected to mammillary body, fornix. It is incorporated with Papez circuit of limbic system
D. Medial geniculate bodies—It receives auditory fibers from both ears through lateral lemniscus and inferior colliculus. It projects to primary auditory cortex

65. According to Brodmann's, classification for functional areas of cerebral cortex, which area is assigned primary visual area:

A. Area 41.
B. Area 6, 8.
C. Area 43.
D. Area 17.

Ans: D (Refer—Gray's anatomy 41st ed. pg. 381)

D. Area 17 Primary visual area—Situated in the posterior part of calcarine sulcus is the primary visual area. It receives the optic radiation from lateral geniculate body. Lesion of this area results in homonymous hemianopia with macular sparing

A. Area 41—Situated in the transverse temporal (Heschl's) gyrus, It receives auditory radiation from medial geniculate body. It helps to identify the direction, intensity, and distance of the sound

B. Area 6, 8—Premotor area. Situated in front of motor area, in the posterior part of superior, middle and inferior frontal gyri. It contributes for corticospinal fibers. Function of this area is preparation for movements and movements itself. Lesion of premotor area results in difficulty in performing skilled movements

C. Area 43—Situated anterior part of on the insular lobe and the frontal operculum on the inferior frontal gyrus of the frontal lobe.

66. In a telocentric chromosome, the centromere is located in which part of chromatid:

A. Centromere is centrally placed.
B. Centromere is slightly away from the center.
C. Centromere is nearer to one end.
D. Centromere lies at one end.

Ans: D (Refer—Essentials of genetics Dr. Renu Chauhan 1st revised ed. pg. 4)
D. Centromere lies at one end—Telocentric
A. Centromere is centrally placed—Metacentric
B. Centromere is slightly away from the center—Submetacentric
C. Centromere is nearer to one end—Acrocentric

67. Rib fractures are common in:

A. Head of the Rib.
B. Neck of the Rib.
C. Angle of the Rib.
D. Shaft of the Rib.

Ans: C (Refer—Gray's anatomy 41st ed. pg. 938)
C. Angle of the rib—Traumatic stress results in compression of the thorax, and fracture is just in front of the angle, which is the weakest point of the rib.

A. Head of the rib—The head has two facets, articulates with the corresponding and the lower vertebra
B. Neck of the rib—It lies in front of the transverse process of the corresponding vertebra
D. Shaft of the rib—Direct impact may fracture a rib at any point

68. The pulmonary ligament which extends from the side of esophagus to the corresponding lung is an extension of which part of parietal pleura:

A. Costal Pleura.
B. Cervical Pleura.
C. Mediastinal Pleura.
D. Diaphragmatic Pleura.

Ans: C (Refer—Gray's anatomy 41st ed. pg. 954)
C. Mediastinal pleura—The mediastinal pleura extends as a double layer, the pulmonary ligament, inferior to the hilum, from the lateral surface of the esophagus to the mediastinal surface of the lung, and is continuous with the visceral pleura. It is free sickle-shaped fold. Above the ligament, the inferior pulmonary vein is situated. It is a dead space containg areolar tissue. It help for expansion of vein in increased blood flow from lung to left atrium
A. Costal pleura—Lines the thoracic cavity separated by endothoracic fascia.
B. Cervical pleura—The parietal pleura extending to root of neck covering apex of lung. It extends upto neck of first rib
D. Diaphragmatic pleura—It covers the dome of diaphragm

69. Name the structure among the following which is the usual content of anterior mediastinum:

A. Superior and Inferior sterno pericardial Ligaments.
B. Origin of Sternothyroid Muscle.
C. Arch of Aorta with its three Branches.
D. Thymus Gland.

Ans: A (Refer—Gray's anatomy 41st ed. pg. 976)
A. Superior and inferior sterno pericardial ligaments—Anterior mediastinum

contains sterno pericardial ligaments, loose connective tissue, few lymph nodes, and mediastinal branches of internal thoracic artery

B. Origin of sternothyroid muscle—It is a content of superior mediastinum. Superior mediastinum contains the lower ends of sternohyoid, sternothyroid and longus colli; thymic remnants; the internal thoracic arteries and veins, the brachiocephalic veins and the upper half of the superior vena cava, the aortic arch, and the three branches, the left superior intercostal vein; the right and left vagi and phrenic nerves, the left recurrent laryngeal nerve, the cardiac nerves and the superficial part of the cardiac plexus; the trachea, esophagus and thoracic duct.

C. Arch of aorta with its three branches—content of superior mediastinum

D. Thymus gland—content of superior mediastinum

70. Choose the correct statement regarding the boundaries of oblique sinus:

A. Anteriorly, bound by Right Atrium.
B. Posteriorly related to serous Pericardium.
C. Above, bound by upper margin of Right Atrium.
D. On either side, bound by corresponding pair of pulmonary veins.

Ans: D (Refer—Gray's anatomy 40th ed. pg. 995)

D. On either side, bound by corresponding pair of pulmonary veins—Oblique sinus of pericardium is a blind sac lying behind the left atrium. It is inverted "J" shaped.
Boundaries: Left side—Left pulmonary veins. Right side—Right pulmonary veins and Superior and inferior vena cava. Anteriorly—left atrium. Posteriorly—fibrous pericardium and posterior mediastinum. Above—Upper margin of left atrium. Below —Opens downwards and laterally

A. Anteriorly, bound by Right Atrium—Anteriorly, bound by left Atrium

B. Posteriorly related to serous Pericardium—fibrous pericardium and posterior mediastinum

C. Above, bound by upper margin of Right Atrium—Upper margin of left atrium

71. Posterior interventricular groove is a feature of which surface of heart:

A. Diaphragmatic surface.
B. Sternocostal surface.
C. Base.
D. Left Surface.

Ans: A (Refer—Gray's anatomy 41st ed. pg. 999)

A. Diaphragmatic surface—The diaphragmatic surface is contributed by left ventricle (⅔) and right ventricle (⅓). The ventricles are separated by posterior interventricular groove which lodges posterior interventricular artery branch of right coronary artery, accompanied by middle cardiac vein which drains into coronary sinus

B. Sternocostal surface—anterior surface of heart. It is formed by right atrium, right ventricle, left auricle and ventricle. Right atrium and ventricle are separated by anterior coronary sulcus/anterior atrioventricular sulcus. It lodges right coronary artery and small cardiac vein. The right and left ventricles are separated by anterior interventricular sulcus which contains anterior interventricular artery and great cardiac vein

C. Base—It is posterior surface formed ⅔ by left atrium and ⅓ by right atrium. The four pulmonary veins open into the left atrium. The base is separated by the diaphragmatic surface by the posterior part of coronary sulcus containing coronary sinus and circumflex branch of left coronary artery

D. Left surface—It is formed by left ventricle and left auricle

72. Anterior cardiac veins draining the infundibulum of the right ventricle drains into which part of heart:

A. Coronary Sinus
B. Great Cardiac Vein
C. Right Ventricle
D. Right Atrium.

Ans: D (Refer—Gray's anatomy 41st ed. pg. 1021)

D. Right atrium—The anterior cardiac veins drain the anterior region of the right ventricle including the right cardiac border and end in right atrium
A. Coronary sinus—Large vein draining the heart. Lies in the posterior coronary sulcus between left atrium and ventricle. Terminates into the sinus venarum part of right atrium between IVC and right atrioventricular orifice. The opening is guarded by the Thebesian valve. Tributaries: great cardiac vein, middle cardiac vein, small cardiac vein, posterior vein of left ventricle, oblique vein of Marshall/left atrium
B. Great cardiac vein— It is one of the tributary of coronary sinus. Situated in the anterior interventricular sulcus along with anterior interventricular artery. Starts from apex of heart.
C. Right ventricle—drained by anterior cardiac vein and ends in right atrium

73. Structure derived from second branchial arch is:

A. Masseter.
B. Buccinator.
C. Medial Pterygoid.
D. Lateral Pterygoid.

Ans: B (Refer—Langman's embryology 13th ed. pg. 279)
B. Buccinator—Second arch is also called as the hyoid arch. The cartilage of the arch is Reichert's cartilage. The nerve of the arch is facial nerve. The artery of the arch is stapedial artery which disappears later. The muscles developed are stapedius, muscles of facial expression including buccinator, auricular muscles, posterior belly of digastrics, stylohyoid, platysma, and occipitofrontalis.
A. Masseter—muscles of mastication from mandibular arch (first arch)
C. Medial pterygoid—from mandibular arch (first arch)
D. Lateral pterygoid—from mandibular arch (first arch)

74. Structure passing through jugular foramen is:

A. Superior Petrosal Sinus.
B. Inferior Petrosal Sinus.
C. Superior Sagittal Sinus.
D. Inferior Sagittal Sinus.

Ans: B (Refer—Gray's anatomy 41st ed. pg. 431)
B. Inferior petrosal sinus—The structures passing through jugular foramen are inferior petrosal sinus, glossopharyngeal, vagus, accessory nerves, meningeal branch of ascending pharyngeal and occipital artery, sigmoid sinus continued as internal jugular vein, emissary veins.
A. Superior petrosal sinus—drains to transverse sinus
C. Superior sagittal sinus—continues as right transverse sinus
D. Inferior sagittal sinus—drains to straight sinus

75. During thyroidectomy surgery, identification and clamping of inferior thyroid artery carefully is necessary for prevention of injury of which nerve:

A. External Laryngeal Nerve.
B. Superior Laryngeal Nerve.
C. Recurrent Laryngeal Nerve.
D. Internal Laryngeal Nerve.

Ans: C (Refer—Keith and Moore 6th ed. pg. 1043)
C. Recurrent laryngeal nerve—Inferior thyroid artery is ligated away from the gland to save the recurrent laryngeal nerve
A. External laryngeal nerve—Superior thyroid artery is ligated near the apex of the gland as the external laryngeal nerve passes medial to lateral lobe. It supplies cricothyroid muscle
B. Superior laryngeal nerve—It is a branch of vagus, which divides into external and internal laryngeal nerves
D. Internal laryngeal nerve—It is a branch from superior laryngeal, pierces the thyrohyoid membrane. Supplies mucous membrane of larynx above vocal cord.

76. The maxillary paranasal air sinus drains into which part of lateral wall of the nasal cavity:

A. Lateral wall of inferior nasal meatus.
B. Semilunar hiatus on the middle nasal meatus.

C. Lateral wall of the superior nasal meatus.
D. Spheno Ethmoidal recess.

Ans: B (Refer—Gray's anatomy 41st ed. pg. 560)

B. Semilunar hiatus on the middle nasal meatus—Hiatus semilunaris is a curved cleft below bulla formed by the edge of uncinate process. Maxillary sinus opens into the hiatus semilunaris
A. Lateral wall of inferior nasal meatus—It is the largest meatus. The nasolacrimal duct opens into it. The opening is at the junction of anterior 1/3rd and posterior 2/3rd of the meatus. The opening is guarded by a mucous fold called lacrimal fold/Hasner's valve
C. Lateral wall of the superior nasal meatus—The posterior ethmoidal sinus opens into it
D. Spheno ethmoidal recess—The depression above superior concha is called sphenoethmoidal recess. Into this space the sphenoidal sinus opens

77. Name the intrinsic muscle of larynx that acts as a primary abductor of vocal cords:

A. Lateral Crico-Arytenoid.
B. Cricothyroid.
C. Posterior Crico Arytenoid.
D. Vocalis.

Ans: C (Refer—Gray's anatomy 41st ed. pg. 595)

C. Posterior crico arytenoid—It is the only muscle abducts the vocal cord. Hence, it is also known as safety muscle of the larynx. It extends from posterior lamina of the cricoid cartilage to muscular process of arytenoid cartilage. It is supplied by recurrent laryngeal nerve
A. Lateral crico arytenoid—Adducts the vocal cord there by closes the rima glottidis
B. Cricothyroid—It is tensor of vocal cord
D. Vocalis—shortens and relaxes the vocal cord

78. The suspensory ligament for the thyroid gland otherwise known as the "Ligament of Berry" is a derivative of:

A. Investing layer of cervical fascia.
B. Pretracheal layer of deep cervical fascia.
C. Prevertebral layer of deep cervical fascia.
D. Bucco pharyngeal fascia.

Ans: B (Refer—Text Book of Anatomy Vishram Singh Vol III 2nd ed. pg. 157)

B. Pretracheal layer of deep cervical fascia—Forms the false capsule of the thyroid gland. It is attached to the oblique line of thyroid cartilage and to hyoid bone. On the posterior side of the lateral lobe the fascia gets thickened and is attached to the arch of cricoid cartilage, known as Berry's ligament
A. Investing layer of cervical fascia—It is the outermost layer and covers all the structures of neck
C. Prevertebral layer of deep cervical fascia – It is the deep layer
D. Bucco pharyngeal fascia—The fibrous layer supporting pharyngeal mucosa is thickened above the superior constrictor which a gap is called sinus of Morgagni separating the muscle from base of skull

79. Name the muscle that separates the orbital part and the palpebral part of the lacrimal gland:

A. Superior Oblique.
B. Inferior Oblique.
C. Lateral Rectus.
D. Levator Palpabrae Superioris.

Ans: D (Ref—Gray's anatomy 41st ed. pg. 683)

D. Levator palpabrae superioris—Levator palpabrae superioris arises from the orbital surface of the lesser wing of the sphenoid bone above and in front of optic canal. It expands into a wide aponeurosis. It divides the lacrimal gland into two which is situated in the anterolateral part of roof of the orbit. It is inserted medially to medial palpebral ligament, laterally to Whitnall's tubercle, middle part passes through orbicularis oculi fibers and is inserted to the skin of upper eyelid. Few fibers to the anterior surface of tarsal plate.
A. Superior oblique—It is an extra ocular muscle arises from roof of orbit and runs along the medial wall of the orbit
B. Inferior oblique— It is an extra ocular muscle origin is from floor of the orbit
C. Lateral rectus—extra ocular muscle origin is from common tendinous ring

80. Name the structure that separates the anterior cranial fossa from the nasal cavity:

A. Orbital plate of frontal bone.
B. Greater wing of sphenoid.
C. Cribriform plate of ethmoid bone.
D. Lesser wing of sphenoid.

Ans: C (Refer—Gray's anatomy 41st ed. pg. 429)

C. Cribriform plate of ethmoid bone—It separates the anterior cranial fossa from nasal cavity
A. Orbital plate of frontal bone—It seperates the anterior cranial fossa from orbit
B. Greater wing of sphenoid—It seperates the middle cranial fossa from infratemporal fossa
D. Lesser wing of sphenoid—It seperates the anterior cranial fossa from orbit

Topic-wise University Questions

1. General Anatomy

- Blood supply of long bone (2009, 2010, 2012, 2013, 2016)
  - Nutrient artery (2017, 2019)
- Cartilaginous joints (2010)
- Classification of joints of body (2014)
- Fibrous joint (2019)
- Epiphysis
  - Types with examples (2007)
  - Epiphysis of fibula (2013)
- Hilton's law (2019)
- Ossifications – type (2013, 2015)
- Pivot joint (2017)
- Pneumatic bones (2020)
- Sesamoid bone (2007, 2012, 2020)
- Syndesmosis (2012)
- Synovial joint (2014, 2015)

2. General Histology

- Aorta/elastic artery (2011, 2012, 2020)
- Bone (compact) (2003, 2005, 2006, 2013, 2021)
- Cardiac muscle (2011, 2015)
- Cartilages (2014)
- Ganglions (2006)
- Hyaline cartilage (2006, 2010, 2020)
- Lymph node (2011, 2015, 2018)
- Skeletal muscle (2010, 2016)
- Skin (2011, 2014, 2016)
- Simple squamous epithelium (2012)

3. General Embryology

- Allantois (2011, 2012)
- Amnion (2005)
- Blastocyst (2011)
- Bilaminar germ disc (2016)
- Conjoint twin (2020)
- Ectoderm derivatives (2009, 2019)
- Erythroblastosis foetalis (2020)
- Fertilization and its results (2014)
- Intraembryonic mesoderm (2003)
- Oogenesis (2016)
- Primitive streak/Notochord (2005, 2015, 2017)
  - Remnants of notochord (2011)
- Somites (2014, 2016)
- Spermatogenesis (2007, 2015)
- Yolk sac (2004, 2006)

4. Genetics

- Barr body (2010)
- Down's syndrome/Trisomy 21 (2005, 2008, 2012, 2020)
- Karyotyping chromosomes (2008, 2009, 2021)
- Klinefelter's syndrome (2005, 2010, 2011)
- Sex linked inheritance (2013)
- Turner's syndrome (2006, 2009, 2010)
- Types of chromosome (2010)

5. Upper limb

- Anatomical snuff box (2018)
  - Floor of anatomical (2018) snuff box (2013)
- Axilla (2011)
- Axillary artery (2007, 2015, 2016)
  - Branches (2011, 2012)
  - 3rd part of axillary artery (2016)
- Axillary lymph nodes (2009)
- Axillary nerve (2013, 2021)
- Axillary vein (2014)
- Biceps brachii (2013, 2015)
- Brachial artery (2003, 2017)
  - Arteria profunda brachii (2009)
- Brachial plexus (2005, 2011, 2013, 2019)
  - Erb's palsy/point (2008, 2009, 2012, 2013, 2017, 2018, 2021)
  - Formation and branches of brachial plexus (2015)
  - Posterior cord (2008, 2010, 2016)
  - Lateral cord (2010)

- Brachialis muscle (2011)
- Brachioradialis muscle (2011)
- Cephalic vein (2012, 2017)
- Clavipectoral fascia (2006, 2013, 2014)
  - Structures piercing (2009, 2010, 2011, 2018, 2020)
- Cubital fossa (2008, 2010, 2018, 2021)
  - Contents of cubital fossa (2012)
- Deltoid muscle (2012, 2016)
  - Structures under cover (2004)
- Elbow
  - Anastomosis around elbow (2006, 2007)
  - Carrying angle (2019)
  - Elbow joint (2014)
  - Supracondylar fracture (2013)
- Extensor digital expansion
  - Buttonhole deformity (2011)
  - Mallet finger (2017)
  - Muscles attached to extensor expansion (2011, 2013)
  - Extensor expansion of middle finger (2014)
- Extensor retinaculum
  - 4th compartment structures (2018)
- First carpometacarpal joint/joint of thumb (2005, 2007)
  - Bones forming the 1st carpometacarpal joint (2014)
- Flexor retinaculum (2012, 2014, 2015, 2018)
  - Carpal tunnel and syndrome (2010, 2015)
  - Structures passing deep to retinaculum (2009, 2012, 2017)
- Hand
  - Applied aspects of hand (2013)
  - Claw hand (2020)
  - Cutaneous nerve supply of hand (2008)
  - Dorsal spaces in hand (2011)
  - Fascial spaces of hand (2020)
  - Intrinsic muscles of hand (2021)
  - Lumbricals of hand (2008, 2009, 2012, 2013)
  - Median nerve in hand (2007, 2015)
  - Mid palmar space (2014)
  - Palmar arch (2011, 2019)
  - Palmar space (2017)
  - Palmaris brevis (2013)
  - Radial bursa (2018)
  - Thenar muscles (2014, 2016)
  - Ulnar nerve in hand (2004)
  - Ulnar claw hand (2016)
- Humerus
  - Lower end of humerus (2008)
  - Nerves related to humerus (2008, 2013)
- Intercostobrachial nerve (2016)
- Mammary gland/breast (2006, 2009, 2019, 2021)
  - Lymphatic drainage (2005, 2012, 2013, 2018, 2020)
- Median nerve (2008)
- Musculocutaneous nerve (2014)
  - Root value and muscles supplied (2012)
- Quadrangular space (2007, 2014)
- Radial nerve (2010)
  - In spiral groove (2005, 2014, 2017)
  - Saturday night palsy (2020)
- Radio-ulnar joint (2015)
  - Pronation and supination (2005, 2013, 2015, 2018)
  - Superior radio-ulnar joint (2012)
- Scapula
  - Anastomosis around scapula (2019)
  - Medial border-muscles attached (2013)
  - Winging of scapula (2015)
- Shoulder joint (2006, 2010, 2013, 2014, 2017, 2020)
  - Rotator cuff (2003, 2010, 2013, 2015, 2021)
  - Lateral rotation of shoulder joint (2011)
  - Movements of shoulder joint (2012)
- Superficial veins of upper limb (2013)
- Triangle of auscultation (2011, 2020)
- Triceps brachii (2006)
- Wrist joint
  - Abductors of wrist (2008, 2010)
  - Muscles involved in movements of joint (2019)
  - Wrist drop (2014, 2018)

6. Lower limb

- Adductor canal (2006, 2007, 2011, 2014)
  - Contents (2017)
- Adductor magnus (2018, 2021)
- Ankle joint (2016)
- Arches of foot (2003, 2005, 2007, 2011, 2013, 2019)

- Club foot (2020)
- Medial longitudinal arch (2010, 2012, 2017)
- Pes planus (2018)
- Cruciate anastomosis (2013, 2015)
- Deep peroneal nerve (2006, 2015)
- Dorsalis pedis artery (2008, 2009, 2019)
- Extensor retinaculum of leg (2011)
- Femoral artery (2014, 2020)
- Femoral hernia (2019)
- Femoral nerve (2011)
- Femoral ring (2014)
- Femoral sheath (2005, 2006, 2007, 2009)
  - Contents of femoral sheath (2012)
- Femoral triangle (2012, 2014, 2018, 2019, 2021)
- Foot
  - Cutaneous nerve supply (2005)
  - Flexor retinaculum of foot (2017, 2019)
  - Foot drop (2013, 2017)
  - Inversion and eversion of foot/leg (2012, 2013, 2019)
- Gluteus maximus
  - Structures under cover (2013, 2018, 2021)
- Gluteus medius muscle (2013, 2014)
  - Trendelenberg's sign (2019)
- Gracilis muscle (2011)
- Great saphenous vein (2005, 2006, 2008, 2009, 2011, 2013, 2014, 2015, 2017, 2021)
- Guy rope muscles (2017)
- Hamstring muscles (2015)
  - Name the hamstring muscles (2010)
- Hip joint (2004, 2008, 2009, 2015)
  - Abductors of hip and gait (2008)
  - Iliofemoral ligament (2016)
  - Ligaments around (2010, 2013)
  - Lateral rotation of hip (2011)
  - Lateral rotators of hip/thigh (2010, 2012, 2014)
- Inguinal lymph nodes (2004, 2020)
  - Superficial inguinal lymph nodes (2013)
- Iliotibial tract
  - Muscles attached (2012)
- Knee joint (2018)
  - Anastomosis around knee joint (2016, 2021)
  - Bursae around patella (2008)
  - Cruciate ligaments (2007)
  - Ligaments within joint (2010, 2012)
  - Ligaments and bursae around joint (2012, 2015, 2021)
  - Locking and unlocking of knee joint (2011)
  - Menisci of knee joint (2010)
    - Bucket handle injury (2013)
  - Oblique popliteal ligament structures piercing (2009)
  - Tibial collateral ligament (2003)
- Lateral compartment of leg (2021)
- Obturator nerve (2010, 2013)
  - Muscles supplied (2009)
- Palthi posture (2011)
- Peroneal artery (2016)
- Peroneal retinaculum (2010)
- Peripheral heart (2015)
- Piriformis muscle (2012)
- Popliteal fossa (2009, 2012, 2013, 2014, 2017)
- Popliteus muscle (2009, 2010, 2013, 2015)
  - Peculiarities of popliteus muscle (2013)
- Quadriceps femoris
  - Parts (2012, 2013, 2014)
- Retzius space (2019)
- Saphenous nerve (2018)
- Sciatic nerve (2007, 2012, 2014, 2015, 2021)
- Shoe makers line (2019)
- Sole
  - 1st layer of sole (2010)
  - 2nd layer of sole (2008)
  - Cutaneous innervation of sole (2019)
  - Layers of sole/foot (2013)
  - Medial plantar nerve (2016)
- Subtalar joint (2009)
- Subsartorial plexus (2012)
- Superficial veins of lower limb (2012)
- Sural nerve (2017)
- Tarsal bones (2010)
- Triceps surae (2013, 2018)
- Trochanteric anastomosis (2009, 2018)

7. Abdomen and Pelvis

- Anal canal (2005, 2014)
  - Anal fissure (2011)
- Anterior abdominal wall

- Cutaneous nerves of anterior abdominal wall (2013)
- Internal oblique muscle (2011)
- Quadrants of abdomen (2013)
- Rectus sheath (2003, 2008, 2015, 2021)
- Appendix/Vermiform appendix (2005, 2015)
  - Positions of appendix (2008, 2010)
- Celiac trunk (2009, 2021)
- Cloaca and its derivatives (2015)
- Coeliac ganglion (2008)
- Corpus luteum (2005)
- Deep perineal pouch muscles (2010)
- Diaphragms
  - Pelvic diaphragm (2005, 2021)
  - Thoracic diaphragm (2005)
    - Development (2008)
    - Openings of diaphragm (2013)
- Duodenum (2007, 2009)
  - Microscopic structure (2004, 2009, 2014)
  - Parts and blood supply of duodenum (2013)
  - Second part of duodenum (2006, 2011, 2015)
    - Interior of second part (2017)
- Epiploic foramen (2009, 2010, 2013, 2014, 2016)
- External iliac artery (2009)
- Extra hepatic biliary apparatus (2005, 2012)
- Gonads – blood supply (2014)
- Hymenal membrane (2013)
- Inguinal canal (2008, 2010, 2014, 2019, 2020)
  - Superficial inguinal ring (2018, 2020)
- Inguinal hernia (2013)
- Inguinal ligament (2008)
- Inferior mesenteric artery (2005, 2017)
- Inferior vena cava tributaries (2009)
- Internal iliac artery (2018)
- Internal pudendal artery branches (2017)
- Ischiorectal fossa (2003, 2008, 2013, 2014, 2020)
- Kehr's sign (2018)
- Kidney
  - Congenital anomalies of kidney (2006, 2014)
  - Coronal section of kidney (2013)
  - Coverings of kidney (2010)
  - Development (2004, 2015)
  - Left renal vein (2008)
  - Left kidney anterior relations (2009)
  - Microscopic structure (2007, 2008, 2011, 2012, 2015)
  - Juxtaglomerular apparatus (2013, 2020)
- Lesser omentum
  - Contents of lesser omentum (2020)
  - Free border (2008, 2017)
- Lesser sac/Omental bursa (2005, 2008, 2009, 2010, 2011, 2013)
- Levator ani muscle (2013)
- Liver
  - Histology of liver (2016, 2018)
  - Ligaments of liver (2008)
  - Bare areas of liver (2009, 2012)
  - Hepatorenal pouch (2010)
  - Inferior surface of liver (2011)
  - Vascular segments of liver (2014)
- Lumbar plexus (2021)
- Meckel's diverticulum (2005, 2014, 2016, 2020)
- Menstrual cycle (2008)
- Mesentery (2008, 2014)
  - Structures crossed-root of mesentry (2014)
- Midgut rotation (2005, 2018)
- Midgut derivatives (2012, 2018, 2020)
- Ovary
  - Microscopic structure (2007, 2014)
- Pancreas (2006, 2008, 2013, 2021)
  - Annular pancreas (2009, 2015)
  - Blood supply of pancreas (2015)
  - Development of pancreas (2005, 2007, 2017, 2021)
  - Head of pancreas (2012)
  - Microscopic structure (2003)
- Paramesonephric duct (2006)
- Perineal body (2004, 2011, 2013, 2014, 2020)
- Perineal membrane (2005, 2019)
- PIN structures (2011)
- Portal vein (2004, 2006, 2012, 2013, 2014, 2017, 2020)
  - Caput medusae (2020)
  - Portocaval anastomosis (2011, 2013, 2018)
  - Tributaries of portal vein (2013)

- Pouch of Douglas/rectouterine (2009, 2015, 2017, 2020)
- Prostate (2008)
  - Lobes of prostate (2019)
  - Prostatic urethra (2006, 2012)
- Pudendal canal contents (2011, 2012)
- Pudendal nerve (2014)
- Rectum blood supply (2012)
- Sacral plexus (2011, 2016, 2020)
- Scrotum layers (2017)
  - Dartos muscle (2018)
- Spermatic cord (2015, 2021)
  - Arteries of spermatic cord (2008)
  - Contents of spermatic cord (2009, 2018)
- Spleen (2003)
  - Microscopic structure (2005, 2009, 2017, 2019)
  - Ligaments attached to spleen (2011, 2012)
- Stomach (2007, 2010, 2012, 2013, 2017)
  - Blood supply (2011, 2016, 2019)
  - Lymphatic drainage (2007, 2016)
  - Microscopic structure of fundus (2006)
  - Stomach bed (2014)
- Superficial perineal pouch (2009, 2018)
- Superior mesenteric artery (2015)
  - Branches (2011)
- Suprarenal gland
  - Blood supply of left suprarenal (2018)
  - Microscopic structure (2010, 2011, 2013, 2015)
- Taenia coli (2017)
- Testis
  - Coverings of testis (2010)
  - Cremastric muscle (2019)
  - Cryptorchism (2014)
  - Descent of testis (2007, 2011, 2012, 2017)
  - Development (2003)
  - Histology (2010)
  - Varicocele (2019)
- Thoracolumbar fascia (2009, 2020)
- Transpyloric plane (2008, 2011)
- Transverse colon blood supply (2010)
- Urachus (2018)
- Ureter (2004)
  - Histology of ureter (2012)
- Urethra male (2011, 2019)
- Urinary bladder (2003, 2010, 2011, 2015)
  - Development of bladder (2007, 2009, 2019)
  - Microscopic structure (2019)
  - Nerve supply, blood supply (2013)
  - Suprapubic cystostomy (2020)
  - Trigone of bladder (2005, 2006, 2012, 2013, 2021)
- Uterine/Fallopian tube (2010, 2014, 2019, 2020)
- Uterus (2004, 2006, 2009, 2013, 2015, 2017, 2020)
  - Ligaments of uterus (2014)
  - Supports of uterus (2010, 2012, 2015, 2017)
  - Broad ligament (2011)
    - Contents of broad ligament (2913)
    - Epoophoron and paroophoron (2016)
- Vulva (2013)

8. Thorax

- Arch of aorta (2004, 2016)
  - Relations of arch of aorta (2011)
  - Branches of arch (2013)
- Ascending aorta branches (2013)
- Azygos vein (2011, 2014, 2016)
- Brachiocephalic vein (2011, 2017)
  - Left brachiocephalic vein (2014)
- Bronchus
  - Right principal bronchus (2012)
- Descending thoracic aorta (2015)
- Esophagus (2003, 2012, 2018)
  - Histology (2008, 2021)
  - Thoracic part of esophagus (2021)
- Flail chest (2020)
- Heart
  - Apex beat of heart – surface marking (2013, 2014)
  - Blood supply/Coronary circulation (2005, 2008, 2015, 2017, 2018, 2021)
    - Arterial supply of heart (2013)
    - Coronary sinus (2007, 2008, 2016)
    - Right coronary artery (2010, 2013)
    - Left coronary artery (2011, 2015, 2016)

- Venous drainage of heart (2013, 2019)
- Conducting and skeletal system (2006, 2019)
- Congenital anomalies of heart (2010)
  - Fallot's tetralogy (2012, 2015, 2017, 2020)
  - Patent ductus arteriosus (2014)
- Development of interatrial septum (2006, 2010, 2015)
- Development of atria (2011)
- Internal features (2006)
  - Inter atrial septum (2012)
  - Interior of right atrium (2009, 2013, 2014, 2015, 2018)
  - Interventricular septum (2011, 2014)
  - Left ventricle (2018)
  - Moderator band (2012)
  - Tendon of Todaro (2020)
  - Triangle of Koch (2012)
  - Tricuspid valve (2011)
- Nerve supply/Cardiac plexus (2007, 2010, 2014, 2017)
- Pericardium/Coverings (2006, 2007, 2013)
  - Sinuses of pericardium (2008, 2012, 2017, 2020)
- Right atrium (2009)
- Ligamentum arteriosum (2009, 2020)

- Internal thoracic artery (2014, 2020)
  - Terminal branches (2013)
- Intercostal space (2009, 2019)
  - 1st intercostal nerve peculiarities (2012)
  - Cross section diagram of typical intercostal space (2015)
  - Left superior intercostal vein
  - Typical intercostal nerve (2006, 2011, 2013, 2014)
- Internal thoracic artery (2008, 2019)
- Lungs (2004, 2019)
  - Blood supply of lung (2013)
  - Bronchopulmonary segments (2006, 2007, 2009, 2015, 2017)
  - Difference between right and left lungs (2019)
  - Development of lung (2011)
  - Hilum of lungs (2005, 2010, 2011, 2018)
    - Hilum of right lung (2014)
  - Lobe of azygos (2013)
  - Medial surface of right lung (2007)
  - Mediastinal surface of left lung (2010, 2013, 2021)
  - Microscopic structure (2005)
  - Oblique fissure of lung (2011)
  - Right lung (2008, 2012)
  - Root of lungs (2013)
- Mediastinum
  - Posterior mediastinum (2012, 2013, 2015, 2019)
  - Subdivisions of mediastinum (2009, 2012)
  - Superior mediastinum (2012, 2014, 2016, 2017, 2021)
- Middle cervical ganglion (2011)
- Pleura (2003, 2021)
  - Applied aspects of pleura (2013)
  - Costodiaphragmatic recess (2011)
  - Pleural diaphragm (2012)
  - Pleural recesses (2005, 2009, 201, 2014, 2015, 2017, 2018, 2020)
  - Suprapleural membrane/Sibson's fascia (2009, 2017)
- Splanchnic nerves (2009)
- Sternal angle
  - Section at the level of T4 (2014, 2018)
- Superior vena cava (2003, 2020)
  - Formation of SVC (2013, 2019)
- Suprasternal space of burns (2013)
- Trachea
  - Microscopic structure (2005, 2009, 2021)
  - Thoracic part of trachea (2016)
  - Tracheoesophageal fistula (2020)
- Thoracic duct (2013, 2018)
  - Areas drained by thoracic duct (2015)
- Thymus
  - Hassall's corpuscles (2009)
  - Histology of thymus (2014, 2021)

9. Head and Neck

- Ansa cervicalis (2008, 2009, 2013, 2014, 2017)
- Aortic arches fate (2006)
  - 3rd aortic arch (2011)
- Arch of aorta (2010)
- Atlantoaxial joint (2010)

- Branchial apparatus
  - 3rd and 4th Pharyngeal pouches (2004)
  - 2nd branchial arch (2005, 2007, 2008, 2010, 2011, 2012, 2019)
  - 1st pharyngeal arch (2007, 2008, 2020)
  - Cervical sinus (2016)
  - Endodermal/Pharyngeal pouches (2021)
- Buccinator (2007, 2015)
- Carotid sheath (2010, 2014, 2017)
- Carotid triangle (2011, 2012, 2013, 2018)
- Cavernous sinus (2008, 2011, 2012, 2015, 2019)
  - Lateral wall of cavernous sinus (2009, 2017, 2018)
  - Tributaries of cavernous sinus (2014)
- Ciliary ganglion (2009, 2014, 2020)
- Cornea histology (2009, 2011, 2015, 2017, 2020)
- Cranial nerves
  - Abducent nerve (2015)
  - Nuclei special somatic afferent (2011)
  - Facial nerve (2003, 2007, 2018)
    - Bell's palsy (2015, 2017, 2019)
    - Chorda tympani (2005)
  - Hypoglossal nerve (2015)
  - Oculomotor nerve (2004)
  - Ophthalmic nerve (2018)
  - Spinal accessory nerve (2014)
  - Trigeminal nerve-sensory nuclei (2013)
  - Trigeminal neuralgia (2018)
  - Trochlear nerve (2016)
- Cricoid cartilage (2015)
  - Muscles attached (2008)
- Digastric triangle (2012, 2014)
- Dural venous sinuses list (2016)
- Emissary veins (2010)
- Extra ocular muscles (2005, 2009, 2014, 2019)
- External acoustic meatus (2012)
- External carotid artery branches (2012, 2014, 2019)
  - Terminal branches (2013)
- Eyeball sagittal section (2013)
- External jugular vein (2006, 2012, 2018, 2021)
- Face
  - Cutaneous innervation of face (2017)
  - Development of face (2007, 2009, 2019, 2021)
  - Facial artery (2007, 2009, 2010)
    - Facial artery in face (2013, 2018)
  - Venous drainage of face (2010)
  - Danger area of face (2009, 2012, 2013, 2018)
- Falx cerebelli (2011)
- Falx cerebri (2007, 2015, 2021)
  - Venous sinuses related (2008)
- Foramen ovale (2009, 2013)
- Foramen spinosum (2010)
- Horner's syndrome (2010)
- Infrahyoid muscles (2010, 2018)
- Internal acoustic meatus (2008)
- Internal carotid artery branches (2018)
- Internal jugular vein
  - Formation and termination (2013)
- Internal thoracic/mammary artery (2014)
- Lacrimal apparatus (2006, 2008, 2015)
  - Parts of lacrimal apparatus (2010, 2012)
  - Nerve supply of lacrimal gland (2010)
  - Lacus lacrimalis (2010)
- Larynx
  - Cartilages of larynx (2021)
  - Inlet of larynx (2012, 2013)
  - Intrinsic muscles of larynx (2012, 2018)
    - Cricothyroid muscle (2013)
  - Nerve supply of larynx (2009)
  - Superior laryngeal nerve (2015)
  - Unpaired cartilages of larynx
  - Vocal cords (2005, 2008, 2010, 2015)
    - Attachment of vocal cords (2013)
- Lymphatic drainage of face (2010)
- Maxillary artery
  - Branches of first part (2009)
- Middle meningeal artery (2008, 2012)
- Midline structures of neck (2009)
- Muscles of mastication (2008, 2015)
  - Lateral pterygoid muscle (2005, 2013)
- Nasal cavity
  - Nasal Septum (2003, 2005, 2012, 2015, 2020)
    - Area of epistaxis/Little's area (2015, 2016, 2017)
    - Bones forming septum (2010)
  - Lateral wall of nasal cavity (2004, 2006, 2014, 2020, 2021)
  - Middle meatus of nose (2010, 2016)
- Orbicularis oculi (2008, 2014, 2016)

- Orbicularis oris (2020)
- Otic ganglion (2009, 2015)
- Palate
  - Development (2003)
  - Muscles of palate (2011, 2020)
- Palatine tonsil (2008, 2009)
  - Blood supply (2013)
  - Development (2005, 2016)
  - Microscopic structure (2005, 2006, 2015)
  - Paratonsillar abscess (2020)
  - Tonsillar bed (2018)
- Paranasal air sinuses (2008, 2013)
  - Maxillary sinus (2005, 2008, 201, 2015, 2016)
    - Opening of maxillary sinus (2013)
- Parathyroid gland histology (2010)
- Parotid gland (2004, 2006, 2010, 2017, 2019)
  - Parotid duct (2010, 2011, 2018)
    - Structures pierced by duct (2012)
  - Histology of parotid gland (2011)
  - Nerve supply of parotid gland (2018, 2021)
  - Structures inside parotid gland (2019)
- Pinna of ear (2018)
- Pharynx (2006, 2021)
  - Piriform fossa (2009, 2013, 2017)
  - Inferior constrictor of pharynx (2014)
  - Killian's dehiscence (2019)
- Phrenic nerve (2013, 2020)
- Pituitary/Hypophysis cerebri gland
  - Arterial supply (2013)
  - Development (2012, 2014, 2017, 2019)
    - Rathke's pouch (2016)
  - Histology (2005, 2007, 2010, 2020)
- Posterior triangle (2021)
  - Contents of triangle (2011)
- Pterion (2008, 2012, 2013, 2019)
- Pterygopalatine ganglion (2012, 2014, 2019)
- Recurrent laryngeal nerve (2017, 2019)
- Retina histology (2008, 2012, 2018)
- Scalp
  - Blood supply of scalp (2006, 2012)
  - Danger area of scalp (2013, 2014)
  - Epicranial aponeurosis (2011)
  - Nerve supply of scalp (2006, 2012)
- Sternocleidomastoid muscle (2006, 2013, 2016)
- Styloid process/Apparatus (2005, 2007, 2010, 2013)
- Subclavian artery
  - 1st part (2017)
- Subclavian triangle (2009)
- Subclavian vein (2015)
- Submandibular/Mixed salivary gland (2003, 2011)
  - Microscopic structure (2004, 2007)
  - Demilunes (2011)
  - Wharton's duct (2018)
- Submental triangle (2011)
- Suboccipital triangle (2014, 2017)
- Suboccipital nerve (2012)
- Superior orbital fissure (2018, 2019)
- Superior sagittal sinus (2013)
- Temporomandibular joint (2003, 2013, 2021)
- Tentorium cerebelli (2012)
- Thyroid gland (2004, 2007, 2009, 2012, 2015, 2020)
  - Blood supply (2008, 2011, 2014, 2015)
  - Development of thyroid gland/Thyroglossal duct (2009, 2015, 2018)
    - Thyroglossal fistula (2017)
  - Microscopic structure of thyroid gland (2014, 2016, 2019)
  - Relations of thyroid gland (2019)
  - Surfaces and borders of thyroid gland (2013)
- Tongue (2007, 2009, 2013, 2015)
  - Development (2003, 2006, 2010, 2014, 2017)
  - Hyoglossus muscle (2004, 2006, 2008, 2010, 2020)
  - Lingual papillae (2008)
  - Lymphatic drainage (2011)
  - Microscopic structure of tongue (2019)
  - Muscles of tongue (2005, 2011, 2012, 2013, 2015)
  - Nerve supply of tongue (2009)
- Torticollis/Wry neck (2017, 2019)
- Tympanic/Middle ear cavity (2013, 2014)
  - Auditory/Eustachian tube (2014, 2020)
    - Openings of auditory tube (2013)
  - Bones of middle ear cavity (2012)
  - Boundaries of tympanic cavity (2005)

- Fenestra vestibule (2011)
- Medial wall (2008)
- Tympanic membrane (2005, 2009, 2020)
- Waldeyer's ring (2011, 2015, 2018, 2019)

10. Neuroanatomy

- Basilar artery (2015)
- Blood supply of brain (2011, 2015)
  - Circle of Willis (2005, 2006, 2007, 2012, 2016, 2021)
  - Charcot's artery of haemorrhage (2020)
  - Basal vein formation (2014)
- Cerebrum
  - Functional areas – superolateral surface (2007, 2008, 2010)
  - Lateral sulcus – structures lodged (2012)
  - Microscopic structure (2003, 2011, 2017, 2018)
  - Sulci and gyri – superolateral surface (2007, 2008, 2010, 2014, 2015)
  - Sulci gyri of medial surface of brain (2021)
  - Superior temporal gyrus functional area (2011)
  - White fibers of cerebrum (2012, 2014, 2018)
- Cerebellum (2011)
  - Arterial supply (2013)
  - Microscopic structure (2004, 2006, 2015)
  - Dentate nucleus (2005)
  - Cerebellar peduncles (2006, 2009, 2020)
  - Nuclei of cerebellum (2012, 2013, 2017, 2019)
  - Paleocerebellar nuclei (2008)
- Corpus callosum (2011, 2015, 2016, 2020)
  - Parts (2009, 2012, 2013)
- Basal ganglion (2011)
  - Caudate nucleus (2014)
  - Components of basal ganglia (2019)
  - Corpus striatum (2004)
  - Parkinsonism (2014)
- Diencephalon parts (2010)
- Fourth ventricle (2012, 2013, 2016)
  - Rhomboid fossa/Floor (2008, 2015, 2021)
- Insula (2009)
- Internal capsule (2005, 2006, 2011, 2012, 2013, 2014)
  - Blood supply of internal capsule (2013, 2014)
- Interpeduncular fossa (2009, 2017, 2020)
- Lateral ventricle
  - Horns of lateral ventricle (2011)
- Limbic system formation (2019)
- Lumbar puncture (2008, 2012, 2013, 2014)
- Medulla oblongata
  - Olive (2013)
  - Lateral medullary/Wallenberg syndrome (2009, 2012, 2014, 2019)
  - Section at mid olivary level (2014)
  - Section at sensory Decussation (2019)
- Meninges
  - Cranial pia mater modifications (2018)
  - Meninges and meningeal spaces
  - Meninges of spinal cord (2021)
  - Ligamentum denticulatum (2012)
- Metathalamus (2003)
- Midbrain
  - Cerebral aqueduct (2020)
  - Section at the level of superior colliculus (2009, 2014, 2016)
  - Section of at the level of inferior colliculus (2017)
  - Substantia nigra (2011)
  - Weber's syndrome (2020)
- Neural tube
  - Development of neural tube (2004, 2009)
  - Derivatives of neural tube (2015)
- Pineal gland (2014)
- Pons
  - Section at the level of facial colliculus/ Lower pons (2004, 2007, 2016, 2017)
  - Millard Gubler syndrome (2018)
- Reticular formation (2020)
- Spinal cord (2013)
  - Arteries of spinal cord (2011)
  - Blood supply (2008, 2010, 2013, 2014)
  - Section at thoracic level (2020)
- Thalamus
  - Sensory nuclei (2008)
- Third ventricle (2003, 2014, 2017)
- Visual reflexes pathway (2012)
- Visual stria (2009)

11. MCQ

- 2021 Questions
- General anatomy – Q 14, 34
  - General embryology – Q 1, 7, 8, 21, 27, 28, 33
- General histology – Q 10, 29, 30
  - Genetics – Q 57, 66
  - Upper limb – Q 18–20, 38–40
  - Lower limb – Q 9, 15–17, 35–37
  - Abdomen and pelvis – Q 2–6, 11–13, 22–26, 31, 32, 45
- Thorax – Q 41–44, 46, 67–72
  - Head and neck – Q 47–54, 73–80
  - Neuroanatomy – Q 55, 56, 58–65